AF449295

The Therapeutic Use of N-Acetylcysteine (NAC) in Medicine

Richard Eugene Frye • Michael Berk

Editors

The Therapeutic Use of N-Acetylcysteine (NAC) in Medicine

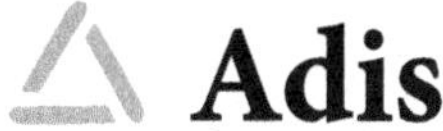

Editors
Richard Eugene Frye
Barrow Neurological Institute
Phoenix Children's Hospital
University of Arizona
College of Medicine – Phoenix
Phoenix, AZ
USA

Michael Berk
IMPACT SRC
Deakin University & Barwon Health
Geelong
Victoria
Australia

ISBN 978-981-10-5310-8   ISBN 978-981-10-5311-5   (eBook)
https://doi.org/10.1007/978-981-10-5311-5

Library of Congress Control Number: 2018941104

Printed on acid-free paper

This Adis imprint is published by the registered company Springer Nature Singapore Pte Ltd.
The registered company address is: 152 Beach Road, #21-01/04 Gateway East, Singapore 189721, Singapore

This book is dedicated to my wife Cara and children Mairin and Quinn, for their daily support and endless joy and to my family, friends, and colleagues who encouraged me to continue forward even when the path ahead was opaque and uncertain.

Richard Eugene Frye, MD, PhD Editor

Preface

I work in the field of autism where effective treatments are few and treatment targets are still ill defined. One principle when looking for a potential effective treatment, especially for children, is to assure safety of the treatment because the young body is vulnerable and because the treatment, if effective, could be required lifelong. My journey into treating children with autism led me to an interest in metabolic disorders that affect the nervous system. I met Dr. S. Jill James and Dr. Stephen Kahler at a scientific think-tank on autism. They introduced me to redox regulation abnormalities associated with autism as well as treatments to improve these abnormalities. We were very excited when Dr. Antonio Hardan published his double-blind clinical trial on the use of N-Acetylcysteine (NAC) in autism that supported our premise that targeting redox metabolism could improve important symptoms associated with autism. Dr. Hardan's article showed that NAC could reduce a common symptom associated with autism called irritability. This is extremely important since the primary treatments for irritability are antipsychotic medications, which can have significant adverse effects to general health both in the short and long term. As I began to learn more about NAC, I found the wide variety of diseases it could treat, leading to our collaboration with Dr. Michael Berk and the systematic review published in *Neuroscience and Biobehavioral Reviews* on the use of NAC in neurology and psychiatry. One of the amazing things that we noticed when reviewing the clinical literature was the safety of NAC, allowing it to be applied to many disorders. This led to a more expanded work that is this book.

This book is divided into three parts. First, we have the honor to have Dr. Leonore A Herzenberg, one of the pioneers of redox physiology and NAC, to write a history of the use and development of NAC from her perspective. Second is a series of chapters on the role of NAC in important physiological processes, including redox metabolism, neurotransmitter systems, mitochondrial function, apoptosis, and inflammation, from a basic science point of view. Lastly the book has a series of clinically oriented chapters that comprehensively review the literature on important disorders in which NAC has been found to be effective, including toxicity and neurological, psychiatric, renal, pulmonary, cardiovascular, and gastrointestinal disorders. The clinical evidence that NAC alters biological processes in the clinical setting is also reviewed. Another chapter led by Dr. Leonore A Herzenberg is also presented to suggest that the effectiveness of NAC may signal a new medical phenomenon that may be an important part of many diseases, glutathione deficiency.

Lastly we review the studies on the pharmacology and adverse effects of NAC. Overall we hope this book will give the reader a broad introduction into this interesting medical treatment.

Phoenix, AZ, USA   Richard Eugene Frye

Contents

About the Editors

Michael Berk is an NHMRC Senior Principal Research Fellow and is the Alfred Deakin Chair of Psychiatry at Deakin University and Barwon Health, where he heads the IMPACT Strategic Research Centre. He is also an Honorary Professorial Research Fellow in the Department of Psychiatry, the Florey Institute for Neuroscience and Mental Health and Orygen Youth Health at Melbourne University, as well as in the School of Public Health and Preventive Medicine at Monash University. His major interests are in the discovery and implementation of novel therapies, and risk factors and prevention of psychiatric disorders.

Richard Eugene Frye is the Chief of Neurodevelopmental Disorders at the Barrow Neurological Institute at Phoenix Children's Hospital and Professor of Child Health at the University of Arizona College of Medicine—Phoenix. He is also the Director of the Autism, Down Syndrome and Fragile X Programs at the Barrow Neurological Institute at Phoenix Children's Hospital and the Director of the Laboratory for the Biological Basis of Neurodevelopmental Disorders at University of Arizona College of Medicine—Phoenix. Dr. Frye received his MD and PhD degrees from Georgetown University Medical Center in Washington DC. He completed a Residency in Pediatrics at the University of Miami/Jackson Memorial Hospital, Residency in Child Neurology and Fellowship in Behavioral Neurology and Learning Disabilities at Harvard University/Children's Hospital Boston, and Fellowship in Psychology at Boston University. He holds board certifications in General Pediatrics and in Neurology with Special Competence in Child Neurology.

Dr. Frye is a leader in autism research. He has authored over 200 peer-reviewed publications and book chapters, and serves on several editorial boards. Over the past several years Dr. Frye has completed several clinical studies on children with autism spectrum disorder (ASD), including studies focusing on defining the clinical, behavioral, cognitive, and genetic characteristics of children with ASD with metabolic disorders, particularly those affected by folate, cobalamin, or mitochondrial metabolism abnormalities. Dr. Frye has completed several clinical trials demonstrating the efficacy of safe and novel treatments that address underlying physiological abnormalities in children with ASD, including open-label trials on tetrahydrobiopterin, cobalamin, and folinic acid and a recent double-blind placebo controlled trial on folinic acid. His research also concentrates on the contribution of the microbiome and the immune system to the pathophysiology of ASD. Future research efforts focus on defining physiological endophenotypes in individuals with ASD and developing targeted treatments.

Part I

Introduction

History of N-Acetylcysteine

1

Leonore A. Herzenberg

1.1 N-Acetylcysteine, the Antidote to Acetaminophen Overdose

N-Acetylcysteine (NAC)[1] is a well-known and universally accepted antidote to acetaminophen (APAP; Tylenol, paracetamol) poisoning. Currently in stock in virtually all hospitals and emergency medical facilities throughout the world, NAC has been administered to literally thousands of patients who walked out of their care facilities alive and healthy despite having intentionally or accidentally ingested lethal amounts of APAP.

However, because NAC is readily oxidized to foul-tasting products, it can develop a foul smell that patients commonly find repulsive. I've lost count of the number of physicians who told me "horror stories" about having to convince people who have overdosed on APAP to swallow this life-saving brew.

Nowadays, this scenario is avoided for most APAP overdose patients by giving them NAC intravenously under controlled conditions that allow ready treatment of side effects due to introduction of NAC in this manner. Further, NAC manufacturers have succeeded in producing and packaging NAC under conditions that are fairly successful in minimizing its oxidation, and the oxidation of any impurities, to decrease the foul-tasting contaminants in the product when it has to be given orally. These improvements have greatly simplified and improved the treatment of accidental and intentional APAP overdose, which unfortunately still continue to be a serious public health hazard (Green et al. 2013).

---

[1] Pronounced either as the homophone for the word "knack" or spelled out as the letters "N-A-C"

L. A. Herzenberg
Department of Genetics, Stanford University, Stanford, CA, USA
e-mail: leeherz@stanford.edu

© Springer Nature Singapore Pte Ltd. 2019
R. E. Frye, M. Berk (eds.), *The Therapeutic Use of N-Acetylcysteine (NAC) in Medicine*, https://doi.org/10.1007/978-981-10-5311-5_1

1.2   Unintentional Acetaminophen Overdose

Intentional overdosing with APAP is relatively common, particularly among teenagers. However, such overdosing is only a part of the APAP overdose problem. Several years ago, I was alerted to this when James Andrus, then a young pediatric intensive care physician with whom we did collaborative studies, came into our laboratory looking thoroughly miserable. He told me that he had just admitted the "sweetest little girl," who was rapidly losing liver function for unknown reasons and was likely to die in less than a week unless he could figure out what was going wrong. A few hours later, Jim came back and told me he had decided that although there was no obvious justification, he was going to put the patient on NAC therapy, treating her as if she was suffering from APAP overdose. The therapy started, the child began rapidly began to recover, and was out of the hospital in a week or two.

Jim was delighted, but he really wanted to know what actually caused the liver disease. After a little detective work speaking with the child's family, he ascertained that she was accidentally overdosed with APAP, which is present in most of the over-the-counter (OTC) cold, cough, fever, and headache medications that her family had given her. In essence, she had been suffering from a fairly intense flu-like illness and her parents and grandparents had, over several days, successively given her a large number of APAP-containing OTC medications, individually labeled as useful for reducing one or another of the symptoms of the illness (fever, sore throat, headache, etc.). After several days of this well-intentioned treatment, the child's liver began to fail. She quickly wound up in the hospital with unexplained liver failure, from which Jim's guess about unintentional APAP overdose and his treatment with NAC rescued her.

This is an extreme example. However, the widespread presence of APAP in common OTC medications means that inadvertent overdosing with this drug may be far more common than recognized. Basically, while most physicians are well aware of the dangers of APAP overdose, few recognize how ubiquitous APAP is in OTC medications, how important it is to maintain the *total* APAP exposure within allowable limits, and how low those allowable doses should be. Thus, one important outcome of the publication of this volume should be to sound the call for focus on glutathione (GSH)-depleting medications and diseases and to make pediatricians and physicians in general more aware of both the serious consequences of APAP overdose and the value of treating with NAC where appropriate.

This kind of thinking also raises the question of whether the increase in pediatric APAP use in the United States (US) and several other countries over the last several decades might have contributed to the increased incidence of autism (Tirouvanziam et al. 2012) and other diseases to which "oxidative stress," a corollary of decreased GSH, may contribute (Atkuri et al. 2007). I have seen several studies focused in this way. However, there is certainly good reason to put more effort into examining and documenting the relationship(s) between APAP usage and APAP-caused diseases and conditions.

1.3   Over-the-Counter NAC

Ingested NAC is rapidly deacetylated by first-pass metabolism to yield the amino acid cysteine, which accumulates in the liver as such and is also incorporated into a key tripeptide, GSH (γ-glutamylcysteinylglycine). GSH, cysteine, and methionine (which can be converted to cysteine) then accumulate in the liver and are doled out to the rest of the body as needed for protein synthesis and for maintenance of GSH levels in cells. Thus, the Food and Drug Administration (FDA) classifies NAC as a nutraceutical, even though it is clearly used for medicinal purposes.

Much of the NAC sold in health food and similar food or drug stores today is packaged in containers that are not designed to protect NAC from air oxidation, and hence deliver increasingly more di-NAC as packages age, particularly when opened. I know of two companies, Zambon Pharma (Italy) and BioAdvantex (Canada and US) that currently produce and package NAC in ways to minimize oxidation. Zambon offers NAC as Fluimucil tablets, packaged in relatively small tubes that minimize NAC exposure to air; BioAdvantex offers NAC as PharmaNAC, effervescent "fizzy tabs" that readily dissolve in water, juice, or soda and are individually packaged in sealed foil packets to minimize exposure to air. Both companies have supplied NAC and placebo for clinical trials in our laboratory and elsewhere.[2]

To my knowledge, despite the growing use of NAC in medical practice discussed in this volume, neither these nor any other NAC-producing company has yet mounted a serious NAC-APAP production effort aimed at providing a safer APAP product.

1.4   NAC-Acetaminophen: Formulate the Antidote Along with the Drug?

The FDA, of course, is well aware that APAP overdose is a public health hazard. On at least two occasions, they have decreed a reduction in the allowable APAP dosage in OTC medications. This has certainly been helpful, but unintentional overdose is still a problem.

Of course, one could ask, since NAC has been found to be a safe antidote to APAP toxicity, "why not prevent acetaminophen overdose problems altogether by mandating that each acetaminophen tablet be formulated with enough NAC to prevent the ingested acetaminophen from significantly decreasing patient glutathione levels?" I'm not sure whether this issue has been discussed by any of the major APAP producers, who perhaps lack an incentive to point out that their APAP products may be toxic at doses that fall far short of typical toxic APAP overdosing.

---

[2] Disclaimer: In accord with our university policy, we have cooperated with BioAdvantex in the development of several patents for NAC use in HIV and other diseases and have worked on clinical trials with both Zambon and BioAdvantex. Some of these patents have been issued; none have as yet secured FDA approval for clinical (or other) uses. Other groups conducting studies discussed in this volume have worked, I believe, with other NAC sources

The failure to field (or mandate) marketing of a NAC-APAP product may also be explained by a relatively short shelf life of *reduced* NAC, which, unless properly sequestered, is rapidly oxidized in air to "di-NAC" (NAC-S-S-NAC). Di-NAC has been reported to be highly pro-inflammatory, and hence its presence, even at low levels in unprotected NAC formulations, could subvert the anti-inflammatory activity of the NAC monomer. Unfortunately, the larger medical community has not embraced this understanding of NAC. For example, in a recent very large clinical trial using NAC, this aspect of protecting the product from oxidation was not addressed (Weisbord et al. 2018).

The failure to create and market a NAC-APAP product could be due to the bad sulfurous smell/taste that accumulates when NAC is not properly sequestered and can often be detected when typical off-the-shelf NAC packages are opened. Any or all of these reasons could account for reluctance on the part of APAP producers to coformulate their product with NAC.

Going in the other direction, I raised this coformulation idea with a small company (BioAdvantex.com) that produces and safely packages NAC to protect it from becoming oxidized. They package the NAC in individually sealed foil packets that minimize NAC exposure to air and thereby prevent significant NAC oxidation and/or generation of foul smells or tastes. The company has sold NAC in such protective packaging for many years and is the mainstay of many people who depend on NAC for medical reasons. However, although this company recognizes the importance of fielding a combined NAC-APAP OTC medication, they have not yet been able to develop the resources to mount the extensive effort required to generate and get approval for this NAC-APAP[3] product. Thus, at present, there is no viable source for a properly protected product designed to provide normal APAP doses along with sufficient NAC to prevent the toxic effects of the ingested APAP.

1.5 How Did We, Two Basic Scientists, Get Involved with Considering the Clinical Uses of NAC?

Having studied at Caltech in the mid-1950s, when biochemical genetics was king, Len (my late husband) and I started out being more familiar with GSH than most of our current medical and genetics colleagues. Len's thesis work (and my "tagalong") brought us into contact with cytochromes, mitochondria, respiratory pathways, and the like, and his postdoctoral work (and again, my tagalong work) with Jacques Monod in Paris studying enzyme (β-galactosidase) induction in *Escherichia coli* taught us more basic biochemistry, cell physiology, and genetics.

When we moved to the National Institutes of Health (NIH) so Len could complete his required "military" service, I continued with bacterial genetics/physiology work

---

[3] In accord with our university policy, we have been joined by this company (BioAdvantex) in the development of several patents for NAC use in HIV and other diseases. However, neither we nor BioAdvantex have secured FDA approval for any clinical (or other) uses.

in Bruce Ames laboratory. Len, however, followed his "dream" and moved to Harry Eagle's laboratory, where mammalian cells were being put into culture for the first time. Joining the effort to craft culture media for these cells, Len found that the cultured cells had a curious need for a metabolite (pyruvate) that they were quite capable of making. Understanding the biochemistry surrounding this "oddity" and other such findings in Eagle's laboratory gave us a solid background for our later explorations of the interplay between biochemical and genetic mechanisms (including redox) and the survival, growth, genetics, and function of mammalian cells. Thus, by the time Len was appointed (and I tagged along) to the faculty of Joshua Lederberg's newly founded Genetics Department at Stanford, we were well primed to begin the mammalian genetics and cell biology studies that have occupied us ever since.

Len initially focused on biochemical and drug sensitivity markers expressed by mammalian cell lines. However, soon after we arrived at Stanford, Lederberg lodged us in a laboratory next door to where Gus Nossal and Olli Makela were engaged in proving that "one cell makes only one antibody." This idea is at the heart of the Lederberg-Burnet theory of antigen-based selection of cells. At this time, medical science believed that all antibodies had the same structure, which then folded in different ways to combine with different antigens.

The work going on in the lab next door was too exciting to just pass by. Len suggested that I learn how to immunize mice and measure antibodies. I did, and within a short time, we were both seduced into in vivo immunology and mouse immunogenetic studies. In the ensuing years, this led to our building the fluorescence-activated cell sorter (FACS), making monoclonal antibodies to identify, sort, and test immunologically relevant mammalian cells, and to using these antibodies and the cell sorter to clone CD5, CD8, and other immunologically relevant mammalian genes.

Relevant to the redox focus of this article, Len and his fellows developed a FACS-detectable reporter gene assay in which they introduced *Escherichia coli* β-galactosidase gene (lacZ) under the control of various genetic regulatory elements (e.g., NF-κB) into cell lines. They then used FACS to measure lacZ cleavage of a fluorogenic substrate in individual cells as an index of promoter efficacy, enhancer activity, trans-acting factors, etc. Thus, we were well prepared to determine the sensitivity of the promoter elements to various stimuli and/or stimulatory conditions, including oxidative stress. Indeed, we later showed, the expression β-galactosidase (lacZ) reporter gene under the control of NF-κB in these various promoter constructs increases in cell lines grown under oxidative stress and decreases when NAC was added to the cultures to reduce oxidative stress (Nolan et al. 1988).

1.6   Growing Cells at Physiological Oxygen Levels

In our early studies we were not equipped to alter our incubator oxygen levels. However, modern ("Tri-Gas") incubators that are now commonly available have the ability to mix and maintain the concentrations of three gases (O_2, CO_2, and nitrogen). Nevertheless, most incubators today are still run with only two gases, 5% CO_2

and air, which results in continuously exposing cells to oxygen levels of about 20%. Since, except for skin and other tissues exposed to air, mammalian cells live at oxygen levels considerably below this (roughly 2–12% oxygen), much of the work with mammalian cells and cell lines has been done with cells growing under significant oxidative stress.

Thus, not surprisingly, when cells are grown in incubators maintained at physiological oxygen levels (5–10% O_2 in a 5% CO_2 "Tri-Gas" incubator), their responses differ in key ways from that are cells grown in incubators maintained at room air oxygen levels. For example, sensitivity to apoptosis induction by HIV-Tat, a widely studied apoptosis inducer, is markedly decreased in cells grown at 5% O_2 versus cells grown at typical incubator oxygen levels (20%). These findings underscore the importance of taking incubator oxygen levels into account when interpreting data from cell culture studies, which today unfortunately are largely conducted at room air.

Adding NAC to cells cultured at 20% O_2 can decrease the oxidative stress, as our early findings with the human immunodeficiency virus (HIV) promoter demonstrated. However, preventing the stress in the first place by lowering the incubator oxygen levels that approximate those the cultured cells encounter in vivo (generally 5–10%) is likely better in the long run. In fact, in vivo *veritas* is probably still a good rule to follow, if experimental goals permit. Keeping incubator oxygen levels in an appropriate range for the cells being cultured is likely to provide findings more suitable for predicting in vivo behavior of the cultured cells.

1.7   NAC and HIV

Some time after we had developed these constructs discussed above, Len and I chanced to hear a seminar by the National Institute of Allergy and Infectious Disease (NIAID) director Anthony Fauci, who reported work done with Mary Anderson and Alton Meister demonstrating NAC's interference with HIV replication in cell lines. Since NF-κB was already known to be an important regulatory element in the HIV promoter, we were immediately energized to use our NF-κB lacZ reporter line to determine whether NAC would decrease lacZ expression upregulated in the cell line under oxidative stress. Indeed, as predicted, we found that adding NAC to the culture downregulated the activity of the NF-κB transcription factor in several reporter constructs, including those in which the HIV promoter controlled lacZ expression.

These findings suggested that ingesting NAC might downregulate HIV expression in HIV-infected individuals. And so began our long and still continuing romance with NAC as a supplementary source of dietary cysteine necessary not only for protein synthesis but also for synthesis and maintenance of reduced intracellular GSH, the primary intracellular antioxidant, a key regulator of intracellular redox status and, in vitro at least, a key regulator of the HIV activity (Staal et al. 1990).

On hearing the above findings, Fauci and his group rapidly decided to run a quick (2-week) trial to determine whether NAC would be an antiretroviral drug and hence would decrease viral load very rapidly. It did not. Further, although administered at a high dose, NAC proved to be minimally detectable in circulation shortly after dosing. This failure to detect NAC in the circulation is not surprising, since orally administered NAC is rapidly metabolized to cysteine once it leaves the digestive tract and enters the liver. However, together with the failure to rapidly achieve the desired antiretroviral effect, this apparent lack of NAC's ability to "get in" was sufficient for Fauci's group to rapidly cross NAC of the list of potential therapeutics in HIV infection. This decision paid off, since it ultimately led to the discovery of the antiretroviral azidothymidine (AZT), which of course went on to become the first of a series of progressively more effective and less toxic therapeutics for treating HIV infection.

Of course, orally administered NAC "gets in" since, as indicated above, its administration is the standard of care for treating toxic APAP overdose. Therefore, although NAC failed as a rapid antiretroviral, we mustered our resources and established a small, short-term (8-week) placebo-controlled double-blind study to determine what benefit, if any, NAC therapy could bring to HIV-infected patients.

Results from this trial were largely eclipsed by the spectacular results obtained with AZT, which were published about the time we were ready to publish our findings. However, our findings established that HIV-infection progressively decreases intracellular GSH levels, that subjects with CD4 T-cell counts below 200 had the lowest GSH levels, and that NAC restores the diminished GSH by the end of the 8-week trial period (Herzenberg et al. 1997; Herzenberg et al. 1998; De Rosa et al. 2000).

We were not confident, or arrogant, enough to set survival as an endpoint for this trial. However, when we surveyed the survival of the subjects 1–2 years after the trial, we found that none of the participants with T-cell counts above 200 had died, that a sizable number with CD4 T-cell counts below 200 had died, and that within this group, the survival of subjects who received NAC was significantly greater than those who had received the placebo. Kaplan-Meier analysis added that even the NAC-taking subjects who died had survived significantly longer than those who were given placebo.

Our findings with this study were eclipsed by spectacular findings obtained with AZT treatment, which were published before or around the same time. As a result, AZT treatment was prescribed for essentially all HIV patients whose survival was at risk. Therefore, there was no justification for continuing our NAC-HIV studies except as adjunct therapy, for which were unlikely to get support since the HIV research community largely still believed that orally administered NAC "does not get in."

Nevertheless, we were encouraged to go on with our NAC-HIV and other NAC-redox studies based on the results from our in vitro reporter gene studies (Herzenberg et al. 1997; Herzenberg et al. 1998; De Rosa et al. 2000), our clinical trial testing NAC in HIV-infected subjects (Herzenberg et al. 1997; Herzenberg et al. 1998; De Rosa et al. 2000), and a series of positive anecdotal results reported by HIV-infected individuals who took NAC. Ultimately, our work and our interests broadened to include findings with NAC treatment in other diseases, including our collaborative clinical studies showing positive effects for NAC treatment in cystic fibrosis (CF) (Tirouvanziam et al. 2006) and autism (Hardan et al. 2012; Tirouvanziam et al. 2012).

1.8   NAC Treatment in Disease

We had started the above clinical HIV studies in accord with a suggestion by a German T-cell biologist, Wulf Droge (now deceased), who had conducted a long series of in vitro studies characterizing the amino acid and other requirements for T-cell growth and function in vitro. On hearing about this work, a pharmacist who lived next door to Wulf asked him whether he could suggest anything that might help his adult HIV-infected son, whose T-cell counts had already diminished markedly as had his ability to help his father in the pharmacy. Wulf reasoned that some help might be gotten by increasing the dietary intake of certain amino acids that he found were necessary for T-cell growth in vitro, naming the sulfur-containing amino acid cysteine as one of these.

The pharmacist, knowing that oral NAC is administered to counter cysteine and GSH loss in APAP toxicity, responded by questioning whether administration of the medicinal grade NAC he had in his pharmacy might be useful in restoring his son's health. Wulf was not sure, but he agreed that since NAC is not known to be toxic, the pharmacist should try administering it to his son. Surprisingly, within a short time of initiating this NAC treatment, the pharmacist's son regained strength, got back to work, and remained relatively healthy for some years until other aspects of HIV disease caught up with him.

Seeing this "miracle," Wulf decided to tell this story in an open letter to 100 immunologists, with the hope that someone would be encouraged to investigate NAC as a potential therapeutic for HIV disease. So far as we know, only one laboratory (ours) took this idea seriously at the time. Working, as we were, only a short distance from San Francisco, we were seeing and hearing close at hand the mounting numbers of HIV deaths in the city. Anything that could help should be considered.

Bringing this plague even closer to home, we had recently learned that a close friend, a gay man working as central engineer/investigator on our FACS development staff, was infected with HIV. Therefore, we were very attuned to Wulf's message suggesting that a nontoxic treatment, NAC, might comfortably contribute to prolonging life in HIV infection and gratefully accepted Wulf's offer to send a "care package" with enough NAC for several months' treatment for our friend and his partner.

At the time, our friend was helping his domestic partner through the last stages of an opportunistic infection and did not want to try anything new for himself or his partner. However, at his suggestion, we gave the NAC to another gay couple, mutual friends also moving toward end-stage acquired immune deficiency syndrome (AIDS). We were surprised and very pleased to see that after a few weeks on NAC (in addition to their medically approved treatment), both friends felt healthier and resumed folk dancing and other activities that their disease had forced them to curtail. When last heard, they had set out on a world tour to "see the places they thought they would never get to see."

Our staff member continued to care for his partner through a sad and immensely painful passing, and was then cut adrift to face his own likely demise. Being quite knowledgeable about the horrendous effects of the then early HIV drugs, he decided not to use any at all. We understood and said we would support him and help him face the potentially painful consequences of this nonstandard response. However, we asked him to take NAC regularly and continued to monitor his T-cell counts as he went along (he had 300–400 CD4 T-cells at the time). His physician was not so sanguine about his choice, but could do nothing to convince him to do otherwise.

Once our friend started taking NAC, his CD4 T-cell counts stabilized in the 300–400 range and only fell to around 200 several years later. By that time, less toxic HIV drugs were available and he decided to take these. Currently, having shifted to better and better drugs in the intervening years, his CD4 T-cell counts are in the very desirable 600 range, and he has ridden his Harley to Canada and Alaska multiple times over the last few years (at this writing he is in Canada enjoying another such ride). Importantly, those of us using FACS have all benefited from his continued good health, since over the years, he has developed FACS/Desk and other innovative mathematics and software that collectively underlie the current FlowJo FACS/CyTOF data analysis program (FlowJo.com) and his/our own CytoGenie software, which provides innovative, statistically based software for FACS/CyTOF data analysis and visualization.

Anecdotal stories like this of course mean very little. Clearly, we would love to see whether a properly controlled trial for NAC as adjunct therapy for HIV would confirm our observations. However, the likelihood of such a trial happening in the near future seems slim indeed in the current world. Therefore, since NAC is not toxic, we content ourselves with recommending that HIV-infected individual supplement a good diet and medication regime with NAC, properly packaged to prevent it from being oxidized while "waiting on the shelf" to be ingested.

Nevertheless, we still continued to measure GSH levels in T-cells from HIV-infected people and to correlate these levels with disease parameters. We also developed a more facile test for determining GSH levels in HIV-infected patients and correlating the measured levels with survival. Using this test, we found again that GSH levels decrease as patient conditions deteriorate.

1.9 Contrast Nephropathy

Several years ago, our colleagues and us attempted to put together a comprehensive review of NAC uses in the clinic. It proved to be a gargantuan task, well beyond what we could manage, and the data available at the time was far too sparse. Nevertheless, we did learn some useful things, particularly about what has now become the fairly routine use of NAC to prevent the development of contrast dye-induced nephropathy in patients scheduled for various radiological procedures.

A survey of the literature available at the time (ca 2010) revealed a striking dichotomy in the reported results, some studies showing clear success in the NAC versus placebo groups, while others showed no differences at all. Broken down further into the study locale, we surprisingly found that studies conducted in Europe were far more likely to show that NAC is successful in preventing nephropathy than studies conducted in the US.

We never arrived at a satisfactory explanation for this observed difference. The patient groups and the trial protocols seemed comparable in the two locales. However, there was likely to have been key differences in the source of the NAC used in the two studies. That is, NAC is commonly used in Europe to treat asthma and a variety of other conditions and hence is packaged and sold under stringent conditions that mitigate against inclusion of oxidized NAC in the product. In contrast, in the US, relatively palatable NAC is commonly sold in health food and other stores that pay little attention to whether care is taken to prevent oxidation of the NAC, either before or after packaging. Since oxidized NAC can be expected to act antithetically to reduced NAC, the differences in study results could well be explained by differences in the oxidative state of the NAC at the time of treatment. Because of this, we used NAC that was properly packaged according to European standards in our studies.

This explanation occurred to us as we collated the data for the contrast nephropathy section of the review we were trying to write. However, although we sent letters and made phone calls requesting specification of the source of the NAC used in the various studies, and although we followed up on most of these requests, we did not receive useful answers from most of the authors of the published studies. Thus, while we believe the source of the NAC and its likelihood of being oxidized may explain the differences in outcomes in these studies, we have no direct evidence to substantiate this claim.

Nowadays, despite the earlier conflicting results, physicians in the US commonly recommend taking NAC some hours prior to exposure to contrast dyes. Fortunately, because they tend to actually prescribe the NAC, it will usually be obtained from a reputable pharmacy that will fill the prescription with pharmaceutical grade NAC used also to treat APAP overdose. Thus, the prescribed NAC may taste terrible, but will likely be safe and efficacious. In Europe, in contrast, NAC is routinely produced under European standards and packaged to prevent or at least minimize oxidation. Thus, it is available from reputable companies (e.g., Zambon, Inc.). In the US, BioAdvantex sells European-produced NAC, mainly via mail or web order.

1.10 Cystic Fibrosis

Some time ago, Dr. Rabindra (Rabin) Tirouvanziam, working in our laboratory, decided to determine whether NAC would be useful for treating cystic fibrosis (CF). Teaming up with Drs. Richard (Rick) Moss and Carol Conrad from the Stanford Medical School CF Clinic, Rabin initially organized a Phase 1 trial that was supported by the US FDA orphan drug unit. Using NAC supplied by BioAdvantex, Rabin and Carol obtained positive Phase I results and embarked on organizing a Phase 2 trial testing NAC efficacy in treating CF.

Here, the story becomes more complex. Carol Conrad, who leads the CF clinic at the Stanford Medical School, became the principal investigator for the planned multicenter trial, with Rick Moss as consultant. Carol and Rabin went to visit the CF foundation to request help and advice in setting the trial guidelines and determining the trial endpoint(s). Richard Moss, who has led the Stanford clinical effort in CF for years, and I (a non-clinician) were pleased that our younger colleagues were "carrying the ball" and left them to it. We did not visit the foundation with them.

At the end of the day, Carol and Rabin sifted the advice they received from the foundation and established a defined magnitude change in sputum human neutrophil elastase (HNE) activity as the primary endpoint. As secondary endpoints, they specified a change in forced expiratory volume in 1 s (FEV1) and other clinical lung function measures that are commonly considered unlikely to change significantly during trials. They also specified the safety and tolerability of NAC and the potential of NAC to promote pulmonary hypertension in subjects with CF as additional endpoints.

The results from this trial proved to be quite surprising. Although HNE is considered to be a good CF clinical endpoint, there was no significant difference between the NAC-treated and placebo control groups. On the other hand, FEV1 increased significantly in the treated group but stayed constant or fell somewhat in the placebo control (Conrad et al. 2015). Since an increase in FEV1 is extremely rare in CF patients, this latter finding suggests that NAC is indeed beneficial for the treated patients.

Ideally, this study should be repeated with FEV1 as the primary endpoint. However, CF is classified by the FDA as an orphan disease, meaning there are too few patients to be able to conduct and repeat trials. In essence, the CF patient pool is probably not large enough to enable recruitment for a second trial, particularly since many CF patients heard about our results and are now "self-dosing" with NAC, which is available OTC in the precise individually sealed packaging used for the trial.

We plan to query the FDA to determine how to move forward within the confines of this result. However, the likelihood is that NAC treatment in CF will be left up to individual physicians and their patients, who will have to find and purchase properly packaged NAC and find the funds to support NAC treatment in the absence of FDA approval and hence the consequent lack of insurance funding for the treatment.

1.11 Autism

One day, as our NAC studies proceeded, a senior administrator in the Stanford Immunology Program came by and asked me whether I thought NAC treatment could be useful in autism. Knowing that she had two autistic children, I didn't simply brush off the query but discussed the issue with her. She told me about another Stanford Medical School professor who had a child who was much less affected than her boys and suggested he might be interested in trying NAC with his son. Since NAC is not known to be toxic, I suggested that I could procure European-style NAC (as it has come to be known) if the faculty member she spoke about was interested. She then invited this professor to meet me to discuss the issue.

When we met, I outlined what I knew about NAC and said that I would be willing to procure the NAC if the NAC treatment were done under the eyes of an autism specialist. This was readily arranged since the child's current physician was just such a specialist. Over time, the NAC treatment appeared to have beneficial effects for the child, leading Dr. Antonio Hardan in the Stanford Pediatrics autism group to establish a serious placebo-controlled, double-blind clinical trial testing NAC for efficacy in autism, which proved successful in that the treatment group showing improvement in key widely used assays of behavioral function (Hardan et al. 2012).

The trial was successful for me in other ways, too, in that Dr. Hardan introduced me to Dr. Michael Berk, the coeditor of this volume, who, together with his coeditor Dr. Richard Frye, invited me to wander through my laboratory's interest in NAC and redox, and to lightly summarize our path as an introduction to this wonderful volume.

1.12 Summary

In the sections above, I have outlined some basic and some clinically related findings from the NAC studies we have conducted in our laboratory or encountered in our travels. The chapters that follow in this book tell a surprising and far broader story of NAC's uses than my husband and I would have ever thought possible when we first began thinking about NAC and NF-κB years ago. Actually, though, we all should be surprised—surprised that it took us, as a scientific and medical community, so long to recognize the importance of the complex relationship between the air we breathe and the life we lead. Just because we don't see air and the oxygen it contains does not mean we should forget that it is there. This book reminds us of this, and brings home to us how far we have come, and how much farther we have to go to understand the processes that together serve the living organism. At least we, a research and medical community, have now made a strong beginning.

References

Atkuri KR, Mantovani JJ, Herzenberg LA, Herzenberg LA (2007) N-acetylcysteine-a safe antidote for cysteine/glutathione deficiency. Curr Opin Pharmacol 7(4):355–359

Conrad C, Lymp J, Thompson V, Dunn C, Davies Z, Chatfield B, Nichols D, Clancy J, Vender R, Egan ME, Quittell L, Michelson P, Antony V, Spahr J, Rubenstein RC, Moss RB, Herzenberg LA, Goss CH, Tirouvanziam R (2015) Long-term treatment with oral N-acetylcysteine: affects lung function but not sputum inflammation in cystic fibrosis subjects. A phase II randomized placebo-controlled trial. J Cyst Fibros 14(2):219–227. https://doi.org/10.1016/j.jcf.2014.08.008

De Rosa SC, Zaretsky MD, Dubs JG, Roederer M, Anderson M, Green A, Mitra D, Watanabe N, Nakamura H, Tjioe I, Deresinski SC, Moore WA, Ela SW, Parks D, Herzenberg LA, Herzenberg LA (2000) N-acetylcysteine (NAC) replenishes glutathione in HIV infection. Eur J Clin Investig 30(10):841–856

Green JL, Heard KJ, Reynolds KM, Albert D (2013) Oral and intravenous acetylcysteine for treatment of acetaminophen toxicity: a systematic review and meta-analysis. West J Emerg Med 14(3):218–226. https://doi.org/10.5811/westjem.2012.4.6885

Hardan AY, Fung LK, Libove RA, Obukhanych TV, Nair S, Herzenberg LA, Frazier TW, Tirouvanziam R (2012) A randomized controlled pilot trial of oral N-acetylcysteine in children with autism. Biol Psychiatry 71(11):956–961. https://doi.org/10.1016/j.biopsych.2012.01.014

Herzenberg LA, De Rosa SC, Dubs JG, Roederer M, Anderson MT, Ela SW, Deresinski SC (1997) Glutathione deficiency is associated with impaired survival in HIV disease. Proc Natl Acad Sci U S A 94(5):1967–1972

Herzenberg LA, De Rosa SC, Herzenberg LA (1998) Low glutathione levels in CD4 T cells predict poor survival in AIDS; N-acetylcysteine may improve survival. In: Monatagnier LOR, Pasquier C (eds) Oxidative stress in cancer, AIDS and neurodegenerative diseases, vol 1. Marcel Dekker, Inc., Stanford, pp 379–387

Nolan GP, Fiering S, Nicolas JF, Herzenberg LA (1988) Fluorescence-activated cell analysis and sorting of viable mammalian cells based on beta-D-galactosidase activity after transduction of Escherichia coli lacZ. Proc Natl Acad Sci U S A 85(8):2603–2607

Staal FJ, Roederer M, Herzenberg LA, Herzenberg LA (1990) Intracellular thiols regulate activation of nuclear factor kappa B and transcription of human immunodeficiency virus. Proc Natl Acad Sci U S A 87(24):9943–9947

Tirouvanziam R, Conrad CK, Bottiglieri T, Herzenberg LA, Moss RB (2006) High-dose oral N-acetylcysteine, a glutathione prodrug, modulates inflammation in cystic fibrosis. Proc Natl Acad Sci U S A 103(12):4628–4633. https://doi.org/10.1073/pnas.0511304103

Tirouvanziam R, Obukhanych TV, Laval J, Aronov PA, Libove R, Banerjee AG, Parker KJ, O'Hara R, Herzenberg LA, Herzenberg LA, Hardan AY (2012) Distinct plasma profile of polar neutral amino acids, leucine, and glutamate in children with autism Spectrum disorders. J Autism Dev Disord 42(5):827–836. https://doi.org/10.1007/s10803-011-1314-x

Weisbord SD, Gallagher M, Jneid H, Garcia S, Cass A, Thwin S-S, Conner TA, Chertow GM, Bhatt DL, Shunk K, Parikh CR, McFalls EO, Brophy M, Ferguson R, Hongsheng W, Androsenko M, Myles J, Kaufman J, Palevsky PM (2018) Outcomes after angiography with sodium bicarbonate and acetylcysteine. N Engl J Med 378(7):603–614

The Basic Science of N-Acetylcysteine (NAC)

M. Foster Olive, Gregory Powell, Erin McClure, and Cassandra D. Gipson

2.1 Overview of Glutamatergic Neurotransmission

Glutamate is the most abundant excitatory neurotransmitter in the central nervous system (CNS) and is vital for a wide variety of CNS functions. It has been estimated that up to 70–80% of all synapses in the CNS utilize glutamate for intercellular communication (Niciu et al. 2012; Zhou and Danbolt 2014) and extracellular concentrations of this amino acid are found in the low millimolar range (Rodriguez et al. 2013; Bridges et al. 2012). In a typical glutamatergic synapse, glutamate is packaged into presynaptic terminal vesicles by one of three different vesicular glutamate transporters (vGluT1-3) (Shigeri et al. 2004). Upon arrival of an action potential at the terminal and mobilization of synaptic vesicles to the active zone, an estimated 3000–10,000 molecules of glutamate are released into the synaptic cleft (Clements 1996; Pendyam et al. 2009).

Released glutamate binds with high affinity to one of the three different types of ionotropic glutamate receptors (iGluRs) that mediate fast excitatory neurotransmission or metabotropic glutamate receptors (mGluRs) that mediate slower, modulatory transmission (Fig. 2.1). iGluRs include the N-methyl-D-aspartate (NMDA), α-amino-3-hydroxy-5-methylisoxazole-4-propionic acid (AMPA), and kainic acid (kainate, KA) receptor subtypes, each of which are multimeric pore-forming structures composed of varying combinations of individual protein subunits. It has been estimated that approximately 50–100 iGluRs populate a typical synapse (Takumi et al. 1999). mGluRs are seven transmembrane domain-spanning G-protein-coupled receptors

M. Foster Olive · G. Powell (✉) · C. D. Gipson
Department of Psychology, Arizona State University,
Tempe, AZ, USA
e-mail: gregory.powell.1@asu.edu; gpowell6@asu.edu

E. McClure
Department of Psychiatry, Medical University of South Carolina,
Charleston, SC, USA

© Springer Nature Singapore Pte Ltd. 2019
R. E. Frye, M. Berk (eds.), *The Therapeutic Use of N-Acetylcysteine (NAC) in Medicine*, https://doi.org/10.1007/978-981-10-5311-5_2

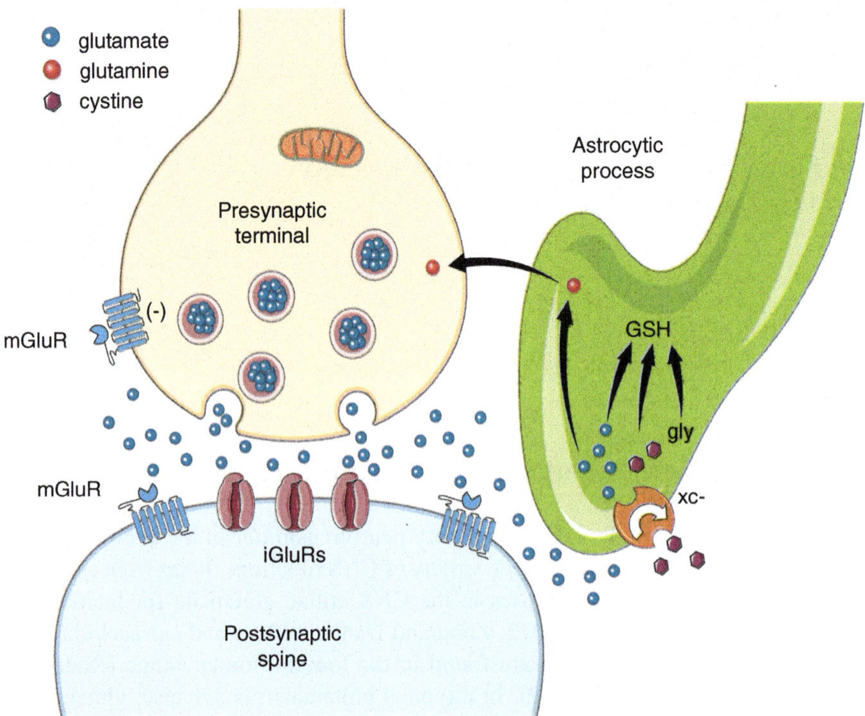

Fig. 2.1 Schematic of a classical glutamatergic synapse. Release of glutamate from presynaptic terminals and/or glial cells binds to and activates iGluRs (NMDA, AMPA, or KA receptors), which in turn allows the influx of Na^+ and Ca^{2+} ions into the postsynaptic dendritic spine and increases the likelihood of depolarization. Presynaptic mGluRs, particularly mGluR2/3, regulate the exocytosis of glutamate via inhibition (−) of second messenger systems such as adenylyl cyclase, and also respond to non-synaptic sources of extracellular glutamate such as system xc- located on astrocytes. Once transported into astroglia, glutamate is enzymatically converted to glutamine, after which it is transported to the presynaptic terminal for conversion back to glutamate. Intracellular cystine can also be reduced to cysteine, which promotes the formation of GSH in both neurons and glia, the latter of which is depicted here

(GPCRs) that are subcategorized into Group I (mGluR 1, 5), Group II (mGluR 2, 3), or Group III (mGluR 4, 6, 7, 8) based on their sequence homologies, pharmacology, and signal transduction mechanisms. In general, iGluRs tend to be localized on postsynaptic membranes of dendritic spines directly opposed to presynaptic release sites, whereas mGluRs tend to be located either on the perisynaptic annulus of the spine or on presynaptic terminals as inhibitory autoreceptors or heteroreceptors (Fig. 2.1). It should be noted that the mGluR6 receptor subtype is not found in the brain or spinal cord but is exclusively expressed in the retina. While traditionally it was believed that glutamate receptors were primarily localized to regions immediately surrounding sites of synaptic glutamate release, there is now clear evidence for localization of iGluRs and mGluRs on extrasynaptic sites as well as glial cells such as astrocytes (Fan et al. 2014; Garcia-Junco-Clemente et al. 2005; Huganir and Nicoll 2013; Parpura and Verkhratsky 2013), making up the tripartite synapse (Fig. 2.1).

It should be mentioned that both neurons and glia synthesize considerable amounts of the endogenous antioxidant glutathione (GSH). This thiol-containing tripeptide exerts neuroprotective effects against damage from reactive oxygen and nitrogen species such as hydrogen peroxide and peroxynitrite and is synthesized from glutamate, glycine, and the rate-limiting substrate cysteine (Bridges et al. 2012). As will be discussed below, in addition to its ability to regulate glutamatergic neurotransmission, NAC elevates brain cysteine levels that promote the formation of GSH.

2.2 Regulation of Extracellular Glutamate Levels by Autoreceptors and Glutamate Uptake

Glutamatergic signaling requires a high level of coordinated activity between neurons and astrocytes, and it has been established that the vast majority of extracellular glutamate is derived from vesicular and non-vesicular release from astrocytes rather than neurons (Rodriguez et al. 2013; Baker et al. 2002a; Danbolt et al. 2016; Baker et al. 2002b; Bridges et al. 2012; Moussawi et al. 2011). Its obligatory role in fast excitatory transmission, as well as the need to safeguard cells against excitotoxicity, requires numerous mechanisms to regulate extracellular glutamate concentrations and achieve glutamate homeostasis (Kalivas 2009). One such mechanism is via activation of presynaptic inhibitory metabotropic autoreceptors, typically mGluR2/3 receptors, but also through various members of the Group III mGluR family (Fig. 2.1). Upon stimulation by extracellular glutamate, these receptors inhibit the activity of adenylyl cyclase (AC), leading to the reduced formation of cyclic adenosine monophosphate (cAMP), which affects numerous downstream targets (e.g., potassium channels and vesicular release machinery) that ultimately reduce subsequent presynaptic glutamate release.

Another key player in the regulation of glutamate homeostasis is the family of sodium-dependent excitatory amino acid transporters (EAATs) (Shigeri et al. 2004; Divito and Underhill 2014; Danbolt et al. 2016; Moussawi et al. 2011). It has been estimated that collectively, EAATs are expressed in a density of 10,000 transporters per μm^2 in the brain, resulting in an uptake capacity of 10 μM/ms (Lehre and Danbolt 1998). This high level of glutamate uptake results in spatially compartmentalized extracellular glutamate that limits activation of, or toxicity to, neighboring cells and synapses. To date, five EAAT isoforms have been identified and are termed EAAT 1–5. However, alternative nomenclatures are frequently used in the literature, such that EAAT1 is often referred to as glutamate aspartate transporter (GLAST), EAAT2 is referred to as glutamate type 1 transporter (GLT-1), and EAAT3 is referred to as excitatory amino acid carrier 1 (EAAC1). Different EAAT isoforms are expressed in different cell types (Fig. 2.2). EAAT1 is primarily localized to glial cells, EAAT2 is primarily localized to glial cells and presynaptic sites, EAAT3 and EAAT4 are primarily localized to postsynaptic neuronal elements, and EAAT5 expression is largely restricted to the retina. It is believed that up to 95% of extracellular

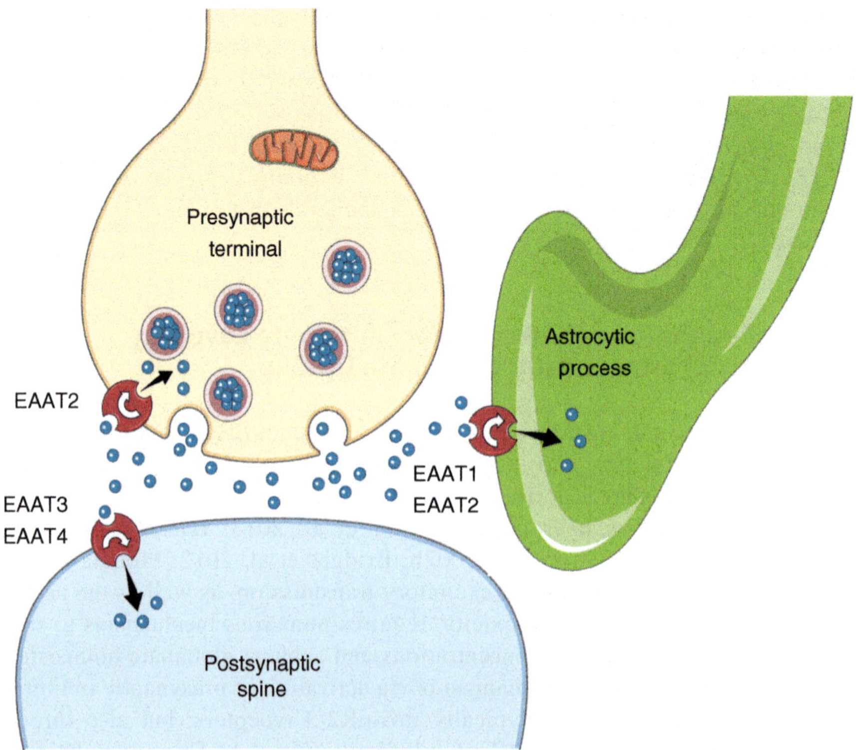

Fig. 2.2 Localization of different glutamate transporter subtypes at a typical tripartite synapse. EAAT1 is expressed predominantly in astrocytes, EAAT2 is expressed on astrocytes as well as presynaptic terminals, and EAAT3 and EAAT4 are primarily localized to postsynaptic elements

glutamate is regulated by EAAT2, which constitutes 1% of the total forebrain protein content (Danbolt et al. 2016).

2.3 Regulation of Glutamate Homeostasis by Cystine-Glutamate Exchangers (System xc-) and NAC

Efflux of glutamate into the synaptic cleft and extrasynaptic space is derived from several sources. Glutamate release into the synaptic cleft is primarily derived from presynaptic vesicles (Fig. 2.1), while extrasynaptic glutamate is primarily derived from non-neuronal cells such as astrocytes, either via calcium-independent vesicular exocytosis (Hamilton and Attwell 2010) or non-vesicular release via the cystine/glutamate exchanger (system xc-) (Bridges et al. 2012; Massie et al. 2015). Also known as the cystine-glutamate antiporter, system xc- is comprised of two functional proteins, xCT which serves as the primary molecular exchanger and an

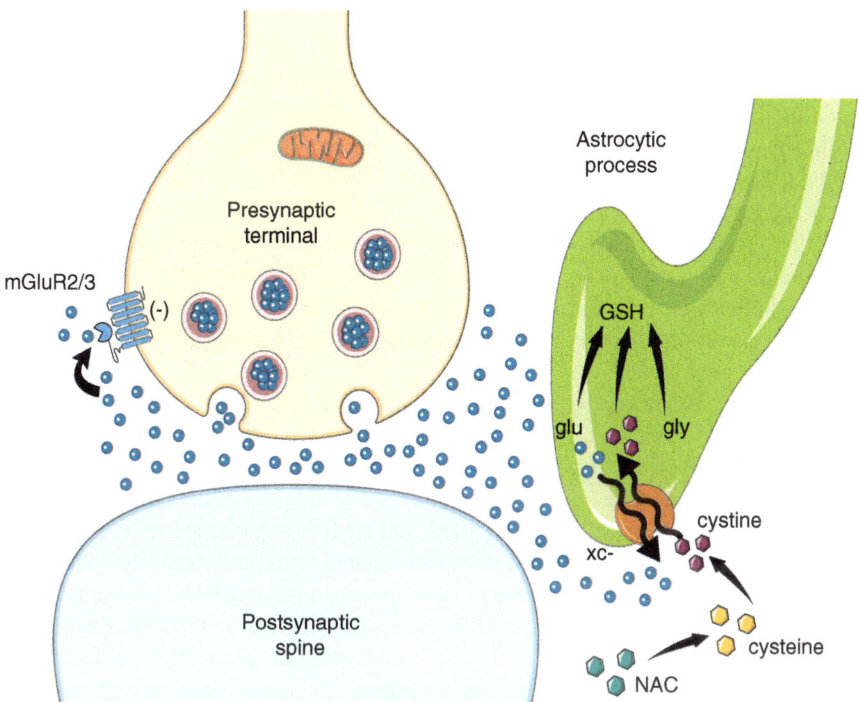

Fig. 2.3 Actions of NAC on system xc- and its effects on glutamate homeostasis. As a cystine prodrug, NAC indirectly activates the antiporter to drive glutamate from glial stores into the extracellular space. The resulting increases in extracellular glutamate can then interact with extrasynaptic iGluRs and/or mGluRs. Under conditions of low levels of extracellular glutamate, basal stimulation of presynaptically localized mGluR2/3 receptors is reduced, resulting in excessive synaptic release of glutamate. Thus, NAC indirectly activates system xc- to increase extracellular levels of glutamate, which restores the inhibitory tone on presynaptic mGluR2/3 receptors and thus reduces presynaptic release of glutamate. As a result of increased system xc- activity, NAC also increases intracellular cystine levels, which can be reduced to cysteine and thus promote GSH formation in both glia (shown here) and neurons

auxiliary heavy chain protein termed 4F2hc. System xc- is primarily expressed by glia and exchanges cystine and glutamate with a 1:1 stoichiometry, transporting one molecule of cystine into the glial cell in exchange for one molecule of glutamate transported into the extracellular environment (Fig. 2.3). It is believed that up to 90% of extracellular glutamate, particular that found in extrasynaptic regions, results from system xc- activity (Massie et al. 2015; Bridges et al. 2012; Baker et al. 2002a). Other endogenous substrates of system xc- include cystathionine and homocysteic acid.

NAC interacts with system xc- via acting as a cystine prodrug in the CNS, where it is converted into cysteine followed by dimerization into the more stable cystine, which then activates the antiporter and drives glutamate from glial stores into the extracellular space (Fig. 2.3). In turn, system xc- derived glutamate can then interact with extrasynaptic iGluRs and/or mGluRs. It is thought that under conditions of low levels of extracellular glutamate, basal stimulation of presynaptically localized mGluR2/3 receptors is reduced, resulting in excessive synaptic release of glutamate. Thus, by serving as a cystine prodrug, NAC activates system xc- to increase extracellular levels of glutamate, which restores the inhibitory tone on presynaptic mGluR2/3 receptors and thus reduces presynaptic release of glutamate (Fig. 2.3). Via this mechanism, NAC has been proposed and tested as a possible pharmacotherapeutic for various neuropsychiatric disorders associated with dysregulated glutamate homeostasis, including drug addiction, pathological gambling, psychotic, mood, and anxiety disorders (Massie et al. 2015; Javitt et al. 2011; Bridges et al. 2012; Berk et al. 2013).

Although NAC primarily influences glutamate homeostasis via acting on system xc-, there is evidence that NAC also interacts directly with iGluRs. In vitro studies have revealed that the NAC by-product GSH, particularly in its oxidized form, inhibits NMDA-mediated increases in intracellular calcium (Gilbert et al. 1991) and can displace ligand binding from NMDA and AMPA receptors (Leslie et al. 1992; Varga et al. 1997). However, NAC may not interact with these receptors under normal (non-perturbed) conditions since they appear to be dependent on the presence of oxidant species and redox state of the receptor (Steullet et al. 2006). Finally, due to its ability to increase brain levels of cysteine and thus promote GSH formation, NAC has been proposed as a therapeutic option for treatment of neuropsychiatric disorders associated with oxidative stress and inflammation such as bipolar disorder, schizophrenia, autism, and perhaps even neurodegenerative diseases including Alzheimer's disease (Massie et al. 2015).

2.4 Regulation of Glial Glutamate Transporters by NAC

As mentioned in Sect. 2.3 above, the highly expressed EAAT2 is believed to be responsible for clearance for up to 95% of glutamate in the extracellular space. Recently it has come to light that many clinically utilized medications, in addition to their therapeutic mechanisms of action, also modulate the expression of EAAT2, thus indirectly affecting glutamate homeostasis (reviewed in Fontana 2015; Takahashi et al. 2015). Such medications include steroid hormones (dexamethasone, estradiol), anticonvulsants (valproate), antidepressants (amitriptyline), and β-lactam and other classes of antibiotics (minocycline, ceftriaxone).

Recently, it has been demonstrated that NAC also increases EAAT2 expression. Knackstedt et al. (2010) found that following self-administration of cocaine, rats demonstrated reduced glutamate uptake corresponding with decreased EAAT2 expression in the nucleus accumbens, which were restored by repeated treatment with NAC or ceftriaxone, resulting in reduced relapse-like reinstatement of cocaine-seeking behavior. Follow-up studies by Reissner et al. demonstrated that upregulation of EAAT2 in the nucleus accumbens by repeated NAC administration was necessary for the ability of this drug to prevent relapse-like behavior (Reissner et al. 2015) and that similar effects were also observed following repeated administration of the glial modulator propentofylline (Reissner et al. 2014). The mechanisms underlying the ability of NAC to increase EAAT2 expression are unclear but appear to be via transcriptional regulation of the EAAT2 gene (Fontana 2015; Takahashi et al. 2015). Similar effects have been found in experimental models of stroke and neurodegenerative diseases, suggesting that NAC and other medications that restore glutamate homeostasis via modulating EAAT2 expression hold promise as therapeutics for CNS disorders that are either caused by or result in dysregulated glutamate homeostasis.

2.5 Possible Regulation of Glutamate Homeostasis by NAC Analogues

While NAC was originally developed over 50 years ago, it has relatively poor oral bioavailability, thus requiring higher doses and longer treatment times in order to produce therapeutic effects. Clinically, this limits its use as a pharmacotherapeutic, and reports of gastrointestinal upset occur due to necessary higher oral dosing regimens (Berk et al. 2013; Deepmala et al. 2015; Chiew et al. 2016). As a result, newer structurally related analogues have recently been developed to circumvent these clinical limitations. These analogues include, but are not limited to, N-Acetylcysteine amide (NACA, also known as AD4), N-Acetylcysteine ethyl ester (NACET), and N-Acetylcysteine methyl ester (NACMT) (Fig. 2.4). Similar to NAC, it has been demonstrated that NACA protects neuronal cells from glutamate-induced excitotoxicity (Penugonda and Ercal 2011; Penugonda et al. 2005; Penugonda et al. 2006), and a recent report indicates that NACA reduces cocaine-seeking behavior in rodents (Jastrzebska et al. 2016). However, the ability of these NAC derivatives to serve as cystine prodrugs and thus exert effects on system xc- in the CNS, while likely, has not yet fully been established. As with NAC, these derivatives also have numerous additional mechanisms of action including copper chelation, GSH formation, and interactions with various intracellular enzymes. Thus, their ability to modulate glutamate homeostasis via actions on system xc- requires further study.

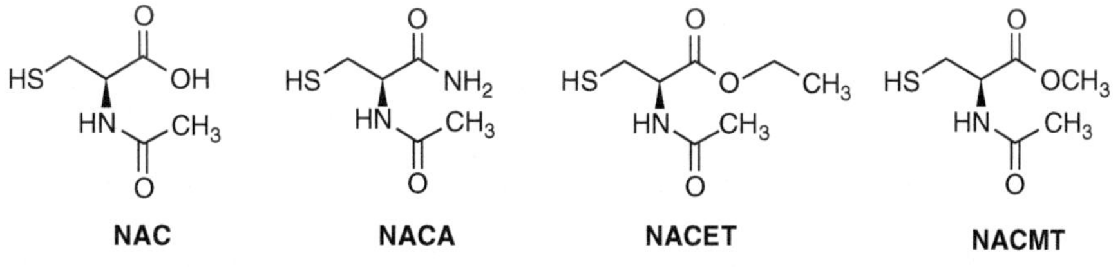

NAC NACA NACET NACMT

Fig. 2.4 Chemical structures of NAC and newer derivatives

2.6 Summary

NAC affects glutamatergic transmission in the CNS via a multistep indirect process. NAC is biotransformed into cysteine followed by cystine, which is an endogenous activator of system xc-, which transports cystine into glial cells in a 1:1 stoichiometry with glutamate transport into the extracellular environment. Under conditions of dysregulated glutamate signaling, such as when extracellular glutamate levels are low, NAC can therefore raise extracellular glutamate levels and restore tone on presynaptic mGluR2/3 autoreceptors to dampen neuronal release of synaptic glutamate. While this mechanism has been studied in detail, less is known about mechanisms that do not involve system xc-, such as GSH formation and/or direct interactions with iGluRs. The development of pharmacological and other tools that selectively activate or inactive system xc- vs. other aspects of glutamatergic transmission will therefore provide valuable information on the precise molecular mechanisms underlying the clinical efficacy of NAC in psychiatric and neurological disorders.

References

Baker DA, Shen H, Kalivas PW (2002a) Cystine/glutamate exchange serves as the source for extracellular glutamate: modifications by repeated cocaine administration. Amino Acids 23(1–3):161–162

Baker DA, Xi ZX, Shen H, Swanson CJ, Kalivas PW (2002b) The origin and neuronal function of in vivo nonsynaptic glutamate. J Neurosci 22(20):9134–9141

Berk M, Malhi GS, Gray LJ, Dean OM (2013) The promise of N-acetylcysteine in neuropsychiatry. Trends Pharmacol Sci 34(3):167–177. https://doi.org/10.1016/j.tips.2013.01.001

Bridges R, Lutgen V, Lobner D, Baker DA (2012) Thinking outside the cleft to understand synaptic activity: contribution of the cystine-glutamate antiporter (System xc-) to normal and pathological glutamatergic signaling. Pharmacol Rev 64(3):780–802. https://doi.org/10.1124/pr.110.003889

Chiew AL, Isbister GK, Duffull SB, Buckley NA (2016) Evidence for the changing regimens of acetylcysteine. Br J Clin Pharmacol 81(3):471–481. https://doi.org/10.1111/bcp.12789

Clements JD (1996) Transmitter timecourse in the synaptic cleft: its role in central synaptic function. Trends Neurosci 19(5):163–171

Danbolt NC, Furness DN, Zhou Y (2016) Neuronal vs glial glutamate uptake: resolving the conundrum. Neurochem Int 98:29–45. https://doi.org/10.1016/j.neuint.2016.05.009

Deepmala, Slattery J, Kumar N, Delhey L, Berk M, Dean O, Spielholz C, Frye R (2015) Clinical trials of N-acetylcysteine in psychiatry and neurology: a systematic review. Neurosci Biobehav Rev 55:294–321. https://doi.org/10.1016/j.neubiorev.2015.04.015

Divito CB, Underhill SM (2014) Excitatory amino acid transporters: roles in glutamatergic neurotransmission. Neurochem Int 73:172–180. https://doi.org/10.1016/j.neuint.2013.12.008

Fan X, Jun WY, Wang YT (2014) The NMDA receptor complex: a multifunctional machine at the glutamatergic synapse. Front Cell Neurosci 8:160

Fontana AC (2015) Current approaches to enhance glutamate transporter function and expression. J Neurochem 134(6):982–1007. https://doi.org/10.1111/jnc.13200

Garcia-Junco-Clemente P, Linares-Clemente P, Fernandez-Chacon R (2005) Active zones for presynaptic plasticity in the brain. Mol Psychiatry 10(2):185–200

Gilbert KR, Aizenman E, Reynolds IJ (1991) Oxidized glutathione modulates N-methyl-D-aspartate- and depolarization-induced increases in intracellular Ca2+ in cultured rat forebrain neurons. Neurosci Lett 133(1):11–14

Hamilton NB, Attwell D (2010) Do astrocytes really exocytose neurotransmitters? Nat Rev Neurosci 11(4):227–238. https://doi.org/10.1038/nrn2803

Huganir RL, Nicoll RA (2013) AMPARs and synaptic plasticity: the last 25 years. Neuron 80(3):704–717. https://doi.org/10.1016/j.neuron.2013.10.025

Jastrzebska J, Frankowska M, Filip M, Atlas D (2016) N-acetylcysteine amide (AD4) reduces cocaine-induced reinstatement. Psychopharmacology 233(18):3437–3448. https://doi.org/10.1007/s00213-016-4388-5

Javitt DC, Schoepp D, Kalivas PW, Volkow ND, Zarate C, Merchant K, Bear MF, Umbricht D, Hajos M, Potter WZ, Lee CM (2011) Translating glutamate: from pathophysiology to treatment. Sci Transl Med 3(102):102mr102. https://doi.org/10.1126/scitranslmed.3002804

Kalivas PW (2009) The glutamate homeostasis hypothesis of addiction. Nat Rev Neurosci 10(8):561–572

Knackstedt LA, Melendez RI, Kalivas PW (2010) Ceftriaxone restores glutamate homeostasis and prevents relapse to cocaine seeking. Biol Psychiatry 67(1):81–84. https://doi.org/10.1016/j.biopsych.2009.07.018

Lehre KP, Danbolt NC (1998) The number of glutamate transporter subtype molecules at glutamatergic synapses: chemical and stereological quantification in young adult rat brain. J Neurosci 18(21):8751–8757

Leslie SW, Brown LM, Trent RD, Lee YH, Morris JL, Jones TW, Randall PK, Lau SS, Monks TJ (1992) Stimulation of N-methyl-D-aspartate receptor-mediated calcium entry into dissociated neurons by reduced and oxidized glutathione. Mol Pharmacol 41(2):308–314

Massie A, Boillee S, Hewett S, Knackstedt L, Lewerenz J (2015) Main path and byways: nonvesicular glutamate release by system xc(-) as an important modifier of glutamatergic neurotransmission. J Neurochem 135(6):1062–1079. https://doi.org/10.1111/jnc.13348

Moussawi K, Riegel A, Nair S, Kalivas PW (2011) Extracellular glutamate: functional compartments operate in different concentration ranges. Front Syst Neurosci 5:94. https://doi.org/10.3389/fnsys.2011.00094

Niciu MJ, Kelmendi B, Sanacora G (2012) Overview of glutamatergic neurotransmission in the nervous system. Pharmacol Biochem Behav 100(4):656–664. https://doi.org/10.1016/j.pbb.2011.08.008

Parpura V, Verkhratsky A (2013) Astroglial amino acid-based transmitter receptors. Amino Acids 44(4):1151–1158. https://doi.org/10.1007/s00726-013-1458-4

Pendyam S, Mohan A, Kalivas PW, Nair SS (2009) Computational model of extracellular glutamate in the nucleus accumbens incorporates neuroadaptations by chronic cocaine. Neuroscience 158(4):1266–1276. https://doi.org/10.1016/j.neuroscience.2008.11.014

Penugonda S, Ercal N (2011) Comparative evaluation of N-acetylcysteine (NAC) and N-acetylcysteine amide (NACA) on glutamate and lead-induced toxicity in CD-1 mice. Toxicol Lett 201(1):1–7. https://doi.org/10.1016/j.toxlet.2010.11.013

Penugonda S, Mare S, Goldstein G, Banks WA, Ercal N (2005) Effects of N-acetylcysteine amide (NACA), a novel thiol antioxidant against glutamate-induced cytotoxicity in neuronal cell line PC12. Brain Res 1056(2):132–138. https://doi.org/10.1016/j.brainres.2005.07.032

Penugonda S, Mare S, Lutz P, Banks WA, Ercal N (2006) Potentiation of lead-induced cell death in PC12 cells by glutamate: protection by N-acetylcysteine amide (NACA), a novel thiol antioxidant. Toxicol Appl Pharmacol 216(2):197–205. https://doi.org/10.1016/j.taap.2006.05.002

Reissner KJ, Brown RM, Spencer S, Tran PK, Thomas CA, Kalivas PW (2014) Chronic administration of the methylxanthine propentofylline impairs reinstatement to cocaine by a GLT-1-dependent mechanism. Neuropsychopharmacology 39(2):499–506. https://doi.org/10.1038/npp.2013.223

Reissner KJ, Gipson CD, Tran PK, Knackstedt LA, Scofield MD, Kalivas PW (2015) Glutamate transporter GLT-1 mediates N-acetylcysteine inhibition of cocaine reinstatement. Addict Biol 20(2):316–323. https://doi.org/10.1111/adb.12127

Rodriguez M, Sabate M, Rodriguez-Sabate C, Morales I (2013) The role of non-synaptic extracellular glutamate. Brain Res Bull 93:17–26. https://doi.org/10.1016/j.brainresbull.2012.09.018

Shigeri Y, Seal RP, Shimamoto K (2004) Molecular pharmacology of glutamate transporters, EAATs and VGLUTs. Brain Res Rev 45(3):250–265

Steullet P, Neijt HC, Cuenod M, Do KQ (2006) Synaptic plasticity impairment and hypofunction of NMDA receptors induced by glutathione deficit: relevance to schizophrenia. Neuroscience 137(3):807–819. https://doi.org/10.1016/j.neuroscience.2005.10.014

Takahashi K, Foster JB, Lin CL (2015) Glutamate transporter EAAT2: regulation, function, and potential as a therapeutic target for neurological and psychiatric disease. Cell Mol Life Sci 72(18):3489–3506. https://doi.org/10.1007/s00018-015-1937-8

Takumi Y, Matsubara A, Rinvik E, Ottersen OP (1999) The arrangement of glutamate receptors in excitatory synapses. Ann N Y Acad Sci 868:474–482

Varga V, Jenei Z, Janaky R, Saransaari P, Oja SS (1997) Glutathione is an endogenous ligand of rat brain N-methyl-D-aspartate (NMDA) and 2-amino-3-hydroxy-5-methyl-4-isoxazolepropionate (AMPA) receptors. Neurochem Res 22(9):1165–1171

Zhou Y, Danbolt NC (2014) Glutamate as a neurotransmitter in the healthy brain. J Neural Transm 121(8):799–817. https://doi.org/10.1007/s00702-014-1180-8

Nihit Kumar

3.1   Introduction

Dopamine is a naturally occurring catecholamine, derived from the amino acid tyrosine and formed by decarboxylation of dihydroxyphenylalanine (L-DOPA). Catecholamines are comprised of a catechol group with an amine side chain and include dopamine, norepinephrine, and epinephrine.

Dopamine is a centrally acting catecholamine and is a precursor of norepinephrine and epinephrine. Dopamine exerts its effects via its action on G-coupled dopamine receptors, D1 through D5, which in turn activate or deactivate adenylyl cyclase to produce the second messenger cyclic adenosine monophosphate. After its release from presynaptic vesicles, it either undergoes reuptake or is degraded by synaptic monoamine oxidase (MAO-A and MAO-B) enzymes to 3,4-dihydroxyphenylacetic acid (DOPAC), which is further converted into homovanillic acid (HVA) by the enzyme catechol-O-methyltransferase (COMT) (Fig. 3.1). Reactive oxygen species can convert dopamine into other compounds like dopamine quinones or dopaminochrome which are associated with cytotoxicity and apoptosis.

Dopamine is a major transmitter in the extrapyramidal system of the brain and the basal ganglia and important in regulating movement (MeSH 2016). Aberrant dopaminergic transmission causes problems with memory, attention, and cognition and is implicated in psychotic disorders and schizophrenia. Degeneration of dopaminergic neurons is also associated with diseases like Parkinson's and

Electronic supplementary material The online version of this article (https://doi.org/10.1007/978-981-10-5311-5_3) contains supplementary material, which is available to authorized users.

N. Kumar
Departments of Child & Adolescent and Addiction Psychiatry, University of Arkansas for Medical Sciences, Little Rock, AR, USA
e-mail: nkumar@uams.edu

© Springer Nature Singapore Pte Ltd. 2019   29
R. E. Frye, M. Berk (eds.), *The Therapeutic Use of N-Acetylcysteine (NAC) in Medicine*, https://doi.org/10.1007/978-981-10-5311-5_3

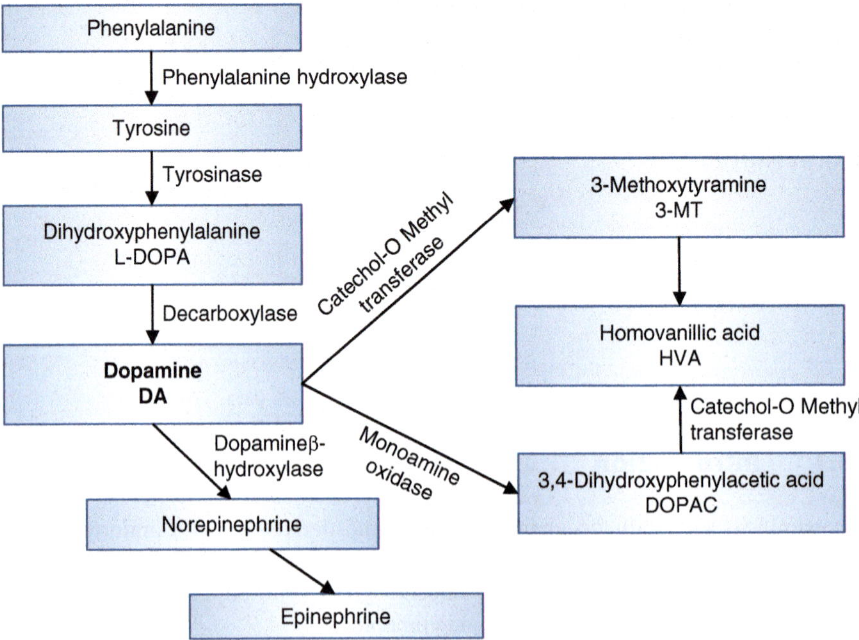

Fig. 3.1 Dopamine metabolism

Alzheimer's. Dopamine plays a significant role in the addiction reward pathway, originating from ventral tegmental area in the striatum and extending to the nucleus accumbens. Dopamine plays an important role in regulating prolactin secretion, processing pain, and mediating nausea in the chemoreceptor trigger zone as well as in mood, cognition, and behavioral reward. Dopamine also has a prominent role in the peripheral circulation where it stimulates adrenergic receptors for the cardiovascular system and peripheral vasculature. Stimulation of dopaminergic receptors in renal vessels leads to renal blood vessel dilation and an increase in glomerular filtration rate, renal blood flow, sodium excretion, and urine output (NCIT 2016).

At a cellular level, however, dopamine and its oxidized metabolites are associated with cytotoxicity, apoptosis, and mitochondrial dysfunction through free radical production and depletion of glutathione. Exposure to exogenous or endogenous toxins may also affect dopamine levels.

N-Acetylcysteine (NAC) acts as an antioxidant and glutathione (GSH) precursor and has been extensively studied as a potential treatment for a number of psychiatric and neurological disorders (Deepmala et al. 2015). However, NAC has received limited research attention as a protective agent against dopamine-induced cell death.

The purpose of this chapter is to examine the association between dopamine and NAC in animal and cellular studies. Below the methodology for the systematic search for this chapter is reviewed.

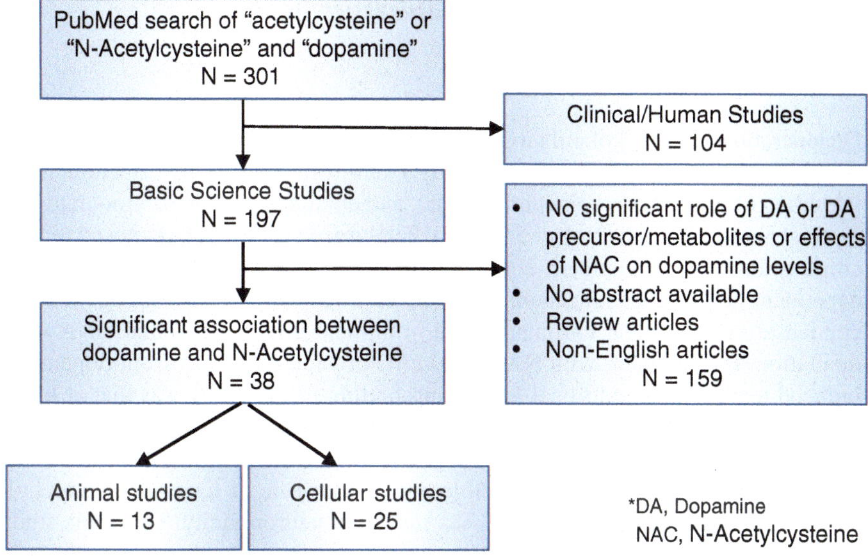

Fig. 3.2 Study selection flowchart

3.2 Methodology

An online literature search of PubMed from inception through October 2016 was conducted using search terms "N-Acetylcysteine" OR "acetylcysteine" AND "dopamine," which yielded 301 studies. Only basic science studies were included for the review using the selection criteria "other animals" under species filter. The resulting 197 studies were screened by title and abstract review to include only those articles with a predominant role of dopamine or its precursor/metabolites and clear evidence of association of dopamine and NAC. Publications which did not add a new or unique perspective, like review articles, along with non-English language publications and publications with no abstract available were excluded. Finally, 38 studies were included in the chapter summary (Fig. 3.2; Online Table 3.1).

For the sake of clinical relevance, this chapter was divided in sections based on each study's potential importance for a certain clinical disorder. Two studies identified potential implications for two syndromes, the first study (Noh et al. 1999) for Parkinson's and Alzheimer's and the second (Bauzo et al. 2012) for amphetamine and cocaine, and were included in both sections. Each section is further classified based on the cellular or animal model of the study.

Some of the literature in this chapter may overlap with those in other chapters, specifically with oxidative stress/redox metabolism, apoptosis, and mitochondrial disorders. This is due to the basic science nature of these publications, where multiple cellular hypotheses may be explored within a single study.

3.3   Summary of Systematic Literature Review

3.3.1   Alzheimer's Disease

Degeneration of catecholaminergic neurons is implicated in the pathogenesis of Alzheimer's disease. This cellular study examined the role of catecholamines including dopamine, norepinephrine (NE), and epinephrine (EP) as modulators of cortical neuronal death (Noh et al. 1999). Fetal mice cortical cells exposed to high concentrations of dopamine (>100 µM) and EP/NE (~1000 µM) underwent dose-dependent neuronal death accompanied by cell body shrinkage, aggregation and condensation of nuclear chromatin, and prominent internucleosomal DNA fragmentation. Pretreatment with NAC (100 µM) protected neurons from dopamine-induced toxicity. An additional interesting finding in this study was that at lower doses, all catecholamines (1–30 µM) mitigated free radical-mediated (ferrous iron, Fe^{2+}, or hydrogen peroxide, H_2O_2) necrotic death of cortical neurons. The results of this study suggest a possible antioxidant role of lower-dose catecholamines, while exposure to higher doses results in neurotoxicity. Thus, this study explores further the mechanism of action of dopamine and other free radicals in the pathogenesis of Alzheimer's disease and the potential role of NAC in preventing these changes.

3.3.2   Environmental Toxin

The following two studies explore the neurotoxic effects of environmental toxins and their impact on biogenic amines.

3.3.2.1 Polychlorinated Biphenyls (PCBs)

This cellular study investigated the role of polychlorinated biphenyls (PCBs) in altering vesicular storage of dopamine, leading to increased levels of unsequestered dopamine and dopamine metabolism, ultimately resulting in increased oxidative stress (Lyng and Seegal 2008). A 24-h exposure of developing rat striatum and ventral mesencephalon (VM) to environmentally relevant mixture of PCBs (8 µM) resulted in significant reduction in dopamine and GABA levels. Also, H_2O_2-treated positive control cocultures resulted in significant depletion of both dopamine and GABA. NAC (10 mM) pretreatment alone did not alter PCB-induced dopamine levels. However, NAC did reverse PCB-induced GABA reduction and H_2O_2-induced reduction in both dopamine and GABA. NAC pretreatment also attenuated PCB- and H_2O_2-induced increase in rhodamine (RH-123) fluorescence in both striatum and VM, a marker of oxidative stress. Reduction in total GSH (reduced glutathione, GSH + oxidized glutathione, GSSG) induced by PCBs and H_2O_2 exposure was completely eliminated by prior treatment with NAC. These results suggest the protective role of NAC in PCB-induced alterations in GABA levels, oxidative stress, and GSH depletion, but not in PCB-induced depletion of tissue dopamine.

3.3.2.2 Tungsten

The effect of sodium tungstate on rat brain biogenic amines as well as on other neurological alterations was examined in this animal study, along with the ability of NAC to prevent these changes (Sachdeva et al. 2015). Rats were treated with sodium tungstate (100 ppm in drinking water) with and without NAC (0.30 mM) orally for 3 months and their brains were dissected and analyzed. Measures of oxidative stress in rat brain were elevated by administration of tungstate, as indicated by increase in brain reactive oxygen species (ROS), tissue thiobarbituric acid reactive substances (TBARS), and GSSG as well as decrease in GSH. Sodium tungstate exposure also resulted in significant increase in glutathione peroxidase (GPx) and significant decrease in glutathione-S-transferase (GST) activity, suggesting increased lipid peroxidation in brain regions. These effects were reversed by co-administration of NAC. Treatment with NAC also resulted in restoration of depleted levels of dopamine, 5-hydroxytryptamine, norepinephrine, and acetylcholinesterase activity induced by sodium tungstate. Thus, tungsten-induced neurotoxicity mediated by increase in oxidative stress in rats was prevented by co-treatment with the antioxidant and GSH precursor NAC.

Thus, these two studies examined the dopamine-depleting effects of environmental toxins like PCBs and tungsten, which may be reversed by administration of NAC.

3.3.3   Ischemic Brain Injury

NAC has been proposed as a neuroprotective agent due to its role as an antioxidant and reactive oxygen species scavenger. This section reviews two cellular studies implicating dopamine in the pathogenesis of ischemic brain injury and the role of NAC in preventing these changes.

The first study assessed the cytotoxic effects of catecholamines, including dopamine on cultured oligodendrocytes, thought to be preferentially damaged during ischemic brain insults (Khorchid et al. 2002). Exposure of both oligodendrocyte progenitors and 12-day differentiated oligodendrocytes to dopamine (150 or 500 µM) resulted in a significant decrease in cell viability as measured by MTT assay, a marker of mitochondrial integrity, and also resulted in marked decreases in intracellular GSH levels. Pretreatment with NAC (1 mM) 30 min prior to dopamine exposure prevented cell death as assessed by MTT reduction and reversed the decrease in GSH levels, thus suggesting a role of oxidative stress and ROS generation in dopamine-induced cytotoxicity. Dopamine-mediated oxidative stress, as measured by expression of HO-1 protein in both oligodendrocyte progenitors and mature cells, was reversed by pretreatment with NAC (1 mM). NAC also prevented dopamine-mediated activation of caspase-3 and caspase-9 and cleavage of poly(ADP-ribose) polymerase (PARP; caspase-3 substrate), which are molecular signals of apoptosis of oligodendrocyte progenitor cells, thus pointing toward a role of ROS generation in apoptosis. These effects were more pronounced in oligodendrocyte progenitors as compared to mature cells. TUNEL assay allows for quantification of apoptotic cells. Exposure of progenitors and differentiated oligodendrocytes to dopamine resulted in an increase in TUNEL-positive cells. However, treatment with NAC (1 mM) prior to dopamine exposure abolished this increase in TUNEL-positive cells, thus implicating the role of oxidative stress in dopamine-induced apoptosis.

Another study examined mechanisms of cell death in cultured rat forebrain neurons by dopamine and glutamate since increased levels of these neurotransmitters are seen during ischemic damage to the brain (Hoyt et al. 1997). Dopamine (250 µM for 2 h)-induced apoptosis as measured by changes in nuclear morphology was completely prevented by pretreatment with NAC (100 µM). NAC attenuated toxicity, even when it was administered after dopamine exposure. However, glutamate (100 µM for 5 min)-induced excitotoxicity was not prevented by NAC (100 µM) treatment. NAC (100 µM) also did not prevent toxicity when administered after combined dopamine and glutamate exposure. Exposure of neurons to neurotoxic concentrations of dopamine resulted in dopamine being covalently bound to cellular proteins, and treatment with NAC (100 µM) completely inhibited this reaction. The ability of NAC to inhibit toxicity, even after dopamine-induced modification of cellular protein, suggests that NAC is able to reverse dopamine-induced cell death or that NAC is able to prevent other downstream events that result in toxicity. Exposure to dopamine induced increased intracellular Ca^{2+} in a subset of responsive neurons. The presence of NAC (100 µM) did not inhibit dopamine-induced increase in intracellular Ca^{2+}, suggesting that dopamine-induced neurotoxicity is mediated by mechanisms other than increase in intracellular Ca^{2+} levels.

Thus, NAC was able to mitigate the damage to cultured brain cells induced by ischemia in the above two cellular studies.

3.3.4 Parkinson's Disease

3.3.4.1 Animal Studies

Parkinson's disease involves degeneration of the nigrostriatal dopaminergic neurons. Various toxins are implicated in this neurodegenerative process. This section explores the impact on dopamine levels of exposure to various endogenous or external toxins in animal model of Parkinson's disease and the potential role of NAC in attenuating these effects.

A recent study examined the role of 2,3,5,4′-tetrahydroxystilbene-2-*O*-beta-D-glucoside (TSG) in preventing MPTP-induced neurotoxicity in mice, an action similar to NAC (He et al. 2015). Co-administration of either TSG or intragastric NAC (32 mg/kg for 14 days) significantly improved behavioral performance of MPTP-treated mice in pole test and open field test. TSG and NAC also reversed MPTP-induced decrease in dopamine, DOPAC, and HVA levels. In addition, treatment with MPTP resulted in loss of TH-positive cells, increased generation of ROS, phosphorylation of JNK and P38, increased bax to bcl-2 ratio, increased protein expression of cytochrome c and smac, and increased levels of cleaved caspase-3, caspase-6, and caspase-9. Co-treatment with TSG or NAC prevented these cytotoxic effects of MPTP. NAC was used as a positive control in this study, and TSG showed similar protective effects as NAC in attenuating MPTP-induced neuronal damage.

Another study published the same year investigated the role of NAC in reversing rotenone-induced changes in dopaminergic areas of rat brain in an animal model of Parkinson's disease (Rahimmi et al. 2015). Rotenone induced motor dysfunction in rats as measured by rotarod, rearing, and bar tests; these behavioral effects were reversed by pretreatment with NAC (25 and 50 mg/kg/48 h, i.p.). Administration of NAC also reversed the decrease in dopamine levels in rat brain substantia nigra seen with administration of rotenone, but this effect of NAC was not significant in the striatum. Cytosolic proteins like parkin and Drp 1 (dynamin-related protein-1) are involved in mitochondrial dysfunction and are implicated in the neurodegenerative process in Parkinson's. The control group showed a significant decrease in parkin levels in both substantia nigra and striatum and significant elevation of Drp 1 in the striatum as compared to the rotenone-treated group. NAC (25 and 50 mg/kg/48 h, i.p.) pretreatment reversed the decrease in parkin and elevation in Drp 1 levels in rat dopaminergic neurons. This study demonstrates the potential neuroprotective role of NAC in an animal model of Parkinson's disease.

A study investigated the involvement of zinc (Zn)- and/or paraquat (PQ)-induced dopaminergic neurodegeneration in a rat model of Parkinson's disease (Kumar et al. 2012). Male Wistar rats were treated with Zn (20 mg/kg, i.p.) which resulted in a significant elevation of Zn in nigrostriatal tissue. Exposure to Zn or PQ for 8 weeks reduced spontaneous locomotor activity (SLA) and time of stay on rotarod, as well as significantly reduced the levels of dopamine and its metabolites, DOPAC and HVA, in the striatum. Pretreatment with NAC (200 mg/kg, i.p., GSH precursor) and/or apocyanin (10 mg/kg, i.p., NADPH oxidase inhibitor) alleviated the neurobehavioral deficits and restored dopamine and DOPAC levels in Zn- and PQ-treated rats. Treatment of rats with Zn and PQ also resulted in reductions in tyrosine hydroxylase (TH) immunoreactivity, number of TH-positive cells, NeuN-/TH-positive cells, expression of TH protein, and GSH content in nigrostriatal tissue, which were all restored significantly by pretreatment with NAC. Elevation of lipid peroxidation (LPO) and SOD, translocation of p67 phox subunit of NADPH oxidase from cytosol to membrane, increased protein expression of gp91 phox subunit, increased gp91 mRNA expression, mitochondrial cytochrome c release, increased caspase-9 and cleaved caspase-3 in cytosol, and CD11b expression were mediated by Zn and PQ treatment, and exposure to NAC or apocyanin resulted in significant reversal of these effects. Combination treatment with NAC and apocyanin showed more pronounced protective effects in all of these neurodegenerative changes induced by Zn or PQ. These results point toward the role of oxidative stress and GSH depletion in Zn-induced apoptotic and neurodegenerative changes, similar to those induced by PQ, which are prevented by pretreatment with NAC.

Another study examined the mechanism of neuroprotection by NAC in a mouse model of Parkinson's disease (Chen et al. 2007). The decrease in striatal dopamine and DOPAC induced by 1-methyl-4-phenyl-1,2,3,6-tetrahydropyridine (MPTP) were significantly attenuated by a 3-week pre-intake of mice drinking water supplemented with NAC (1 g/L). Pre-intake of NAC also attenuated MPTP-induced glutathione loss, reinstated the activity of GPx and superoxide dismutase (SOD), alleviated MPTP-induced elevation of IL-6 and TNF-alpha, significantly upregulated the expression of GPx mRNA, and downregulated TNF-alpha mRNA expression. Thus NAC was able to effectively prevent dopamine loss and decrease markers of oxidative stress and inflammatory damage in this animal model of Parkinson's.

A previous study published during the same year examined the effects on dopamine levels on exposure of mice dopaminergic neurons to MPTP (Sharma et al. 2007). Treatment with MPTP resulted in about 80 percent reduction in striatal dopamine concentration, whereas no change in dopamine level was seen with NAC treatment alone. When NAC (150 mg/kg, i.p., three injections every 12 h) was co-administered with MPTP, dopamine levels decreased slightly, but this change was not significant compared to control. NAC also attenuated MPTP-induced increase in lipid peroxidation and decrease in substantia nigra glutathione levels as well as total tissue thiol levels. Treatment with MPTP caused a decrease in GPx (glutathione peroxidase) and increase in superoxide dismutase activity; however, both changes were partly reversed with co-administration of NAC. Thus, NAC appears to protect against the neurodegenerative and oxidative effects of MPTP in mice dopaminergic neurons.

A further study examined the effects of nitric oxide (NO) donor S-nitroso-N-acetylpenicillamine (SNAP) on dopamine levels in the striatum of freely moving rats (Serra et al. 2001). SNAP administration at lower dose (0.2 mM for 180 min) resulted in moderate increase in dopamine and decrease in ascorbic acid dialysate levels. At higher dose of SNAP (1 mM), however, both dopamine and ascorbic acid concentrations decreased. Co-infusion of ascorbic acid (0.1 mM) with SNAP (1 mM) did not result in changes in dialysate dopamine levels. However, when NAC (0.1 mM) was added to SNAP (1 mM) for 180 min, levels of dopamine in dialysate significantly increased. NAC administration also reversed SNAP-induced decrease in ascorbic acid levels. Thus, this study showed that SNAP at higher doses induced nonenzymatic dopamine oxidation which was prevented by co-administration of NAC. Addition of ascorbic acid did not prevent oxidation of dopamine; hence, dopamine levels remained the same.

Another study by the same author investigated the effects of manganese (Mn) on L-DOPA-induced toxicity in the striatum of freely moving rats using in vivo microdialysis (Serra et al. 2000). Administration of L-DOPA (25 mg/kg) intraperitoneally significantly decreased dopamine and ascorbic acid levels and significantly increased concentrations of L-DOPA, DOPAC, HVA, and uric acid in the dialysate, suggesting that systemic administration of L-DOPA results in increased dopamine auto-oxidation. L-DOPA administration intraperitoneally or in the striatum resulted in detection of L-DOPA oxidation product, L-DOPA semiquinone, in the dialysate. Treatment with continuous infusion of NAC (0.1 mM for 220 min) in rats given L-DOPA resulted in fivefold increase in L-DOPA dialysate concentrations, as well as significant inhibition of L-DOPA semiquinone production. NAC also significantly reversed L-DOPA-induced decrease in dopamine concentration as well as increase in DOPAC + HVA and uric acid concentrations in the dialysate. Treatment with NAC did not affect ascorbic acid levels. Administration of $MnCl_2$ (30 mM for 15 min) intrastriatally in L-DOPA-treated rats significantly decreased L-DOPA concentrations and increased L-DOPA semiquinone concentrations in the dialysate. NAC infusion significantly inhibited $MnCl_2$-induced changes. NAC also reversed $MnCl_2$-induced biphasic changes in DOPAC + HVA (initial short-lasting increase followed by a significant and long-lasting decrease) and increase in uric acid dialysate concentrations. These findings suggest that the auto-oxidation of administered L-DOPA via production of ROS is enhanced by manganese and abolished by NAC.

Finally, a study investigated the neurodegenerative effects of an environmental toxin, MPTP, on dopaminergic nigrostriatal neurons in C57 black mice as an animal model for Parkinson's disease (Perry et al. 1985). MPTP was converted to one or more toxic metabolites by monoamine oxidase B (MAO-B) that caused about a 90% reduction in striatal dopamine content, along with reductions in dopamine metabolites, DOPAC, and HVA. Pretreatment with pargyline, an MAO-B inhibitor, prevented the reduction in dopamine levels, and pretreatment with NAC (500 mg/kg daily) reversed significantly the decrease in levels of dopamine and its metabolites caused by MPTP. This study examines potential environmental risk factors for development of idiopathic Parkinson's disease and the protective role of antioxidants like NAC in reversing these changes.

Thus, a diverse group of toxins produced neurodegenerative changes in animal model of Parkinson's disease by altering dopamine levels, and NAC was able to protect against or reverse these changes.

3.3.4.2 Cellular Studies

Dopamine (Toxin)

In contrast to the animal studies seen above, dopamine has been directly implicated in cell damage mediated by oxidative stress leading to apoptosis, cytotoxicity, and mitochondrial dysfunction. This section reviews several cellular studies exploring the cytotoxic and neurodegenerative actions of dopamine and the role of NAC in reversing these changes.

A study assessed the potential neuroprotective role of the botanical Z-ligustilide, used in the treatment of Parkinson's, to reduce dopamine-induced cytotoxicity (Qi et al. 2012). The addition of Z-ligustilide (50 µM) to dopamine (500 µM) in rat PC12 cells potentiated dopamine-mediated cell death as measured by MTT assay. The reduction in cell viability with this combination was beyond the toxicity seen with using Z-ligustilide or dopamine alone. The cytotoxic effects of Z-ligustilide on dopamine were specific to dopaminergic cells only. Dopamine- and Z-ligustilide-induced cell toxicity appeared to be mediated by decrease in intracellular GSH and production of intracellular ROS, and combining these agents had more severe effects compared to treatment with either agent. Thiol antioxidant NAC (0.5 mM) and GSH (0.5 mM) pretreatment 0.5 h before exposure to Z-ligustilide-dopamine combination almost completely protected against loss of cell viability in a concentration-dependent manner; however, non-thiol antioxidants ascorbic acid and trolox only had slight protective effects. This suggests that the reduction of GSH plays a role in Z-ligustilide-dopamine-mediated cytotoxicity and is not simply mediated by production of ROS.

A few years earlier, a study examined dopamine-induced non-apoptotic cell death in PC12 cells by overexpression of human mutant A53T alpha-synuclein (α-syn) (Zhou et al. 2009). α-syn expression is highly related to the pathogenesis of Parkinson's disease. Transfection of PC12 cells with A53T plasmids resulted in an expression level- and time-dependent loss of cell viability, and this was further enhanced by addition of 200 μM exogenous dopamine. In cells overexpressing A53T α-syn gene, considerable amount of yellow cells was observed (yellow color observed by increase in red propidium iodide-positive cells in green fluorescent protein-positive PC12 cells), but no cells with condensed/fragmented and bright nuclei were found, suggesting that transfection and overexpression of A53T α-syn may cause non-apoptotic cell death. Treatment with NAC (10 mM) significantly reversed loss of cell viability in PC12 cells overexpressing mutant A53T α-syn. Similarly, administration of nerve growth factor (NGF) and L-cysteine, but not tyrosinase inhibitors and ER stress alleviator, could also improve cell viability. Treatment with NAC (10 mM) or GSH (10 mM) alleviated dopamine auto-oxidation and tyrosinase-catalyzed dopamine oxidation. PC12 cells overexpressing mutant A53T α-syn increased oxidized GSH levels and decreased total and reduced GSH levels, but treatment with NAC (10 mM) or L-cysteine (10 mM) completely reversed these changes in GSH levels. These data collectively suggest that dopamine causes non-apoptotic cell death in PC12 cells by auto-oxidation and overexpression of human mutant A53T α-syn and these changes can be abolished by treatment with NAC.

The ROS scavenging properties of NAC and its effect on dopamine induced mitochondrial electron transport chain (ETC) inactivation, and Na^+, K^+-ATPase inhibition in rat brain was examined, all changes that have been implicated in the pathogenesis of Parkinson's disease (Bagh et al. 2008). Slow auto-oxidation of dopamine resulted in production of H_2O_2 and quinones, both of which were effectively scavenged by addition of NAC (0.25–1 mM). Dopamine induced a dose-dependent inhibition of mitochondrial ETC complex I and complex IV and a decrease in mitochondrial MTT reduction ability; these changes were also reversed by NAC (0.25–1 mM). Addition of NAC alone, without dopamine, had no effects on ETC activity. Similarly, pretreatment with NAC (0.25–1 mM) prevented dopamine-induced inhibition of synaptosomal Na^+, K^+-ATPase activity. This study demonstrates the antioxidant and quinone scavenging properties of NAC, thus highlighting its potential role as a neuroprotective agent, particularly in the treatment of sporadic Parkinson's disease.

Another study published the same year compared the effects of dopamine and the proteasome inhibitor MG132 on apoptosis in N27 rat mesencephalic cells (Zafar et al. 2007). Treatment with both dopamine (100–500 μM/L, 6–24 h) and MG132 (1–5 μM/L, 6–24 h) resulted in apoptosis as well as loss of mitochondrial membrane potential (MMP) in a time- and concentration-dependent manner. Pretreatment with NAC (5 mM/L) protected against dopamine-induced cell death and loss of MMP, implicating the role of quinone and ROS production in dopamine-mediated apoptosis. However, NAC was unable to prevent MG132-induced apoptosis, suggesting a more direct effect of MG132. Administration of dopamine to N27 cells also inhibited proteasomal activity independent of cell death, and inhibition of proteasome occurred prior to toxicity. Pretreatment with NAC prevented dopamine-induced proteasome inhibition, suggesting dopamine-mediated ROS production involvement in inhibition of proteasome. Proteasome inhibition by MG132 was not reversed by NAC, pointing toward a more specific action of MG132 on proteasome.

A study investigated the effects of co-addition of 1-methyl-4-phenylpyridinium (MPP$^+$) and dopamine on cell viability in PC12 cells and the role of NAC in preventing these changes (Lee et al. 2003). Dopamine alone as well as dopamine + MPP$^+$ induced significant production of ROS, as measured by increase in DCF fluorescence. NAC (1 mM) reversed this dopamine + MPP$^+$-mediated increase in DCF fluorescence, but not significantly. Similarly, dopamine + MPP$^+$ more so than dopamine or MPP$^+$ alone resulted in loss of cell viability, as measured by the MTT assay. This cytotoxic effect of dopamine + MPP$^+$ was mediated by the production of dopamine quinone and melanin in PC12 cells, and addition of NAC (1 mM) decreased the production of dopamine quinone and melanin. Cell death from combined dopamine + MPP$^+$ was not prevented by other antioxidants (rutin or ascorbate), pointing away from a mediating role of ROS in this process. This study suggests that dopamine oxidation products, rather than ROS, are involved in the cytotoxicity associated with combined dopamine + MPP$^+$ administration.

Another study examined the evidence for non-oxidative mechanism of cytotoxicity by intracellular dopamine via activation of NF-κB in genetically modified dopamine-producing Chinese hamster ovary (CHO) cell line to model dopamine-producing neurons (Weingarten et al. 2001). Unlike dopamine, L-DOPA is quite permeable to cells and allows for differentiation of intracellular and extracellular toxicity. L-DOPA induced decrease in cell viability, which was not prevented by NAC (500 µM) in either wild-type or modified CHO cells. Intracellular administration of dopamine also activated the stress-induced transcription factor NF-κB, and this change was only minimally inhibited by other antioxidants like ascorbic acid (AA). The lack of protective effect of antioxidants against L-DOPA suggests a non-oxidative mechanism of action for intracellular dopamine toxicity. AA, however, was able to prevent externally applied dopamine toxicity in both wild-type and modified CHO cells, thus pointing toward an oxidative mechanism of action of externally applied dopamine.

As mentioned above in the section for Alzheimer's disease, this study examined the role of catecholamines including dopamine, NE, and EP as modulators of cortical neuronal death, thought to be associated with Parkinson's disease (Noh et al. 1999). Fetal mice cortical cells exposed to high concentrations of dopamine (>100 µM) and EP/NE (~1000 µM) underwent dose-dependent neuronal death accompanied by cell body shrinkage, aggregation and condensation of nuclear chromatin, and prominent internucleosomal DNA fragmentation. Pretreatment with NAC (100 µM) protected neurons from dopamine-induced toxicity. An additional interesting finding in this study was that at lower doses, all catecholamines (1–30 µM) mitigated free radical-mediated (Fe^{2+} or H$_2$O$_2$) necrotic death of cortical neurons. The results of this study suggest a possible antioxidant role of lower-dose catecholamines, while exposure to higher doses results in neurotoxicity.

A few years earlier, a study investigated the role of NAC in preventing dopamine-induced apoptosis using 293 cell line and primary neonatal rat postmitotic striatal neuron cultures (Luo et al. 1998). Cells exposed to dopamine (100–500 μM) underwent apoptotic changes in a time- and concentration-dependent manner. Dopamine auto-oxidation and enzyme catalysis produce free radicals which subsequently activate the JNK pathway, including increases in JNK activity, phosphorylation of c-Jun, and increase in the protein product of c-Jun, contributing to apoptosis. Preincubation of cells with NAC (1 mM) completely abolished dopamine-induced JNK activity and cell death.

Another study investigated the apoptotic effects of dopamine in a clonal catecholaminergic cell line (CATH.a) derived from the central nervous system (Masserano et al. 1996). Administration of dopamine (50–500 μM) to CATH.a cells produced dose-dependent and time-dependent cell death over 48 h. Dopamine-induced cell death was mediated by DNA fragmentation, a hallmark of apoptosis. Dopamine (50–500 μM) also increased formation of peroxide in CATH.a cells in a dose-dependent manner, suggesting free radical production as a mechanism of action. Pretreatment with antioxidant NAC (1 mM) prevented dopamine-induced cytotoxicity in CATH.a cells in a dose-dependent manner, and this also correlated with decrease in peroxide formation. Incubation of CATH.a cells with antisense of anti-apoptotic protein bcl-2 resulted in decrease in bcl-2 levels by 40% and enhanced dopamine-induced loss of cell viability.

Finally, a study published the same year examined the cytotoxic effects of dopamine in PC12 cells as a cellular model for Parkinson's disease (Offen et al. 1996). Dopamine induced a dose-dependent loss of cell viability as measured by increase in thymidine uptake. Co-incubation with thiol antioxidants NAC (10 mM) and GSH (10 mM) protected against dopamine-induced cytotoxicity. Pretreatment with NAC and GSH also reversed dopamine-induced toxicity, indicating the protective effects of these antioxidants may also be achieved by increasing their intracellular concentrations. NAC prevented oxidation of dopamine and production of dopamine-melanin (DA-M). Depletion of cellular GSH by phoron (0.5 mM) or buthionine sulfoximine (BSO) enhanced dopamine-induced cell death. Addition of NAC reversed dopamine-, dopamine + phoron-, and dopamine + BSO-mediated cytotoxicity. Treatment with NAC and GSH also prevented DNA fragmentation as measured by TUNEL assay. These results suggest the role of oxidative stress and GSH depletion in dopamine-induced cell toxicity and the ability of NAC to prevent these changes.

Thus, these cellular studies examined the role of dopamine as a cytotoxic and apoptotic agent and the impact of NAC in protecting against dopamine-induced toxicity.

Dopamine-Related Compounds (Toxin)

Dopamine precursor, L-DOPA, or immediate metabolites of dopamine (auto-oxidized dopamine, ODA; dopaminochrome, DAC; and DOPAC) may also affect levels of biologic amines or cell viability. This section reviews the toxic effects of dopamine-related compounds in cellular studies related to Parkinson's disease.

A study investigated the concerted action of a major dopamine metabolite, DOPAC, and nitric oxide (•NO) on mitochondrial dysfunction and cell death in rat pheochromocytoma-derived PC12 cells as a model for Parkinson's disease (Nunes et al. 2011). DOPAC and the •NO donor, S-nitroso-N-acetylpenicillamine (SNAP), increased the production of free radicals synergistically compared to their individual effects, measured directly by electron paramagnetic resonance (EPR) technique. DOPAC + SNAP also significantly increased GSSG/GSH ratio, a measure of cellular redox status, mainly by depleting GSH. Mitochondrial complex I activity was significantly reduced, and an increase in Bax/Bcl-2 ratio was seen by incubation with DOPAC + SNAP. Pretreatment with NAC (1 mM) significantly enhanced intracellular GSH content. Incubation of PC12 cells with NAC (1 mM) for 3 h before exposure to DOPAC + SNAP prevented loss of cell viability and membrane integrity as determined by MTT assay and intracellular LDH leakage, respectively. DOPAC + SNAP-mediated apoptotic changes in morphology of cells were completely reversed by pretreatment with NAC. NAC also reversed DOPAC + SNAP-induced reduction in cellular ATP, a measure of mitochondrial function back to control levels. These suggest an oxidative stress model involving generation of free radicals in the mechanism of action of DOPAC + SNAP, as well as the critical role of GSH in maintaining mitochondrial function.

Another study investigated the effects of dopaminochrome (DAC), an oxidized product of dopamine, on cell death in murine mesencephalic cell line, MN9D, as a model for neurodegeneration in Parkinson's disease (Linsenbardt et al. 2009). DAC (50–250 μM) treatment for 24 h induced a concentration-dependent decrease in cell viability in MN9D cells; however, this effect was only seen when MN9D cells were incubated with the highest concentration of dopachrome (DPC, 50–250 μM), an oxidized product of L-DOPA. Exposure to DAC (175 μM) for as little as 1 h resulted in significant loss of cell viability when observed at 24 h, suggesting rapid initiation of cell toxicity. When exposed chronically to nontoxic or moderately toxic concentrations of DAC (50–100 μM), MN9D cells exhibited cytotoxicity over a period of 96 h. DAC (175 μM) treatment for 2 h enhanced dihydroethidium (DHE, fluorescent redox indicator for O_2^-) fluorescence in MN9D cells, thus suggesting the role of oxidative stress. NAC (5 mM) prevented DAC-induced increase in DHE fluorescence. Pretreatment with NAC (1–5 mM) also inhibited DAC (175 μM)-induced cell death, demonstrating the role of DAC-mediated superoxide production in cytotoxicity. Since exogenously administered NAC is similar to endogenous glutathione, the role of glutathione in MN9D cytotoxicity by DAC was also examined. Pretreatment of cells with buthionine sulfoximine (BSO, 50 and 100 μM), an intracellular glutathione depletor, significantly enhanced DAC-mediated cell death. DAC (175 μM) administration also resulted in a loss of total glutathione, as well as an increase in GSSG in MN9D cells. These results suggest the integral role of exogenous NAC as well as glutathione in maintaining cell viability in MN9D cells exposed to DAC.

The synergistic effects of the dopamine precursor, L-DOPA, and manganese (Mn) on oxidative stress-mediated apoptosis in catecholaminergic PC12 cells were examined (Migheli et al. 1999). Lower concentrations of L-DOPA (10 and 20 mM) as well as fixed concentration of $MnCl_2$ (0.2 mM) alone did not affect cell viability; however, a significant concentration-dependent decrease in cell viability was noted when L-DOPA was combined with $MnCl_2$. Addition of NAC (0.1 mM) antagonized the L-DOPA + $MnCl_2$-induced decrease in cell viability. The exposure of PC12 cells to nontoxic concentrations of L-DOPA (20 mM) resulted in increase in levels of dopamine and its metabolites, DOPAC and HVA. The presence of $MnCl_2$ inhibited L-DOPA-induced increase in dopamine and DOPAC + HVA concentrations in both cell lysate and incubation medium. Addition of NAC (0.1 mM) to L-DOPA + $MnCl_2$ resulted in reversal of $MnCl_2$-induced decrease in dopamine and DOPAC + HVA levels. Apoptotic nuclear changes in PC12 cells, as measured by TUNEL assay, flow cytometry, and fluorescence microscopy, were noted when L-DOPA (10 and 20 mM) was associated with $MnCl_2$ (0.2 mM), and this was completely abolished by addition of NAC (0.1 mM). Thus this study suggests the protective role of NAC on combined L-DOPA + $MnCl_2$ toxicity on catecholaminergic PC12 cells.

Finally, another study examined the apoptotic effects of auto-oxidized dopamine (ODA) on PC12 cells as a model for Parkinson's disease toxicity (Kang et al. 1998). Treatment with ODA (100 μM), but not dopamine (100 μM), resulted in DNA fragmentation, a hallmark of apoptosis. Activation of c-Jun N-terminal kinase (JNK)/ stress-activated protein kinase (SAPK) and p38 kinase is prerequisite for apoptosis. ODA induced 11.6-fold activation of JNK/SAPK and 7.7-fold activation of p38 kinase, suggesting the role of JNK/SAPK and p38 kinase in dopamine-induced apoptosis. ODA-induced apoptosis also appears to be mediated by initial increase of the pro-apoptotic protein Bax and delayed decrease of anti-apoptotic protein Bcl-2. The role of ROS generation in dopamine-induced apoptosis is suggested by the ability of NAC (400 μM) to prevent ODA-induced SAPK activation and apoptosis.

Thus, these studies examined the cellular degenerative processes or alterations of dopamine levels induced by dopamine-related compounds and the ability of NAC in preventing these changes.

3.3.5 Pituitary Tumor

Dopamine, a major hypothalamic neurotransmitter acting via D2 receptors, inhibits secretion of prolactin from anterior pituitary. The absence of D2 receptors in transgenic mice resulted in abnormal pituitary development (Baik et al. 1995; Kelly et al. 1997). A cellular study investigated the cytotoxic effects of dopamine on rat pituitary tumor cell lines expressing dopamine receptors (An et al. 2003). Dopamine (10 nM–100 μM) induced dose-dependent decrease in cell viability in GH3D2L and GH3D2S cells, but this effect was not observed in GH3 cells. This was mediated specifically by D2 receptors as evidenced by the ability of quinpirole to induce toxicity in GH3D2L and GH3D2S cells, but not in GH3 cells, and the ability of haloperidol, a D2 receptor antagonist, to prevent dopamine-induced cytotoxicity. Dopamine also inhibited DNA synthesis via D2 receptors in these cells measured by significant decrease in BrdU-labeling index, an indicator of DNA proliferation rate.

Cell morphology changes including change from elongated to spherical and shrunken shape were observed in GH3D2L and GH3D2S cells after treatment with dopamine, but such changes were not seen in GH3 cells. Dopamine also induced DNA laddering and caspase-3 activation in GH3D2L and GH3D2S cells, along with increase in activity of ERK 1/2 and p38 MAPK. Pretreatment with NAC (10 mM) inhibited dopamine-induced activation of ERKs and p38 MAPK and reversed decrease in cell viability as well as caspase-3 activation and DNA laddering. The ability of NAC to reverse changes in pituitary tumor GH3D2L and GH3D2S cells suggests a role of reactive oxygen species in dopamine-induced cytotoxicity.

3.3.6 Renal Pathology

Dopamine plays a critical role in renal physiology regulating blood flow in the renal vasculature and urine output. It is synthesized in the renal proximal tubule and is also released from the renal nerves that contain dopamine. At a cellular level, however, exposure to dopamine can be toxic to renal cells. The following two cellular studies investigated the mechanism of action of dopamine-induced cell death in renal proximal tubule cells.

The first study examined the mechanism of dopamine-induced apoptosis in rat renal proximal tubule cells and in MAO-B-transfected HEK 293 cells, mediated by internalization of dopamine in cells, and degradation by the MAO enzyme, resulting in the production of H_2O_2 (Bianchi et al. 2003). Pretreatment with NAC (1 mM) prevented increases in dopamine (50–200 μM)-induced SYTO-13 and TUNEL staining and DNA laddering in rat proximal tubule cells, markers of apoptosis. Similarly, in HEK-MAO-B cells, NAC abolished the increase in SYTO-13 staining associated with dopamine-induced production of MAO-dependent H_2O_2. Incubation of proximal tubule cells in the presence of dopamine induced an increase in the pro-apoptotic protein *Bax* and decrease in anti-apoptotic protein *Bcl-2*, leading to release of mitochondrial cytochrome c and activation of caspase-3 indicating that dopamine needs to be internalized and metabolized by MAO to activate the pro-apoptotic cascade. These effects were effectively prevented by NAC, thus indicating the protective effects of NAC on dopamine-induced oxidative damage in rat renal cells.

Another study investigated the effects of dopamine on ERK activation in rat renal proximal tubule cells and HEK 293 MAO-B cells via MAO-mediated H_2O_2 production (Vindis et al. 2001). In proximal tubule cells rich in MAO-A, dopamine (5 μM/L) induced increase in DNA synthesis, ERK activation, and Shc phosphorylation which were prevented by NAC (1 mM/L) pretreatment, suggesting the role of H_2O_2 production in MAO-A-mediated dopamine oxidation. Similarly, in HEK 293 cells stably transfected with human MAO-B cDNA as compared to wild-type HEK 293 cells (lacking MAO activity), incubation with dopamine (5 μM/L) resulted in tyrosine phosphorylation of p42/44 ERKs and p52 Shc, as well as dose-dependent increase in cell proliferation and cell counting. These effects were reversed by anti-oxidant NAC, suggesting similar mechanism of action of MAO-B-dependent dopamine degradation and H_2O_2 production.

Thus, these two cellular studies examined the effects of NAC in preventing dopamine-induced damage in rat renal tubule cells.

3.3.7 Schizophrenia

Alterations in the mesocortical and mesolimbic dopaminergic pathways, among others, are implicated in the pathogenesis of schizophrenia. The following two studies examine effects of social isolation rearing on dopamine levels in an animal model of schizophrenia.

This study evaluated the mitochondrial, immunological, neurochemical, and behavioral deficits associated with social isolation rearing (SIR) in rats, a valid neurodevelopmental animal model of schizophrenia (Moller et al. 2013a). SIR rats showed significant decrease in social interactive behaviors (rearing, approaching, staying together, and anogenital sniffing), increase in self-directed behaviors (square crossing and self-grooming), and pronounced deficits in object recognition memory and prepulse inhibition (PPI). NAC (150 mg/kg/day) alone significantly reversed these changes but was only partially effective in some parameters; however, NAC + clozapine (150 mg/kg/day and 5 mg/kg/day × 14 days) and clozapine alone (5 mg/kg/day × 14 days) successfully reversed all of these behavioral effects of SIR. Cytokine alterations induced by SIR in peripheral blood included significant decreases in IL-6 and IL-4 as well as increases in TNF-alpha and IFN-gamma. NAC (150 mg/kg) partially reversed changes in IL-6 and IL-4 and fully reversed changes in TNF-alpha and IFN-gamma. Clozapine treatment fully reversed alterations in IL-6, TNF-alpha, and IFN-gamma, and clozapine + NAC was superior to clozapine alone in reversing SIR-induced changes in IL-4. Similarly, SIR induced alterations in tryptophan-kynurenine metabolites including a significant increase in kynurenine and QA and a significant decrease in KYNA and neuroprotective ratio. NAC (150 mg/kg) partially reversed changes in kynurenine, QA, KYNA, and neuroprotective ratio, but both clozapine alone and clozapine + NAC were able to fully reverse these changes. Clozapine + NAC was superior to clozapine alone in reversing changes to KYNA, QA, and neuroprotective ratio. SIR induced decrease in levels of ATP and dopamine in the frontal cortex as well as increase in levels of ATP and dopamine in the striatum in rat brains. NAC (150 mg/kg) partially reversed changes in dopamine in both frontal cortex and striatum, whereas NAC + clozapine fully reversed changes in ATP as well as dopamine in both brain regions. Thus, NAC or clozapine attenuated SIR-induced behavioral deficits, possibly mediated by immunological and neurochemical changes, with combination treatment superior to treatment with NAC or clozapine alone.

A similar study investigated the role of NAC in reversing social isolation rearing (SIR)-induced changes in cortico-striatal monoamines in an animal model of schizophrenia (Moller et al. 2013b). SIR induced significant decrease in the frontal cortex and significant increase in striatal dopamine and its metabolites, DOPAC and HVA. NAC (50, 150, and 250 mg/kg) was used in a dose-dependent manner to reverse these changes. Decreases of dopamine and DOPAC in the frontal cortex were significantly but not fully reversed by 150 and 250 mg/kg of NAC; however, decreases in HVA were significantly reversed by 150 mg/kg NAC and fully reversed by 250 mg/kg NAC. SIR-induced increase in dopamine and HVA in the striatum was significantly reversed by 150 mg/kg NAC and fully reversed by 250 mg/kg NAC. Similarly, the increase in DOPAC in the striatum was fully reversed by both 150 and 250 mg/kg NAC. Treatment with lower dose of NAC 50 mg/kg was ineffective in reversing SIR-induced changes in dopamine or its metabolites. Similar to dopamine and its metabolites, SIR induced increase in striatal 5-HT, 5-HIAA, NA, and MHPG, increase in frontal cortical NA, and decrease in frontal cortical 5-HT, 5-HIAA, and MHPG. NAC dose dependently reversed all cortico-striatal alterations in 5-HT, 5-HIAA, and NA, with NAC 250 mg/kg also reversing MHPG alterations in both the frontal cortex and striatum. Thus, NAC was able to dose dependently reverse changes in cortico-striatal monoamines induced by SIR in rats.

Thus, the above two studies investigated changes in levels of dopamine and its metabolites induced by social isolation rearing in an animal model of schizophrenia and the ability of NAC to attenuate these changes.

3.3.8 Substance Use Disorders

Dopamine is one of the major neurotransmitters implicated in development of addictions and mediates the neural reward pathway from the ventral tegmental area in the ventral striatum to the nucleus accumbens. The following studies explore the impact of substances of abuse on dopamine levels in animal and cellular studies and the potential role of NAC in reversing these changes.

3.3.8.1 Amphetamine

Animal Studies
The effects of manipulating the glutamatergic system on the neurochemical and behavioral effects of cocaine and amphetamine administration in the caudate nucleus of adult male squirrel monkeys were examined using in vivo microdialysis (Bauzo et al. 2012). Cysteine-glutamate enhancer NAC (3 or 10 mg/kg, i.m.), given as a pretreatment 3 h prior to cocaine administration, significantly attenuated cocaine-induced increase in extracellular dopamine without altering baseline extracellular dopamine concentration. This effect was independent of NAC dose. Surprisingly, NAC at lower dose (3 mg/kg, i.m.) actually enhanced amphetamine-induced dopamine increase; however, at higher dose of NAC (10 mg/kg, i.m.), amphetamine effects on dopamine were similar to that of cocaine, resulting in decreases in dopamine levels. Overall, the effects of NAC on amphetamine-induced changes in extracellular dopamine were not significant. To examine the behavioral-stimulant and reinforcing effect of stimulants, squirrel monkeys were trained on fixed-interval stimulus termination and second-order schedule of self-administration, respectively. Behavioral-stimulant effects of cocaine and amphetamine were not influenced by pretreatment with NAC (3.0–17 mg/kg, i.m.) 30 min or 3 h prior to

stimulant administration. Thus NAC pretreatment neither resulted in significant attenuation of amphetamine-induced dopamine increase, nor did it affect behavioral-stimulant response of amphetamine in squirrel monkeys.

Another study examined the effects of NAC on dopamine levels and free radical formation during D-amphetamine (AMPH)-induced neurotoxicity in rat brain striatum (Wan et al. 2006). AMPH (7.5 mg/kg, i.p.) administration for 7 days resulted in decrease in striatal dopamine concentration, and this was significantly reversed by treatment with NAC (326 mg/kg). NAC treatment also inhibited AMPH-induced lipid peroxidation formation, as measured by significant decrease in striatal malondialdehyde (MDA) content. Direct intrastriatal administration of AMPH (10 µM) significantly increased 2,3-DHBA levels, an indicator of hydroxyl radical formation. Treatment with NAC significantly reduced this effect of AMPH. Thus NAC, via its free radical scavenging properties, could act as a potential neuroprotective agent during AMPH toxicity.

Cellular Studies

This cellular study investigated the role of ROS and protein phosphatases in acute amphetamine (AMPH)-mediated dopamine release in rat PC12 cells (Paszti-Gere and Jakus 2013). Application of two different fluorescent dyes confirmed the lack of involvement of ROS formation in acute AMPH-mediated dopamine release. However, double AMPH challenge (DAC) was utilized to standardize differences in striatal slices, and pretreatment with 10 mM of NAC for 60 min prior to second AMPH bolus significantly reduced dopamine release. This effect of NAC on quenching AMPH-mediated dopamine release remains to be explained.

A previous study by the same author investigated the role of NAC as an antioxidant in AMPH-mediated dopamine release by using a novel chromatographic measurement protocol (Gere-Paszti and Jakus 2009). AMPH-mediated production of H_2O_2 along with nonenzymatic auto-oxidation of dopamine is major precipitants of striatal degeneration and neurotoxicity in stimulant overuse. Pretreatment with 10 mM NAC 1 h before AMPH administration almost completely blocked the dopamine release in rat brain striatal slices. In further experiments, Reserpine, an irreversible vesicular monoamine depletor, was used to localize the intracellular origin of NAC-induced dopamine release. Reserpine-depleted striatum could not respond to 10 mM of NAC in the same manner as vehicle brain slices, thus pointing toward the vesicular dopamine mobilizing properties of NAC. NAC in lower concentrations (0.3, 1, and 3 mM) actually enhanced AMPH-induced dopamine release, presumably due to its free radical scavenging properties preventing dopamine from being a substrate of oxidative metabolism.

3.3.8.2 Cocaine

As described above, an animal study examined the effects of manipulating the glutamatergic system on the neurochemical and behavioral effects of cocaine and amphetamine administration in the caudate nucleus of adult male squirrel monkeys using in vivo microdialysis (Bauzo et al. 2012). NAC (3 or 10 mg/kg, i.m.), given as a pretreatment 3 h prior to cocaine administration, significantly attenuated cocaine-induced increase in extracellular dopamine without altering baseline extracellular dopamine concentration. This effect was independent of NAC dose. Surprisingly, NAC at lower dose (3 mg/kg, i.m.) actually enhanced amphetamine-induced dopamine increase; however, at higher dose of NAC (10 mg/kg, i.m.), amphetamine effects on dopamine were similar to that of cocaine, resulting in decreases in dopamine levels. Overall, the effects of NAC on amphetamine-induced changes in extracellular dopamine were not significant. To examine the behavioral-stimulant and reinforcing effect of stimulants, squirrel monkeys were trained on fixed-interval stimulus termination and second-order schedule of self-administration, respectively. Behavioral-stimulant effects of cocaine and amphetamine were not influenced by pretreatment with NAC (3.0–17 mg/kg, i.m.) 30 min or 3 h prior to stimulant administration. Prior NAC treatment also did not alter cocaine self-administration or reinstatement of previously extinguished cocaine self-administration. Thus, effects of NAC on attenuation of cocaine-induced increase in dopamine did not result in altered behavioral effects of cocaine in squirrel monkeys.

3.3.8.3 Methamphetamine

This animal study investigated the effects of NAC on methamphetamine (MAP)-induced behavioral changes and neurotoxicity in rat brain dopaminergic neurons (Fukami et al. 2004). Rats were pretreated with NAC (1, 3, 10, and 30 mg/kg, i.p.) 30 min before each MAP injection (7.5 mg/kg × 4, 2-h intervals), and their striatum was dissected and analyzed for dopamine levels by high-performance liquid chromatography (HPLC). Pretreatment with NAC significantly attenuated the reduction in dopamine levels by repeated administration of MAP in a dose-dependent fashion. NAC also attenuated MAP-induced elevation of rectal temperature, an indicator of neurotoxicity. There was significant attenuation of MAP (2 mg/kg, i.p.)-induced hyperlocomotion with NAC pretreatment (30, 100, or 300 mg/kg, i.p.) in a dose-dependent manner. NAC pretreatment (100 mg/kg, i.p.) also significantly attenuated the development of behavioral sensitization in rats after repeated injection of MAP (2 mg/kg).

Thus, these studies demonstrated the potential protective role of NAC by reversing dopamine levels induced by various substances of abuse.

3.3.9 Vitiligo

Increased levels of catecholamines in plasma and urine of patients are associated with the onset and progression phase of vitiligo (Cucchi et al. 2003). Dopamine has been implicated in neurotoxicity in brain cells, which are derived from the same ectoderm that give rise to melanin containing dermatocytes. The following two cellular studies looked at the potential role of dopamine cytotoxicity in the pathogenesis of vitiligo.

A study demonstrated the apoptotic pathway in Mel-Ab cells induced by dopamine mediated by the chronic activation of Akt and increased oxidative stress (Choi et al. 2010). Pretreatment with 10 mM NAC prevents the loss of cell viability and melanocyte death as measured by decrease in annexin V-positive cells. Anti-apoptotic effects of NAC in this study were possibly mediated by inhibiting dopamine-induced chronic activation of Akt and Bad, mediators of cell death.

Additionally, the cytotoxic effects of dopamine on mouse Mel-Ab cells and cultured normal human melanocytes were investigated, as well as the role of NAC in preventing this toxicity (Park et al. 2007). Dopamine induced a dose-dependent and time-dependent reduction in cell viability in cultured Mel-Ab cells and human melanocytes, with about 50% decrease in viability with addition of 500 µM of dopamine. This dopamine-induced cytotoxicity was prevented by pretreatment with 1 and 10 mM NAC and 1 mM GSH. Using flow cytometry, it was demonstrated that dopamine-induced Mel-Ab cell death was due to apoptosis as measured by increase in annexin V staining, and this was mediated by phosphorylation of JNK and p38 MAPK. Pretreatment with NAC or GSH inhibited JNK and p38 MAPK activation and protected against dopamine-induced apoptotic cell death. This study demonstrates the protective role of thiol antioxidants like NAC and GSH against dopamine-induced cytotoxicity in the pathogenesis of vitiligo.

Thus, these two studies explored the mechanism of action of cell damage induced by exposure to dopamine and the role of NAC in mitigating these effects.

3.4 Summary

Dopamine plays a critical role as a neurotransmitter in the human brain and is implicated in a number of peripheral physiological processes. At the cellular level, a number of substances of abuse, exogenous as well as endogenous toxins, affect the level of dopamine and its metabolites. As seen in animal models of schizophrenia, behavioral interventions also affect dopamine concentrations in the brain. On the other hand, dopamine itself, along with its oxidized metabolites, acts as cytotoxic or neurotoxic agent in cells exposed to oxidative stress.

NAC is able to prevent or reverse many of these effects of dopamine mediated by an oxidative stress mechanism. NAC is also able to reverse changes in dopamine levels induced by social isolation rearing, as seen in schizophrenia studies above, as well as those induced by exposure to toxins. These protective effects of NAC are mediated by its action as an antioxidant as well as a GSH precursor.

References

An JJ, Cho SR, Jeong DW, Park KW, Ahn YS, Baik JH (2003) Anti-proliferative effects and cell death mediated by two isoforms of dopamine D2 receptors in pituitary tumor cells. Mol Cell Endocrinol 206(1–2):49–62

Bagh MB, Maiti AK, Jana S, Banerjee K, Roy A, Chakrabarti S (2008) Quinone and oxyradical scavenging properties of N-acetylcysteine prevent dopamine mediated inhibition of Na+, K+-ATPase and mitochondrial electron transport chain activity in rat brain: implications in the neuroprotective therapy of Parkinson's disease. Free Radic Res 42(6):574–581

Baik JH, Picetti R, Saiardi A, Thiriet G, Dierich A, Depaulis A, Le Meur M, Borrelli E (1995) Parkinsonian-like locomotor impairment in mice lacking dopamine D2 receptors. Nature 377(6548):424–428. https://doi.org/10.1038/377424a0

Bauzo RM, Kimmel HL, Howell LL (2012) The cystine-glutamate transporter enhancer N-acetyl-L-cysteine attenuates cocaine-induced changes in striatal dopamine but not self-administration in squirrel monkeys. Pharmacol Biochem Behav 101(2):288–296

Bianchi P, Seguelas MH, Parini A, Cambon C (2003) Activation of pro-apoptotic cascade by dopamine in renal epithelial cells is fully dependent on hydrogen peroxide generation by monoamine oxidases. J Am Soc Nephrol 14(4):855–862

Chen CM, Yin MC, Hsu CC, Liu TC (2007) Antioxidative and anti-inflammatory effects of four cysteine-containing agents in striatum of MPTP-treated mice. Nutrition 23(7–8):589–597

Choi HR, Shin JW, Lee HK, Kim JY, Huh CH, Youn SW, Park KC (2010) Potential redox-sensitive Akt activation by dopamine activates Bad and promotes cell death in melanocytes. Oxidative Med Cell Longev 3(3):219–224

Cucchi ML, Frattini P, Santagostino G, Preda S, Orecchia G (2003) Catecholamines increase in the urine of non-segmental vitiligo especially during its active phase. Pigment Cell Res 16(2):111–116

Deepmala, Slattery J, Kumar N, Delhey L, Berk M, Dean O, Spielholz C, Frye R (2015) Clinical trials of N-acetylcysteine in psychiatry and neurology: a systematic review. Neurosci Biobehav Rev 55:294–321. https://doi.org/10.1016/j.neubiorev.2015.04.015

Fukami G, Hashimoto K, Koike K, Okamura N, Shimizu E, Iyo M (2004) Effect of antioxidant N-acetyl-L-cysteine on behavioral changes and neurotoxicity in rats after administration of methamphetamine. Brain Res 30(1):90–95

Gere-Paszti E, Jakus J (2009) The effect of N-acetylcysteine on amphetamine-mediated dopamine release in rat brain striatal slices by ion-pair reversed-phase high performance liquid chromatography. Biomed Chromatogr 23(6):658–664

He H, Wang S, Tian J, Chen L, Zhang W, Zhao J, Tang H, Zhang X, Chen J (2015) Protective effects of 2,3,5,4′-tetrahydroxystilbene-2-O-beta-D-glucoside in the MPTP-induced mouse model of Parkinson's disease: involvement of reactive oxygen species-mediated JNK, P38 and mitochondrial pathways. Eur J Pharmacol 767:175–182. https://doi.org/10.1016/j.ejphar.2015.10.023

Hoyt KR, Reynolds IJ, Hastings TG (1997) Mechanisms of dopamine-induced cell death in cultured rat forebrain neurons: interactions with and differences from glutamate-induced cell death. Exp Neurol 143(2):269–281

Kang CD, Jang JH, Kim KW, Lee HJ, Jeong CS, Kim CM, Kim SH, Chung BS (1998) Activation of c-jun N-terminal kinase/stress-activated protein kinase and the decreased ratio of Bcl-2 to Bax are associated with the auto-oxidized dopamine-induced apoptosis in PC12 cells. Neurosci Lett 256(1):37–40

Kelly MA, Rubinstein M, Asa SL, Zhang G, Saez C, Bunzow JR, Allen RG, Hnasko R, Ben-Jonathan N, Grandy DK, Low MJ (1997) Pituitary lactotroph hyperplasia and chronic hyperprolactinemia in dopamine D2 receptor-deficient mice. Neuron 19(1):103–113

Khorchid A, Fragoso G, Shore G, Almazan G (2002) Catecholamine-induced oligodendrocyte cell death in culture is developmentally regulated and involves free radical generation and differential activation of caspase-3. Glia 40(3):283–299

Kumar A, Singh BK, Ahmad I, Shukla S, Patel DK, Srivastava G, Kumar V, Pandey HP, Singh C (2012) Involvement of NADPH oxidase and glutathione in zinc-induced dopaminergic neurodegeneration in rats: similarity with paraquat neurotoxicity. Brain Res 15:48–64

Lee CS, Song EH, Park SY, Han ES (2003) Combined effect of dopamine and MPP+ on membrane permeability in mitochondria and cell viability in PC12 cells. Neurochem Int 43(2):147–154

Linsenbardt AJ, Wilken GH, Westfall TC, Macarthur H (2009) Cytotoxicity of dopaminochrome in the mesencephalic cell line, MN9D, is dependent upon oxidative stress. Neurotoxicology 30(6):1030–1035

Luo Y, Umegaki H, Wang X, Abe R, Roth GS (1998) Dopamine induces apoptosis through an oxidation-involved SAPK/JNK activation pathway. J Biol Chem 273(6):3756–3764

Lyng GD, Seegal RF (2008) Polychlorinated biphenyl-induced oxidative stress in organotypic co-cultures: experimental dopamine depletion prevents reductions in GABA. Neurotoxicology 29(2):301–308

Masserano JM, Gong L, Kulaga H, Baker I, Wyatt RJ (1996) Dopamine induces apoptotic cell death of a catecholaminergic cell line derived from the central nervous system. Mol Pharmacol 50(5):1309–1315

MeSH (2016) Dopamine D004298. MeSH Database. National Center for Biotechnology Information, US National Library of Medicine, Bethesda

Migheli R, Godani C, Sciola L, Delogu MR, Serra PA, Zangani D, De Natale G, Miele E, Desole MS (1999) Enhancing effect of manganese on L-DOPA-induced apoptosis in PC12 cells: role of oxidative stress. J Neurochem 73(3):1155–1163

Moller M, Du Preez JL, Viljoen FP, Berk M, Emsley R, Harvey BH (2013a) Social isolation rearing induces mitochondrial, immunological, neurochemical and behavioural deficits in rats, and is reversed by clozapine or N-acetyl cysteine. Brain Behav Immun 30:156–167

Moller M, Du Preez JL, Viljoen FP, Berk M, Harvey BH (2013b) N-acetyl cysteine reverses social isolation rearing induced changes in cortico-striatal monoamines in rats. Metab Brain Dis 28(4):687–696

NCIT (2016) Dopamine C62025. National Cancer Institute Thesaurus, US National Institutes of Health, Bethesda. Version 16.07d

Noh JS, Kim EY, Kang JS, Kim HR, Oh YJ, Gwag BJ (1999) Neurotoxic and neuroprotective actions of catecholamines in cortical neurons. Exp Neurol 159(1):217–224

Nunes C, Barbosa RM, Almeida L, Laranjinha J (2011) Nitric oxide and DOPAC-induced cell death: from GSH depletion to mitochondrial energy crisis. Mol Cell Neurosci 48(1):94–103

Offen D, Ziv I, Sternin H, Melamed E, Hochman A (1996) Prevention of dopamine-induced cell death by thiol antioxidants: possible implications for treatment of Parkinson's disease. Exp Neurol 141(1):32–39

Park ES, Kim SY, Na JI, Ryu HS, Youn SW, Kim DS, Yun HY, Park KC (2007) Glutathione prevented dopamine-induced apoptosis of melanocytes and its signaling. J Dermatol Sci 47(2):141–149

Paszti-Gere E, Jakus J (2013) Protein phosphatases but not reactive oxygen species play functional role in acute amphetamine-mediated dopamine release. Cell Biochem Biophys 66(3):831–841

Perry TL, Yong VW, Clavier RM, Jones K, Wright JM, Foulks JG, Wall RA (1985) Partial protection from the dopaminergic neurotoxin N-methyl-4-phenyl-1,2,3,6-tetrahydropyridine by four different antioxidants in the mouse. Neurosci Lett 60(2):109–114

Qi H, Zhao J, Han Y, Lau AS, Rong J (2012) Z-ligustilide potentiates the cytotoxicity of dopamine in rat dopaminergic PC12 cells. Neurotox Res 22(4):345–354

Rahimmi A, Khosrobakhsh F, Izadpanah E, Moloudi MR, Hassanzadeh K (2015) N-acetylcysteine prevents rotenone-induced Parkinson's disease in rat: an investigation into the interaction of parkin and Drp1 proteins. Brain Res Bull 113:34–40

Sachdeva S, Pant SC, Kushwaha P, Bhargava R, Flora SJ (2015) Sodium tungstate induced neurological alterations in rat brain regions and their response to antioxidants. Food Chem Toxicol 82:64–71

Serra PA, Esposito G, Enrico P, Mura MA, Migheli R, Delogu MR, Miele M, Desole MS, Grella G, Miele E (2000) Manganese increases L-DOPA auto-oxidation in the striatum of the freely moving rat: potential implications to L-DOPA long-term therapy of Parkinson's disease. Br J Pharmacol 130(4):937–945

Serra PA, Esposito G, Delogu MR, Migheli R, Rocchitta G, Miele E, Desole MS, Miele M (2001) Analysis of S-nitroso-N-acetylpenicillamine effects on dopamine release in the striatum of freely moving rats: role of endogenous ascorbic acid and oxidative stress. Br J Pharmacol 132(4):941–949

Sharma A, Kaur P, Kumar V, Gill KD (2007) Attenuation of 1-methyl-4-phenyl-1, 2,3,6-tetrahydropyridine induced nigrostriatal toxicity in mice by N-acetyl cysteine. Cell Mol Biol 53(1):48–55

Vindis C, Seguelas MH, Lanier S, Parini A, Cambon C (2001) Dopamine induces ERK activation in renal epithelial cells through H2O2 produced by monoamine oxidase. Kidney Int 59(1):76–86

Wan FJ, Tung CS, Shiah IS, Lin HC (2006) Effects of alpha-phenyl-N-tert-butyl nitrone and N-acetylcysteine on hydroxyl radical formation and dopamine depletion in the rat striatum produced by d-amphetamine. European Neuropsychopharmacol 16(2):147–153

Weingarten P, Bermak J, Zhou QY (2001) Evidence for non-oxidative dopamine cytotoxicity: potent activation of NF-kappa B and lack of protection by anti-oxidants. J Neurochem 76(6):1794–1804

Zafar KS, Inayat-Hussain SH, Ross D (2007) A comparative study of proteasomal inhibition and apoptosis induced in N27 mesencephalic cells by dopamine and MG132. J Neurochem 102(3):913–921

Zhou ZD, Kerk SY, Xiong GG, Lim TM (2009) Dopamine auto-oxidation aggravates non-apoptotic cell death induced by over-expression of human A53T mutant alpha-synuclein in dopaminergic PC12 cells. J Neurochem 108(3):601–610

Oxidative Stress in Psychiatric Disorders

Lawrence Fung and Antonio Hardan

4.1 Introduction

Oxidative stress has been postulated as one of the pathophysiologic mechanisms implicated in various medical conditions, including neurologic and psychiatric disorders. In this chapter, we will start with the definition of oxidative stress, sources of cellular oxidative stress, and key components of the anti-oxidation system in the body. Then, we will summarize the evidence supporting the role of oxidative stress in various psychiatric disorders. We will also describe the molecular pharmacology of N-Acetylcysteine (NAC), a medication that has been shown to reduce oxidative stress. Finally, we will conclude by explaining the role of NAC in decreasing oxidative stress in psychiatric disorders.

4.2 Oxidative Stress and the Anti-oxidation System

4.2.1 Oxidative Stress

Oxidative stress is defined as an imbalance between the levels of prooxidants and antioxidants. This phenomenon is known to result in damage to macromolecules (i.e., proteins and DNA) and activation of redox-sensitive signals. The reactions to macromolecules are generally caused by prooxidant reactive chemicals containing oxygen or nitrogen and are called reactive oxygen species (ROS) and reactive nitrogen species (RNS), respectively.

One main source of ROS is the nicotinamide adenine dinucleotide phosphate (NADPH) oxidase (NOX) complexes in cell membranes and other cell organelles including mitochondria, peroxisomes, and endoplasmic reticulum. Mitochondria

L. Fung (⊠) · A. Hardan
Stanford University School of Medicine, Stanford, CA, USA
e-mail: lkfung@stanford.edu

© Springer Nature Singapore Pte Ltd. 2019
R. E. Frye, M. Berk (eds.), *The Therapeutic Use of N-Acetylcysteine (NAC) in Medicine*, https://doi.org/10.1007/978-981-10-5311-5_4

convert energy for the cell into a usable form, adenosine triphosphate (ATP), by oxidative phosphorylation. This process involves reduction of oxygen to water. However, this process does not occur perfectly all the time. A small percentage of oxidative phosphorylation will reduce the oxygen prematurely and form superoxide radical ($O_2^{-\bullet}$). The superoxide radical can then initiate lipid peroxidation. The lipid hydroperoxide will then be transformed to lipid radicals, which can further cause damage in cell membranes and even trigger a cascade of events leading to apoptosis. Other examples of ROS include singlet oxygen ($^1O_2$), hydroperoxyl radical ($HO_2^{\bullet}$), hydrogen peroxide (H_2O_2), hydroxyl radical ($HO^{\bullet}$), hydroxyl anion (OH^-), peroxyl radical ($ROO^{\bullet}$), lipid peroxyl radical ($LOO^{\bullet}$), hypochlorous acid (HOCl), hypobromous acid (HOBr), and hypothiocyanous acid (HOSCN) (Moniczewski et al. 2015). In regard to RNS, the key source is nitric oxide ($NO^{\bullet}$). Other examples of RNS include nitrogen dioxide ($NO_2^{\bullet}$), peroxynitrite ($ONOO^-$), nitrite (NO_2^-), nitrate (NO_3^-), and nitronium ion (NO_2^+). Nitrite is often used as a marker of NO activity. In addition to endogenous sources, ROS and RNS can also come from exogenous sources such as medications and environmental toxicants.

4.2.2 Antioxidant Systems in the Body

Under normal physiologic conditions, the body can neutralize ROS and RNS by anti-oxidation systems before significant cellular damage occurs. These systems can reverse oxidative damage by supplying electrons to ROS, RNS, proteins, and electrophilic xenobiotics, thereby maintaining redox balance. Superoxide radicals are typically transformed to hydrogen peroxide by superoxide dismutase (SOD). The resulting hydrogen peroxide is then converted to water by either catalase (CAT) or glutathione peroxidase (GPX). The glutathione system is the predominant antioxidant system in our body. Glutathione exists in two forms: reduced glutathione (GSH) and oxidized glutathione (GSSG) (see Fig. 4.1). The biotransformation between the two forms is central to the regulation of redox balance in the brain. The oxidation of GSH to GSSG is catalyzed by GPX, the same enzyme that converts hydrogen peroxide to water. This GSH→GSSG reaction is key in protecting proteins by coupling with the reduction of thiol groups in proteins via glutaredoxins (GRXs). The reduction of GSSG back to GSH is catalyzed by glutathione reductase (GR), which uses NADPH as a cofactor. In addition to the above biochemical functions, GSH plays a key role in neutralizing electrophilic xenobiotic compounds by conjugating to them via glutathione-*S*-transferases (GSTs). Other endogenous antioxidants include vitamin E and vitamin C, which convert lipid peroxyl radicals to stable vitamin radicals. Collectively, the anti-oxidation system plays a key role in cellular redox homeostasis and has special relevance to pathophysiology of several psychiatric disorders (e.g., schizophrenia and autism) and neurologic diseases (e.g., Alzheimer's disease and Parkinson's disease).

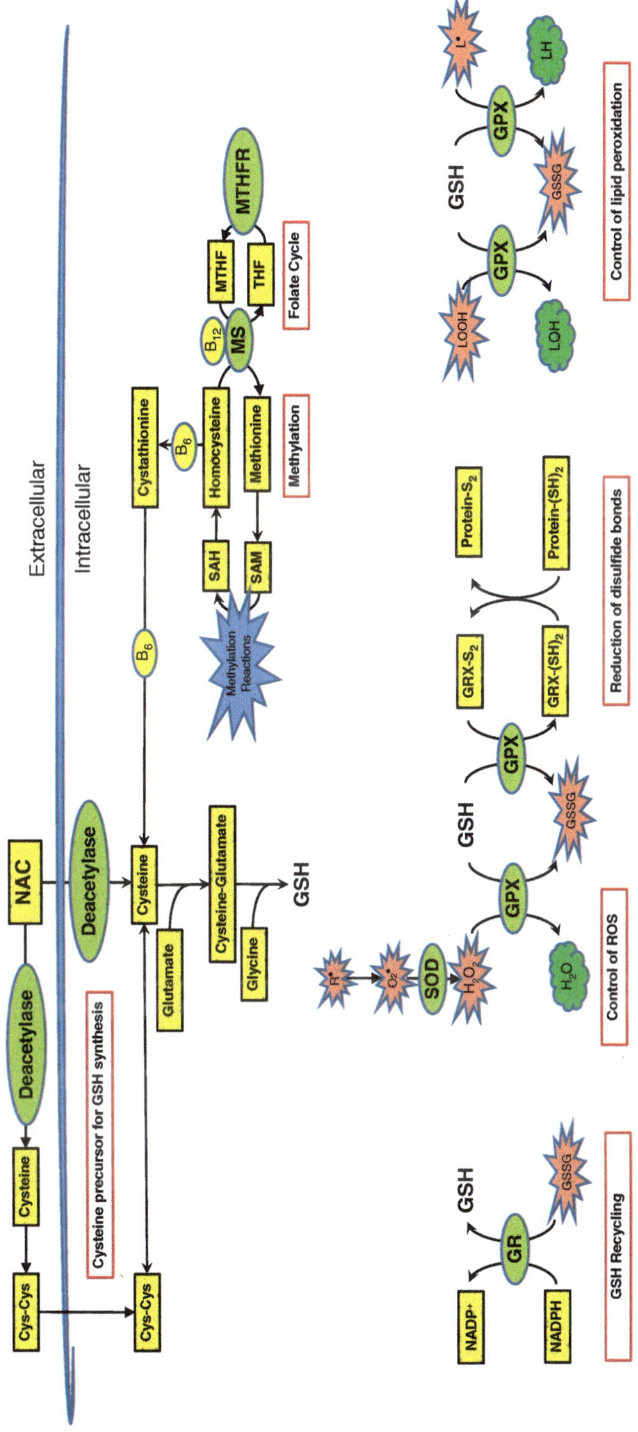

Fig. 4.1 Anti-oxidation systems of the body involving glutathione and the role of N-Acetylcysteine (NAC) in restoring glutathione

4.2.3 Biomarkers of Oxidative Stress

The level of oxidative stress can be assessed peripherally by measuring the concentrations of GSH and GSSG using high-performance liquid chromatography (HPLC) and fluorimetric assays and in the central nervous system using proton magnetic resonance spectroscopy (^{1}H MRS). Other common biomarkers of oxidative stress include the enzyme activities of CAT, GPX, and SOD. In addition to oxidative stress, downstream processes such as lipid peroxidation, oxidative protein damage, and oxidative DNA damage can also be monitored. Aconitase activity has been employed as a biomarker of mitochondrial superoxide production. Thiobarbituric acid reactive substances (TBARS) are common biomarkers for lipid peroxidation. 3-nitrotyrosine (3-NT) has been used to assess oxidative protein damage. 8-oxo-deoxyguanosine (8-oxo-dG) is a biomarker of oxidative DNA damage. 3-chlorotyrosine (3-CT) is an established biomarker of a chronic inflammatory response.

4.2.4 Oxidative Stress in the Developing Brain

Neurons are highly susceptible to oxidative damage due to high levels of ROS and RNS production, relatively low amounts of antioxidant enzymes, the high brain's lipid content and metabolic rate, and the non-regenerative nature of neurons. Of particular interest is the developing brain that has a high metabolic rate. When low levels of antioxidants and high levels of heavy metal ions are present, ROS levels will become elevated. The developing brain at an early age is sensitive to even small changes to redox balance, which can affect the signaling pathways and processes involved in neurogenesis, neuronal differentiation, and myelination. Therefore, oxidative stress is associated with neuronal injury in the developing brain when subjected to hypoxia, ischemia, and traumatic brain injury. Consequently, these insults may derail brain development and result in neurodevelopmental disorders such as autism spectrum disorder (ASD) and schizophrenia.

4.3 Oxidative Stress and Psychiatric Disorders

Oxidative stress has been implicated in various psychiatric disorders including ASD, schizophrenia, bipolar disorder, and major depressive disorder (MDD). Here we will summarize the evidence of oxidative stress in these disorders (Table 4.1).

4.3.1 Oxidative Stress and Autism Spectrum Disorder

4.3.1.1 Peripheral Biomarkers of Redox Balance in ASD

ASD is characterized by deficits in socio-communicative abilities, stereotypic behaviors, restricted interests, cognitive inflexibility, and sensory aberrations. Like

Table 4.1 Summary of oxidation status assessed in the systemic circulation and brain for representative psychiatric disorders

Disorder	Systemic circulation		Brain
	Individual studies	Meta-analysis	
Autism spectrum disorder	Decreased GSH (Han et al. 2015; Geier et al. 2009; James et al. 2006) Decreased GSH/GSSG (Han et al. 2015) Increased GSSG (Geier et al. 2009; James et al. 2006) Increased homocysteine (Han et al. 2015) Increased SOD (Al-Gadani et al. 2009; Zoroglu et al. 2004), decreased SOD (Meguid et al. 2011; Yorbik et al. 2002), no difference in SOD (Ghezzo et al. 2013) Decreased CAT (Zoroglu et al. 2004), no difference in CAT (Al-Gadani et al. 2009; Ghezzo et al. 2013) Decreased GPX (Meguid et al. 2011; El-Ansary and Al-Ayadhi 2012; Laszlo et al. 2013), increased GPX (Al-Gadani et al. 2009)	Decreased GSH (Frustaci et al. 2012) Increased GSSG (Frustaci et al. 2012) No difference in homocysteine (Frustaci et al. 2012) No difference in SOD (Frustaci et al. 2012) Decreased GPX (Frustaci et al. 2012)	*MRS* No difference in GSH in basal ganglia and dorsomedial PFC in adults (Durieux et al. 2016) *Postmortem* Decreased GSH in cerebellum and temporal cortex (Rose et al. 2012) Increased 3-NT and 3-CT in cerebellum and temporal cortex (Rose et al. 2012) Decreased aconitase in cerebellum and temporal cortex (Rose et al. 2012)
Schizophrenia	Decreased GSH (Altuntas et al. 2000; Mico et al. 2011; Raffa et al. 2009; Raffa et al. 2011) Increased GSSG (Raffa et al. 2009; Raffa et al. 2011)	Decreased TAS in FEP but increased in chronic patients (Flatow et al. 2013) Decreased CAT in FEP but increased in chronic patients (Flatow et al. 2013) Increased nitrite in FEP but decreased in chronic patients (Flatow et al. 2013)	*MRS* Decreased GSH in PFC (Do et al. 2000; Matsuzawa and Hashimoto 2011) No difference in GSH in ACC (Terpstra et al. 2005) No difference in GSH in posterior medial frontal cortex (Matsuzawa et al. 2008) Increased GSH in medial temporal lobe (Wood et al. 2009) Positive correlation between GSH in medial PFC and FA in patients with schizophrenia (Monin et al. 2015) No correlation between GSH in medial PFC and rsFC in patients with schizophrenia (Monin et al. 2015) *Postmortem* Decreased GSH in PFC (Gawryluk et al. 2011) and striatum (Yao et al. 2006)

(continued)

Table 4.1 (continued)

Disorder	Systemic circulation		Brain
	Individual studies	Meta-analysis	
Bipolar disorder	Decreased GSH (Rosa et al. 2014), no difference in GSH (Tuncel et al. 2015) Increased GSSG (Rosa et al. 2014), no difference in GSSG (Tuncel et al. 2015) No difference in SOD (Tuncel et al. 2015; Tsai and Huang 2015) Decreased GPX (Tsai and Huang 2015) No difference in CAT (Tsai and Huang 2015) Increased TBARS only in manic patients after treatment (Tsai and Huang 2015) No difference in 3-NT in older bipolar patients	No difference in SOD (Brown et al. 2014) No difference in GPX (Brown et al. 2014) No difference in CAT (Brown et al. 2014)	*MRS* No difference in GSH in PFC (Godlewska et al. 2014), ACC (Soeiro-de-Souza et al. 2016; Lagopoulos et al. 2013), and occipital cortex (Godlewska et al. 2014) Increased lactate in dorsal ACC (Soeiro-de-Souza et al. 2016) Correlation between GSH and lactate in dorsal ACC (Soeiro-de-Souza et al. 2016) *Postmortem* Increased 3-NT in PFC (Andreazza et al. 2013)
Major depressive disorder	Decreased SOD (Wei et al. 2009; Selek et al. 2008), increased SOD (Kodydkova et al. 2009; Khanzode et al. 2003; Sarandol et al. 2007; Bilici et al. 2001) Decreased GPX (Ozcan et al. 2004; Kodydkova et al. 2009), no difference in GPX (Andreazza et al. 2009) Decreased CAT (Ozcan et al. 2004; Wei et al. 2009) Increased GR (Kodydkova et al. 2009; Andreazza et al. 2009) Increased GST (Andreazza et al. 2009; Galecki et al. 2009)		*MRS* Decreased GSH in occipital cortex (Godlewska et al. 2015) Negative correlation between GSH and anhedonia in patients with MDD (Lapidus et al. 2014) Escitalopram did not change brain GSH levels (Godlewska et al. 2015) Increased GSH in ACC of elderly at risk for MDD (Godlewska et al. 2015) In elderly at risk for MDD, GSH correlates positively with depression and negatively with cognitive function (Godlewska et al. 2015) *Postmortem* Increased SOD in PFC (Michel et al. 2007) No difference in SOD in the hippocampus (Michel et al. 2007)

All findings are relative to controls

3-CT 3-chlorotyrosine, *3-NT* 3-nitrotyrosine, *ACC* anterior cingulate cortex, *CAT* catalase, *MDD* major depressive disorder, *FA* fractional anisotropy, *FEP* first-episode psychosis, *GSH* reduced glutathione, *GPX* glutathione peroxidase, *GR* glutathione reductase, *GSSG* oxidized glutathione, *GST* glutathione-S-transferase, *PFC* prefrontal cortex, *rsFC* resting-state functional connectivity, *SOD* superoxide dismutase, *TAS* total antioxidant status, *TBARS* thiobarbituric acid reactive substances schizophrenia, many investigators in the field of autism have studied oxidative stress. Han et al. reported that GSH levels as well as the GSH/GSSG ratio showed significantly lower values in children with ASD compared to control subjects (Han et al. 2015). Other investigators showed that children with ASD had lower levels of plasma GSH but higher levels of GSSG than typically developing children (Geier et al. 2009; James et al. 2006). Furthermore, homocysteine and GSSG levels were significantly higher in children with ASD (Han et al. 2015). Finally, homocysteine levels were found to correlate positively with Childhood Autism Rating Scale (CARS) scores in children with ASD. The associations between other oxidative stress parameters and ASD have not been consistent. The SOD activity was either increased in erythrocytes (Al-Gadani et al. 2009; Zoroglu et al. 2004) or decreased in plasma and erythrocytes (Meguid et al. 2011; Yorbik et al. 2002). The CAT activity was reduced in erythrocytes (Zoroglu et al. 2004) but unchanged in plasma (Al-Gadani et al. 2009). The GPX activity was reduced in plasma (El-Ansary and Al-Ayadhi 2012; Laszlo et al. 2013) and erythrocytes (Meguid et al. 2011) but increased in plasma (Al-Gadani et al. 2009).

Ghezzo et al. evaluated oxidative stress parameters in children with ASD and neurotypical controls. While some oxidative stress biomarkers including TBARS, urinary isoprostane, and hexanoyl-lysine adduct levels in RBC were found to be elevated in ASD, many others (RBC SOD and CAT activities, urinary 8-oxo-dG, plasma radical absorbance capacity, and carbonyl groups) were not different between the two groups (Ghezzo et al. 2013). Interestingly, Na^+/K^+-ATPase activity and RBC membrane fluidity were found to be reduced in ASD compared to TD (Ghezzo et al. 2013). Furthermore, fatty acid membrane profile was altered in ASD; children with ASD demonstrated an increase in monounsaturated fatty acids, decrease in eicosapentaenoic acid (EPA), decrease in docosahexaenoic acid (DHA)-ω3, and increase in the ω6/ω3 ratio as compared to controls (Ghezzo et al. 2013).

Existing evidence is not consistent and small sample sizes and effects limit many studies. Frustaci and his colleagues, who completed a recent systematic review and meta-analyses of oxidative stress-related biomarkers in autism, recognized this problem. This meta-analysis showed the children with autism consistently demonstrated decreased blood levels of reduced GSH, GPX, methionine, and cysteine and increased concentrations of GSSG relative to controls across multiple studies, whereas SOD, homocysteine, and cystathionine were not consistently different between ASD and controls across published studies (Frustaci et al. 2012).

Building on the above findings, Frye and his colleagues studied the connection between oxidative stress and mitochondrial dysfunction in children with ASD. Compared to typically developing controls, children with ASD [with or without comorbid mitochondrial disease (MD)] showed lower GSH and GSH/GSSG. Compared to children with ASD only, children with ASD + MD were found to have significantly higher GSH/GSSG and lower levels of GSSG. Furthermore, the authors demonstrated that signs of chronic inflammation were present in both groups of children with ASD, as evidenced by higher levels of 3-chlorotyrosine (3-CT). Finally, children with ASD + MD were found to have lower scores on the daily living skill and communication subscales of the Vineland Adaptive Behavior

Scale (VABS) despite having similar language and ASD symptoms. This study suggested that different subgroups of children with ASD have different abnormalities in their redox balance, which may arise from different etiologies.

4.3.1.2 Evaluation of Brain GSH Levels in Individuals with ASD by ^{1}H MRS

Using ^{1}H MRS, no difference in brain GSH was found in either basal ganglia or dorsomedial prefrontal cortex in adults with ASD (Durieux et al. 2016).

4.3.1.3 Assessing Redox Balance from Postmortem Brain Samples of Individuals with ASD

Using postmortem brain samples of individuals with ASD, central nervous system levels of oxidative stress biomarkers were measured (Rose et al. 2012). Consistent with previous studies on plasma and immune cells, the oxidative stress biomarkers GSH and GSH/GSSG, as measured by HPLC, were significantly decreased in both ASD cerebellum and temporal cortex as compared to controls.

A significant increase in 3-NT, a biomarker of oxidative protein damage, in the cerebellum and temporal cortex was found in ASD (Rose et al. 2012). Similarly, 8-oxo-dG, a biomarker of oxidative DNA damage, was elevated in cerebellar and temporal cortices in individuals with ASD in comparison to controls and was inversely correlated with GSH/GSSG in the cerebellum (Rose et al. 2012). An increase in levels of 3-CT, a biomarker of chronic inflammatory response, in both brain regions was also observed. Finally, the activity of aconitase, a biomarker of mitochondrial superoxide production, was significantly decreased in cerebellar tissue of individuals with ASD cerebellum and was negatively correlated with GSH/GSSG (Rose et al. 2012). Together, these results indicate that decreased GSH/GSSG redox/antioxidant capacity and increased oxidative stress in the brain tissue from individuals with ASD may have functional consequence in terms of a chronic inflammatory response, increased mitochondrial superoxide production, and oxidative protein and DNA damage. Finally, in a similar study, cerebellar tissues from individuals with ASD were examined, and the activities of GSH-related enzymes GPX, GST, GR, and glutamate-cysteine ligase (GCL) were measured (Gu et al. 2013). Compared to that of the control group, the activities of GPX, GST, and GCL were significantly decreased in ASD.

4.3.1.4 Oxidative Stress and Mitochondrial Dysfunction in ASD

The relationship of oxidative stress and mitochondrial dysfunction was also demonstrated in a subset of individuals with ASD (Rose et al. 2014, 2015). Using lymphoblastoid cell lines (LCLs) derived from children with ASD, Rose et al. reported that this subset of ASD children had an abnormal mitochondrial reserve capacity before and after exposure to ROS. LCLs from a subset of children with ASD displayed high reserve capacity at baseline but a precipitous drop in reserve capacity when challenged with ROS. In a recent study, this group demonstrated that this metabolic phenotype was related to worse repetitive and stereotyped behaviors (Rose et al. 2017). Interestingly, in this ASD LCL subgroup, pretreatment with NAC prevented this sharp decline of anti-oxidation reserve capacity and improved GSH metabolism, suggesting a role for altered GSH metabolism associated with this type of mitochondrial dysfunction (Rose et al. 2015). Collectively, these results suggested that a subgroup of children with ASD might have alterations in mitochondrial function, which could cause increased vulnerability to prooxidants.

4.3.2 Oxidative Stress and Schizophrenia

4.3.2.1 Peripheral Biomarkers of Redox Balance in Schizophrenia

Schizophrenia is a psychiatric disorder characterized by hallucinations, delusions, and cognitive dysfunction. This disorder has been viewed as a neurodevelopmental disorder due to the known risk factors of early life insult and genetic loading. Redox regulation has been hypothesized as one of the components of a "central hub" in the pathophysiology of schizophrenia (Steullet et al. 2010). Redox dysregulation, NMDA hypofunction, and neuroinflammation were hypothesized as the three components of this hub, which mediates the impairment of microcircuits and macrocircuits, thereby causing aberrations in circuit connectivity and psychopathologic findings in schizophrenia (Steullet et al. 2010). Peripheral (blood and plasma) GSH levels in patients with schizophrenia have been found to be lower than in healthy volunteers (Altuntas et al. 2000; Mico et al. 2011; Raffa et al. 2009, 2011). Further, blood GSSG concentrations were found to be higher in patients with schizophrenia (Raffa et al. 2009, 2011). GSH levels correlated positively with the Scale for the Assessment of Positive Symptoms (SAPS) (Raffa et al. 2011).

In addition to GSH and GSSG levels, the disorder was found to be associated with aberrations in other oxidative stress parameters based on a recent meta-analysis of oxidative stress of 44 studies involving individuals with schizophrenia (Flatow et al. 2013). Compared to control subjects, serum or plasma total antioxidant status (TAS) levels were significantly lower in patients who underwent first episodes of psychosis (FEP). However, TAS levels were found to be significantly higher in patients who have been treated with antipsychotic medications after acute exacerbations of psychosis. Similarly, cross-sectional studies revealed that red blood cell (RBC) CAT and plasma nitrite were significantly decreased in FEP and significantly increased in stable outpatients. Based on these results, the authors concluded that plasma or serum TAS, plasma nitrite, and RBC CAT were state-related biomarker of oxidative stress in individuals with schizophrenia. In contrast, compared to control subjects, RBC SOD was found to be lower in FEP, acutely relapsed inpatients, and stable outpatients, and therefore, SOD appeared to be a trait-related biomarker for schizophrenia. Collectively, these findings supported that abnormalities in oxidative stress in FEP might be independent of antipsychotic medications.

One genetic factor that has been reported to influence GSH concentrations in the systemic circulation is the GAG trinucleotide repeat (TNR) polymorphism in the gene coding for the catalytic subunit of glutamate-cysteine ligase (GCL), the rate-limiting enzyme for GSH synthesis. Importantly, polymorphism of this catalytic subunit of GCL (GCLC) was associated with schizophrenia in two case-control studies. As compared with GCLC low-risk genotypes, GCLC high-risk genotypes were more frequent in patients with schizophrenia and were associated with lower GCLC protein expression, GCL activity, and GSH levels in fibroblasts when challenged with oxidative stress conditions. In their recent studies in patients with early psychosis, Xin et al. found that glutamate concentrations in the mPFC as measured by MRS were lower in patients with low-risk GCLC genotypes, but this was not the case for patients with high-risk genotypes (Xin et al. 2016). Furthermore, the authors revealed that the GSH levels in the mPFC, as measured by ^{1}H MRS, correlated negatively with GPX levels in RBC in patients with schizophrenia. In contrast to individuals with early psychosis, GSH levels in the mPFC of healthy volunteers correlated positively with GPX levels in RBC (Xin et al. 2016).

4.3.2.2 Evaluation of Brain GSH Levels in Individuals with Schizophrenia by ^{1}H MRS

Regarding GSH levels in the brain, Do and her colleagues found that the GSH concentrations in cerebrospinal fluid (CSF) of inpatients with schizophrenia or schizophreniform disorder were lower than those of age- and gender-matched healthy controls (Do et al. 2000). They examined the prefrontal cortex (PFC) of these participants by proton magnetic resonance spectroscopy (^{1}H MRS), which revealed the GSH levels in the PFC to be lower in patients with schizophrenia than healthy volunteers (Do et al. 2000). This finding was replicated by ^{1}H MRS of the frontal cortex in patients with schizophrenia (Matsuzawa and Hashimoto 2011).

Despite the consistent findings of reduced GSH in the frontal cortex, decreased GSH levels were not found in other areas of the brain. For example, a ^{1}H MRS study detected no changes in GSH levels in the anterior cingulate (Terpstra et al. 2005) and posterior medial frontal cortex (Matsuzawa et al. 2008), whereas GSH concentrations in the medial temporal lobe were increased in patients with their first episode of schizophrenia (Wood et al. 2009). Collectively, these results suggested that perturbation in the GSH levels may be regionally specific in schizophrenia.

4.3.2.3 Assessing Redox Balance from Postmortem Brain Samples of Individuals with Schizophrenia

According to postmortem studies, the concentrations of GSH in the prefrontal cortex (Gawryluk et al. 2011) and striatum (Yao et al. 2006) of schizophrenic patients were lower than controls. Such decreases were linked with lowered activity of related enzymes, such as GPX, GSH-R, and GSH-S-transferase mu isoform (Gawryluk et al. 2011; Yao et al. 2006). Furthermore, increased oxidation and nitration was also found in the postmortem PFC samples of patients with schizophrenia (Kim et al. 2014).

Among brain cells, oligodendrocytes are known to be highly vulnerable to oxidative stress. Monin and his colleagues investigated the interplay between glutathione and myelin (Monin et al. 2015). In control subjects, a positive association was found between mPFC GSH levels as assessed by MRS and both fractional anisotropy (FA) and resting-state functional connectivity along the cingulum bundle. In contrast, in early psychosis patients, mPFC GSH levels were correlated only with FA measures.

Therefore, redox regulation has a critical role in myelination processes and white matter maturation in the mPFC of patients with schizophrenia.

4.3.2.4 Oxidative Stress and Other Pathophysiologic Mechanisms of Schizophrenia

On one hand, oxidative stress can cause damage in the cellular machinery for neurotransmission. On the other hand, abnormalities in the neurotransmission system can trigger changes in oxidative stress. For example, hypofunction of the NMDA receptor (NMDAR) can trigger the downregulation of antioxidant genes, leading to ROS generation through the activation of NADPH oxidase (NOX). NMDAR hypofunction can also result in circuit-level disinhibition of cortical networks. These events cause GSH depletion, which in turn can further repress NMDAR activity. Consequently, during brain development, oxidative stress and GSH deficits caused by NMDAR hypofunction can cause cellular impairment of specific neurons including parvalbumin-expressing interneurons (PVIs), leading to excitation-inhibition (E/I) imbalance (Do et al. 2015; Morishita et al. 2015). The E/I imbalance may lead to the alterations in sensory processing, cognition, and behavior in individuals with schizophrenia.

4.3.3 Oxidative Stress and Bipolar Disorder

4.3.3.1 Peripheral Biomarkers of Redox Balance in Bipolar Disorder

Bipolar disorder is a mood disorder characterized by discrete episodes of manic and depressive symptoms. The findings on redox status are mixed and are mostly from data obtained from studies of adult individuals with bipolar disorder. Rosa et al. found that bipolar patients had significantly lower plasma levels of GSH and higher levels of GSSG, compared to controls (Rosa et al. 2014). This investigation also revealed a correlation between total GSH levels and age of illness onset, so that lower plasma levels of GSH were associated with later onset of disease, not length of illness. Interestingly, Tuncel et al. however could not replicate the difference in plasma GSH levels between bipolar patients and control subjects (Tuncel et al. 2015). Additionally, the activity of SOD was found to be similar between bipolar patients and healthy volunteers (Tuncel et al. 2015; Tsai and Huang 2015). Serum GPX activity in bipolar patients was found to be significantly lower than that of control subjects and correlated negatively with severity of manic symptoms as measured by the Young Mania Rating Scale (YMRS) (Tsai and Huang 2015). No difference in CAT activity was found between bipolar patients and control subjects. However, serum CAT activity was associated positively with YMRS (Tsai and Huang 2015).

Tuncel et al. also examined other oxidation markers of lipid peroxidation, protein oxidation, and total oxidized guanine species, in adult bipolar patients during manic and euthymic episodes (Tuncel et al. 2015). Significant increase in the level of lipid peroxidation was found in the bipolar disorder manic episode group compared to the control group. Furthermore, the level of total oxidized guanine species was statistically higher in bipolar groups compared to the control group. Tsai and colleagues replicated the increased lipid peroxidation (Tsai and Huang 2015). Serum levels of TBARS in bipolar patients in a manic phase were significantly higher than those of healthy volunteers. Furthermore, these authors found significantly decreased changes in TBARS levels only in bipolar manic patients after treatment, suggesting that TBARS levels might be a state biomarker of oxidative stress in bipolar patients (Tsai and Huang 2015).

Brown et al. conducted a meta-analysis of studies that examined markers of oxidative stress in bipolar patients compared to healthy volunteers (Brown et al. 2014). Bipolar disorder patients were found to have significantly higher markers of lipid peroxidation and DNA/RNA damage, as compared to healthy controls. While the effect size for lipid peroxidation was very high, GPX, SOD, and CAT in bipolar patients were not different from that of healthy volunteers.

The evidence of oxidative stress appears to persist into later life in individuals with bipolar disorder (Andreazza et al. 2015). Andreazza et al. compared the levels of oxidative damage to proteins and lipids in plasma from 110 euthymic older patients with bipolar disorder (mean age, 62 years) and found that these patients showed higher levels of lipid hydroperoxide (LPH) and 4-hydroxynonenal (4-HNE) than age-matched healthy volunteers. However, no significant differences for PC, 3-NT, and 4-HNE were found between the two groups. These results support the persistent effect of oxidative stress in patients with bipolar disorder into later life.

4.3.3.2 Brain GSH Levels in Individuals with Bipolar Disorder by ^{1}H MRS

GSH levels were assessed in prefrontal (Godlewska et al. 2014), anterior cingulate (Soeiro-de-Souza et al. 2016; Lagopoulos et al. 2013), and occipital (Godlewska et al. 2014) cortices of patients with euthymic bipolar disorder. No difference in GSH levels between bipolar participants and controls was found. Similarly, participants showed no difference from controls in other measured cortical metabolites including GABA, glutamate, and NAA. Although no difference in GSH levels was found in the brain regions studied, lactate levels in the dorsal anterior cingulate cortex were found to be higher in bipolar disorder patients, as compared to healthy controls. Interestingly, lactate and GSH levels in the dorsal anterior cingulate cortex correlated positively in euthymic bipolar patients only (Soeiro-de-Souza et al. 2016). While no alterations of markers of the oxidative system were observed in euthymic individuals with bipolar disorder, it remains to be determined whether abnormalities in this system might be observed during active clinical activities, either manic or depressive.

4.3.3.3 Assessing Redox Balance from Postmortem Brain Samples of Individuals with Bipolar Disorder

Pathologic studies have also examined the antioxidant system in individuals with bipolar disorder. Andreazza et al. examined the postmortem PFC samples from patients with bipolar disorder and isolated mitochondria, synaptosomes, and myelin

(Andreazza et al. 2013). They found decreased complex I subunit levels in bipolar subjects compared with healthy volunteers, but no difference in complex III subunits. Additionally, carbonylation was increased in synaptosomes from the bipolar group, while 3-NT was increased in mitochondria from the bipolar group. These results suggest that mitochondrial proteins in the PFC of bipolar patients are more susceptible to potentially reversible nitrosative damage, while more long-standing oxidative damage occurs to synaptic proteins.

Kim et al. found increased oxidation of dopamine transporter (DAT)-immunoreactive regions and decreased nitration of tyrosine hydroxylase (TH)-immunoreactive regions in the PFC of patients with bipolar disorder (Kim et al. 2014). On the other hand, these authors found increased global levels of oxidation in patients with bipolar disorder. (Kim et al. 2014) These findings suggest alterations in levels of protein oxidation and nitration in DA-rich regions of the prefrontal cortex in patients with bipolar disorder.

4.3.4 Oxidative Stress and Major Depressive Disorder

4.3.4.1 Peripheral Biomarkers of Redox Balance in Major Depressive Disorder (MDD)

Major depressive disorder is a psychiatric disorder characterized by discrete episodes of low mood, sadness, and hopelessness accompanied by vegetative symptoms of depression involving alterations of sleep and appetite. Several lines of evidence support that the redox balance in patients with MDD is perturbed. However, findings of oxidative stress parameters are mixed. While various studies revealed that systemic levels of GPX (Ozcan et al. 2004; Kodydkova et al. 2009), CAT (Ozcan et al. 2004; Wei et al. 2009), and SOD (Wei et al. 2009; Selek et al. 2008) were lower in MDD patients than healthy volunteers, opposite results were also published. Some reports indicated the rise of activities of GR (Kodydkova et al. 2009; Andreazza et al. 2009) and GST (Andreazza et al. 2009) in the late stage of MDD, without alteration in GPX activity (Andreazza et al. 2009; Galecki et al. 2009). Higher levels of SOD activities were also found in serum and erythrocytes of patients with MDD (Kodydkova et al. 2009; Khanzode et al. 2003; Sarandol et al. 2007; Bilici et al. 2001).

4.3.4.2 Evaluation of Brain GSH Levels in Individuals with Major Depressive Disorder by ^{1}H MRS

GSH concentration in the occipital cortex of patients with MDD was determined by ^{1}H MRS (Lapidus et al. 2014; Godlewska et al. 2015). Patients with MDD were found to have lower GSH levels in the occipital cortex than control participants; however, GABA and glutamate levels between MDD patients and controls were similar (Godlewska et al. 2015). Furthermore, the severity of anhedonia was found to correlate negatively with occipital GSH levels (Lapidus et al. 2014). Effects of the selective serotonin reuptake inhibitor, escitalopram, on GSH levels were also examined in one study. After a 6-week escitalopram treatment, brain levels of GSH, GABA, and glutamate in the occipital cortex remained unchanged (Godlewska et al. 2015).

Oxidative stress and depressive symptoms were investigated in one study of older adults at risk for depression (Duffy et al. 2015). Compared to age-matched controls, the elderly "at-risk" individuals had increased GSH levels in the anterior cingulate cortex (ACC). Additionally, the increased GSH levels were associated with greater symptoms of depression and worse cognitive performance.

4.3.4.3 Assessing Redox Balance from Postmortem Brain Samples of Individuals with MDD

A limited number of studies examined the redox balance in postmortem brain tissue in individuals with MDD. In one study, the concentration of SOD was found to be increased in the prefrontal cortex, but not in the hippocampus in postmortem brain samples of individuals with depression in comparison to controls (Michel et al. 2007).

4.3.5 Summary

While several investigations have assessed the antioxidant defense system in neuropsychiatric disorders, findings have not been very consistent. Additional studies are warranted to examine large sample sizes in a developmental approach and longitudinally to determine the stability of some of the observations over time and the effect of age and treatment on the abnormalities observed. Using a multimodal approach is also needed where markers of oxidative system are examined peripherally and centrally by innovative imaging methodologies.

4.4 Pharmacology of N-Acetylcysteine

N-Acetylcysteine (NAC) is a well-known antidote against acetaminophen overdose, which works by increasing the concentrations of GSH through supplementation of cysteine. Cysteine can also be oxidized to cystine, which is a substrate for the glutamate-cystine antiporter. In exchange of the cystine taken by the glial cells, the antiporter transports glutamate into the extracellular space. The non-vesicular glutamate released into the extracellular space activates the type 2/3 metabotropic glutamate receptors, which inhibit the release of vesicular glutamate, thereby decreasing glutamatergic neurotransmission.

NAC has been shown to prevent oxidative damage in animal models, such as the *Gclm* knockout mice which have impaired synthesis of GSH (Cabungcal et al. 2013). Without supplementation of NAC, the redox dysregulation in the *Gclm* knockout mice was found to cause oxidative stress in the brain. In particular, parvalbumin (PV)-containing GABAergic interneurons, but not GABAergic interneurons containing calbindin or calretinin, were found to be especially vulnerable to oxidative damage. This effect was revealed to persist into adulthood of the *Gclm* knockout mice and could be prevented with NAC.

4.5 Role of NAC in Relieving Oxidative Stress in Patient Population

NAC has been tested as adjunctive treatments for patients with ASD (Hardan et al. 2012; Dean et al. 2016), schizophrenia (Berk et al. 2008a; Farokhnia et al. 2013; Lavoie et al. 2008), bipolar disorder (Berk et al. 2008b, 2012), depression (Berk et al. 2014), and other psychiatric disorders. While many of these studies found that NAC resulted in behavioral improvements, only one study had confirmed the mechanism of action of NAC in patient populations (Lavoie et al. 2008). Here we will summarize the evidence for the modulation of the redox system in the brain as demonstrated by clinical trials of NAC.

As discussed above, redox dysregulation and NMDA hypofunction have been demonstrated in patients with schizophrenia. Based on these pathophysiologic mechanisms of schizophrenia, several investigators had conducted randomized, double-blind trials of NAC. Lavoie et al. performed the only study to date that measured the GSH levels in the systemic circulation (Lavoie et al. 2008). After a 6-week treatment of NAC, the mean concentration of GSH in whole blood was 0.89 μmol/mL, which was significantly higher than the mean GSH concentration after placebo treatment (0.81 μmol/mL).

One study has also been completed to examine the effect of NAC on the antioxidant system in mood disorders. Das and her colleagues conducted a multicenter, randomized, double-blind, placebo-controlled study of MDD patients treated with NAC (Das et al. 2013). Participants ($n = 76$) from one site completed ^{1}H MRS of the ACC at the end of treatment (12 weeks). MR spectra from the ACC yielded absolute concentrations of glutamate (Glu), glutamate+glutamine (Glx), N-acetyl-aspartate (NAA), and myoinositol (mI), but not GSH. Binary logistic regression analysis was performed to determine whether metabolite profiles could predict NAC versus placebo group. While controlling for the severity of depression and gender, the regression model including concentrations of Glx, NAA, and mI resulted in 75% accuracy in predicting group outcome (NAC or placebo). The finding of higher Glx and NAA levels being predictive of the NAC group provides preliminary support for the putative anti-oxidative role of NAC in MDD. The authors stated that the links between Glx and GSH synthesis (Dodd et al. 2008) and between NAA and GSH levels (Heales et al. 1995) would support that GSH levels were likely elevated by NAC.

Despite the overwhelming evidence of GSH depletion in multiple psychiatric disorders, monitoring of brain levels of GSH before and after oral NAC treatment has not been conducted to date. The closest attempt to this strategy was performed by Holmay et al., who showed that a single-dose, intravenous administration of NAC resulted in an increase in GSH in the occipital cortices of patients with Gaucher and Parkinson diseases (Holmay et al. 2013). Clearly, the use of ^{1}H MRS is at its infancy.

4.6 Future Directions

The evidence supporting the role of the antioxidant system in the pathophysiology in neuropsychiatric disorders is mounting. Treatment studies examining the effect of NAC on behavioral improvement are of interest to many investigators, and attempts are being made to replicate existing findings in larger trials. More importantly, there is a dire need to examine the direct effect of NAC on the antioxidant system either peripherally or centrally. Therefore, measuring GSH concentrations in the brain before and after NAC treatment is essential not only important to confirm the mechanism of action of NAC but also provide a potential avenue to develop biomarkers that can track disease progression and predict response to treatment. This strategy will be facilitated by the development of advanced MRS methodologies to allow the reliable measurement of GSH in the brain using acquisition sequences that are of short duration to facilitate the participation of individuals with severe neuropsychiatric disorders.

References

Al-Gadani Y, El-Ansary A, Attas O, Al-Ayadhi L (2009) Metabolic biomarkers related to oxidative stress and antioxidant status in Saudi autistic children. Clin Biochem 42(10–11):1032–1040. https://doi.org/10.1016/j.clinbiochem.2009.03.011

Altuntas I, Aksoy H, Coskun I, Caykoylu A, Akcay F (2000) Erythrocyte superoxide dismutase and glutathione peroxidase activities, and malondialdehyde and reduced glutathione levels in schizophrenic patients. Clin Chem Lab Med 38(12):1277–1281. https://doi.org/10.1515/CCLM.2000.201

Andreazza AC, Kapczinski F, Kauer-Sant'Anna M, Walz JC, Bond DJ, Goncalves CA, Young LT, Yatham LN (2009) 3-Nitrotyrosine and glutathione antioxidant system in patients in the early and late stages of bipolar disorder. J Psychiatry Neurosci 34(4):263–271

Andreazza AC, Wang JF, Salmasi F, Shao L, Young LT (2013) Specific subcellular changes in oxidative stress in prefrontal cortex from patients with bipolar disorder. J Neurochem 127(4):552–561. https://doi.org/10.1111/jnc.12316

Andreazza AC, Gildengers A, Rajji TK, Zuzarte PM, Mulsant BH, Young LT (2015) Oxidative stress in older patients with bipolar disorder. Am J Geriatr Psychiatry 23(3):314–319. https://doi.org/10.1016/j.jagp.2014.05.008

Berk M, Copolov D, Dean O, Lu K, Jeavons S, Schapkaitz I, Anderson-Hunt M, Judd F, Katz F, Katz P, Ording-Jespersen S, Little J, Conus P, Cuenod M, Do KQ, Bush AI (2008a) N-acetyl cysteine as a glutathione precursor for schizophrenia--a double-blind, randomized, placebo-controlled trial. Biol Psychiatry 64(5):361–368. https://doi.org/10.1016/j.biopsych.2008.03.004

Berk M, Copolov DL, Dean O, Lu K, Jeavons S, Schapkaitz I, Anderson-Hunt M, Bush AI (2008b) N-acetyl cysteine for depressive symptoms in bipolar disorder--a double-blind randomized placebo-controlled trial. Biol Psychiatry 64(6):468–475. https://doi.org/10.1016/j.biopsych.2008.04.022

Berk M, Dean OM, Cotton SM, Gama CS, Kapczinski F, Fernandes B, Kohlmann K, Jeavons S, Hewitt K, Moss K, Allwang C, Schapkaitz I, Cobb H, Bush AI, Dodd S, Malhi GS (2012) Maintenance N-acetyl cysteine treatment for bipolar disorder: a double-blind randomized placebo controlled trial. BMC Med 10:91. https://doi.org/10.1186/1741-7015-10-91

Berk M, Dean OM, Cotton SM, Jeavons S, Tanious M, Kohlmann K, Hewitt K, Moss K, Allwang C, Schapkaitz I, Robbins J, Cobb H, Ng F, Dodd S, Bush AI, Malhi GS (2014) The efficacy of adjunctive N-acetylcysteine in major depressive disorder: a double-blind, randomized, placebo-controlled trial. J Clin Psychiatry 75(6):628–636. https://doi.org/10.4088/JCP.13m08454

Bilici M, Efe H, Koroglu MA, Uydu HA, Bekaroglu M, Deger O (2001) Antioxidative enzyme activities and lipid peroxidation in major depression: alterations by antidepressant treatments. J Affect Disord 64(1):43–51

Brown NC, Andreazza AC, Young LT (2014) An updated meta-analysis of oxidative stress markers in bipolar disorder. Psychiatry Res 218(1–2):61–68. https://doi.org/10.1016/j.psychres.2014.04.005

Cabungcal JH, Steullet P, Kraftsik R, Cuenod M, Do KQ (2013) Early-life insults impair parvalbumin interneurons via oxidative stress: reversal by N-acetylcysteine. Biol Psychiatry 73(6):574–582. https://doi.org/10.1016/j.biopsych.2012.09.020

Das P, Tanious M, Fritz K, Dodd S, Dean OM, Berk M, Malhi GS (2013) Metabolite profiles in the anterior cingulate cortex of depressed patients differentiate those taking N-acetyl-cysteine versus placebo. Aust N Z J Psychiatry 47(4):347–354. https://doi.org/10.1177/0004867412474074

Dean OM, Gray KM, Villagonzalo KA, Dodd S, Mohebbi M, Vick T, Tonge BJ, Berk M (2016) A randomised, double blind, placebo-controlled trial of a fixed dose of N-acetyl cysteine in children with autistic disorder. Aust N Z J Psychiatry 51(3):241–249. https://doi.org/10.1177/0004867416652735

Do KQ, Trabesinger AH, Kirsten-Kruger M, Lauer CJ, Dydak U, Hell D, Holsboer F, Boesiger P, Cuenod M (2000) Schizophrenia: glutathione deficit in cerebrospinal fluid and prefrontal cortex in vivo. Eur J Neurosci 12(10):3721–3728

Do KQ, Cuenod M, Hensch TK (2015) Targeting oxidative stress and aberrant critical period plasticity in the developmental trajectory to schizophrenia. Schizophr Bull 41(4):835–846. https://doi.org/10.1093/schbul/sbv065

Dodd S, Dean O, Copolov DL, Malhi GS, Berk M (2008) N-acetylcysteine for antioxidant therapy: pharmacology and clinical utility. Expert Opin Biol Ther 8(12):1955–1962. https://doi.org/10.1517/14728220802517901

Duffy SL, Lagopoulos J, Cockayne N, Hermens DF, Hickie IB, Naismith SL (2015) Oxidative stress and depressive symptoms in older adults: a magnetic resonance spectroscopy study. J Affect Disord 180:29–35. https://doi.org/10.1016/j.jad.2015.03.007

Durieux AM, Horder J, Mendez MA, Egerton A, Williams SC, Wilson CE, Spain D, Murphy C, Robertson D, Barker GJ, Murphy DG, McAlonan GM (2016) Cortical and subcortical glutathione levels in adults with autism spectrum disorder. Autism Res 9(4):429–435. https://doi.org/10.1002/aur.1522

El-Ansary A, Al-Ayadhi L (2012) Lipid mediators in plasma of autism spectrum disorders. Lipids Health Dis 11:160. https://doi.org/10.1186/1476-511X-11-160

Farokhnia M, Azarkolah A, Adinehfar F, Khodaie-Ardakani MR, Hosseini SM, Yekehtaz H, Tabrizi M, Rezaei F, Salehi B, Sadeghi SM, Moghadam M, Gharibi F, Mirshafiee O, Akhondzadeh S (2013) N-acetylcysteine as an adjunct to risperidone for treatment of negative symptoms in patients with chronic schizophrenia: a randomized, double-blind, placebo-controlled study. Clin Neuropharmacol 36(6):185–192. https://doi.org/10.1097/WNF.0000000000000001

Flatow J, Buckley P, Miller BJ (2013) Meta-analysis of oxidative stress in schizophrenia. Biol Psychiatry 74(6):400–409. https://doi.org/10.1016/j.biopsych.2013.03.018

Frustaci A, Neri M, Cesario A, Adams JB, Domenici E, Dalla Bernardina B, Bonassi S (2012) Oxidative stress-related biomarkers in autism: systematic review and meta-analyses. Free Radic Biol Med 52(10):2128–2141. https://doi.org/10.1016/j.freeradbiomed.2012.03.011

Galecki P, Szemraj J, Bienkiewicz M, Florkowski A, Galecka E (2009) Lipid peroxidation and antioxidant protection in patients during acute depressive episodes and in remission after fluoxetine treatment. Pharmacol Rep 61(3):436–447

Gawryluk JW, Wang JF, Andreazza AC, Shao L, Young LT (2011) Decreased levels of glutathione, the major brain antioxidant, in post-mortem prefrontal cortex from patients with psychiatric disorders. Int J Neuropsychopharmacol 14(1):123–130. https://doi.org/10.1017/S1461145710000805

Geier DA, Kern JK, Garver CR, Adams JB, Audhya T, Geier MR (2009) A prospective study of transsulfuration biomarkers in autistic disorders. Neurochem Res 34(2):386–393. https://doi.org/10.1007/s11064-008-9782-x

Ghezzo A, Visconti P, Abruzzo PM, Bolotta A, Ferreri C, Gobbi G, Malisardi G, Manfredini S, Marini M, Nanetti L, Pipitone E, Raffaelli F, Resca F, Vignini A, Mazzanti L (2013) Oxidative stress and erythrocyte membrane alterations in children with autism: correlation with clinical features. PLoS One 8(6):e66418. https://doi.org/10.1371/journal.pone.0066418

Godlewska BR, Yip SW, Near J, Goodwin GM, Cowen PJ (2014) Cortical glutathione levels in young people with bipolar disorder: a pilot study using magnetic resonance spectroscopy. Psychopharmacology 231(2):327–332. https://doi.org/10.1007/s00213-013-3244-0

Godlewska BR, Near J, Cowen PJ (2015) Neurochemistry of major depression: a study using magnetic resonance spectroscopy. Psychopharmacology 232(3):501–507. https://doi.org/10.1007/s00213-014-3687-y

Gu F, Chauhan V, Chauhan A (2013) Impaired synthesis and antioxidant defense of glutathione in the cerebellum of autistic subjects: alterations in the activities and protein expression of glutathione-related enzymes. Free Radic Biol Med 65:488–496. https://doi.org/10.1016/j.freeradbiomed.2013.07.021

Han Y, Xi QQ, Dai W, Yang SH, Gao L, Su YY, Zhang X (2015) Abnormal transsulfuration metabolism and reduced antioxidant capacity in Chinese children with autism spectrum disorders. Int J Dev Neurosci 46:27–32. https://doi.org/10.1016/j.ijdevneu.2015.06.006

Hardan AY, Fung LK, Libove RA, Obukhanych TV, Nair S, Herzenberg LA, Frazier TW, Tirouvanziam R (2012) A randomized controlled pilot trial of oral N-acetylcysteine in children with autism. Biol Psychiatry 71(11):956–961. https://doi.org/10.1016/j.biopsych.2012.01.014

Heales SJ, Davies SE, Bates TE, Clark JB (1995) Depletion of brain glutathione is accompanied by impaired mitochondrial function and decreased N-acetyl aspartate concentration. Neurochem Res 20(1):31–38

Holmay MJ, Terpstra M, Coles LD, Mishra U, Ahlskog M, Oz G, Cloyd JC, Tuite PJ (2013) N-acetylcysteine boosts brain and blood glutathione in Gaucher and Parkinson diseases. Clin Neuropharmacol 36(4):103–106. https://doi.org/10.1097/WNF.0b013e31829ae713

James SJ, Melnyk S, Jernigan S, Cleves MA, Halsted CH, Wong DH, Cutler P, Bock K, Boris M, Bradstreet JJ, Baker SM, Gaylor DW (2006) Metabolic endophenotype and related genotypes are associated with oxidative stress in children with autism. Am J Med Genet B Neuropsychiatr Genet 141B(8):947–956. https://doi.org/10.1002/ajmg.b.30366

Khanzode SD, Dakhale GN, Khanzode SS, Saoji A, Palasodkar R (2003) Oxidative damage and major depression: the potential antioxidant action of selective serotonin re-uptake inhibitors. Redox Rep 8(6):365–370. https://doi.org/10.1179/135100003225003393

Kim HK, Andreazza AC, Yeung PY, Isaacs-Trepanier C, Young LT (2014) Oxidation and nitration in dopaminergic areas of the prefrontal cortex from patients with bipolar disorder and schizophrenia. J Psychiatry Neurosci 39(4):276–285

Kodydkova J, Vavrova L, Zeman M, Jirak R, Macasek J, Stankova B, Tvrzicka E, Zak A (2009) Antioxidative enzymes and increased oxidative stress in depressive women. Clin Biochem 42(13-14):1368–1374. https://doi.org/10.1016/j.clinbiochem.2009.06.006

Lagopoulos J, Hermens DF, Tobias-Webb J, Duffy S, Naismith SL, White D, Scott E, Hickie IB (2013) In vivo glutathione levels in young persons with bipolar disorder: a magnetic resonance spectroscopy study. J Psychiatr Res 47(3):412–417. https://doi.org/10.1016/j.jpsychires.2012.12.006

Lapidus KA, Gabbay V, Mao X, Johnson A, Murrough JW, Mathew SJ, Shungu DC (2014) In vivo (1)H MRS study of potential associations between glutathione, oxidative stress and anhedonia in major depressive disorder. Neurosci Lett 569:74–79. https://doi.org/10.1016/j.neulet.2014.03.056

Laszlo A, Novak Z, Szollosi-Varga I, Hai du Q, Vetro A, Kovacs A (2013) Blood lipid peroxidation, antioxidant enzyme activities and hemorheological changes in autistic children. Ideggyogy Sz 66(1–2):23–28

Lavoie S, Murray MM, Deppen P, Knyazeva MG, Berk M, Boulat O, Bovet P, Bush AI, Conus P, Copolov D, Fornari E, Meuli R, Solida A, Vianin P, Cuenod M, Buclin T, Do KQ (2008) Glutathione precursor, N-acetyl-cysteine, improves mismatch negativity in schizophrenia patients. Neuropsychopharmacology 33(9):2187–2199. https://doi.org/10.1038/sj.npp.1301624

Matsuzawa D, Hashimoto K (2011) Magnetic resonance spectroscopy study of the antioxidant defense system in schizophrenia. Antioxid Redox Signal 15(7):2057–2065. https://doi.org/10.1089/ars.2010.3453

Matsuzawa D, Obata T, Shirayama Y, Nonaka H, Kanazawa Y, Yoshitome E, Takanashi J, Matsuda T, Shimizu E, Ikehira H, Iyo M, Hashimoto K (2008) Negative correlation between brain glutathione level and negative symptoms in schizophrenia: a 3T 1H-MRS study. PLoS One 3(4):e1944. https://doi.org/10.1371/journal.pone.0001944

Meguid NA, Dardir AA, Abdel-Raouf ER, Hashish A (2011) Evaluation of oxidative stress in autism: defective antioxidant enzymes and increased lipid peroxidation. Biol Trace Elem Res 143(1):58–65. https://doi.org/10.1007/s12011-010-8840-9

Michel TM, Frangou S, Thiemeyer D, Camara S, Jecel J, Nara K, Brunklaus A, Zoechling R, Riederer P (2007) Evidence for oxidative stress in the frontal cortex in patients with recurrent depressive disorder—a postmortem study. Psychiatry Res 151(1-2):145–150. https://doi.org/10.1016/j.psychres.2006.04.013

Mico JA, Rojas-Corrales MO, Gibert-Rahola J, Parellada M, Moreno D, Fraguas D, Graell M, Gil J, Irazusta J, Castro-Fornieles J, Soutullo C, Arango C, Otero S, Navarro A, Baeza I, Martinez-Cengotitabengoa M, Gonzalez-Pinto A (2011) Reduced antioxidant defense in early onset first-episode psychosis: a case-control study. BMC Psychiatry 11:26. https://doi.org/10.1186/1471-244X-11-26

Moniczewski A, Gawlik M, Smaga I, Niedzielska E, Krzek J, Przegalinski E, Pera J, Filip M (2015) Oxidative stress as an etiological factor and a potential treatment target of psychiatric disorders. Part 1. Chemical aspects and biological sources of oxidative stress in the brain. Pharmacol Rep 67(3):560–568. https://doi.org/10.1016/j.pharep.2014.12.014

Monin A, Baumann PS, Griffa A, Xin L, Mekle R, Fournier M, Butticaz C, Klaey M, Cabungcal JH, Steullet P, Ferrari C, Cuenod M, Gruetter R, Thiran JP, Hagmann P, Conus P, Do KQ (2015) Glutathione deficit impairs myelin maturation: relevance for white matter integrity in schizophrenia patients. Mol Psychiatry 20(7):827–838. https://doi.org/10.1038/mp.2014.88

Morishita H, Cabungcal JH, Chen Y, Do KQ, Hensch TK (2015) Prolonged period of cortical plasticity upon redox dysregulation in fast-spiking interneurons. Biol Psychiatry 78(6):396–402. https://doi.org/10.1016/j.biopsych.2014.12.026

Ozcan ME, Gulec M, Ozerol E, Polat R, Akyol O (2004) Antioxidant enzyme activities and oxidative stress in affective disorders. Int Clin Psychopharmacol 19(2):89–95

Raffa M, Mechri A, Othman LB, Fendri C, Gaha L, Kerkeni A (2009) Decreased glutathione levels and antioxidant enzyme activities in untreated and treated schizophrenic patients. Prog Neuro-Psychopharmacol Biol Psychiatry 33(7):1178–1183. https://doi.org/10.1016/j.pnpbp.2009.06.018

Raffa M, Atig F, Mhalla A, Kerkeni A, Mechri A (2011) Decreased glutathione levels and impaired antioxidant enzyme activities in drug-naive first-episode schizophrenic patients. BMC Psychiatry 11:124. https://doi.org/10.1186/1471-244X-11-124

Rosa AR, Singh N, Whitaker E, de Brito M, Lewis AM, Vieta E, Churchill GC, Geddes JR, Goodwin GM (2014) Altered plasma glutathione levels in bipolar disorder indicates higher oxidative stress; a possible risk factor for illness onset despite normal brain-derived neurotrophic factor (BDNF) levels. Psychol Med 44(11):2409–2418. https://doi.org/10.1017/S0033291714000014

Rose S, Melnyk S, Pavliv O, Bai S, Nick TG, Frye RE, James SJ (2012) Evidence of oxidative damage and inflammation associated with low glutathione redox status in the autism brain. Transl Psychiatry 2:e134. https://doi.org/10.1038/tp.2012.61

Rose S, Frye RE, Slattery J, Wynne R, Tippett M, Pavliv O, Melnyk S, James SJ (2014) Oxidative stress induces mitochondrial dysfunction in a subset of autism lymphoblastoid cell lines in a well-matched case control cohort. PLoS One 9(1):e85436. https://doi.org/10.1371/journal.pone.0085436

Rose S, Frye RE, Slattery J, Wynne R, Tippett M, Melnyk S, James SJ (2015) Oxidative stress induces mitochondrial dysfunction in a subset of autistic lymphoblastoid cell lines. Transl Psychiatry 5:e526. https://doi.org/10.1038/tp.2015.29

Rose S, Bennuri SC, Wynne R, Melnyk S, James SJ, Frye RE (2017) Mitochondrial and redox abnormalities in autism lymphoblastoid cells: a sibling control study. FASEB J 31(3):904–909. https://doi.org/10.1096/fj.201601004R

Sarandol A, Sarandol E, Eker SS, Erdinc S, Vatansever E, Kirli S (2007) Major depressive disorder is accompanied with oxidative stress: short-term antidepressant treatment does not alter oxidative-antioxidative systems. Hum Psychopharmacol 22(2):67–73. https://doi.org/10.1002/hup.829

Selek S, Savas HA, Gergerlioglu HS, Bulbul F, Uz E, Yumru M (2008) The course of nitric oxide and superoxide dismutase during treatment of bipolar depressive episode. J Affect Disord 107(1-3):89–94. https://doi.org/10.1016/j.jad.2007.08.006

Soeiro-de-Souza MG, Pastorello BF, Leite Cda C, Henning A, Moreno RA, Garcia Otaduy MC (2016) Dorsal anterior cingulate lactate and glutathione levels in euthymic bipolar I disorder: 1H-MRS study. Int J Neuropsychopharmacol 19(8):pyw032. https://doi.org/10.1093/ijnp/pyw032

Steullet P, Cabungcal JH, Kulak A, Kraftsik R, Chen Y, Dalton TP, Cuenod M, Do KQ (2010) Redox dysregulation affects the ventral but not dorsal hippocampus: impairment of parvalbumin neurons, gamma oscillations, and related behaviors. J Neurosci 30(7):2547–2558. https://doi.org/10.1523/JNEUROSCI.3857-09.2010

Terpstra M, Vaughan TJ, Ugurbil K, Lim KO, Schulz SC, Gruetter R (2005) Validation of glutathione quantitation from STEAM spectra against edited 1H NMR spectroscopy at 4T: application to schizophrenia. MAGMA 18(5):276–282. https://doi.org/10.1007/s10334-005-0012-0

Tsai MC, Huang TL (2015) Thiobarbituric acid reactive substances (TBARS) is a state biomarker of oxidative stress in bipolar patients in a manic phase. J Affect Disord 173:22–26. https://doi.org/10.1016/j.jad.2014.10.045

Tuncel OK, Sarisoy G, Bilgici B, Pazvantoglu O, Cetin E, Unverdi E, Avci B, Boke O (2015) Oxidative stress in bipolar and schizophrenia patients. Psychiatry Res 228(3):688–694. https://doi.org/10.1016/j.psychres.2015.04.046

Wei YC, Zhou FL, He DL, Bai JR, Hui LY, Wang XY, Nan KJ (2009) The level of oxidative stress and the expression of genes involved in DNA-damage signaling pathways in depressive patients with colorectal carcinoma. J Psychosom Res 66(3):259–266. https://doi.org/10.1016/j.jpsychores.2008.09.001

Wood SJ, Berger GE, Wellard RM, Proffitt TM, McConchie M, Berk M, McGorry PD, Pantelis C (2009) Medial temporal lobe glutathione concentration in first episode psychosis: a 1H-MRS investigation. Neurobiol Dis 33(3):354–357. https://doi.org/10.1016/j.nbd.2008.11.018

Xin L, Mekle R, Fournier M, Baumann PS, Ferrari C, Alameda L, Jenni R, Lu H, Schaller B, Cuenod M, Conus P, Gruetter R, Do KQ (2016) Genetic polymorphism associated prefrontal glutathione and its coupling with brain glutamate and peripheral redox status in early psychosis. Schizophr Bull 42(5):1185–1196. https://doi.org/10.1093/schbul/sbw038

Yao JK, Leonard S, Reddy R (2006) Altered glutathione redox state in schizophrenia. Dis Markers 22(1–2):83–93

Yorbik O, Sayal A, Akay C, Akbiyik DI, Sohmen T (2002) Investigation of antioxidant enzymes in children with autistic disorder. Prostaglandins Leukot Essent Fatty Acids 67(5):341–343

Zoroglu SS, Armutcu F, Ozen S, Gurel A, Sivasli E, Yetkin O, Meram I (2004) Increased oxidative stress and altered activities of erythrocyte free radical scavenging enzymes in autism. Eur Arch Psychiatry Clin Neurosci 254(3):143–147. https://doi.org/10.1007/s00406-004-0456-7

Mitochondrial Metabolism

5

Shannon Rose and Sirish C. Bennuri

5.1 Introduction

Mitochondria are unique organelles containing a double membrane as well as their own genome. The distinctive structural components of mitochondria include the outer membrane, matrix, inner membrane, and intermembrane space. The inner mitochondrial membrane is folded into cristae and densely packed with the five multi-subunit enzyme complexes of the electron transport chain (ETC), as well as two electron carriers, cytochrome c and ubiquinone, also known as coenzyme Q10 (Fig. 5.1). The mitochondrial DNA (mtDNA) contains 37 genes that code for its own transcription and translation machinery as well as 13 subunits of the energy-generating ETC.

Mitochondria are best known for their role in generating adenosine triphosphate (ATP) from adenosine diphosphate (ADP) through the oxidation of substrates including glucose and fatty acids. The process used by the mitochondria to produce ATP is known as oxidative phosphorylation. The oxidation of glucose and fatty acids generates acetyl-CoA, which is metabolized by the citric acid cycle (also known as the tricarboxylic acid (TCA) cycle) to generate the electron donors, nicotinamide adenine dinucleotide (NADH) and flavin adenine dinucleotide (FADH$_2$), which transfer energy to the ETC. Electrons flow through the ETC from electron donors to electron acceptors, with each step incrementally releasing energy that is used to pump protons across the inner membrane from the matrix into the intermembrane space, creating an electrochemical gradient. The protons flow down the gradient through ATP synthase, and the energy released is used to phosphorylate ADP to generate ATP, and O$_2$, the final electron acceptor, is reduced to H$_2$O.

Electronic supplementary material The online version of this article (https://doi.org/10.1007/978-981-10-5311-5_5) contains supplementary material, which is available to authorized users.

S. Rose (✉) · S. C. Bennuri
Department of Pediatrics, Arkansas Children's Research Institute, University of Arkansas for Medical Sciences, Little Rock, AR, USA
e-mail: SRose@uams.edu

© Springer Nature Singapore Pte Ltd. 2019
R. E. Frye, M. Berk (eds.), *The Therapeutic Use of N-Acetylcysteine (NAC) in Medicine*, https://doi.org/10.1007/978-981-10-5311-5_5

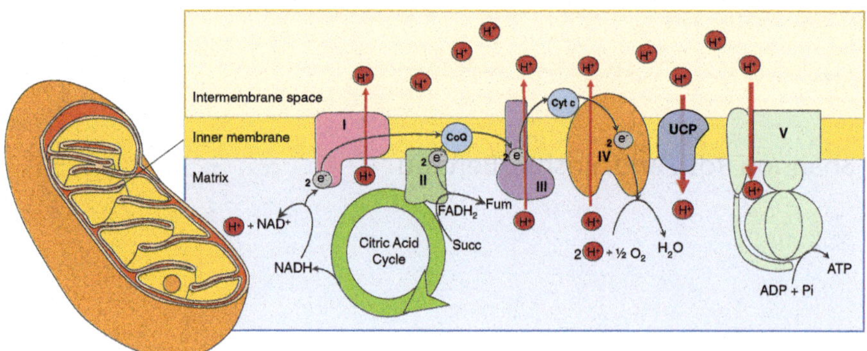

Fig. 5.1 The electron transport chain. The electron transport chain (ETC) consists of five multi-subunit enzyme complexes (denoted I, II, III, IV, and V), as well as two electron carriers, cytochrome c and ubiquinone, also known as coenzyme Q10. Electron carriers, nicotinamide adenine dinucleotide (NADH) and flavin adenine dinucleotide ($FADH_2$), are generated by the citric acid cycle and donate electrons to ETC complexes I and II, respectively. ETC complex II, also called succinate dehydrogenase, is the only enzyme that is a component of both the ETC and the citric acid cycle. Succinate (Succ) is oxidized to fumarate (Fum) to generate $FADH_2$. Electrons from NADH and $FADH_2$ flow to ETC complex III through ubiquinone (CoQ) and then to ETC complex IV through cytochrome c (Cyt c), which reduces O_2 to H_2O. Each of these electron transfers generates energy used to pump protons (H^+) across the inner membrane from the matrix to the intermembrane space, generating an electrochemical gradient. The flow of protons down the gradient through ETC complex V (ATP synthase) generates the energy to phosphorylate ADP to generate ATP. Uncoupling proteins (UCP) act as a release valve, allowing protons to flow through the membrane.

Because the process of oxidative phosphorylation is imperfect, leakage of electrons results in the formation of reactive oxygen species (ROS). Indeed, a continuous low-level generation of superoxide (~1%) accompanies inner membrane electron transfer resulting in the mitochondria being both the predominant source and the major target of ROS in most cells. Mitochondria possess several mechanisms to combat and protect themselves from oxidative damage including the tripeptide glutathione (GSH) and antioxidant enzymes such as manganese superoxide dismutase (MnSOD), glutathione peroxidase (GPx), peroxiredoxins (Prx), and thioredoxins (TRx).

Mitochondria lack the enzymes for GSH synthesis; thus, the mitochondrial redox state is dependent upon cytosolic GSH production and the transport of reduced and oxidized glutathione across the mitochondrial membrane. Depletion of mitochondrial GSH increases vulnerability to oxidative damage from ETC-derived ROS. Additionally, exogenous agents that damage mitochondrial proteins can lead to ETC dysfunction and increased mitochondrial ROS production, which can deplete mitochondrial GSH.

Several key bioenergetic enzymes including aconitase, oxoglutarate dehydrogenase, and ETC complexes I, II, and III are particularly susceptible to oxidative damage and inactivation as they contain labile iron-sulfur (Fe-S) clusters, which are targets of superoxide (Welter et al. 1996). Through Fenton chemistry, displaced Fe^{+2}

from oxidized Fe-S clusters reacts with H_2O_2, forming the damaging hydroxyl radical. Thus, mitochondrial ROS production coupled with a fragile redox state can lead to decreased ETC function, initiating a vicious cycle leading to ATP depletion and activation of the apoptosis cascade.

Mitochondrial-mediated apoptosis, also known as the intrinsic apoptosis pathway, is initiated by the release of cytochrome c, a component of the ETC that is loosely associated with the mitochondrial inner membrane. Cytochrome c release from the mitochondria results in activation of caspase 9, initiating the caspase activation cascade that results in cleavage of multiple substrates and ultimately death of the cell. Pro-apoptotic proteins of the Bcl (B cell leukemia) family and depolarization of the mitochondrial membrane potential ($\Delta\Psi_M$) promote cytochrome c release. Mitochondrial-mediated apoptosis can also be induced by the p38 mitogen-activated protein kinase (MAPK) signaling pathway that includes c-Jun NH_2-terminal kinase (JNK) and extracellular signal-regulated kinase (ERK). Phosphorylation of pro-survival proteins of the Bcl family by MAPKs leads to loss of $\Delta\Psi_M$ and cytochrome c release (Farley et al. 2006; Kim and Choi 2010).

Mitochondria are dynamic organelles, responding to changing cellular physiology, nutrient availability, and energy demands. The shape, size, distribution, and number of mitochondria vary among different types of cells according to their function and energy demands. For example, skin cells, which have a relatively low energy demand, have fewer mitochondria than cells with higher energy demands, such as muscle, liver, and brain cells. Individual mitochondria are connected through an interconnected tubular network, the morphology of which is responsive to changes in nutrient availability and metabolic stress and demands. The mitochondrial network is shaped by balanced coordination of fusion and fission events. The machinery primarily responsible for fusion includes mitofusin (Mfn) 1 and Mfn2 and optic atrophy (OPA) 1 and OPA3, while fission machinery includes dynamin-related protein 1 (DRP1), mitochondrial fission factor (MFF), and mitochondrial fission 1 protein (FIS1). For a detailed review, see Wai and Langer (2016) and Lackner (2014).

Mitoplasticity refers to the adaptive changes in mitochondrial structure and function in response to cellular stress and changes in energy demand and nutrient availability. Mitoplasticity is regulated and carried out by multiple energy sensing and cell signaling mechanisms. Major regulators of mitoplasticity include AMP-activated protein kinase (AMPK), peroxisome proliferator-activated receptor-c coactivator 1-α (PGC1α), mammalian target of rapamycin complex 1 (mTORC1), and uncoupling protein 2 (UCP2) (Jose et al. 2013). AMPK is considered a master regulator of energy metabolism that is activated by an increase in the adenosine monophosphate (AMP)/ATP ratio, and it downregulates energy consumption and upregulates energy production. PGC1α is a transcriptional coactivator that induces mitochondrial biogenesis. Uncoupling proteins such as UCP2 are activated by superoxide, and they decrease the mitochondrial membrane potential to decrease ROS production by the ETC. Mitophagy is a process whereby damaged mitochondria are removed from the cell. Mitophagy is regulated by multiple signaling mechanisms, with two well-described regulators being PTEN-induced kinase 1 (PINK1) and Parkin (McWilliams and Muqit 2017). Interestingly, mTORC1, a serine/theonine kinase, enhances oxidative phosphorylation but inhibits mitophagy.

In addition to their major roles in producing energy for the cell and initiating apoptosis, mitochondria also contribute to redox signaling, steroid synthesis, lipid metabolism, and intracellular calcium homeostasis by rapid uptake and storage of cytosolic calcium. Given the many important roles of the mitochondria for normal cellular function, it stands to reason that mitochondrial dysfunction is involved in a wide variety of diseases and medical disorders.

Mitochondrial dysfunction has been implicated in multiple psychiatric disorders (Anglin et al. 2012; Jou et al. 2009; Manji et al. 2012; Rezin et al. 2009; Scaglia 2010; Clay et al. 2011), neurodevelopmental disorders including autism spectrum disorder (Rossignol and Frye 2012, 2014; Goh et al. 2014; Valenti et al. 2014; Giulivi et al. 2010; Palmieri and Persico 2010; Oliveira et al. 2005), neurodegenerative disorders (Mattson and Liu 2002; Federico et al. 2012), cardiovascular disease (Dai et al. 2012; Lopez-Crisosto et al. 2017; Vasquez-Trincado et al. 2016; Ballinger 2005; Dominic et al. 2014), obesity and diabetes (Civitarese and Ravussin 2008; Patti and Corvera 2010; Simoneau and Kelley 1997; Ritov et al. 2005; Naudi et al. 2012), cancer (Weinberg and Chandel 2009; Samudio et al. 2009; Vyas et al. 2016; Boland et al. 2013; Wallace 2012), and aging (Balaban et al. 2005; Sun et al. 2016; Shigenaga et al. 1994).

Given that mitochondria are the primary producers and targets of ROS and their importance in health and disease, the effects of the antioxidant and glutathione precursor, NAC, on mitochondrial function have been examined in many studies of a wide variety of medical conditions. NAC has also been used as a tool to investigate the role of ROS in normal biological processes as well as pathological conditions. The purpose of this review is to conduct a systematic review of the literature on the effects of NAC on mitochondrial metabolism.

5.2   Methods

A PubMed search conducted in April 2016 using the terms "acetylcysteine" and "mitochondria" or "mitochondrial" returned 1122 results. The authors screened the titles and abstracts for relevance. Reviews, articles not available in English, and studies using nonmammalian models were excluded. Full-text manuscripts were obtained for 1035 results and were further reviewed for inclusion. Manuscripts were included if the effect of NAC on a mitochondrial endpoint was directly measured and reported, and studies in which apoptosis was the only mitochondrial-related endpoint were included if apoptosis was clearly mitochondrial mediated.

5.3   Results

After screening, 623 articles were determined to be relevant to this review and were subcategorized into specific research areas and are discussed below.

5.3.1 Aging

Mitochondrial function declines with age and likely contributes to age-related medical conditions (Balaban et al. 2005; Sun et al. 2016; Shigenaga et al. 1994). Several groups have examined the effects of long-term dietary supplementation with NAC on mitochondrial function in animal models with limited success. After 12–16 months of dietary NAC supplementation (0.3% w/w), isolated brain and heart mitochondria from 28-month-old rats exhibited increased activities of ETC complexes I, II, III, and IV and decreased protein carbonyls, and ETC complex I gene and protein expression was increased in the cortex and hippocampus (Cocco et al. 2005; Nicoletti et al. 2005). Another study demonstrated that liver mitochondria from aged rats supplemented with NAC exhibited increased oxygen consumption, decreased oxidative and nitrosative damage, and increased mitochondrial GSH and GPx (Grattagliano et al. 2004). It is important to note that in these studies, while there was a noted increase in mitochondrial activity in the NAC-supplemented animals, the activities were still significantly lower as compared to young mice. In a study of 71-week-old mice supplemented with dietary NAC for 23 weeks, there was decreased oxidative damage to lipids and proteins in synaptic mitochondria, but no significant improvement of synaptic mitochondrial activity was noted (Martinez et al. 2000). NAC has also been shown to improve mitochondrial function of aged mitochondria when applied in vitro. Synaptic mitochondria from aged mice treated in vitro with NAC (1–20 mM) demonstrated increased ETC complex IV activity at concentrations of NAC <20 mM, whereas 20 mM NAC actually decreased ETC complex IV activity (Martinez Banaclocha and Martinez 1999). In a study of cultured oocytes from aged mice, 1 mM NAC supplementation (along with alpha lipoic acid, tocopherol, hypotaurine, and sirtuin) increased $\Delta\Psi_M$ (Silva et al. 2015).

5.3.2 Cardiovascular

Cardiovascular diseases including cardiomyopathies, myocardial infarction, and heart failure all involve cardiac mitochondrial dysfunction. Five out of six studies that examined the ability of NAC to protect mitochondria in cardiovascular disease animal models were positive. In the streptozotocin (STZ)-induced diabetes rat model of diabetic cardiomyopathy, NAC (150 mg/kg/day intragastrically for 4 weeks post diabetes onset) preserved myocardium mitochondrial size and morphology and decreased cardiac apoptosis in two studies (Yildirim et al. 2013; Cicek et al. 2014), and NAC increased cardiac MnSOD activity in a third study by a separate group (Wang et al. 2011). In a monocrotaline-induced cardiac heart failure (CHF) rat model of CHF-induced cachexia, NAC (3 mmol/kg/day by gavage for 30 days post onset) increased ETC complex I activity in gastrocnemius muscle (Barreiro et al. 2016). In a permanent left coronary artery ligation-induced myocardial infarction rat model, NAC (75 mg/day in drinking water from 8 to 12 weeks post ligation) decreased mitochondrial superoxide production and increased ETC complex I and IV activities in subendocardial cardiomyocytes (Andre et al. 2013).

In an isoproterenol-induced myocardial infarction rat model, isolated heart mitochondria from rats pretreated for 14 days with NAC (10 mg/kg/day p.o.) exhibited decreased lipid peroxidation, increased MnSOD and mitochondrial GPx activity, increased mitochondrial GSH, and increased ETC complex I–V activities and had normal mitochondrial morphology as compared to rats without NAC (Basha and Priscilla 2013). On the other hand, in an angiotensin II-induced hypertensive cardiomyopathy mouse model, concurrent treatment with NAC (500 mg/kg/day in drinking water) did not decrease cardiac mitochondrial protein oxidative damage nor did it decrease cardiac PGC-1α and NRF upregulation or cardiac apoptosis (Dai et al. 2011).

NAC has been shown to be effective in numerous in vitro models of cardiomyopathies, cardiac ischemia-reperfusion, hearth failure, and various other heart pathologies (see Online Table 5.1). NAC improves mitochondrial calcium handling, decreases mitochondrial superoxide production, protects against loss of $\Delta\Psi_M$, and prevents mitochondrial permeability transition and apoptosis induction. Interestingly, in two studies NAC also improved mitochondrial fusion and fission abnormalities (Loor et al. 2011; Redpath et al. 2013). NAC was not effective at decreasing mitochondrial superoxide production, oxidative damage to mitochondrial proteins, or apoptosis induction in angiotensin II-stimulated neonatal cardiomyocytes when applied at a concentration of 0.5 mM, while a mitochondrial-targeted antioxidant, Szeto-Schiller (SS)-31 peptide, was effective (Dai et al. 2011). It is possible that a higher concentration of NAC may have been effective, but this was not tested.

In an interesting study, Korge and Weiss (2006) demonstrated that isolated cardiac mitochondria could run on their own fatty acids when substrates are limited, providing the mitochondrial redox microenvironment was maintained in a reduced state. Specifically, they determined that the oxidation of endogenous fatty acids requires both NAC and catalase (Korge and Weiss 2006) as catalase allowed the efflux of H_2O_2 from the mitochondrial matrix and, along with NAC, maintained a reduced redox environment in the matrix.

5.3.3 Obesity and Diabetes

Obesity and the development of type 2 diabetes are associated with oxidative stress and mitochondrial dysfunction (Ritov et al. 2005). Wang et al. (2010) demonstrated that rat adipocytes have no mitochondrial respiratory reserve capacity and that the addition of NAC increases mitochondrial oxygen consumption of adipocytes in vitro. Interestingly NAC was also found to stimulate respiration in vivo in an animal model of obesity. Rats fed a high-fat diet (HFD) and treated with NAC for 15 days (3 mg/mL in drinking water) exhibited increased O_2 consumption and CO_2 production and decreased body fat as compared to HFD-fed rats not given NAC (Wang et al. 2010). NAC increases cellular and whole-body respiration in HFD-fed rats by either directly scavenging excess free radicals or by supplying cysteine, the rate-limiting amino acid for GSH synthesis.

In the rat model of STZ-induced diabetes, NAC treatment after onset of diabetes has been shown by several groups to protect mitochondria. NAC treatment after diabetes onset preserved cardiac mitochondrial morphology in three studies (Cicek et al. 2014; Yildirim et al. 2013; Wang et al. 2011). Kamboj and Sandhir (2011) demonstrated that NAC is also effective at protecting brain mitochondria in this model. Specifically they found that isolated cerebral cortex mitochondria from mice treated with NAC (1.4 g/kg/day in drinking water for 7 weeks beginning 1 week after diabetes onset) exhibited decreased lipid peroxidation and oxidant production; increased MnSOD activity; increased mitochondrial thiols; increased activities of ETC complex I, II, and IV; and decreased mitochondrial swelling as compared to diabetic rats not treated with NAC (Kamboj and Sandhir 2011).

Many groups have also tested the ability of NAC to protect mitochondria in cell culture models of diabetes (see Online Table 5.2). NAC, especially when used as a pretreatment, has been shown to protect mitochondria primarily by preventing loss of $\Delta\Psi_M$ and decreasing apoptosis in numerous cell types cultured under diabetes-like conditions including high glucose (Hung et al. 2009; Kumar and Sitasawad 2009; Liu et al. 2013; Park et al. 2015; Recchioni et al. 2002), serum from diabetic subjects (Feng et al. 2013), the reducing sugar 2-deoxy-D-ribose (Kletsas et al. 1998; Suh et al. 2012), and methylglyoxal-induced carbonyl stress (Okouchi et al. 2009), as well as in pancreatic β cells stressed with antimycin A (Wu et al. 2011). Co-treatment with NAC prevented apoptosis but failed to normalize (decrease) mitochondrial respiration and metabolic flux in 4IIEC3 rat hepatocytes cultured with excess palmitate, indicating that palmitate-induced activation of mitochondrial metabolism is independent of ROS accumulation and apoptosis initiation (Egnatchik et al. 2014). In rat pancreatic islets cultured with high glucose, NAC failed to prevent mitochondrial-mediated apoptosis, oxidation of the mitochondrial redox potential, and increased cytosolic calcium (Roma et al. 2012).

5.3.4 Central Nervous System Conditions and Disorders

The metabolic rate of the central nervous system (CNS) is incredibly high due to the large amounts of ATP required by neurons for neurotransmission and the maintenance of ion gradients (Sokoloff 1960). Thus, the CNS is critically dependent on mitochondrial function, and many neurological conditions have been associated with mitochondrial dysfunction. NAC protects mitochondria in animal and in vitro models of CNS conditions including nerve injury, cerebral ischemia, stroke, spinal muscular atrophy, and autism (see Online Table 5.3). NAC was not mito-protective in an animal model of status epilepticus as it failed to improve the activities of several bioenergetic enzymes (Sleven et al. 2006). NAC has been shown to be protective of neuronal mitochondrial function in in vitro models of neurogenesis. In primary rat hippocampal neurons, NAC prevented loss of $\Delta\Psi_M$ induced by sigma-1 receptor knockdown (Tsai et al. 2009), and it prevented mitochondrial-mediated apoptosis in nerve growth factor-deprived embryonic rat neurons (Kirkland and Franklin 2001).

Neurodegenerative disorders including Alzheimer's disease, Parkinson's disease, and Huntington's disease have all been linked to oxidative stress and mitochondrial dysfunction (Mattson and Liu 2002; Federico et al. 2012); thus, it is not surprising that antioxidants including NAC have been examined for their potential to improve mitochondrial function in animal and in vitro models of neurodegenerative disorders (see Online Table 5.4). In 95% (21/22) of studies, NAC was mito-protective, improving mitochondrial respiration and increasing activities of individual ETC complexes, as well as decreasing apoptosis and mitochondrial fragmentation, and preserving $\Delta\Psi_M$ and ATP. Contrarily, a study of glutamate excitotoxicity found that glutamate-induced mitophagy was enhanced by NAC in rat cortical neurons (Van Laar et al. 2015). The authors suggest that NAC conserves critical cysteines on the mitophagy protein, Parkin, and increases the availability of functional Parkin.

5.3.5　Genetic Disorders

NAC has been used in several in vitro models of genetic diseases. In skin fibroblast cybrids established from a patient with chronic progressive external ophthalmoplegia (CPEO), a mitochondrial encephalomyopathy associated with the 4977 base pair deletion of mitochondrial DNA, 1 mM NAC for 18 h decreased mitochondrial sensitivity to UV-induced apoptosis (Liu et al. 2009). In fibroblasts from patients with combined mitochondrial respiratory chain deficiency caused by defects in nuclear-encoded mitochondrial genes, treatment with 4 mM NAC for 72 h preserved ATP, prevented loss of $\Delta\Psi_M$, and increased ETC complex IV activity (Soiferman et al. 2014). In primary lymphocytes and fibroblasts from patients with Fanconi anemia, treatment with 500 μM NAC for 3–5 days increased mitochondrial respiration, ETC complex I activity, and ATP and decreased cytosolic calcium, but failed to normalize mitochondrial morphology (Columbaro et al. 2014; Ravera et al. 2013; Usai et al. 2015). Trisomy 21, or Down syndrome, is a complex genetic and metabolic disease associated with oxidative stress and impaired glutathione (Pogribna et al. 2001). Human embryonic kidney 293 cells transfected with Down syndrome candidate region 1 (DSCR1) exhibited increased mitochondrial superoxide production, which was dampened by 2 mM NAC (Ko et al. 2014). Malignant hyperthermia susceptibility, an autosomal dominant inherited pharmacogenetic disorder, can arise from mutations in ryanodine receptor type-1 (RYR1), the gene that encodes the Ca^{+2} release channel of the skeletal muscle sarcoplasmic reticulum (Denborough 1998). In a rodent model of this disorder, mice lacking calsequestrin-1 (CASQ1), a calcium-binding protein that interacts RYR1, develop malignant hyperthermia crisis upon exposure to the anesthetic halothane. However, Michelucci et al. (2015) reported that NAC supplementation (1% w/v in drinking water) protected these mice from death following halothane, and examination of hind limb muscle revealed that NAC decreased mitochondrial superoxide production and decreased cytosolic calcium.

5.3.6　Inflammatory Conditions

Polycystic ovary syndrome (PCOS) is a common inflammatory disease with unknown etiology associated with oxidative stress and apoptosis and linked to obesity (Zuo et al. 2016). In an open-label trial, 600 mg NAC was administered daily for 6 weeks to 17 women with PCOS, and neutrophil mitochondrial function was examined (Kose and Naziroglu 2015). Neutrophils from PCOS patients treated with NAC exhibited decreased apoptosis and increased $\Delta\Psi_M$ as compared to untreated PCOS patients.

Atherosclerosis is a chronic inflammatory condition involving endothelial dysfunction, thickening of artery walls, and accumulation of macrophages which become foam cells upon the uptake of lipids. In a study of mouse macrophages treated with triacylglycerol (TG), co-treatment with 0.5 mM NAC prevented TG-induced downregulation of PGC1α and ETC complexes I and III, and it prevented the accumulation of a complex IV precursor protein (Aronis et al. 2009). The mito-protective effects of NAC in this model were attributed to the fact that NAC attenuated lipid accumulation in the TG-treated macrophages. In atherosclerosis, the endothelium is exposed to nitric oxide and reactive oxygen species. In a bovine aortic endothelial cell (BAEC) model, NAC co-treatment prevented the depletion of ATP and NAD^+ upon exposure to the redox-cycling agent and superoxide generator, DMNQ; however, NAC was not protective when BAECs were exposed to a combination of DMNQ and the S-nitrosothiol, S-nitrosocysteine (CysNO) (Diers et al. 2013). Inducing macrophage apoptosis has been investigated as a potential treatment for atherosclerosis. Several groups have employed NAC in in vitro studies to demonstrate that sonodynamic therapy (SDT)-induced macrophage cell death is mediated by the mitochondrial apoptosis pathway (Li et al. 2015b; Zheng et al. 2014; Zheng et al. 2016; Wang et al. 2014a). In each of these studies, pretreatment of human THP-1 macrophages with NAC prevented SDT-induced $\Delta\Psi_M$ depolarization and apoptosis.

Psoriasis is a chronic inflammatory condition of the skin characterized by keratinocyte hyperproliferation, and defects in epidermal apoptosis have been found (Zhang et al. 2015; Laporte et al. 2000). Thus, inducing epidermal apoptosis has been examined as a potential therapeutic avenue. Shen et al. (2012) demonstrated that a combination of the flavonoid quercetin and inorganic arsenic induced depolarization of $\Delta\Psi_M$ and mitochondrial-mediated apoptosis of normal human HaCat keratinocytes which was prevented by NAC pretreatment.

The chronic inflammatory autoimmune disease, systemic lupus erythematosus (SLE), is associated with oxidative stress, mitochondrial hyperpolarization and resistance to apoptosis in T cells, and a deficiency of regulatory T cells (Perl 2013; Moulton and Tsokos 2015). A double-blind placebo-controlled trial of NAC (1.2–2.4 g daily for 3 months) was carried out in 36 SLE patients, and NAC was found to be safe and improved disease activity and fatigue (Lai et al. 2012). NAC had some very interesting effects on T cell metabolism. NAC increased mitochondrial hyperpolarization, mitochondrial mass, H_2O_2 production, and spontaneous apoptosis of T cells. Interestingly, the effect of NAC considered most important was its ability to decrease T cell mTOR activity, disconnecting mTOR activation from mitochondrial hyperpolarization, which resulted in increased numbers of regulatory T cells. A follow-up in vitro study demonstrated that an overnight incubation with 3 mM NAC also increased mitochondrial hyperpolarization in peripheral blood lymphocytes

(PBLs) from patients with SLE and controls (Doherty et al. 2014). SLE T cells exhibited increased respiration driven primarily through complex I, and this was decreased by NAC. Nitric oxide treatment increased mitochondrial mass and mitochondrial Ca^{+2} levels, but co-treatment with NAC prevented these effects. NAC was unable to prevent nitric oxide-induced complex I inhibition, and additional studies revealed that NAC alone inhibits respiration driven by complex I substrates. Thus, the mechanism of action of NAC in SLE may be decreasing ETC activity at complex I and decreasing mTOR activation.

5.3.7 Immune

NAC has been applied in studies of immune disorders, viral and bacterial infections, as well as immune cell development and death. Several groups have reported mitoprotective effects of NAC in in vitro studies of viral and bacterial infection. Cossarizza et al. (1997) found that NAC prevented the loss of $\Delta\Psi_M$ and spontaneous apoptosis in PBLs from individuals with symptomatic, acute HIV-1 primary infection. In human U937 cells infected with HIV, NAC prevented $TNF\alpha$-induced mitochondrial damage including mitochondrial swelling and distortion of cristae (Malorni et al. 1994). In human neuronal SH-Sy5Y cells treated with the HIV-derived peptide, lentivirus lytic peptide 1, NAC co-treatment prevented the loss of $\Delta\Psi_M$ (Sung et al. 2001). Furthermore, NAC pretreatment prevented cytochrome c release in two human intestinal cell lines treated with HIV-1 transactivator factor (Buccigrossi et al. 2011).

Similarly, NAC has been shown to prevent loss of $\Delta\Psi_M$ and to prevent mitochondrial-mediated apoptosis in both human hepatoma Huh-7.5 cells and Raji cells infected with hepatitis c virus (HCV) (Deng et al. 2015; Machida et al. 2006), as well as in epithelial PK-15 cells infected with transmissible gastroenteritis virus (Ding et al. 2013), and in neuroblastoma Neuro2a cells infected with Japanese encephalitis virus (Mishra et al. 2009). In primary mouse bone marrow macrophages infected with the pathogenic bacteria, *Pseudomonas aeruginosa*, NAC pretreatment decreased mitochondrial superoxide production (Jabir et al. 2015). Likewise, in aspirin-sensitized mouse macrophages and in human hepatoma HepG2 cells, NAC protected mitochondria during lipopolysaccharide (LPS)-induced toxicity (Raza et al. 2014, 2016). Specifically, NAC pretreatment increased mitochondrial glutathione, increased activities of ETC complexes I and IV, increased ATP, and prevented LPS-induced mitochondrial-mediated apoptosis.

In a study examining thymocyte development, pretreatment of dexamethasone-treated mice with NAC (400 mg/kg i.p. at 1 and 6 h prior) prevented thymocyte apoptosis and loss of $\Delta\Psi_M$ (Tonomura et al. 2003). Similarly in in vitro studies, NAC prevented dexamethasone-induced loss of $\Delta\Psi_M$ and apoptosis in cultured mouse thymocytes (Tonomura et al. 2003), CD95-induced loss of $\Delta\Psi_M$ and apoptosis in Jurkat cells (Ziegler et al. 2016), as well as spontaneous apoptosis of human tonsillar B lymphocytes (Rosati et al. 2004).

5.3.8 Sepsis

Sepsis results from an exaggerated inflammatory response to infection that can lead to multi-organ failure and has been associated with mitochondrial dysfunction (Singer 2014). In a rat model of sepsis-induced muscle contractile dysfunction, NAC pretreatment (3 mmol/kg p.o. for 7 days) induced increased MnSOD activity and content in the diaphragm, likely by scavenging peroxynitrite and thus preventing MnSOD inactivation (Barreiro et al. 2005). In a cecal ligation and perforation (CLP) rat sepsis model, a single injection of NAC with deferoxamine (20 mg/kg NAC+ 20 mg/kg deferoxamine, s.c.) immediately after CLP improved activities of ETC complexes I and II in several brain regions (Cassol et al. 2010). Finally, NAC pretreatment for 1 h at 1 mM protected human alveolar epithelial A549 cells from mitochondrial-mediated apoptosis following LPS exposure (Chuang et al. 2011). On the other hand, in a co-exposure animal model of chronic ethanol consumption and sepsis, a NAC-supplemented diet did not preserve mitochondrial glutathione and failed to decrease mitochondrial superoxide production and apoptosis in alveolar type II cells isolated from these animals (Brown et al. 2001).

5.3.9 Pulmonary

NAC has long been used in pulmonary medicine for decreasing mucous viscosity. The use of NAC in pulmonary medicine is reviewed in detail elsewhere in this book. NAC has also been tested for its potential to protect mitochondria during hyperoxia/ mechanical ventilation-induced lung injury. In two animal models of hyperoxic lung injury, NAC pretreatment was found to be mito-protective in lung tissue by preventing apoptosis (Makena et al. 2011) and increasing MnSOD expression (Nagata et al. 2007). NAC has also been shown to protect lung mitochondria during various exposures. In an animal model of meconium aspiration, NAC (10 mg/kg i.v.) given 30 min after aspiration decreased mitochondrial oxidative damage as evidenced by decreased mitochondrial thiobarbituric acid reactive substances (TBARS), dityrosine and thiol groups, and improved the activity of ETC complex IV (Mokra et al. 2015). In cultured lung cells, NAC pretreatment prevented inflammatory cytokine-induced upregulation of MnSOD gene expression (Das et al. 1995) and H_2O_2-induced apoptosis and loss of $\Delta\Psi_M$ (Park 2013a, b).

5.3.10 Reproductive

NAC has been used in a few studies of infertility and reproductive health. In a congenital toxoplasmosis mouse model, NAC pretreatment (100 mg/kg i.p.) protected placental trophoblast mitochondria by preserving $\Delta\Psi_M$ and mitochondrial ultrastructure and preventing apoptosis (Xu et al. 2015). In an infertility study of human endometrial epithelial RL95-2 cells, NAC pretreatment (1 h, 5 mm) prevented X-irradiation-induced apoptosis and loss of $\Delta\Psi_M$ (Gao et al. 2015). Mixed effects of

NAC have been reported in studies of freeze/thaw-induced damage to semen, with NAC preventing loss of $\Delta\Psi_M$ in semen from rams (Mata-Campuzano et al. 2012a), but not in red deer spermatozoa (Mata-Campuzano et al. 2012b) when present during freeze/thaw at concentrations ranging between 0.1 and 1 mM. In human spermatozoa treated with a STAT inhibitor to decrease mobility, NAC co-treatment effectively prevented the loss of $\Delta\Psi_M$ and decreased mitochondrial superoxide production (Lachance et al. 2016). Interestingly, NAC has been shown to decrease $\Delta\Psi_M$ and impair survival of steroidogenic luteal cells isolated from bovine ovaries (Lohrke et al. 2010), likely by disrupting the fragile redox balance that supports mitochondrial steroidogenesis.

5.3.11 Liver

GSH is synthesized in all cells; however, the liver is essential to maintaining appropriate circulating GSH levels (Lu 1999). In a study examining the kinetics of a single 5 mM/kg i.p. injection of NAC on rat liver GSH content, it was observed that liver mitochondrial cysteine content increased 1.6-fold at 60 min and returned to baseline at 2 h after NAC while GSH content was unaffected (Yao et al. 1994). However, these were healthy rats with assumedly normal liver mitochondrial GSH. In gamma-glutamyl-transpeptidase-deficient mice which exhibit liver GSH deficiency, supplementation of 1 mg/mL NAC in drinking water from 3 to 10 weeks of age increased liver mitochondrial GSH as well as improved liver mitochondrial respiration, structure, and morphology (Will et al. 2000). NAC was found to be mito-protective in animal models of liver conditions including hepatic encephalopathy, liver disease, obstructive jaundice, and cirrhosis and in cell culture models of liver disease and fibrosis (see Online Table 5.5). On the other hand, in a mouse model of steatohepatitis, NAC administration along with a methionine- and choline-deficient diet was not effective at preserving liver mitochondrial GSH; however, the details of NAC administration were not reported (von Montfort et al. 2012).

5.3.12 Kidney

Hyperoxaluria is a disease of the kidney where there is excessive urination of oxalate and can be caused by mis-targeting of serine-pyruvate aminotransferase (AGXT), a protein that is involved in the breakdown of oxalate, to the mitochondria instead of peroxisomes (Purdue et al. 1991). In a rat model of ethylene glycol and ammonium chloride-induced hyperoxaluria, isolated renal mitochondria exhibited abnormal mitochondrial structure and morphology characterized by swelling and diffuse cristae, as well as decreased $\Delta\Psi_M$, and proteomics analysis revealed differential expression of multiple mitochondrial proteins (Sharma et al. 2016). These mitochondrial abnormalities were improved with concurrent treatment with NAC (50 mg/kg/day i.p.) and ameliorated with a combination of NAC and apocynin.

Renal failure may arise from damage due to trauma or infection or as a result of chronic diseases such as diabetes and cardiovascular diseases. Uremic encephalopathy is an organic brain disorder caused by elevated toxins in the blood due to renal failure. In a rat model of uremic encephalopathy, NAC pretreatment (20 mg/kg i.p.) failed to prevent complex I and IV inhibition in several affected brain regions, but NAC plus deferoxamine pretreatment effectively prevented complex I and IV inhibition (Barbosa et al. 2010). Dialysis and transplant remain the primary treatments for kidney disease. In two in vitro models of peritoneal dialysis treatment of end-stage renal failure, human peritoneal mesothelial cells were protected by NAC from loss of $\Delta\Psi_M$ by conventional 1.5% dextrose bio-incompatible peritoneal dialysate fluids (Kuo et al. 2009) and from increased mitochondrial superoxide production, mitochondrial fragmentation, loss of $\Delta\Psi_M$, and induction of apoptosis by high dialysate glucose (Hung et al. 2014).

5.3.13 Pancreas

The induction of acute pancreatitis, inflammation of the pancreas, has been associated with oxidative stress (Fu et al. 1997; Leung and Chan 2009). In a rat model of caerulein-induced pancreatitis, co-administration of NAC (181 mg/kg i.p.) and ascorbate (14.3 mg/kg) prevented pancreatic mitochondrial structural damage including swelling, loss of cristae, and vacuolation (Esrefoglu et al. 2006). The effects of NAC alone were not examined. In an in vitro study of pancreatitis, ethanol-induced loss of $\Delta\Psi_M$ in dog pancreatic ductal epithelial cells was prevented by NAC pretreatment (Seo et al. 2013b).

Pancreatic β cells are insulin-secreting cells, and death of pancreatic β cells contributes to diabetes development. NAC pretreatment of insulin-secreting HIT-T15 pancreatic β cells has been shown to prevent 2-deoxy-D-ribose-induced loss of $\Delta\Psi_M$ and induction of apoptosis (Suh et al. 2012). In rat insulinoma pancreatic β RIN-m5F cells, NAC pretreatment prevented copper-induced apoptosis and loss of $\Delta\Psi_M$ (Wu et al. 2012).

5.3.14 Gastrointestinal

NAC has been applied to the study of inflammatory digestive diseases colitis and gastritis. In a rat model of dextran sulfate sodium-induced colitis, concurrent treatment with NAC (20 mg/kg s.c. twice daily) resulted in increased activity of ETC complex IV in the colon as compared to animals not treated with NAC (Damiani et al. 2007), while the same dose of NAC used for 7 days prior to indomethacin-induced gastritis increased the activity of ETC complex II–III (Rezin et al. 2011) and decreased mitochondrial superoxide production (Petronilho et al. 2009) in stomach tissue as compared to animals not treated with NAC. Finally, NAC (500 mg/kg) provided in the diet to weaning piglets preserved intestinal mitochondrial structure and morphology but did not decrease weaning-induced apoptosis (Zhu et al.

2013). The role of β-hydroxybutyrate (β-HB) in stomach diseases was investigated in bovine abomasum smooth muscle cells, and it was found that β-HB-induced apoptosis could be inhibited by pretreatment with 1 mM NAC, but not the β-HB-induced elevation in cytosolic Ca^{+2}, indicating that toxic effects of β-HB are both ER and mitochondrial mediated (Tian et al. 2014).

5.3.15 Cartilage and Bone

Disorders of bones, joints, and cartilage are often associated with oxidative stress (Henrotin et al. 2003). In disease states such as osteoarthritis, the already relatively hypoxic environment in cartilage becomes more hypoxic and acidic (Wilkins et al. 2000; Collins et al. 2013). In a study examining normal equine articular chondrocytes cultured under very low O_2, low pH, and the inflammatory cytokine (IL1β), the addition of NAC (2 mM) to the cultures protected $\Delta\Psi_M$ and induction of apoptosis by dramatically enhancing cellular GSH (Collins et al. 2015). Chondrocytes cultured under 20% O_2 exhibited increased mitochondrial mass and respiration linked to ATP production, and the addition of 2 mM NAC prevented these adaptive changes, thereby maintaining the metabolic phenotype and increasing the proliferative rate (Heywood and Lee 2016). Furthermore, pretreatment of rabbit chondrocytes with 5 mM NAC prevented advanced glycation end product-induced loss of $\Delta\Psi_M$ and induction of apoptosis (Yang et al. 2015), as well as thymoquinone-induced mitochondrial-mediated apoptosis (Yu and Kim 2013). Monosodium iodoacetate (MIA)-induced loss of $\Delta\Psi_M$ and induction of apoptosis in primary rat chondrocytes were also prevented by 5 mM NAC (Jiang et al. 2013). In a cell model of osteoarthropathy, thioredoxin reductase 2 (TrxR2) knockdown in cultured chondrocytes resulted in increased mitochondrial superoxide production and apoptosis, which was prevented with 2.5 mM NAC (Yan et al. 2016). NAC (10 mM) has also been shown to protect mouse osteoblasts from H_2O_2 and 2-deoxy-D-ribose-induced loss of $\Delta\Psi_M$ and induction of apoptosis (Jung 2014; Kim et al. 2013). Despite these positive findings of NAC in cell models, there are no reports of the use of NAC in animal models of these bone and joint disorders.

5.3.16 Eye

Three in vitro models of eye disorders have reported positive effects of NAC on mitochondrial function. In a model of Fuchs endothelial corneal dystrophy, pretreatment of human corneal endothelial cells with 5 mM NAC prevented menadione-induced mitochondrial DNA damage, mitochondrial superoxide production, as well as loss of $\Delta\Psi_M$ and ATP (Halilovic et al. 2016). In primary trabecular meshwork cells from primary open-angle glaucoma patients, pretreatment with 10 mM NAC prevented rotenone-induced apoptosis (He et al. 2008). In human retinal pigment epithelial cells (ARPE-19) treated with carotenoid-derived aldehydes, NAC pre-treatment (1 mM) protected against apoptosis induction as well as loss of $\Delta\Psi_M$ (Kalariya et al. 2008).

5.3.17 Dental

Periodontal disease is an inflammatory condition linked to other serious health conditions such as coronary heart disease (Hujoel et al. 2000) and characterized by neutrophil-mediated oxidative stress-induced damage to surrounding tissues. Several studies have examined the ability of NAC to protect mitochondria in in vitro models of periodontal disease. Pretreatment of Jurkat T cells with 1–5 mM NAC prevented butyric acid-induced apoptosis and loss of $\Delta\Psi_M$ (Kurita-Ochiai and Ochiai 2010). Lipopolysaccharide-treated primary human gingival fibroblasts exhibited increased mitochondrial superoxide production, decreased mitochondrial respiration, and increased apoptosis, all of which were alleviated by co-treatment with 10 mM NAC (Bullon et al. 2015). On the other hand, pretreatment of human gingival fibroblast HGF-1 cells with 1.5 mM NAC did not prevent H_2O_2-induced loss of mitochondrial respiratory reserve capacity (Orihuela-Campos et al. 2015). In a study of dental pulp inflammation, pretreatment of human dental pulp cells with 5 mM NAC prevented nitric oxide-induced mitochondrial-mediated apoptosis induction (Park et al. 2014). In a model of dental fluorosis, fluoride-induced apoptosis in mouse ameloblast-derived LS8 cells was prevented by pretreatment with 5–10 mM NAC (Suzuki et al. 2015). Agents used during dental procedures including several dental monomers and resins have been shown to be toxic to human dental pulp cells; however, co-treatment with NAC protected mitochondria by preserving mitochondrial morphology and preventing the loss of $\Delta\Psi_M$ and ATP and the induction of apoptosis (Jiao et al. 2015, 2016; Paranjpe et al. 2008).

5.3.18 Stem Cells

Prevention of in vitro stress is important in stem cell culture due to the length of time in culture during differentiation protocols, and the addition of NAC to stem cell cultures has been shown to protect mitochondria from various in vitro stressors (Berniakovich et al. 2012; Cai et al. 2013; Li et al. 2015a; Seo et al. 2013a). Human induced pluripotent stem cells (iPSCs) differentiated toward hematopoietic cells in the presence of NAC had decreased loss of $\Delta\Psi_M$ and decreased apoptosis over time as compared to iPSCs differentiated without NAC (Berniakovich et al. 2012). NAC also protected bone marrow mesenchymal stem cells from homocysteine-induced loss of $\Delta\Psi_M$ and induction of apoptosis (Cai et al. 2013); human adipose tissue-derived mesenchymal stem cells from H_2O_2-induced loss of $\Delta\Psi_M$, induction of apoptosis, mitochondrial superoxide production, and fusion and fission abnormalities (Li et al. 2015a); and mouse embryonic stem cells from hypoxia-induced apoptosis (Seo et al. 2013a).

5.3.19 Hypoxia

Hypoxia has been shown to induce oxidative stress and cellular damage (Cobb et al. 1996; Davies 1995), and the mitochondria as the major producers of ROS in the cell are an obvious target to decrease hypoxia-induced ROS. Eleven studies have utilized NAC to protect mitochondria during hypoxic conditions (see Online Table 5.6). In all the in vitro models of hypoxia, NAC at concentrations ranging from as low as 10 µM to as high as 5 mM protected mitochondria from hypoxic injury, usually by preserving $\Delta\Psi_M$ and preventing apoptosis. In animal models, however, NAC was not universally effective as it improved ETC complex IV activity in the liver, heart, and lung, but not the brain in a guinea pig model of fetal hypoxia (Al-Hasan et al. 2013), and it failed to prevent mitochondrial structural damage in ovarian epithelium in a rat model of laparoscopic surgery-induced ovarian hypoxia (Kiray et al. 2011).

5.3.20 Exercise and Fasting

In addition to pathological conditions, NAC has been investigated for its ability to protect mitochondria under conditions including exercise and fasting. In a double-blind placebo-controlled trial, healthy men were treated prophylactically with 1800 mg NAC daily for 14 days prior to a single bout of eccentric exercise (Kerksick et al. 2010). Those treated with NAC reported decreased perceived soreness; however, intramuscular markers of mitochondrial apoptosis were not significantly different between the placebo and NAC group.

Several animal studies have examined the effects of NAC supplementation on muscle mitochondria. Mice supplemented with NAC for 6 weeks exhibited decreased $\Delta\Psi_M$ in muscle fibers which was attenuated by a bout of eccentric exercise (Lo Verso et al. 2014). Interestingly, in muscle-specific autophagy-deficient mice, the mitochondrial depolarizing effect of NAC was not improved by exercise, indicating that exercise induces mitophagy to clear damaged mitochondria and that some oxidant production is necessary for basal mitophagy and mitochondrial quality control (Lo Verso et al. 2014). Mitochondrial quality control also requires biogenesis to replace damaged mitochondria eliminated through mitophagy, and aerobic exercise-induced mitochondrial biogenesis is also thought to be initiated by oxidative stress (Steinbacher and Eckl 2015). Indeed, NAC treatment (0.1 mg/g/2 days i.p.) for 3 weeks in mice undergoing a treadmill exercise training protocol reversed exercise-induced increased mitochondrial biogenesis as well as ATP, ETC complex IV activity, and mitochondrial DNA in subsarcolemmal and intermyofibrillar mitochondria from gastrocnemius muscle (Sun et al. 2015). NAC decreased exercise-induced mitochondrial oxidative stress in this model as evidenced by decreased mitochondrial malondialdehyde (MDA) levels, increased mitochondrial GSH, and increased MnSOD activity (Sun et al. 2015).

To determine whether ROS is essential for fasting-induced muscle mitophagy, Qi et al. (2014) subjected mice treated with NAC (100 mg/kg/2 days i.p. for 3 weeks) to a 24 h fast. Examination of gastrocnemius muscle mitochondria revealed that NAC alone decreased the expression of several autophagy genes but that NAC failed to prevent fasting-induced upregulation of these genes. NAC improved mitochondrial GSH and decreased ROS in both fed and fasted animals, but NAC also decreased the activity and content of MnSOD and failed to protect mitochondria against fasting-induced lipid peroxidation (Qi et al. 2014). Thus, while ROS is required for basal constitutive muscle mitophagy and exercise-induced mitophagy, muscle mitophagy during starvation is ROS-independent. In an in vitro study of HeLa cervical cancer cells, starvation-induced autophagy was inhibited by NAC, which was found to be due to decreased AMPK phosphorylation and increased mTOR signaling (Li et al. 2013). In addition to mitochondrial quality control through mitophagy and biogenesis, normal muscle mitochondrial function is also maintained through mitochondrial fusion (Westermann 2012). Wang et al. (2014a) demonstrated that the fusion protein OPA1 is activated in differentiated C2C12 myotubes by mitochondrial-generated ROS and that NAC can inhibit this activation (Wang et al. 2014b). Thus, NAC may improve mitochondrial function in pathological conditions driven by excess oxidative stress, but it may impair normal mitochondrial quality control.

Intense exercise is associated with post-exercise immunosuppression and is thought to be due to exercise-induced lymphocyte apoptosis (Mooren et al. 2002; Phaneuf and Leeuwenburgh 2001). In mice subjected to exhaustive exercise, it has been shown that pretreatment with NAC (1 g/kg i.p. 30 min prior) decreases apoptosis and loss of $\Delta\Psi_M$ in intestinal lymphocytes as well as in thymocytes (Quadrilatero and Hoffman-Goetz 2005a, b, c, 2004). Prolonged strenuous exercise may also induce male reproductive dysfunction, which may be mediated by oxidative stress (Hackney 2001). Indeed an intense swimming exercise protocol was shown to decrease ATP and $\Delta\Psi_M$ and induce apoptosis in epididymal sperm of rats (Jana et al. 2014). Supplementation with NAC and α-lipoic acid orally by gavage (3 and 50 mg/100 g/day, respectively) during the swimming exercise protocol prevented these effects.

5.3.21 Cancer

Hundreds of in vitro cancer studies have utilized NAC as a tool to demonstrate that particular cancer treatments induce death of cancer cells through the induction of ROS. In general, the addition of NAC reverses the cancer-killing effects (usually induction of mitochondrial membrane depolarization and apoptosis), if the particular anticancer agent's effects are mediated through ROS production (see Online Table 5.7).

5.3.22 Toxicity

The approach of using NAC as a tool to investigate the role of ROS in the cytotoxicity of particular agents has been used in many studies (see Online Table 5.8), and a few were selected to be discussed. Doxorubicin, a chemotherapy agent, is well known to be cardiotoxic. In a randomized trial, 10 healthy men were given a 140 mg oral capsule of NAC 1 h prior and 70 mg/kg NAC at 4 h after a single dose of doxorubicin, and cardiac biopsies taken at 4 and 24 h after revealed no protective effects of NAC on mitochondrial swelling (Unverferth et al. 1983) suggesting that doxorubicin-induced cardiac mitochondrial damage is not ROS mediated. However, in an in vitro study, NAC protected bone marrow mesenchymal stem cells, which may be involved in cardiac repair, from doxorubicin-induced loss of $\Delta\Psi_M$ and apoptosis (Yang et al. 2013).

Rosiglitazone is an antidiabetic drug that targets PPARγ and increases the risk of heart failure. In a mouse model, NAC was shown to decrease rosiglitazone cardiotoxicity by protecting mitochondria. Specifically, perfused hearts from animals treated concurrently with rosiglitazone and NAC exhibited improved respiratory function, ETC complex I and IV activity, increased ATP, and decreased mitochondrial superoxide production compared to animals not treated with NAC (He et al. 2014).

In a mouse model of methamphetamine-induced hyperthermia, NAC (1000 mg/kg i.p.) provided 30 min prior or 1, 2, or 4 h after a single dose of methamphetamine was found to prevent hyperthermia (Sanchez-Alavez et al. 2014). Examination of brown adipose tissue from these animals revealed that NAC pretreatment prevented hyperpolarization of $\Delta\Psi_M$ and preserved mitochondrial number despite not decreasing mitochondrial superoxide production (Sanchez-Alavez et al. 2014). NAC's effectiveness even when administered after methamphetamine supports further investigation of the use of NAC in treating methamphetamine-induced hyperthermia.

5.3.23 NAC as a Prooxidant

In some cases NAC has been shown to induce ROS production, depolarization of the mitochondrial membrane potential, and cell death. A study by Lohrke et al. (2010) demonstrated a strong dose dependency of the effect of NAC (0.5–5 mM) on mitochondrial membrane potential and mitochondrial ROS production in bovine luteal cells from midphase corpus luteum. In this case, NAC disrupted the highly sensitive equilibrium between prooxidants and antioxidants in the luteal cells. Similarly, Zhang et al. (2012) demonstrated that NAC-induced reductive stress resulted in a permanently more oxidized mitochondrial redox state in rat myoblast H9c2 cells after treatment for 1 h with 4 mM NAC and increased cell death after 12 h. NAC has also been shown to enhance cadmium-induced loss of $\Delta\Psi_M$ in several studies (Chatterjee et al. 2009; Liu et al. 2011; Wang et al. 2015), and Wang et al. (2015) demonstrated that NAC inhibited autophagy during cadmium toxicity, thereby allowing further mitochondrial damage.

5.4 Summary

Despite possessing several mechanisms to combat the leakage of electrons that accompanies electron transfer during the process of oxidative phosphorylation, mitochondria remain the primary ROS producers in most cell types. Given the importance of mitochondria in health and disease, NAC has been applied in many studies to determine its ability to protect mitochondria in a wide variety of conditions and models of disease. It can be concluded that NAC protects mitochondria in several ways, which are graphically illustrated in Fig. 5.2. First, NAC is a thiol and can directly scavenge free radicals. Mitochondria are both the primary producers and targets of ROS. Thus, the free radical-scavenging properties of NAC can prevent mitochondrial oxidative damage. Second, NAC supports GSH synthesis by supplying the cell with cysteine, the rate-limiting amino acid for GSH synthesis. GSH is the main intracellular redox buffer, and because mitochondria lack the

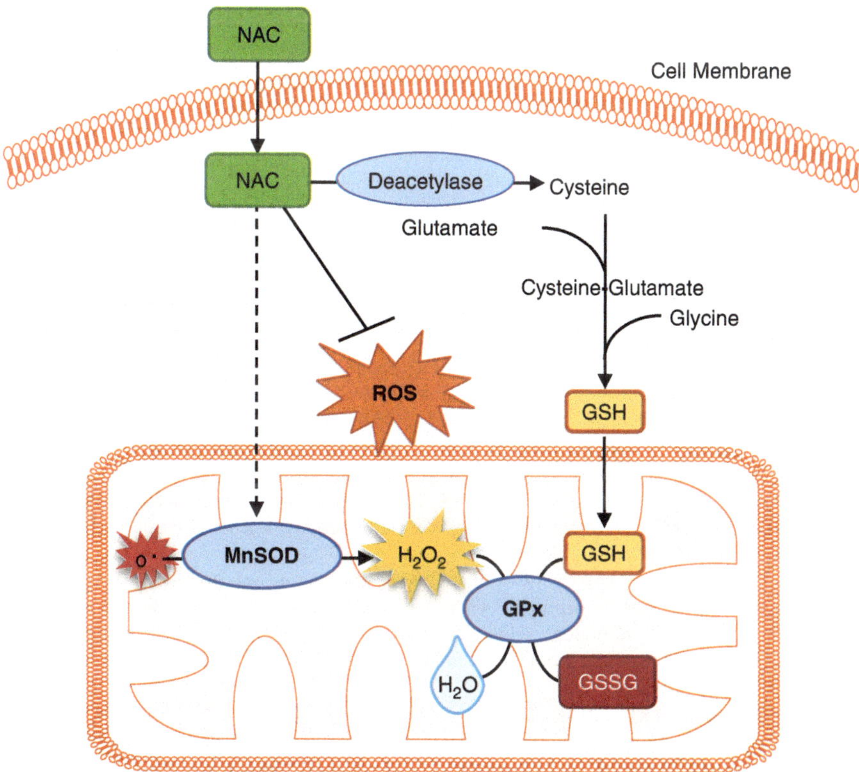

Fig. 5.2 The mito-protective mechanisms of NAC. Upon entering a cell, NAC can directly scavenge reactive oxygen species (ROS). Inside the cell, deacetylation of NAC generates cysteine, the rate-limiting amino acid for glutathione (GSH) synthesis. GSH synthesized in the cytosol is imported into mitochondria where it maintains reduced glutathione peroxidase (GPx) and thereby supports the reduction of H_2O_2 into H_2O. Highly reactive superoxide ($O^\bullet$) generated by the ETC is converted to the less reactive H_2O_2 by manganese superoxide dismutase (MnSOD). By mechanisms that are not well elucidated, NAC can upregulate MnSOD.

enzymes to synthesize GSH, they are reliant upon adequate cytosolic GSH. Furthermore, the mitochondrial permeability transition has been shown to be initiated by GSH depletion and prevented by NAC (Lu and Armstrong 2007). Third, NAC has been shown to directly induce the expression of MnSOD (Warner et al. 1996), a vital mitochondrial antioxidant mechanism. In pathological conditions where oxidants are produced in excess, NAC can also help maintain homeostasis of the mitochondrial network by balancing fusion and fission events as well as mitophagy and biogenesis. However, this homeostasis is tightly linked to the redox state, and thus, as demonstrated by Lohrke et al. (2010), NAC can also disrupt the equilibrium in certain cell types.

References

Al-Hasan YM, Evans LC, Pinkas GA, Dabkowski ER, Stanley WC, Thompson LP (2013) Chronic hypoxia impairs cytochrome oxidase activity via oxidative stress in selected fetal Guinea pig organs. Reprod Sci 20(3):299–307. https://doi.org/10.1177/1933719112453509

Andre L, Fauconnier J, Reboul C, Feillet-Coudray C, Meschin P, Farah C, Fouret G, Richard S, Lacampagne A, Cazorla O (2013) Subendocardial increase in reactive oxygen species production affects regional contractile function in ischemic heart failure. Antioxid Redox Signal 18(9):1009–1020. https://doi.org/10.1089/ars.2012.4534

Anglin RE, Mazurek MF, Tarnopolsky MA, Rosebush PI (2012) The mitochondrial genome and psychiatric illness. Am J Med Genet B Neuropsychiatr Genet 159B(7):749–759. https://doi.org/10.1002/ajmg.b.32086

Aronis A, Aharoni-Simon M, Madar Z, Tirosh O (2009) Triacylglycerol-induced impairment in mitochondrial biogenesis and function in J774.2 and mouse peritoneal macrophage foam cells. Arch Biochem Biophys 492(1–2):74–81. https://doi.org/10.1016/j.abb.2009.09.011

Balaban RS, Nemoto S, Finkel T (2005) Mitochondria, oxidants, and aging. Cell 120(4):483–495. https://doi.org/10.1016/j.cell.2005.02.001

Ballinger SW (2005) Mitochondrial dysfunction in cardiovascular disease. Free Radic Biol Med 38(10):1278–1295. https://doi.org/10.1016/j.freeradbiomed.2005.02.014

Barbosa PR, Cardoso MR, Daufenbach JF, Goncalves CL, Machado RA, Roza CA, Scaini G, Rezin GT, Schuck PF, Dal-Pizzol F, Streck EL (2010) Inhibition of mitochondrial respiratory chain in the brain of rats after renal ischemia is prevented by N-acetylcysteine and deferoxamine. Metab Brain Dis 25(2):219–225. https://doi.org/10.1007/s11011-010-9187-9

Barreiro E, Sanchez D, Galdiz JB, Hussain SN, Gea J (2005) N-acetylcysteine increases manganese superoxide dismutase activity in septic rat diaphragms. Eur Respir J 26(6):1032–1039. https://doi.org/10.1183/09031936.05.00003705

Barreiro E, Puig-Vilanova E, Marin-Corral J, Chacon-Cabrera A, Salazar-Degracia A, Mateu X, Puente-Maestu L, Garcia-Arumi E, Andreu AL, Molina L (2016) Therapeutic approaches in mitochondrial dysfunction, proteolysis, and structural alterations of diaphragm and gastrocnemius in rats with chronic heart failure. J Cell Physiol 231(7):1495–1513. https://doi.org/10.1002/jcp.25241

Basha RH, Priscilla DH (2013) An in vivo and in vitro study on the protective effects of N-acetylcysteine on mitochondrial dysfunction in isoproterenol treated myocardial infarcted rats. Exp Toxicol Pathol 65(1–2):7–14. https://doi.org/10.1016/j.etp.2011.05.002

Berniakovich I, Laricchia-Robbio L, Izpisua Belmonte JC (2012) N-acetylcysteine protects induced pluripotent stem cells from in vitro stress: impact on differentiation outcome. Int J Dev Biol 56(9):729–735. https://doi.org/10.1387/ijdb.120070ji

Boland ML, Chourasia AH, Macleod KF (2013) Mitochondrial dysfunction in cancer. Front Oncol 3:292. https://doi.org/10.3389/fonc.2013.00292

Brown LA, Harris FL, Guidot DM (2001) Chronic ethanol ingestion potentiates TNF-alpha-mediated oxidative stress and apoptosis in rat type II cells. Am J Physiol Lung Cell Mol Physiol 281(2):L377–L386

Buccigrossi V, Laudiero G, Nicastro E, Miele E, Esposito F, Guarino A (2011) The HIV-1 transactivator factor (Tat) induces enterocyte apoptosis through a redox-mediated mechanism. PLoS One 6(12):e29436. https://doi.org/10.1371/journal.pone.0029436

Bullon P, Roman-Malo L, Marin-Aguilar F, Alvarez-Suarez JM, Giampieri F, Battino M, Cordero MD (2015) Lipophilic antioxidants prevent lipopolysaccharide-induced mitochondrial dysfunction through mitochondrial biogenesis improvement. Pharmacol Res 91:1–8. https://doi.org/10.1016/j.phrs.2014.10.007

Cai B, Li X, Wang Y, Liu Y, Yang F, Chen H, Yin K, Tan X, Zhu J, Pan Z, Wang B, Lu Y (2013) Apoptosis of bone marrow mesenchymal stem cells caused by homocysteine via activating JNK signal. PLoS One 8(5):e63561. https://doi.org/10.1371/journal.pone.0063561

Cassol OJ Jr, Rezin GT, Petronilho FC, Scaini G, Goncalves CL, Ferreira GK, Roesler R, Schwartsmann G, Dal-Pizzol F, Streck EL (2010) Effects of N-acetylcysteine/deferoxamine, taurine and RC-3095 on respiratory chain complexes and creatine kinase activities in rat brain after sepsis. Neurochem Res 35(4):515–521. https://doi.org/10.1007/s11064-009-0089-3

Chatterjee S, Kundu S, Sengupta S, Bhattacharyya A (2009) Divergence to apoptosis from ROS induced cell cycle arrest: effect of cadmium. Mutat Res 663(1–2):22–31

Chuang CY, Chen TL, Cherng YG, Tai YT, Chen TG, Chen RM (2011) Lipopolysaccharide induces apoptotic insults to human alveolar epithelial A549 cells through reactive oxygen species-mediated activation of an intrinsic mitochondrion-dependent pathway. Arch Toxicol 85(3):209–218. https://doi.org/10.1007/s00204-010-0585-x

Cicek FA, Toy A, Tuncay E, Can B, Turan B (2014) Beta-blocker timolol alleviates hyperglycemia-induced cardiac damage via inhibition of endoplasmic reticulum stress. J Bioenerg Biomembr 46(5):377–387. https://doi.org/10.1007/s10863-014-9568-6

Civitarese AE, Ravussin E (2008) Mitochondrial energetics and insulin resistance. Endocrinology 149(3):950–954. https://doi.org/10.1210/en.2007-1444

Clay HB, Sillivan S, Konradi C (2011) Mitochondrial dysfunction and pathology in bipolar disorder and schizophrenia. Int J Dev Neurosci 29(3):311–324. https://doi.org/10.1016/j.ijdevneu.2010.08.007

Cobb JP, Hotchkiss RS, Karl IE, Buchman TG (1996) Mechanisms of cell injury and death. Br J Anaesth 77(1):3–10

Cocco T, Sgobbo P, Clemente M, Lopriore B, Grattagliano I, Di Paola M, Villani G (2005) Tissue-specific changes of mitochondrial functions in aged rats: effect of a long-term dietary treatment with N-acetylcysteine. Free Radic Biol Med 38(6):796–805. https://doi.org/10.1016/j.freeradbiomed.2004.11.034

Collins JA, Moots RJ, Winstanley R, Clegg PD, Milner PI (2013) Oxygen and pH-sensitivity of human osteoarthritic chondrocytes in 3-D alginate bead culture system. Osteoarthr Cartil 21(11):1790–1798. https://doi.org/10.1016/j.joca.2013.06.028

Collins JA, Moots RJ, Clegg PD, Milner PI (2015) Resveratrol and N-acetylcysteine influence redox balance in equine articular chondrocytes under acidic and very low oxygen conditions. Free Radic Biol Med 86:57–64. https://doi.org/10.1016/j.freeradbiomed.2015.05.008

Columbaro M, Ravera S, Capanni C, Panfoli I, Cuccarolo P, Stroppiana G, Degan P, Cappelli E (2014) Treatment of FANCA cells with resveratrol and N-acetylcysteine: a comparative study. PLoS One 9(7):e104857. https://doi.org/10.1371/journal.pone.0104857

Cossarizza A, Mussini C, Mongiardo N, Borghi V, Sabbatini A, De Rienzo B, Franceschi C (1997) Mitochondria alterations and dramatic tendency to undergo apoptosis in peripheral blood lymphocytes during acute HIV syndrome. AIDS 11(1):19–26

Dai DF, Chen T, Szeto H, Nieves-Cintron M, Kutyavin V, Santana LF, Rabinovitch PS (2011) Mitochondrial targeted antioxidant peptide ameliorates hypertensive cardiomyopathy. J Am Coll Cardiol 58(1):73–82. https://doi.org/10.1016/j.jacc.2010.12.044

Dai DF, Rabinovitch PS, Ungvari Z (2012) Mitochondria and cardiovascular aging. Circ Res 110(8):1109–1124. https://doi.org/10.1161/CIRCRESAHA.111.246140

Damiani CR, Benetton CA, Stoffel C, Bardini KC, Cardoso VH, Di Giunta G, Pinho RA, Dal-Pizzol F, Streck EL (2007) Oxidative stress and metabolism in animal model of colitis induced by dextran sulfate sodium. J Gastroenterol Hepatol 22(11):1846–1851. https://doi.org/10.1111/j.1440-1746.2007.04890.x

Das KC, Lewis-Molock Y, White CW (1995) Thiol modulation of TNF alpha and IL-1 induced MnSOD gene expression and activation of NF-kappa B. Mol Cell Biochem 148(1):45–57

Davies KJ (1995) Oxidative stress: the paradox of aerobic life. Biochem Soc Symp 61:1–31

Denborough M (1998) Malignant hyperthermia. Lancet 352(9134):1131–1136. https://doi.org/10.1016/S0140-6736(98)03078-5

Deng L, Chen M, Tanaka M, Ku Y, Itoh T, Shoji I, Hotta H (2015) HCV upregulates Bim through the ROS/JNK signalling pathway, leading to Bax-mediated apoptosis. J Gen Virol 96(9):2670–2683. https://doi.org/10.1099/jgv.0.000221

Diers AR, Broniowska KA, Hogg N (2013) Nitrosative stress and redox-cycling agents synergize to cause mitochondrial dysfunction and cell death in endothelial cells. Redox Biol 1:1–7. https://doi.org/10.1016/j.redox.2012.11.003

Ding L, Zhao X, Huang Y, Du Q, Dong F, Zhang H, Song X, Zhang W, Tong D (2013) Regulation of ROS in transmissible gastroenteritis virus-activated apoptotic signaling. Biochem Biophys Res Commun 442(1–2):33–37. https://doi.org/10.1016/j.bbrc.2013.10.164

Doherty E, Oaks Z, Perl A (2014) Increased mitochondrial electron transport chain activity at complex I is regulated by N-acetylcysteine in lymphocytes of patients with systemic lupus erythematosus. Antioxid Redox Signal 21(1):56–65. https://doi.org/10.1089/ars.2013.5702

Dominic EA, Ramezani A, Anker SD, Verma M, Mehta N, Rao M (2014) Mitochondrial cytopathies and cardiovascular disease. Heart 100(8):611–618. https://doi.org/10.1136/heartjnl-2013-304657

Egnatchik RA, Leamy AK, Noguchi Y, Shiota M, Young JD (2014) Palmitate-induced activation of mitochondrial metabolism promotes oxidative stress and apoptosis in H4IIEC3 rat hepatocytes. Metab Clin Exp 63(2):283–295. https://doi.org/10.1016/j.metabol.2013.10.009

Esrefoglu M, Gul M, Ates B, Yilmaz I (2006) Ultrastructural clues for the protective effect of ascorbic acid and N-acetylcysteine against oxidative damage on caerulein-induced pancreatitis. Pancreatology 6(5):477–485. https://doi.org/10.1159/000094665

Farley N, Pedraza-Alva G, Serrano-Gomez D, Nagaleekar V, Aronshtam A, Krahl T, Thornton T, Rincon M (2006) p38 mitogen-activated protein kinase mediates the Fas-induced mitochondrial death pathway in CD8+ T cells. Mol Cell Biol 26(6):2118–2129. https://doi.org/10.1128/MCB.26.6.2118-2129.2006

Federico A, Cardaioli E, Da Pozzo P, Formichi P, Gallus GN, Radi E (2012) Mitochondria, oxidative stress and neurodegeneration. J Neurol Sci 322(1–2):254–262. https://doi.org/10.1016/j.jns.2012.05.030

Feng YF, Wang L, Zhang Y, Li X, Ma ZS, Zou JW, Lei W, Zhang ZY (2013) Effect of reactive oxygen species overproduction on osteogenesis of porous titanium implant in the present of diabetes mellitus. Biomaterials 34(9):2234–2243. https://doi.org/10.1016/j.biomaterials.2012.12.023

Fu K, Sarras MP Jr, De Lisle RC, Andrews GK (1997) Expression of oxidative stress-responsive genes and cytokine genes during caerulein-induced acute pancreatitis. Am J Phys 273(3 Pt 1):G696–G705

Gao W, Liang JX, Liu S, Liu C, Liu XF, Wang XQ, Yan Q (2015) Oxidative damage of DNA induced by X-irradiation decreases the uterine endometrial receptivity which involves mitochondrial and lysosomal dysfunction. Int J Clin Exp Med 8(3):3401–3410

Giulivi C, Zhang YF, Omanska-Klusek A, Ross-Inta C, Wong S, Hertz-Picciotto I, Tassone F, Pessah IN (2010) Mitochondrial dysfunction in autism. JAMA 304(21):2389–2396. https://doi.org/10.1001/jama.2010.1706

Goh S, Dong Z, Zhang Y, DiMauro S, Peterson BS (2014) Mitochondrial dysfunction as a neurobiological subtype of autism spectrum disorder: evidence from brain imaging. JAMA Psychiat 71(6):665–671. https://doi.org/10.1001/jamapsychiatry.2014.179

Grattagliano I, Portincasa P, Cocco T, Moschetta A, Di Paola M, Palmieri VO, Palasciano G (2004) Effect of dietary restriction and N-acetylcysteine supplementation on intestinal mucosa and liver mitochondrial redox status and function in aged rats. Exp Gerontol 39(9):1323–1332. https://doi.org/10.1016/j.exger.2004.06.001

Hackney AC (2001) Endurance exercise training and reproductive endocrine dysfunction in men: alterations in the hypothalamic-pituitary-testicular axis. Curr Pharm Des 7(4):261–273

Halilovic A, Schmedt T, Benischke AS, Hamill C, Chen Y, Santos JH, Jurkunas UV (2016) Menadione-induced DNA damage leads to mitochondrial dysfunction and fragmentation during rosette formation in Fuchs endothelial corneal dystrophy. Antioxid Redox Signal 24(18):1072–1083. https://doi.org/10.1089/ars.2015.6532

He H, Tao H, Xiong H, Duan SZ, McGowan FX Jr, Mortensen RM, Balschi JA (2014) Rosiglitazone causes cardiotoxicity via peroxisome proliferator-activated receptor gamma-independent mitochondrial oxidative stress in mouse hearts. Toxicol Sci 138(2):468–481. https://doi. org/10.1093/toxsci/kfu015

He Y, Leung KW, Zhang YH, Duan S, Zhong XF, Jiang RZ, Peng Z, Tombran-Tink J, Ge J (2008) Mitochondrial complex I defect induces ROS release and degeneration in trabecular meshwork cells of POAG patients: protection by antioxidants. Invest Ophthalmol Vis Sci 49(4):1447–1458. https://doi.org/10.1167/iovs.07-1361

Henrotin YE, Bruckner P, Pujol JP (2003) The role of reactive oxygen species in homeostasis and degradation of cartilage. Osteoarthr Cartil 11(10):747–755

Heywood HK, Lee DA (2016) Bioenergetic reprogramming of articular chondrocytes by exposure to exogenous and endogenous reactive oxygen species and its role in the anabolic response to low oxygen. J Tissue Eng Regen Med 11(8):2286–2294. https://doi.org/10.1002/term.2126

Hujoel PP, Drangsholt M, Spiekerman C, DeRouen TA (2000) Periodontal disease and coronary heart disease risk. JAMA 284(11):1406–1410

Hung KY, Liu SY, Kao SH, Huang JW, Chiang CK, Tsai TJ (2009) N-acetylcysteine-mediated antioxidation prevents hyperglycemia-induced apoptosis and collagen synthesis in rat mesangial cells. Am J Nephrol 29(3):192–202. https://doi.org/10.1159/000155657

Hung KY, Liu SY, Yang TC, Liao TL, Kao SH (2014) High-dialysate-glucose-induced oxidative stress and mitochondrial-mediated apoptosis in human peritoneal mesothelial cells. Oxidative Med Cell Longev 2014:642793. https://doi.org/10.1155/2014/642793

Jabir MS, Hopkins L, Ritchie ND, Ullah I, Bayes HK, Li D, Tourlomousis P, Lupton A, Puleston D, Simon AK, Bryant C, Evans TJ (2015) Mitochondrial damage contributes to Pseudomonas aeruginosa activation of the inflammasome and is downregulated by autophagy. Autophagy 11(1):166–182. https://doi.org/10.4161/15548627.2014.981915

Jana K, Dutta A, Chakraborty P, Manna I, Firdaus SB, Bandyopadhyay D, Chattopadhyay R, Chakravarty B (2014) Alpha-lipoic acid and N-acetylcysteine protects intensive swimming exercise-mediated germ-cell depletion, pro-oxidant generation, and alteration of steroidogenesis in rat testis. Mol Reprod Dev 81(9):833–850. https://doi.org/10.1002/mrd.22354

Jiang L, Li L, Geng C, Gong D, Ishikawa N, Kajima K, Zhong L (2013) Monosodium iodoacetate induces apoptosis via the mitochondrial pathway involving ROS production and caspase activation in rat chondrocytes in vitro. J Orthop Res 31(3):364–369. https://doi.org/10.1002/ jor.22250

Jiao Y, Ma S, Li J, Shan L, Wang Y, Tian M, Yang Y, Sun J, Ban J, Chen J (2015) N-Acetyl Cysteine (NAC)-Directed Detoxification of Methacryloxylethyl Cetyl Ammonium Chloride (DMAE-CB). PLoS One 10(8):e0135815. https://doi.org/10.1371/journal.pone.0135815

Jiao Y, Ma S, Wang Y, Li J, Shan L, Liu Q, Liu Y, Song Q, Yu F, Yu H, Liu H, Huang L, Chen J (2016) N-acetyl cysteine depletes reactive oxygen species and prevents dental monomer-induced intrinsic mitochondrial apoptosis in vitro in human dental pulp cells. PLoS One 11(1):e0147858. https://doi.org/10.1371/journal.pone.0147858

Jose C, Melser S, Benard G, Rossignol R (2013) Mitoplasticity: adaptation biology of the mitochondrion to the cellular redox state in physiology and carcinogenesis. Antioxid Redox Signal 18(7):808–849. https://doi.org/10.1089/ars.2011.4357

Jou SH, Chiu NY, Liu CS (2009) Mitochondrial dysfunction and psychiatric disorders. Chang Gung Med J 32(4):370–379

Jung WW (2014) Protective effect of apigenin against oxidative stress-induced damage in osteo-blastic cells. Int J Mol Med 33(5):1327–1334. https://doi.org/10.3892/ijmm.2014.1666

Kalariya NM, Ramana KV, Srivastava SK, van Kuijk FJ (2008) Carotenoid derived aldehydes-induced oxidative stress causes apoptotic cell death in human retinal pigment epithelial cells. Exp Eye Res 86(1):70–80. https://doi.org/10.1016/j.exer.2007.09.010

Kamboj SS, Sandhir R (2011) Protective effect of N-acetylcysteine supplementation on mitochon-drial oxidative stress and mitochondrial enzymes in cerebral cortex of streptozotocin-treated diabetic rats. Mitochondrion 11(1):214–222. https://doi.org/10.1016/j.mito.2010.09.014

Kerksick CM, Kreider RB, Willoughby DS (2010) Intramuscular adaptations to eccentric exer-cise and antioxidant supplementation. Amino Acids 39(1):219–232. https://doi.org/10.1007/s00726-009-0432-7

Kim EK, Choi EJ (2010) Pathological roles of MAPK signaling pathways in human diseases. Biochim Biophys Acta 1802(4):396–405. https://doi.org/10.1016/j.bbadis.2009.12.009

Kim HS, Suh KS, Ko A, Sul D, Choi D, Lee SK, Jung WW (2013) The flavonoid glabridin attenu-ates 2-deoxy-D-ribose-induced oxidative damage and cellular dysfunction in MC3T3-E1 osteoblastic cells. Int J Mol Med 31(1):243–251. https://doi.org/10.3892/ijmm.2012.1172

Kiray S, Onalan G, Karabay G, Zeyneloglu H, Kuscu E (2011) Antioxidant prophylaxis for cellular injury in ovarian surface epithelium resulting from CO(2) pneumoperitoneum in a laparoscopic rat model. Arch Gynecol Obstet 284(3):765–772. https://doi.org/10.1007/s00404-011-1933-7

Kirkland RA, Franklin JL (2001) Evidence for redox regulation of cytochrome C release during programmed neuronal death: antioxidant effects of protein synthesis and caspase inhibition. J Neurosci 21(6):1949–1963

Kletsas D, Barbieri D, Stathakos D, Botti B, Bergamini S, Tomasi A, Monti D, Malorni W, Franceschi C (1998) The highly reducing sugar 2-deoxy-D-ribose induces apoptosis in human fibroblasts by reduced glutathione depletion and cytoskeletal disruption. Biochem Biophys Res Commun 243(2):416–425. https://doi.org/10.1006/bbrc.1997.7975

Ko JW, Lim SY, Chung KC, Lim JW, Kim H (2014) Reactive oxygen species mediate IL-8 expres-sion in Down syndrome candidate region-1-overexpressed cells. Int J Biochem Cell Biol 55:164–170. https://doi.org/10.1016/j.biocel.2014.08.017

Korge P, Weiss JN (2006) Redox regulation of endogenous substrate oxidation by cardiac mitochondria. Am J Phys Heart Circ Phys 291(3):H1436–H1445. https://doi.org/10.1152/ajpheart.01292.2005

Kose SA, Naziroglu M (2015) N-acetyl cysteine reduces oxidative toxicity, apoptosis, and calcium entry through TRPV1 channels in the neutrophils of patients with polycystic ovary syndrome. Free Radic Res 49(3):338–346. https://doi.org/10.3109/10715762.2015.1006214

Kumar S, Sitasawad SL (2009) N-acetylcysteine prevents glucose/glucose oxidase-induced oxida-tive stress, mitochondrial damage and apoptosis in H9c2 cells. Life Sci 84(11–12):328–336. https://doi.org/10.1016/j.lfs.2008.12.016

Kuo HT, Lee JJ, Hsiao HH, Chen HW, Chen HC (2009) N-acetylcysteine prevents mitochondria from oxidative injury induced by conventional peritoneal dialysate in human peritoneal meso-thelial cells. Am J Nephrol 30(3):179–185. https://doi.org/10.1159/000213502

Kurita-Ochiai T, Ochiai K (2010) Butyric acid induces apoptosis via oxidative stress in Jurkat T-cells. J Dent Res 89(7):689–694. https://doi.org/10.1177/0022034510365456

Lachance C, Goupil S, Tremblay RR, Leclerc P (2016) The immobilization of human spermatozoa by STAT3 inhibitory compound V results from an excessive intracellular amount of reactive oxygen species. Andrology 4(1):133–142. https://doi.org/10.1111/andr.12123

Lackner LL (2014) Shaping the dynamic mitochondrial network. BMC Biol 12:35. https://doi.org/10.1186/1741-7007-12-35

Lai ZW, Hanczko R, Bonilla E, Caza TN, Clair B, Bartos A, Miklossy G, Jimah J, Doherty E, Tily H, Francis L, Garcia R, Dawood M, Yu J, Ramos I, Coman I, Faraone SV, Phillips PE, Perl A (2012) N-acetylcysteine reduces disease activity by blocking mammalian tar-get of rapamycin in T cells from systemic lupus erythematosus patients: a randomized, double-blind, placebo-controlled trial. Arthritis Rheum 64(9):2937–2946. https://doi.org/10.1002/art.34502

Laporte M, Galand P, Fokan D, de Graef C, Heenen M (2000) Apoptosis in established and healing psoriasis. Dermatology 200(4):314–316. https://doi.org/10.1159/000018394

Leung PS, Chan YC (2009) Role of oxidative stress in pancreatic inflammation. Antioxid Redox Signal 11(1):135–165. https://doi.org/10.1089/ars.2008.2109

Li CJ, Sun LY, Pang CY (2015a) Synergistic protection of N-acetylcysteine and ascorbic acid 2-phosphate on human mesenchymal stem cells against mitoptosis, necroptosis and apoptosis. Sci Rep 5:9819. https://doi.org/10.1038/srep09819

Li L, Chen Y, Gibson SB (2013) Starvation-induced autophagy is regulated by mitochondrial reactive oxygen species leading to AMPK activation. Cell Signal 25(1):50–65. https://doi.org/10.1016/j.cellsig.2012.09.020

Li X, Gao L, Zheng L, Kou J, Zhu X, Jiang Y, Zhong Z, Dan J, Xu H, Yang Y, Li H, Shi S, Cao W, Zhao Y, Tian Y, Yang L (2015b) The efficacy and mechanism of apoptosis induction by hypericin-mediated sonodynamic therapy in THP-1 macrophages. Int J Nanomedicine 10:821–838. https://doi.org/10.2147/IJN.S75398

Liu CY, Lee CF, Wei YH (2009) Activation of PKCdelta and ERK1/2 in the sensitivity to UV-induced apoptosis of human cells harboring 4977 bp deletion of mitochondrial DNA. Biochim Biophys Acta 1792(8):783–790. https://doi.org/10.1016/j.bbadis.2009.05.005

Liu D, Zhang H, Gu W, Liu Y, Zhang M (2013) Neuroprotective effects of ginsenoside Rb1 on high glucose-induced neurotoxicity in primary cultured rat hippocampal neurons. PLoS One 8(11):e79399. https://doi.org/10.1371/journal.pone.0079399

Liu T, He W, Yan C, Qi Y, Zhang Y (2011) Roles of reactive oxygen species and mitochondria in cadmium-induced injury of liver cells. Toxicol Ind Health 27(3):249–256. https://doi.org/10.1177/0748233710386408

Lo Verso F, Carnio S, Vainshtein A, Sandri M (2014) Autophagy is not required to sustain exercise and PRKAA1/AMPK activity but is important to prevent mitochondrial damage during physical activity. Autophagy 10(11):1883–1894. https://doi.org/10.4161/auto.32154

Lohrke B, Xu J, Weitzel JM, Kruger B, Goldammer T, Viergutz T (2010) N-acetylcysteine impairs survival of luteal cells through mitochondrial dysfunction. Cytometry A 77(4):310–320. https://doi.org/10.1002/cyto.a.20873

Loor G, Kondapalli J, Iwase H, Chandel NS, Waypa GB, Guzy RD, Vanden Hoek TL, Schumacker PT (2011) Mitochondrial oxidant stress triggers cell death in simulated ischemia-reperfusion. Biochim Biophys Acta 1813(7):1382–1394. https://doi.org/10.1016/j.bbamcr.2010.12.008

Lopez-Crisosto C, Pennanen C, Vasquez-Trincado C, Morales PE, Bravo-Sagua R, Quest AFG, Chiong M, Lavandero S (2017) Sarcoplasmic reticulum-mitochondria communication in cardiovascular pathophysiology. Nat Rev Cardiol 14(6):342–360. https://doi.org/10.1038/nrcardio.2017.23

Lu C, Armstrong JS (2007) Role of calcium and cyclophilin D in the regulation of mitochondrial permeabilization induced by glutathione depletion. Biochem Biophys Res Commun 363(3):572–577. https://doi.org/10.1016/j.bbrc.2007.08.196

Lu SC (1999) Regulation of hepatic glutathione synthesis: current concepts and controversies. FASEB J 13(10):1169–1183

Machida K, Cheng KT, Lai CK, Jeng KS, Sung VM, Lai MM (2006) Hepatitis C virus triggers mitochondrial permeability transition with production of reactive oxygen species, leading to DNA damage and STAT3 activation. J Virol 80(14):7199–7207. https://doi.org/10.1128/JVI.00321-06

Makena PS, Gorantla VK, Ghosh MC, Bezawada L, Balazs L, Luellen C, Parthasarathi K, Waters CM, Sinclair SE (2011) Lung injury caused by high tidal volume mechanical ventilation and hyperoxia is dependent on oxidant-mediated c-Jun NH2-terminal kinase activation. J Appl Physiol 111(5):1467–1476. https://doi.org/10.1152/japplphysiol.00539.2011

Malorni W, Rivabene R, Santini MT, Rainaldi G, Donelli G (1994) N-acetylcysteine prevents TNF-induced mitochondrial damage, apoptosis and viral particle production in HIV-infected U937 cells. Redox Rep 1(1):57–64. https://doi.org/10.1080/13510002.1994.11746957

Manji H, Kato T, Di Prospero NA, Ness S, Beal MF, Krams M, Chen G (2012) Impaired mitochondrial function in psychiatric disorders. Nat Rev Neurosci 13(5):293–307. https://doi.org/10.1038/nrn3229

Martinez Banaclocha M, Martinez N (1999) N-acetylcysteine elicited increase in cytochrome c oxidase activity in mice synaptic mitochondria. Brain Res 842(1):249–251

Martinez M, Hernandez AI, Martinez N (2000) N-Acetylcysteine delays age-associated memory impairment in mice: role in synaptic mitochondria. Brain Res 855(1):100–106

Mata-Campuzano M, Alvarez-Rodriguez M, Alvarez M, Anel L, de Paz P, Garde JJ, Martinez-Pastor F (2012a) Effect of several antioxidants on thawed ram spermatozoa submitted to 37 degrees C up to four hours. Reprod Domest Anim 47(6):907–914. https://doi.org/10.1111/j.1439-0531.2012.01990.x

Mata-Campuzano M, Alvarez-Rodriguez M, del Olmo E, Fernandez-Santos MR, Garde JJ, Martinez-Pastor F (2012b) Quality, oxidative markers and DNA damage (DNA) fragmentation of red deer thawed spermatozoa after incubation at 37 degrees C in presence of several antioxidants. Theriogenology 78(5):1005–1019. https://doi.org/10.1016/j.theriogenology.2011.12.018

Mattson MP, Liu D (2002) Energetics and oxidative stress in synaptic plasticity and neurodegenerative disorders. NeuroMolecular Med 2(2):215–231. https://doi.org/10.1385/NMM:2:2:215

McWilliams TG, Muqit MM (2017) PINK1 and Parkin: emerging themes in mitochondrial homeostasis. Curr Opin Cell Biol 45:83–91. https://doi.org/10.1016/j.ceb.2017.03.013

Michelucci A, Paolini C, Canato M, Wei-Lapierre L, Pietrangelo L, De Marco A, Reggiani C, Dirksen RT, Protasi F (2015) Antioxidants protect calsequestrin-1 knockout mice from halothane- and heat-induced sudden death. Anesthesiology 123(3):603–617. https://doi.org/10.1097/ALN.0000000000000748

Mishra MK, Ghosh D, Duseja R, Basu A (2009) Antioxidant potential of Minocycline in Japanese Encephalitis Virus infection in murine neuroblastoma cells: correlation with membrane fluidity and cell death. Neurochem Int 54(7):464–470. https://doi.org/10.1016/j.neuint.2009.01.022

Mokra D, Drgova A, Mokry J, Antosova M, Durdik P, Calkovska A (2015) N-acetylcysteine effectively diminished meconium-induced oxidative stress in adult rabbits. J Physiol Pharmacol 66(1):101–110

Mooren FC, Bloming D, Lechtermann A, Lerch MM, Volker K (2002) Lymphocyte apoptosis after exhaustive and moderate exercise. J Appl Physiol 93(1):147–153. https://doi.org/10.1152/japplphysiol.01262.2001

Moulton VR, Tsokos GC (2015) T cell signaling abnormalities contribute to aberrant immune cell function and autoimmunity. J Clin Invest 125(6):2220–2227. https://doi.org/10.1172/JCI78087

Nagata K, Iwasaki Y, Yamada T, Yuba T, Kono K, Hosogi S, Ohsugi S, Kuwahara H, Marunaka Y (2007) Overexpression of manganese superoxide dismutase by N-acetylcysteine in hyperoxic lung injury. Respir Med 101(4):800–807. https://doi.org/10.1016/j.rmed.2006.07.017

Naudi A, Jove M, Ayala V, Cassanye A, Serrano J, Gonzalo H, Boada J, Prat J, Portero-Otin M, Pamplona R (2012) Cellular dysfunction in diabetes as maladaptive response to mitochondrial oxidative stress. Exp Diabetes Res 2012:696215. https://doi.org/10.1155/2012/696215

Nicoletti VG, Marino VM, Cuppari C, Licciardello D, Patti D, Purrello VS, Stella AM (2005) Effect of antioxidant diets on mitochondrial gene expression in rat brain during aging. Neurochem Res 30(6–7):737–752. https://doi.org/10.1007/s11064-005-6867-7

Okouchi M, Okayama N, Aw TY (2009) Preservation of cellular glutathione status and mitochondrial membrane potential by N-acetylcysteine and insulin sensitizers prevent carbonyl stress-induced human brain endothelial cell apoptosis. Curr Neurovasc Res 6(4):267–278

Oliveira G, Diogo L, Grazina M, Garcia P, Ataide A, Marques C, Miguel T, Borges L, Vicente AM, Oliveira CR (2005) Mitochondrial dysfunction in autism spectrum disorders: a population-based study. Dev Med Child Neurol 47(3):185–189

Orihuela-Campos RC, Tamaki N, Mukai R, Fukui M, Miki K, Terao J, Ito HO (2015) Biological impacts of resveratrol, quercetin, and N-acetylcysteine on oxidative stress in human gingival fibroblasts. J Clin Biochem Nutr 56(3):220–227. https://doi.org/10.3164/jcbn.14-129

Palmieri L, Persico AM (2010) Mitochondrial dysfunction in autism spectrum disorders: cause or effect? Biochim Biophys Acta 1797(6–7):1130–1137. https://doi.org/10.1016/j.bbabio.2010.04.018

Paranjpe A, Cacalano NA, Hume WR, Jewett A (2008) Mechanisms of N-acetyl cysteine-mediated protection from 2-hydroxyethyl methacrylate-induced apoptosis. J Endod 34(10):1191–1197. https://doi.org/10.1016/j.joen.2008.06.011

Park JH, Kang SS, Kim JY, Tchah H (2015) The antioxidant N-acetylcysteine inhibits inflammatory and apoptotic processes in human conjunctival epithelial cells in a high-glucose environment. Invest Ophthalmol Vis Sci 56(9):5614–5621. https://doi.org/10.1167/iovs.15-16909

Park MY, Jeong YJ, Kang GC, Kim MH, Kim SH, Chung HJ, Jung JY, Kim WJ (2014) Nitric oxide-induced apoptosis of human dental pulp cells is mediated by the mitochondria-dependent pathway. Korean J Physiol Pharmacol 18(1):25–32. https://doi.org/10.4196/kjpp.2014.18.1.25

Park WH (2013a) Effects of antioxidants and MAPK inhibitors on cell death and reactive oxygen species levels in HO-treated human pulmonary fibroblasts. Oncol Lett 5(5):1633–1638. https://doi.org/10.3892/ol.2013.1216

Park WH (2013b) The effects of exogenous H2O2 on cell death, reactive oxygen species and glutathione levels in calf pulmonary artery and human umbilical vein endothelial cells. Int J Mol Med 31(2):471–476. https://doi.org/10.3892/ijmm.2012.1215

Patti ME, Corvera S (2010) The role of mitochondria in the pathogenesis of type 2 diabetes. Endocr Rev 31(3):364–395. https://doi.org/10.1210/er.2009-0027

Perl A (2013) Oxidative stress in the pathology and treatment of systemic lupus erythematosus. Nat Rev Rheumatol 9(11):674–686. https://doi.org/10.1038/nrrheum.2013.147

Petronilho F, Araujo JH, Steckert AV, Rezin GT, Ferreira GK, Roesler R, Schwartsmann G, Dal-Pizzol F, Streck EL (2009) Effect of a gastrin-releasing peptide receptor antagonist and a proton pump inhibitor association in an animal model of gastritis. Peptides 30(8):1460–1465. https://doi.org/10.1016/j.peptides.2009.04.026

Phaneuf S, Leeuwenburgh C (2001) Apoptosis and exercise. Med Sci Sports Exerc 33(3):393–396

Pogribna M, Melnyk S, Pogribny I, Chango A, Yi P, James SJ (2001) Homocysteine metabolism in children with Down syndrome: in vitro modulation. Am J Hum Genet 69(1):88–95. https://doi.org/10.1086/321262

Purdue PE, Allsop J, Isaya G, Rosenberg LE, Danpure CJ (1991) Mistargeting of peroxisomal L-alanine:glyoxylate aminotransferase to mitochondria in primary hyperoxaluria patients depends upon activation of a cryptic mitochondrial targeting sequence by a point mutation. Proc Natl Acad Sci U S A 88(23):10900–10904

Qi Z, He Q, Ji L, Ding S (2014) Antioxidant supplement inhibits skeletal muscle constitutive autophagy rather than fasting-induced autophagy in mice. Oxidative Med Cell Longev 2014:315896. https://doi.org/10.1155/2014/315896

Quadrilatero J, Hoffman-Goetz L (2004) N-acetyl-L-cysteine prevents exercise-induced intestinal lymphocyte apoptosis by maintaining intracellular glutathione levels and reducing mitochondrial membrane depolarization. Biochem Biophys Res Commun 319(3):894–901. https://doi.org/10.1016/j.bbrc.2004.05.068

Quadrilatero J, Hoffman-Goetz L (2005a) Mouse thymocyte apoptosis and cell loss in response to exercise and antioxidant administration. Brain Behav Immun 19(5):436–444. https://doi.org/10.1016/j.bbi.2004.12.004

Quadrilatero J, Hoffman-Goetz L (2005b) N-acetyl-L-cysteine inhibits exercise-induced lymphocyte apoptotic protein alterations. Med Sci Sports Exerc 37(1):53–56

Quadrilatero J, Hoffman-Goetz L (2005c) N-acetyl-l-cysteine protects intestinal lymphocytes from apoptotic death after acute exercise in adrenalectomized mice. Am J Physiol Regul Integr Comp Physiol 288(6):R1664–R1672. https://doi.org/10.1152/ajpregu.00843.2004

Ravera S, Vaccaro D, Cuccarolo P, Columbaro M, Capanni C, Bartolucci M, Panfoli I, Morelli A, Dufour C, Cappelli E, Degan P (2013) Mitochondrial respiratory chain complex I defects in Fanconi anemia complementation group A. Biochimie 95(10):1828–1837. https://doi.org/10.1016/j.biochi.2013.06.006

Raza H, John A, Shafarin J (2014) NAC attenuates LPS-induced toxicity in aspirin-sensitized mouse macrophages via suppression of oxidative stress and mitochondrial dysfunction. PLoS One 9(7):e103379. https://doi.org/10.1371/journal.pone.0103379

Raza H, John A, Shafarin J (2016) Potentiation of LPS-induced apoptotic cell death in human hepatoma HepG2 cells by aspirin via ROS and mitochondrial dysfunction: protection by N-acetyl cysteine. PLoS One 11(7):e0159750. https://doi.org/10.1371/journal.pone.0159750

Recchioni R, Marcheselli F, Moroni F, Pieri C (2002) Apoptosis in human aortic endothelial cells induced by hyperglycemic condition involves mitochondrial depolarization and is prevented by N-acetyl-L-cysteine. Metabolism 51(11):1384–1388

Redpath CJ, Bou Khalil M, Drozdzal G, Radisic M, McBride HM (2013) Mitochondrial hyperfusion during oxidative stress is coupled to a dysregulation in calcium handling within a C2C12 cell model. PLoS One 8(7):e69165. https://doi.org/10.1371/journal.pone.0069165

Rezin GT, Amboni G, Zugno AI, Quevedo J, Streck EL (2009) Mitochondrial dysfunction and psychiatric disorders. Neurochem Res 34(6):1021–1029. https://doi.org/10.1007/s11064-008-9865-8

Rezin GT, Petronilho FC, Araujo JH, Goncalves CL, Daufenbach JF, Cardoso MR, Roesler R, Schwartsmann G, Dal-Pizzol F, Streck EL (2011) Gastrin-releasing peptide receptor antagonist or N-acetylcysteine combined with omeprazol protect against mitochondrial complex II inhibition in a rat model of gastritis. Basic Clin Pharmacol Toxicol 108(3):214–219. https://doi.org/10.1111/j.1742-7843.2010.00645.x

Ritov VB, Menshikova EV, He J, Ferrell RE, Goodpaster BH, Kelley DE (2005) Deficiency of subsarcolemmal mitochondria in obesity and type 2 diabetes. Diabetes 54(1):8–14

Roma LP, Pascal SM, Duprez J, Jonas JC (2012) Mitochondrial oxidative stress contributes differently to rat pancreatic islet cell apoptosis and insulin secretory defects after prolonged culture in a low non-stimulating glucose concentration. Diabetologia 55(8):2226–2237. https://doi.org/10.1007/s00125-012-2581-6

Rosati E, Sabatini R, Ayroldi E, Tabilio A, Bartoli A, Bruscoli S, Simoncelli C, Rossi R, Marconi P (2004) Apoptosis of human primary B lymphocytes is inhibited by N-acetyl-L-cysteine. J Leukoc Biol 76(1):152–161. https://doi.org/10.1189/jlb.0403148

Rossignol DA, Frye RE (2012) Mitochondrial dysfunction in autism spectrum disorders: a systematic review and meta-analysis. Mol Psychiatry 17(3):290–314. https://doi.org/10.1038/mp.2010.136

Rossignol DA, Frye RE (2014) Evidence linking oxidative stress, mitochondrial dysfunction, and inflammation in the brain of individuals with autism. Front Physiol 5:150. https://doi.org/10.3389/fphys.2014.00150

Samudio I, Fiegl M, Andreeff M (2009) Mitochondrial uncoupling and the Warburg effect: molecular basis for the reprogramming of cancer cell metabolism. Cancer Res 69(6):2163–2166. https://doi.org/10.1158/0008-5472.CAN-08-3722

Sanchez-Alavez M, Bortell N, Galmozzi A, Conti B, Marcondes MC (2014) Reactive oxygen species scavenger N-acetyl cysteine reduces methamphetamine-induced hyperthermia without affecting motor activity in mice. Temperature (Austin) 1(3):227–241. https://doi.org/10.4161/23328940.2014.984556

Scaglia F (2010) The role of mitochondrial dysfunction in psychiatric disease. Dev Disabil Res Rev 16(2):136–143. https://doi.org/10.1002/ddrr.115

Seo BN, Ryu JM, Yun SP, Jeon JH, Park SS, Oh KB, Park JK, Han HJ (2013a) Delphinidin prevents hypoxia-induced mouse embryonic stem cell apoptosis through reduction of intracellular reactive oxygen species-mediated activation of JNK and NF-kappaB, and Akt inhibition. Apoptosis 18(7):811–824. https://doi.org/10.1007/s10495-013-0838-2

Seo JB, Gowda GA, Koh DS (2013b) Apoptotic damage of pancreatic ductal epithelia by alcohol and its rescue by an antioxidant. PLoS One 8(11):e81893. https://doi.org/10.1371/journal.pone.0081893

Sharma M, Sud A, Kaur T, Tandon C, Singla SK (2016) N-acetylcysteine with apocynin prevents hyperoxaluria-induced mitochondrial protein perturbations in nephrolithiasis. Free Radic Res 50(9):1–13. https://doi.org/10.1080/10715762.2016.1221507

Shen SC, Lee WR, Yang LY, Tsai HH, Yang LL, Chen YC (2012) Quercetin enhancement of arsenic-induced apoptosis via stimulating ROS-dependent p53 protein ubiquitination in human HaCaT keratinocytes. Exp Dermatol 21(5):370–375. https://doi.org/10.1111/j.1600-0625.2012.01479.x

Shigenaga MK, Hagen TM, Ames BN (1994) Oxidative damage and mitochondrial decay in aging. Proc Natl Acad Sci U S A 91(23):10771–10778

Silva E, Greene AF, Strauss K, Herrick JR, Schoolcraft WB, Krisher RL (2015) Antioxidant supplementation during in vitro culture improves mitochondrial function and development of embryos from aged female mice. Reprod Fertil Dev 27(6):975–983. https://doi.org/10.1071/RD14474

Simoneau JA, Kelley DE (1997) Altered glycolytic and oxidative capacities of skeletal muscle contribute to insulin resistance in NIDDM. J Appl Physiol 83(1):166–171

Singer M (2014) The role of mitochondrial dysfunction in sepsis-induced multi-organ failure. Virulence 5(1):66–72. https://doi.org/10.4161/viru.26907

Sleven HJ, Gibbs JE, Cock HR (2006) The antioxidant N-acetyl-L-cysteine does not prevent hippocampal glutathione loss or mitochondrial dysfunction associated with status epilepticus. Epilepsy Res 69(2):165–169. https://doi.org/10.1016/j.eplepsyres.2006.01.006

Soiferman D, Ayalon O, Weissman S, Saada A (2014) The effect of small molecules on nuclear-encoded translation diseases. Biochimie 100:184–191. https://doi.org/10.1016/j.biochi.2013.08.024

Sokoloff L (1960) The metabolism of the central nervous system in vivo. In: Field J, Magoun HW, Hall VE (eds) Handbook of physiology—neurophysiology, vol 3, pp 1843–1864

Steinbacher P, Eckl P (2015) Impact of oxidative stress on exercising skeletal muscle. Biomol Ther 5(2):356–377. https://doi.org/10.3390/biom5020356

Suh KS, Oh S, Woo JT, Kim SW, Kim JW, Kim YS, Chon S (2012) Apigenin attenuates 2-deoxy-D-ribose-induced oxidative cell damage in HIT-T15 pancreatic beta-cells. Biol Pharm Bull 35(1):121–126

Sun N, Youle RJ, Finkel T (2016) The mitochondrial basis of aging. Mol Cell 61(5):654–666. https://doi.org/10.1016/j.molcel.2016.01.028

Sun Y, Qi Z, He Q, Cui D, Qian S, Ji L, Ding S (2015) The effect of treadmill training and N-acetyl-l-cysteine intervention on biogenesis of cytochrome c oxidase (COX). Free Radic Biol Med 87:326–335. https://doi.org/10.1016/j.freeradbiomed.2015.06.035

Sung JH, Shin SA, Park HK, Montelaro RC, Chong YH (2001) Protective effect of glutathione in HIV-1 lytic peptide 1-induced cell death in human neuronal cells. J Neurovirol 7(5):454–465. https://doi.org/10.1080/135502801753170318

Suzuki M, Bandoski C, Bartlett JD (2015) Fluoride induces oxidative damage and SIRT1/autophagy through ROS-mediated JNK signaling. Free Radic Biol Med 89:369–378. https://doi.org/10.1016/j.freeradbiomed.2015.08.015

Tian W, Wei T, Li B, Wang Z, Zhang N, Xie G (2014) Pathway of programmed cell death and oxidative stress induced by beta-hydroxybutyrate in dairy cow abomasum smooth muscle cells and in mouse gastric smooth muscle. PLoS One 9(5):e96775. https://doi.org/10.1371/journal.pone.0096775

Tonomura N, McLaughlin K, Grimm L, Goldsby RA, Osborne BA (2003) Glucocorticoid-induced apoptosis of thymocytes: requirement of proteasome-dependent mitochondrial activity. J Immunol 170(5):2469–2478

Tsai SY, Hayashi T, Harvey BK, Wang Y, Wu WW, Shen RF, Zhang Y, Becker KG, Hoffer BJ, Su TP (2009) Sigma-1 receptors regulate hippocampal dendritic spine formation via a free radical-sensitive mechanism involving Rac1xGTP pathway. Proc Natl Acad Sci U S A 106(52):22468–22473. https://doi.org/10.1073/pnas.0909089106

Unverferth DV, Jagadeesh JM, Unverferth BJ, Magorien RD, Leier CV, Balcerzak SP (1983) Attempt to prevent doxorubicin-induced acute human myocardial morphologic damage with acetylcysteine. J Natl Cancer Inst 71(5):917–920

Usai C, Ravera S, Cuccarolo P, Panfoli I, Dufour C, Cappelli E, Degan P (2015) Dysregulated Ca2+ homeostasis in Fanconi anemia cells. Sci Rep 5:8088. https://doi.org/10.1038/srep08088

Valenti D, de Bari L, De Filippis B, Henrion-Caude A, Vacca RA (2014) Mitochondrial dysfunction as a central actor in intellectual disability-related diseases: an overview of Down syndrome, autism, Fragile X and Rett syndrome. Neurosci Biobehav Rev 46(Pt 2):202–217. https://doi.org/10.1016/j.neubiorev.2014.01.012

Van Laar VS, Roy N, Liu A, Rajprohat S, Arnold B, Dukes AA, Holbein CD, Berman SB (2015) Glutamate excitotoxicity in neurons triggers mitochondrial and endoplasmic reticulum accumulation of Parkin, and, in the presence of N-acetyl cysteine, mitophagy. Neurobiol Dis 74:180–193. https://doi.org/10.1016/j.nbd.2014.11.015

Vasquez-Trincado C, Garcia-Carvajal I, Pennanen C, Parra V, Hill JA, Rothermel BA, Lavandero S (2016) Mitochondrial dynamics, mitophagy and cardiovascular disease. J Physiol 594(3):509–525. https://doi.org/10.1113/JP271301

von Montfort C, Matias N, Fernandez A, Fucho R, Conde de la Rosa L, Martinez-Chantar ML, Mato JM, Machida K, Tsukamoto H, Murphy MP, Mansouri A, Kaplowitz N, Garcia-Ruiz C, Fernandez-Checa JC (2012) Mitochondrial GSH determines the toxic or therapeutic potential of superoxide scavenging in steatohepatitis. J Hepatol 57(4):852–859. https://doi.org/10.1016/j.jhep.2012.05.024

Vyas S, Zaganjor E, Haigis MC (2016) Mitochondria and cancer. Cell 166(3):555–566. https://doi.org/10.1016/j.cell.2016.07.002

Wai T, Langer T (2016) Mitochondrial dynamics and metabolic regulation. Trends Endocrinol Metab 27(2):105–117. https://doi.org/10.1016/j.tem.2015.12.001

Wallace DC (2012) Mitochondria and cancer. Nat Rev Cancer 12(10):685–698. https://doi.org/10.1038/nrc3365

Wang H, Yang Y, Chen H, Dan J, Cheng J, Guo S, Sun X, Wang W, Ai Y, Li S, Li Z, Peng L, Tian Z, Yang L, Wu J, Zhong X, Zhou Q, Wang P, Zhang Z, Cao W, Tian Y (2014a) The predominant pathway of apoptosis in THP-1 macrophage-derived foam cells induced by 5-aminolevulinic acid-mediated sonodynamic therapy is the mitochondria-caspase pathway despite the participation of endoplasmic reticulum stress. Cell Physiol Biochem 33(6):1789–1801. https://doi.org/10.1159/000362958

Wang J, Wang H, Hao P, Xue L, Wei S, Zhang Y, Chen Y (2011) Inhibition of aldehyde dehydrogenase 2 by oxidative stress is associated with cardiac dysfunction in diabetic rats. Mol Med 17(3–4):172–179. https://doi.org/10.2119/molmed.2010.00114

Wang T, Si Y, Shirihai OS, Si H, Schultz V, Corkey RF, Hu L, Deeney JT, Guo W, Corkey BE (2010) Respiration in adipocytes is inhibited by reactive oxygen species. Obesity (Silver Spring) 18(8):1493–1502. https://doi.org/10.1038/oby.2009.456

Wang T, Wang Q, Song R, Zhang Y, Zhang K, Yuan Y, Bian J, Liu X, Gu J, Liu Z (2015) Autophagy plays a cytoprotective role during cadmium-induced oxidative damage in primary neuronal cultures. Biol Trace Elem Res 168(2):481–489. https://doi.org/10.1007/s12011-015-0390-8

Wang X, Li H, Zheng A, Yang L, Liu J, Chen C, Tang Y, Zou X, Li Y, Long J, Zhang Y, Feng Z (2014b) Mitochondrial dysfunction-associated OPA1 cleavage contributes to muscle degeneration: preventative effect of hydroxytyrosol acetate. Cell Death Dis 5:e1521. https://doi.org/10.1038/cddis.2014.473

Warner BB, Stuart L, Gebb S, Wispe JR (1996) Redox regulation of manganese superoxide dismutase. Am J Phys 271(1 Pt 1):L150–L158

Weinberg F, Chandel NS (2009) Mitochondrial metabolism and cancer. Ann N Y Acad Sci 1177:66–73. https://doi.org/10.1111/j.1749-6632.2009.05039.x

Welter R, Yu L, Yu CA (1996) The effects of nitric oxide on electron transport complexes. Arch Biochem Biophys 331(1):9–14. https://doi.org/10.1006/abbi.1996.0276

Westermann B (2012) Bioenergetic role of mitochondrial fusion and fission. Biochim Biophys Acta 1817(10):1833–1838. https://doi.org/10.1016/j.bbabio.2012.02.033

Wilkins RJ, Browning JA, Ellory JC (2000) Surviving in a matrix: membrane transport in articular chondrocytes. J Membr Biol 177(2):95–108

Will Y, Fischer KA, Horton RA, Kaetzel RS, Brown MK, Hedstrom O, Lieberman MW, Reed DJ (2000) Gamma-glutamyltranspeptidase-deficient knockout mice as a model to study the relationship between glutathione status, mitochondrial function, and cellular function. Hepatology 32(4 Pt 1):740–749. https://doi.org/10.1053/jhep.2000.17913

Wu CC, Yen CC, Lee k I, Su CC, Tang FC, Chen KL, Su YC, Chen YW (2012) Involvement of oxidative stress-induced ERK/JNK activation in the Cu(2+)/pyrrolidine dithiocarbamate complex-triggered mitochondria-regulated apoptosis in pancreatic beta-cells. Toxicol Lett 208(3):275–285. https://doi.org/10.1016/j.toxlet.2011.10.022

Wu H, Jiang C, Gan D, Liao Y, Ren H, Sun Z, Zhang M, Xu G (2011) Different effects of low- and high-dose insulin on ROS production and VEGF expression in bovine retinal microvascular endothelial cells in the presence of high glucose. Graefes Arch Clin Exp Ophthalmol 249(9):1303–1310. https://doi.org/10.1007/s00417-011-1677-x

Xu X, He L, Zhang A, Li Q, Hu W, Chen H, Du J, Shen J (2015) Toxoplasma gondii isolate with genotype Chinese 1 triggers trophoblast apoptosis through oxidative stress and mitochondrial dysfunction in mice. Exp Parasitol 154:51–61. https://doi.org/10.1016/j.exppara.2015.04.008

Yan J, Xu J, Fei Y, Jiang C, Zhu W, Han Y, Lu S (2016) TrxR2 deficiencies promote chondrogenic differentiation and induce apoptosis of chondrocytes through mitochondrial reactive oxygen species. Exp Cell Res 344(1):67–75. https://doi.org/10.1016/j.yexcr.2016.04.014

Yang F, Chen H, Liu Y, Yin K, Wang Y, Li X, Wang G, Wang S, Tan X, Xu C, Lu Y, Cai B (2013) Doxorubicin caused apoptosis of mesenchymal stem cells via p38, JNK and p53 pathway. Cell Physiol Biochem 32(4):1072–1082. https://doi.org/10.1159/000354507

Yang Q, Guo S, Wang S, Qian Y, Tai H, Chen Z (2015) Advanced glycation end products-induced chondrocyte apoptosis through mitochondrial dysfunction in cultured rabbit chondrocyte. Fundam Clin Pharmacol 29(1):54–61. https://doi.org/10.1111/fcp.12094

Yao WB, Zhao YQ, Abe T, Ohta J, Ubuka T (1994) Effect of N-acetylcysteine administration on cysteine and glutathione contents in liver and kidney and in perfused liver of intact and diethyl maleate-treated rats. Amino Acids 7(3):255–266. https://doi.org/10.1007/BF00807701

Yildirim SS, Akman D, Catalucci D, Turan B (2013) Relationship between downregulation of miRNAs and increase of oxidative stress in the development of diabetic cardiac dysfunction: junctin as a target protein of miR-1. Cell Biochem Biophys 67(3):1397–1408. https://doi.org/10.1007/s12013-013-9672-y

Yu SM, Kim SJ (2013) Thymoquinone-induced reactive oxygen species causes apoptosis of chondrocytes via PI3K/Akt and p38kinase pathway. Exp Biol Med (Maywood) 238(7):811–820. https://doi.org/10.1177/1535370213492685

Zhang H, Limphong P, Pieper J, Liu Q, Rodesch CK, Christians E, Benjamin IJ (2012) Glutathione-dependent reductive stress triggers mitochondrial oxidation and cytotoxicity. FASEB J 26(4):1442–1451. https://doi.org/10.1096/fj.11-199869

Zhang Y, Tu C, Zhang D, Zheng Y, Peng Z, Feng Y, Xiao S, Li Z (2015) Wnt/beta-Catenin and Wnt5a/Ca pathways regulate proliferation and apoptosis of keratinocytes in psoriasis lesions. Cell Physiol Biochem 36(5):1890–1902. https://doi.org/10.1159/000430158

Zheng L, Sun X, Zhu X, Lv F, Zhong Z, Zhang F, Guo W, Cao W, Yang L, Tian Y (2014) Apoptosis of THP-1 derived macrophages induced by sonodynamic therapy using a new sonosensitizer hydroxyl acetylated curcumin. PLoS One 9(3):e93133. https://doi.org/10.1371/journal.pone.0093133

Zheng X, Wu J, Shao Q, Li X, Kou J, Zhu X, Zhong Z, Jiang Y, Liu Z, Li H, Tian Y, Yang L (2016) Apoptosis of THP-1 macrophages induced by pseudohypericin-mediated sonodynamic therapy through the mitochondria-caspase pathway. Cell Physiol Biochem 38(2):545–557. https://doi.org/10.1159/000438649

Zhu L, Cai X, Guo Q, Chen X, Zhu S, Xu J (2013) Effect of N-acetyl cysteine on enterocyte apoptosis and intracellular signalling pathways' response to oxidative stress in weaned piglets. Br J Nutr 110(11):1938–1947. https://doi.org/10.1017/S0007114513001608

Ziegler C, Finke J, Grullich C (2016) Features of cell death, mitochondrial activation and caspase dependence of rabbit anti-T-lymphocyte globulin signaling in lymphoblastic Jurkat cells are distinct from classical apoptosis signaling of CD95. Leuk Lymphoma 57(1):177–182. https://doi.org/10.3109/10428194.2015.1044449

Zuo T, Zhu M, Xu W (2016) Roles of oxidative stress in polycystic ovary syndrome and cancers. Oxidative Med Cell Longev 2016:8589318. https://doi.org/10.1155/2016/8589318

Apoptosis

6

Sirish C. Bennuri, Shannon Rose, and Richard Eugene Frye

6.1 Introduction

N-Acetylcysteine (NAC) is a molecule with great therapeutic potential, positively affecting multiple pathways that protect cellular systems. One of the molecular pathways that NAC appears to have a therapeutic effect is through modulation of programed cell death, a process known as apoptosis.

6.2 Apoptosis

Apoptosis refers to the process of programed cell death in which a cascade of molecular events lead to the destruction and dissolution of the cell. Apoptosis is a highly regulated and controlled process that confers advantages during an organism's life cycle. For example, the separation of fingers and toes in a developing human embryo occurs because cells between the digits undergo apoptosis. Another example is the involvement of apoptosis in preventing autoimmune responses by the destruction of immune cells that might cause an autoimmune response in the thymus. Another important function of apoptosis is the destruction of cancer cells.

Apoptosis can be initiated through one of two pathways. In the intrinsic pathway the cell kills itself because it senses cell stress, while in the extrinsic pathway the cell kills itself because of signals from other cells. Both pathways induce cell death by activating caspases, which are proteases, enzymes that degrade proteins. The two

S. C. Bennuri · S. Rose
Arkansas Children's Research Institute and University of Arkansas for Medical Sciences, Little Rock, AR, USA

R. E. Frye (✉)
Barrow Neurological Institute, Phoenix Children's Hospital, University of Arizona College of Medicine – Phoenix, Phoenix, AZ, USA
e-mail: rfrye@phoenixchildrens.com

© Springer Nature Singapore Pte Ltd. 2019
R. E. Frye, M. Berk (eds.), *The Therapeutic Use of N-Acetylcysteine (NAC) in Medicine*, https://doi.org/10.1007/978-981-10-5311-5_6

pathways both activate initiator caspases, which then activate executioner caspases, which then kill the cell by degrading proteins indiscriminately.

Of course apoptosis can become dysfunctional and contribute to the destructive effects of disease. Excessive apoptosis causes atrophy, whereas an insufficient amount results in uncontrolled cell proliferation, such as cancer.

In contrast to apoptosis, in necrosis, cell death results from acute cellular injury. Unlike necrosis, apoptosis produces cell fragments called apoptotic bodies that phagocytic cells are able to engulf and quickly remove before the contents of the cell can spill out onto surrounding cells and cause damage.

Figure 6.1 provides an overview of the major apoptosis pathways. Oxidative stress, the main target of NAC, is a major signal for apoptosis and can affect several pathways. Oxidative stress can affect the mitochondria directly, resulting in initiation of apoptosis through mitochondrial mechanisms that include release of cytochrome c through the mitochondrial permeability transition (MPT) pore. Cytochrome c initiates a cascade including activation of caspase-9 and then caspase-3 that results in the initiation of apoptosis. Mitochondrial-initiated apoptosis also releases apoptosis-inducing factor that causes DNA fragmentation and chromatin condensation resulting in apoptosis that is caspase independent. Endonuclease G is another enzyme released from the mitochondria during apoptosis that also initiates caspase-independent apoptosis through DNA degradation.

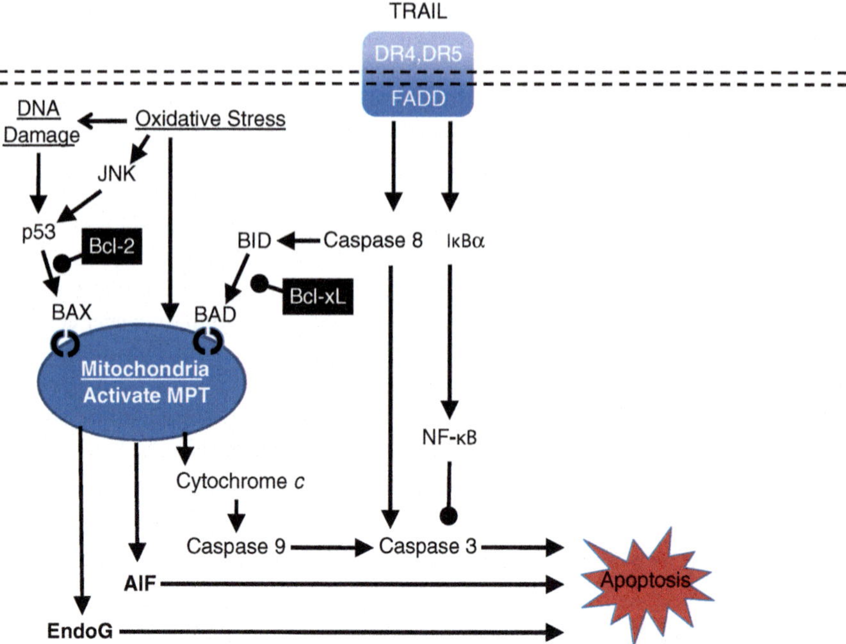

Fig. 6.1 Major pathways involved in cellular apoptosis. Both intrinsic pathways for apoptosis that are activated by internal cellular signals and extrinsic pathways that are activated by signals outside of the cell are depicted

Oxidative stress also damages DNA directly, resulting in activation of p53 that, in turn, promotes Bax to dimerize, causing mitochondrial-mediated apoptosis. Oxidative stress can activate other pathways in the cell associated with apoptosis including c-Jun N-terminal kinase (JNK) which also actives Bax to dimerize and initiate mitochondrial-dependent apoptosis.

Tumor necrosis factor-related apoptosis-inducing ligands (TRAILs) bind to death receptors that initiate apoptosis. These receptors are mitigated by Fas-associated protein with death domain (FADD) which helps produce the death-inducing signaling complex (DISC) to form caspase-8 which, in turn, activates caspase-3 that directly induces apoptosis and also Bid which induces mitochondrial-mediated apoptosis through dimerizing Bad.

TRAILs can also induce the activation of nuclear factor kappa-light-chain-enhancer of activated B cells (NF-κB) that is an important pathway involved in cell survival and response to physiologic and immune stressors. NF-κB is involved in a wide variety of diseases including cancer, autoimmune disease, infection, development of the immune system, as well as optimal function of the nervous system particularly related to synaptic plasticity and memory.

6.3 The Influence of NAC on Apoptosis

NAC has been used to demonstrate that particular molecular manipulations create apoptosis through the induction of reactive oxygen species (ROS). Specifically NAC is commonly used to reverse the apoptotic effect of specific treatments and cellular molecular changes by presumably reducing ROS. A comprehensive literature search of all studies that have investigated NAC and apoptosis in the same study demonstrates that since 1993, there have been 2815 studies (see Fig. 6.2). In this chapter we will review some of the more significant studies that highlight the role of NAC in apoptosis in experimental models of select diseases as well as highlight some of the major molecular pathways influenced by NAC.

6.4 The Role of NAC in Apoptosis in Specific Disorders

6.4.1 Cancer

6.4.1.1 Chemotherapy

NAC has been used to reverse the apoptotic effect of chemotherapy in animal and cell line laboratory studies in order to show that the mechanism of action of these treatments is through increasing ROS. These studies include the chemotherapeutic effect of 5-fluorouracil on HCT-15 tumor xenografts in nude mice (Bach et al. 2001); dexamethasone on myeloma cells (Bera et al. 2010); perifosine, an alkylphospholipid, on head and neck squamous carcinoma cells (Fu et al. 2010a); zoledronic acid, a third-generation bisphosphonate, on salivary adenoid cystic carcinoma cell line SACC-83 xenograft tumors in nude mice (Ge et al. 2014); pure fullerene suspension

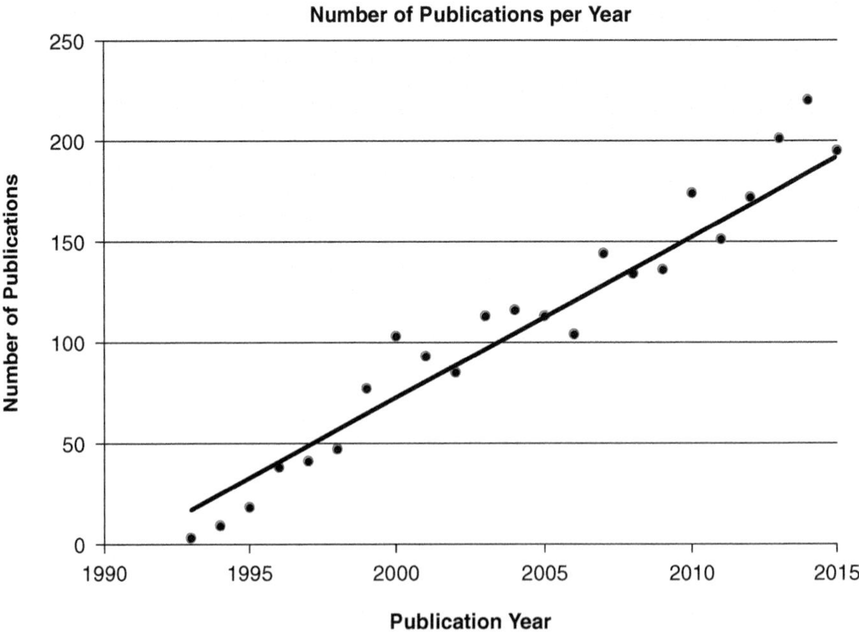

Fig. 6.2 The number of publications studying N-Acetylcysteine and apoptosis by year

(nano-C60) on mouse L929 fibrosarcoma, rat C6 glioma, and U251 human glioma cell lines (Isakovic et al. 2006); niclosamide on acute myelogenous leukemia cells (Jin et al. 2010); LAQ824, a histone deacetylase inhibitor, in combination with 13-*cis*-retinoic acid on HMV-I cells (Kato et al. 2007); anti-Fas receptor monoclonal antibody on a human myeloid HL-60 leukemia cell line (Laouar et al. 1999); AY4, an anti-DR4 agonistic monoclonal antibody, on head and neck cancer cells (Lee et al. 2012); intracellular iodide on NIS/TPO-modified lung cancer cells (Zhang et al. 2003); the combination of dichloroacetate and Adriamycin in HCC-LM3 and SMMC-7721 hepatoma cells (Dai et al. 2014); doxorubicin on cardiomyocytes from metallothionein-I/II null mice (Fu et al. 2010c); synthetic gold(III) dithiocarbamate on intact highly metastatic MDA-MB-231 breast cancer cells (Milacic et al. 2006); piperlongumine on head and neck cancer tumor xenograft mouse models (Roh et al. 2014); and cisplatin on LLC-PK1 cells (Xiao et al. 2003).

In these studies, NAC alters several subcellular pathways, including the NF-κB pathway (Jin et al. 2010), caspase-3/7 (Laouar et al. 1999), and anti-apoptotic molecules of Bcl-xL and X-linked inhibitor of apoptosis without affecting the expression levels of DR4 and Mcl-1 (Lee et al. 2012). Interestingly, in one study NAC reversed elevation of p-c-Jun, DR4, and DR5 even though these effects are believed to be independent of ROS (Fu et al. 2010a).

6.4.1.2 Chemopreventive Therapies

NAC has been used in animal and cell line studies to show that the apoptotic effect of chemopreventive agents on cancer cells involve ROS. These studies include the chemopreventive effect of OSU-A9, a novel derivative of indole-3-carbinol, on acute myeloid leukemia cell lines (Bai et al. 2013); *N*-(4-hydroxyphenyl) retinamide-induced apoptosis in NB4 neuroblastoma cell lines (Cao et al. 2009); baicalein (5,6,7-trihydroxyflavone) on ZR-75-1 human breast cancer cells (Chang et al. 2015) and SW620 colorectal cancer cells (Chen et al. 2012); the protoapigenone analogue WYC02-9, a novel synthetic flavonoid, on DU145 prostate cancer cells (Chen et al. 2011); caffeic acid phenethyl ester on Wt3A CREF cells (Chiao et al. 1995); Aplidin, a novel antitumor agent of marine origin, on human MDA-MB-231 breast cancer cells (Cuadrado et al. 2003); saporin, a plant ribosome-inactivating toxin, on malignant B cells (Daniels-Wells et al. 2013); carmustine on rat bone marrow cells (El-Sayed el et al. 2010); honokiol, an agent derived from the oriental medicinal plant Magnolia officinalis, on PC-3 prostate cancer tumor xenografts from mice (Hahm et al. 2014); brucein D on PANC-1 human pancreatic adenocarcinoma cells (Lau et al. 2010); parthenolide, a component of feverfew (*Tanacetum parthenium*), on melanoma cells (Lesiak et al. 2010); Eriocalyxin B, a diterpenoid isolated from Isodon eriocalyx, on CAPAN-2 pancreatic tumor cells (Li et al. 2014); Longikaurin A, an ent-kaurane diterpenoid isolated from the plant Isodon ternifolius, on human hepatocellular carcinoma cell lines (Liao et al. 2014); T63, a 4-arylidene curcumin analogue, on A549 lung cancer xenograft tumors (Liu et al. 2012); soybean lectin on HeLa cells (Panda et al. 2014); the snake venom toxin from *Vipera lebetina turanica* combined with tumor necrosis factor-related apoptosis-inducing ligand on human colorectal HCT116 carcinoma and HT-29 adenocarcinoma cell lines (Park et al. 2012); QD232, a novel quinazolinediones, on a xenograft mouse model of pancreatic cancer (Pathania et al. 2015); Triphala, a Ayurvedic medicine treatment, on Capan-2 pancreatic cancer cells (Shi et al. 2008); Alternol on prostate cancer cell lines (Tang et al. 2014); macrostemonoside A, an active steroidal saponin from *Allium macrostemon* Bung, on human colorectal SW480 cancer cell lines (Wang et al. 2013c); anthracenymethyl homospermidine on B16 melanoma cells (Xie et al. 2009); and AD-1, a dammarane-type sapogenins derived from the hydrolysates of the saponins extracted from the *P. ginseng* berry, on subcutaneously implanted A549 and H292 lung cancer cells in nude mice (Zhang et al. 2013).

In these studies, NAC normalize several apoptosis-related subcellular pathways, including those involving polyadenosine diphosphate-ribose polymerase (PARP) cleavage (Bai et al. 2013; Chen et al. 2011; Tang et al. 2014); caspase-3, caspase-8, and caspase-9 (Chen et al. 2011, 2012; Daniels-Wells et al. 2013; Lesiak et al. 2010; Liu et al. 2012; Park et al. 2012; Tang et al. 2014; Wang et al. 2013c; Xie et al. 2009); epidermal growth factor receptor (Cuadrado et al. 2003); non-receptor protein-tyrosine kinase Src (Cuadrado et al. 2003); p38 mitogen-activated protein kinase (MAPK) (Cuadrado et al. 2003; Lau et al. 2010; Liu et al. 2012; Li et al. 2014; Zhang et al. 2013); LC3BII (Hahm et al. 2014); mitochondrial membrane depolarization (Lesiak et al. 2010; Xie et al. 2009); NF-κB pathways (Li et al. 2014); FOXO3a cascade (Liu et al. 2012); cyclin D1 (Liu et al. 2012); DR4 and DR5 (Park et al. 2012); Bax protein (Tang et al. 2014; Xie et al. 2009); and Bcl-2 family proteins (Wang et al. 2013c; Xie et al. 2009) as well as phosphorylation of JNK (Cuadrado et al. 2003; Liao et al. 2014), Src/FAK and STAT3 (Pathania et al. 2015), p53 and extracellular signal-regulated kinase (ERK) (Shi et al. 2008), and AKT (Bai et al. 2013; Liu et al. 2012; Cao et al. 2009).

6.4.1.3 NAC Protects Against the Adverse Effects of Cancer Drugs

NAC has been shown to be protective against the apoptotic effect of chemotherapy for non-cancer tissues. NAC inhibited apoptosis caused by carboplatin in murine renal tubular cell (Lin et al. 2010); prevented rat H9c2 cardiomyoblast from apoptosis induced by adriamycin (Arunachalam et al. 2012) and daunorubicin (Guo et al. 2013); protected the outer stripe of the rat outer renal medulla (Luo et al. 2008), mouse dorsal root ganglion neuron-neuroblastoma N18D3 hybrid cell line (Park et al. 2000), and male ICR mice (Wu et al. 2011) from the apoptosis included by cisplatin; and reduced doxorubicin-induced apoptosis in cardiac myocytes in Wistar-Imamichi rats (Nitobe et al. 2003) and Japanese white rabbits (Wu et al. 2014).

6.4.2 Cardiac Disorders

NAC reduced ischemia-reperfusion-associated myocardium apoptosis in male Sprague-Dawley rats with an accompanied reduction in interleukin (IL)-6 (Kin et al. 2006), superoxide, malondialdehyde, and caspase-3 (Kin et al. 2008) and tumor necrosis factor-alpha (TNFα) and NF-κB (Kin et al. 2006, 2008); prevented hydrogen peroxide-induced apoptosis in ischemic-reperfused myocardium in adult Wistar rats (Inserte et al. 2000); attenuated neonatal myocyte apoptosis induced by cytokines IL-1β, TNFα, and interferon-gamma (IFNγ) (Ing et al. 1999) and hydrogen peroxide (Xie et al. 2014); and decreased hypoxia-reoxygenation-induced apoptosis in embryonic rat H9c2 cardiomyocytes (Peng et al. 2011). In one study NAC with or without allopurinol attenuated postischemic myocardial infarction in diabetic-induced Sprague-Dawley rats and normalized cardiac levels of hypoxia-inducible factor 1α (HIF-1α) and heme oxygenase 1 (HO-1) protein expression (Mao et al. 2013).

6.4.3 Gastrointestinal Disorders

6.4.3.1 Colitis

NAC improved apoptosis in animal models of colitis. Epithelial cell apoptosis was reduced in a dextran sulfate sodium male albino NMRI mice chronic colitis model (Amrouche-Mekkioui and Djerdjouri 2012), and apoptosis was attenuated in an acetic acid-induced piglet colitis model (Wang et al. 2013b). NAC significantly reduced immunohistochemical apoptosis as well as severity in a necrotizing enterocolitis in a newborn Sprague-Dawley rat model (Tayman et al. 2012).

However, in a female C57BL/6J mouse model of ulcerative colitis associated colorectal cancer, NAC significantly reduced tumor incidence and multiplicity through significantly inducing apoptosis in both non-cancerous epithelia and colorectal adenocarcinoma (Seril et al. 2002).

6.4.3.2 Liver

Several studies have demonstrated the protective effect of NAC on liver ischemia. NAC prevented liver apoptosis in a liver ischemia-reperfusion injury in a

Wistar-EPM rat model (Galhardo et al. 2007) and reduced apoptosis markers after liver ischemia-reperfusion injury in male C57BL mice along with protein expression of Bcl-2 and Bcl-xL (Sun et al. 2014). NAC reduced apoptosis in a mouse model of segmental hepatic warm ischemia along with decreasing Beclin 1 and LC3 expression and JNK, p-JNK, Bax, TNFα, NF-κB, IL-2, and IL-6 (Wang et al. 2014). Interestingly, NAC has been used to demonstrate that the protective effect of ischemic preconditioning is dependent on increased ROS as NAC reversed the protective effect of ischemic preconditioning in several partial and total hepatic ischemia mouse models (Rudiger et al. 2003).

NAC has also been found to be effective in immune-induced liver injury. NAC was found to abolish Fas mAb-induced acute fulminant liver failure in mice by reducing apoptosis as well as suppressing Valpha14i NK T-cell activation, IFN-γ signaling, and nitrotyrosine formation (Downs et al. 2012). NAC reduced D-galactosamine (GalN)/lipopolysaccharide (LPS)-induced apoptotic liver injury in mice but did not decrease serum TNFα (Wang et al. 2007a).

Other studies have examined the effect of NAC on other models of liver injury. NAC protected male Wistar rat hepatic parenchyma from apoptosis during liver hypothermic preservation as determined by optical microscopy (Risso et al. 2014). NAC had a dual effect on magnesium deficiency-induced apoptosis of human and rat hepatocytes, improving apoptosis and ROS markers in the context of magnesium deficiency but increasing apoptosis and ROS markers when hepatocytes were cultured in physiological concentrations of magnesium (Martin et al. 2006).

6.4.3.3 Pancreas

NAC reversed the effects of aldosterone triggered beta-cell dysfunction, which includes apoptosis, in 12-week-old female diabetic db/db mice, presumably though reducing oxidative stress, as confirmed on the mouse MIN6 pancreatic beta-cell line (Jin et al. 2013). NAC partially reversed apoptosis and inhibited the expression and activity of matrix metalloproteinase 2 in the rat pancreatic beta-cell line INS-1 induced by advanced glycation end products (Liu et al. 2014).

6.4.4 Renal Disorders

6.4.4.1 Contrast-Induced Nephropathy Models

NAC attenuated outer medulla apoptosis in a streptozotocin-induced diabetic male Wistar rat model exposed to iomeprol contrast medium (Ahmad et al. 2012). NAC demonstrated a dose-dependent protective effect on HEK 293 human embryonic kidney cells, LLC-PK1 porcine proximal renal tubular cells, and canine Madin-Darby distal tubular renal cells exposed to either low-osmolality or iso-osmolality contrast medium (Romano et al. 2008). In another study, NAC attenuated iopromide-induced NRK-52E cell apoptosis by inhibiting the overproduction of intracellular ROS, as determined by confocal microscopy with fluorescent CM-H2DCFDA probe, and prevented the increase of glucose-regulated protein 78 (GRP78) and CAAT/enhancer-binding protein homologous protein (CHOP) caused by iopromide exposure (Yang et al. 2014). NAC failed to reduce apoptosis in Madin-Darby canine kidney exposed to the hyperosmolar, ionic radiocontrast agent diatrizoate or hyperosmolar NaCl, suggesting that NAC was not protective against the osmolar effect of contrast agents (Hizoh and Haller 2002).

6.4.4.2 Other Renal Studies

NAC was found to completely block 2,3-dimethoxy-1,4-naphthoquinone (DMNQ)-induced ceramide formation and prevent superoxide-induced apoptosis of microcapillary glomerular endothelial cells (Huwiler et al. 2001). NAC decreased apoptosis pathway activation as evidenced by a decrease in ERK, JNK, Bax, and Bad and an increase in Bcl-2 and Bcl-xL in a male Sprague-Dawley rat model of glycerol-induced rhabdomyolysis (Kim et al. 2010). NAC inhibited high glucose-induced autophagy in podocytes in a Sprague-Dawley model of diabetic nephropathy (Ma et al. 2013). NAC was found to significantly increase Nrf2 and downstream HO-1 expression and decreased cleaved caspase-3, p53, and apoptosis in renal epithelial tubular cells in a renal ischemic injury model in Sprague-Dawley rats (Zhang et al. 2014).

6.4.5 Pulmonary Studies

Studies have demonstrated that NAC prevents apoptotic injury to lung tissue resulting from a wide variety of noxious insults. NAC protects against hypoxic injury as demonstrated in at least two studies. NAC significantly prevented caspase-3 activation in pneumocytes following cardioplegic arrest in a pig model (Klass et al. 2007) and attenuated cardiopulmonary bypass-induced lung injury, including reducing apoptosis, malondialdehyde, and TNF-β1 and upregulated superoxide dismutase activity in mongrel dogs (Qu et al. 2013). NAC protected alveolar type II cells from apoptosis caused by oxidative injury resulting from hydrogen peroxide in Sprague-Dawley rats (Fu et al. 2010b) and cigarette smoke in both C57BL mice and Nrf2 knockout mice (Messier et al. 2013).

NAC also protected lung tissue from inflammatory injury. NAC enhanced the clearance of apoptotic cells and the production of TNF-β1 as well as reduced RhoA activity in alveolar macrophages, proinflammatory mediators, and the accumulation of inflammatory cells in BALB C male mice treated intratracheally with LPS (Moon et al. 2010). NAC reduced the number of apoptotic cells in lung tissue in a Wistar rat model of septic lung injury as a result of cecal ligation and puncture (Ozdulger et al. 2003). NAC significantly improved zymosan-induced lung damage and function and suppressed dendritic cell apoptosis and immune activity in a Balb/c mouse model of early stage of severe sepsis (Wang et al. 2013a).

NAC also protected against the effect of mechanical lung injury. NAC prevented the decrease in lung glutathione and significantly lowered serum isoprostane levels and airway neutrophil infiltration, cytokines, and apoptosis in a Sprague-Dawley rat model of ventilator-induced lung injury (Syrkina et al. 2008).

6.4.6 Neurological Studies

NAC has been used in a wide variety of studies focusing on neural cell injury. A number of studies have examined models of ischemia, so this is addressed in a separate section.

6.4.6.1 Ischemia Models

In a male Wistar rat model of cerebral ischemic injury, NAC reduced infarct size (Wang et al. 2012). Post-resuscitation NAC attenuated cortical apoptosis, as measured by caspase-3, as well as lipid hydroperoxide and improved cerebral oxygen delivery in a subacute swine model of neonatal hypoxia-reoxygenation (Liu et al. 2010). NAC protected neurons from arachidonic acid toxicity and/or ischemia in cultured fetal rat cortical neurons (Pawlas and Malecki 2009). NAC inhibited markers of apoptosis, including caspase-3, calpain, and caspase-1, in a LPS rat model of hypoxia-ischemia-induced perinatal brain injury (Wang et al. 2007b). NAC reduced cerebral apoptosis, infarct area and volume, cytokines TNFα and IL-1β, macrophages and microglia activity, and inducible nitric oxide synthase and improved neurologic scores and glutathione levels in an ischemia-reperfusion injury model of stroke using male Sprague-Dawley rats (Khan et al. 2004). In a 4-vessel occlusion global brain ischemia model using adult male Sprague-Dawley rats, NAC reduced pyramidal layer of CA1 apoptosis (Shen et al. 2003). Finally, NAC was used to demonstrate that the protective effect of remote ischemic post-conditioning on cerebral infarction is dependent on ROS generation using male Sprague-Dawley rats (Wang et al. 2011).

6.4.6.2 Excitotoxicity

NAC has been shown to protect neurons from apoptosis in several models of excitotoxicity. NAC protected rat oligodendrocyte progenitor cultures from alpha-amino-3-hydroxy-5-methylisoxazole-4-propionate receptor-mediated excitotoxicity (Liu et al. 2002). NAC protected glial C6 and MN9D cell lines and a rat model of Parkinson's disease against apoptosis through modulation of group I metabotropic glutamate receptors and modulation of the extracellular signal-regulated kinase (ERK) pathway (Sun et al. 2012), a pathway that is a key integrator of dopamine and glutamate metabolism. In a pilocarpine model of chronic temporal lobe epilepsy, NAC prevented apoptosis as well as thiol oxidation and NR2B subunit overexpression in rat primary hippocampal cultures depending on the timing of application (Di Maio et al. 2013).

6.4.6.3 Cerebral Apoptosis Models

NAC has been shown to protect against apoptosis in neuronal tissue exposed to many other types of stress. In a male Sprague-Dawley rat traumatic brain injury model, NAC decreased apoptosis, cytosolic-free Ca^{2+}, ROS, and caspase-3 and caspase-9 activities in hippocampal neurons (Naziroglu et al. 2014). In rat primary oligodendrocytes, NAC blocked cytokine-mediated ceramide production by TNFα or IL-1β that resulted in glutathione depletion and DNA fragmentation (Singh et al.

1998). NAC prevented apoptosis and maintained long-term survival in serum-deprived PC12 cells, neuronally differentiated PC12 cells and neonatal sympathetic neurons deprived of trophic factors (Ferrari et al. 1995). NAC protected cultured rat hippocampal neurons from staurosporine-induced apoptotic degeneration (Prehn et al. 1997). Finally, NAC promoted neuroprotection of cutaneous sensory neurons through modulation of apoptosis pathways, including upregulation of Bcl-2 and downregulation of both Bax and caspase-3 (Reid et al. 2009).

6.5 Summary

In both cellular and animal model studies, NAC has been shown to protect cells and tissue against apoptotic changes and/or activation of apoptotic molecular pathways. Although there are many studies in which NAC has been investigated with apoptotic markers, this chapter has selected a subset of such studies to provide an example of the tissues and pathways investigated with NAC. This chapter has reviewed studies on cancer, cardiac, gastrointestinal, renal, pulmonary, and neurological tissues.

NAC is used in several studies to demonstrate that the mechanism of action of therapeutic treatments involves modulation of oxidative stress. This includes many of the studies examining the mechanism of action of chemotherapeutic and chemo-protective agents in cancer. This also extends to demonstrating that the effects on ischemic preconditioning and post-conditioning are dependent on ROS.

Several common themes arise in which NAC appears to be therapeutic. NAC has been shown to be protective against apoptosis in hypoxic-ischemic models of the liver, kidney, lung, and brain. Another theme is the protective effect of NAC from inflammation as investigated in models of colitis and inflammatory liver, lung, and neuronal injury. NAC has also been shown to be protective from stressors, both intrinsic stressors such as glycation end products in pancreatic tissue, glucose in renal tissue, and excitotoxicity in neuronal tissue and extrinsic stressors such as hypothermia and magnesium deficiency in liver tissue, contrast agents in kidney tissue, cigarette smoke and mechanical injury in lung tissue, and traumatic injury and depletion of trophic factors in neuronal tissue.

Although the goal of many studies is to use NAC to modulate oxidative stress-mediated apoptosis, the effect of NAC in these studies appears to be related to many other pathways, not typically involved in oxidative stress such as receptor-mediated apoptosis signaling, cellular growth and differentiation pathways, and pathways involved in epigenetic regulation. In addition, NAC appears in many studies to have a role in reducing inflammatory mediators. Overall, there is significant evidence that NAC can provide protection against apoptosis in many cellular and animal models of disease in both pathways directly involved in apoptosis as well as pathways that indirectly modulate molecular apoptosis factors. Of course, the basic research studies outlined here require follow-up with clinical studies to better understand their practical implications.

References

Ahmad A, Mondello S, Di Paola R, Mazzon E, Esposito E, Catania MA, Italiano D, Mondello P, Aloisi C, Cuzzocrea S (2012) Protective effect of apocynin, a NADPH-oxidase inhibitor, against contrast-induced nephropathy in the diabetic rats: a comparison with n-acetylcysteine. Eur J Pharmacol 674(2-3):397–406. https://doi.org/10.1016/j.ejphar.2011.10.041

Amrouche-Mekkioui I, Djerdjouri B (2012) N-acetylcysteine improves redox status, mitochondrial dysfunction, mucin-depleted crypts and epithelial hyperplasia in dextran sulfate sodium-induced oxidative colitis in mice. Eur J Pharmacol 691(1-3):209–217. https://doi.org/10.1016/j.ejphar.2012.06.014

Arunachalam S, Kim SY, Lee SH, Lee YH, Kim MS, Yun BS, Yi HK, Hwang PH (2012) Davallialactone protects against adriamycin-induced cardiotoxicity in vitro and in vivo. J Nat Med 66(1):149–157. https://doi.org/10.1007/s11418-011-0567-1

Bach SP, Williamson SE, Marshman E, Kumar S, O'Dwyer ST, Potten CS, Watson AJ (2001) The antioxidant n-acetylcysteine increases 5-fluorouracil activity against colorectal cancer xenografts in nude mice. J Gastrointest Surg 5(1):91–97

Bai LY, Weng JR, Chiu CF, Wu CY, Yeh SP, Sargeant AM, Lin PH, Liao YM (2013) OSU-A9, an indole-3-carbinol derivative, induces cytotoxicity in acute myeloid leukemia through reactive oxygen species-mediated apoptosis. Biochem Pharmacol 86(10):1430–1440. https://doi.org/10.1016/j.bcp.2013.09.002

Bera S, Greiner S, Choudhury A, Dispenzieri A, Spitz DR, Russell SJ, Goel A (2010) Dexamethasone-induced oxidative stress enhances myeloma cell radiosensitization while sparing normal bone marrow hematopoiesis. Neoplasia 12(12):980–992

Cao J, Xu D, Wang D, Wu R, Zhang L, Zhu H, He Q, Yang B (2009) ROS-driven Akt dephosphorylation at Ser-473 is involved in 4-HPR-mediated apoptosis in NB4 cells. Free Radic Biol Med 47(5):536–547. https://doi.org/10.1016/j.freeradbiomed.2009.05.024

Chang HT, Chou CT, Kuo DH, Shieh P, Jan CR, Liang WZ (2015) The mechanism of Ca(2+) movement in the involvement of baicalein-induced cytotoxicity in ZR-75-1 human breast cancer cells. J Nat Prod 78(7):1624–1634. https://doi.org/10.1021/acs.jnatprod.5b00173

Chen HM, Chang FR, Hsieh YC, Cheng YJ, Hsieh KC, Tsai LM, Lin AS, Wu YC, Yuan SS (2011) A novel synthetic protoapigenone analogue, WYC02-9, induces DNA damage and apoptosis in DU145 prostate cancer cells through generation of reactive oxygen species. Free Radic Biol Med 50(9):1151–1162. https://doi.org/10.1016/j.freeradbiomed.2011.01.015

Chen WC, Kuo TH, Tzeng YS, Tsai YC (2012) Baicalin induces apoptosis in SW620 human colorectal carcinoma cells in vitro and suppresses tumor growth in vivo. Molecules 17(4):3844–3857. https://doi.org/10.3390/molecules17043844

Chiao C, Carothers AM, Grunberger D, Solomon G, Preston GA, Barrett JC (1995) Apoptosis and altered redox state induced by caffeic acid phenethyl ester (CAPE) in transformed rat fibroblast cells. Cancer Res 55(16):3576–3583

Cuadrado A, Garcia-Fernandez LF, Gonzalez L, Suarez Y, Losada A, Alcaide V, Martinez T, Fernandez-Sousa JM, Sanchez-Puelles JM, Munoz A (2003) Aplidin induces apoptosis in human cancer cells via glutathione depletion and sustained activation of the epidermal growth factor receptor, Src, JNK, and p38 MAPK. J Biol Chem 278(1):241–250. https://doi.org/10.1074/jbc.M201010200

Dai Y, Xiong X, Huang G, Liu J, Sheng S, Wang H, Qin W (2014) Dichloroacetate enhances adriamycin-induced hepatoma cell toxicity in vitro and in vivo by increasing reactive oxygen species levels. PLoS One 9(4):e92962. https://doi.org/10.1371/journal.pone.0092962

Daniels-Wells TR, Helguera G, Rodriguez JA, Leoh LS, Erb MA, Diamante G, Casero D, Pellegrini M, Martinez-Maza O, Penichet ML (2013) Insights into the mechanism of cell death induced by saporin delivered into cancer cells by an antibody fusion protein targeting the transferrin receptor 1. Toxicol In Vitro 27(1):220–231. https://doi.org/10.1016/j.tiv.2012.10.006

Di Maio R, Mastroberardino PG, Hu X, Montero LM, Greenamyre JT (2013) Thiol oxidation and altered NR2B/NMDA receptor functions in in vitro and in vivo pilocarpine models: implications for epileptogenesis. Neurobiol Dis 49:87–98. https://doi.org/10.1016/j.nbd.2012.07.013

Downs I, Liu J, Aw TY, Adegboyega PA, Ajuebor MN (2012) The ROS scavenger, NAC, regulates hepatic Valpha14iNKT cells signaling during Fas mAb-dependent fulminant liver failure. PLoS One 7(6):e38051. https://doi.org/10.1371/journal.pone.0038051

El-Sayed el SM, Abdel-Aziz AA, Helal GK, Saleh S, Saad AS (2010) Protective effect of N-acetylcysteine against carmustine-induced myelotoxicity in rats. Food Chem Toxicol 48(6):1576–1580. https://doi.org/10.1016/j.fct.2010.03.027

Ferrari G, Yan CY, Greene LA (1995) N-acetylcysteine (D- and L-stereoisomers) prevents apoptotic death of neuronal cells. J Neurosci 15(4):2857–2866

Fu L, Lin YD, Elrod HA, Yue P, Oh Y, Li B, Tao H, Chen GZ, Shin DM, Khuri FR, Sun SY (2010a) c-Jun NH2-terminal kinase-dependent upregulation of DR5 mediates cooperative induction of apoptosis by perifosine and TRAIL. Mol Cancer 9:315. https://doi.org/10.1186/1476-4598-9-315

Fu YQ, Fang F, Lu ZY, Kuang FW, Xu F (2010b) N-acetylcysteine protects alveolar epithelial cells from hydrogen peroxide-induced apoptosis through scavenging reactive oxygen species and suppressing c-Jun N-terminal kinase. Exp Lung Res 36(6):352–361. https://doi.org/10.3109/01902141003678582

Fu Z, Guo J, Jing L, Li R, Zhang T, Peng S (2010c) Enhanced toxicity and ROS generation by doxorubicin in primary cultures of cardiomyocytes from neonatal metallothionein-I/II null mice. Toxicol In Vitro 24(6):1584–1591. https://doi.org/10.1016/j.tiv.2010.06.009

Galhardo MA, Junior CQ, Riboli Navarro PG, Morello RJ, Simoes Mde J, Montero EF (2007) Liver and lung late alterations following hepatic reperfusion associated to ischemic preconditioning or N-acetylcysteine. Microsurgery 27(4):295–299. https://doi.org/10.1002/micr.20359

Ge XY, Yang LQ, Jiang Y, Yang WW, Fu J, Li SL (2014) Reactive oxygen species and autophagy associated apoptosis and limitation of clonogenic survival induced by zoledronic acid in salivary adenoid cystic carcinoma cell line SACC-83. PLoS One 9(6):e101207. https://doi.org/10.1371/journal.pone.0101207

Guo R, Lin J, Xu W, Shen N, Mo L, Zhang C, Feng J (2013) Hydrogen sulfide attenuates doxorubicin-induced cardiotoxicity by inhibition of the p38 MAPK pathway in H9c2 cells. Int J Mol Med 31(3):644–650. https://doi.org/10.3892/ijmm.2013.1246

Hahm ER, Sakao K, Singh SV (2014) Honokiol activates reactive oxygen species-mediated cytoprotective autophagy in human prostate cancer cells. Prostate 74(12):1209–1221. https://doi.org/10.1002/pros.22837

Hizoh I, Haller C (2002) Radiocontrast-induced renal tubular cell apoptosis: hypertonic versus oxidative stress. Investig Radiol 37(8):428–434

Huwiler A, Boddinghaus B, Pautz A, Dorsch S, Franzen R, Briner VA, Brade V, Pfeilschifter J (2001) Superoxide potently induces ceramide formation in glomerular endothelial cells. Biochem Biophys Res Commun 284(2):404–410. https://doi.org/10.1006/bbrc.2001.4941

Ing DJ, Zang J, Dzau VJ, Webster KA, Bishopric NH (1999) Modulation of cytokine-induced cardiac myocyte apoptosis by nitric oxide, Bak, and Bcl-x. Circ Res 84(1):21–33

Inserte J, Taimor G, Hofstaetter B, Garcia-Dorado D, Piper HM (2000) Influence of simulated ischemia on apoptosis induction by oxidative stress in adult cardiomyocytes of rats. Am J Physiol Heart Circ Physiol 278(1):H94–H99

Isakovic A, Markovic Z, Todorovic-Markovic B, Nikolic N, Vranjes-Djuric S, Mirkovic M, Dramicanin M, Harhaji L, Raicevic N, Nikolic Z, Trajkovic V (2006) Distinct cytotoxic mechanisms of pristine versus hydroxylated fullerene. Toxicol Sci 91(1):173–183. https://doi.org/10.1093/toxsci/kfj127

Jin Y, Lu Z, Ding K, Li J, Du X, Chen C, Sun X, Wu Y, Zhou J, Pan J (2010) Antineoplastic mechanisms of niclosamide in acute myelogenous leukemia stem cells: inactivation of the NF-kappaB pathway and generation of reactive oxygen species. Cancer Res 70(6):2516–2527. https://doi.org/10.1158/0008-5472.can-09-3950

Jin HM, Zhou DC, Gu HF, Qiao QY, Fu SK, Liu XL, Pan Y (2013) Antioxidant N-acetylcysteine protects pancreatic beta-cells against aldosterone-induced oxidative stress and apoptosis in female db/db mice and insulin-producing MIN6 cells. Endocrinology 154(11):4068–4077. https://doi.org/10.1210/en.2013-1115

Kato Y, Salumbides BC, Wang XF, Qian DZ, Williams S, Wei Y, Sanni TB, Atadja P, Pili R (2007) Antitumor effect of the histone deacetylase inhibitor LAQ824 in combination with 13-cis-retinoic acid in human malignant melanoma. Mol Cancer Ther 6(1):70–81. https://doi.org/10.1158/1535-7163.mct-06-0125

Khan M, Sekhon B, Jatana M, Giri S, Gilg AG, Sekhon C, Singh I, Singh AK (2004) Administration of N-acetylcysteine after focal cerebral ischemia protects brain and reduces inflammation in a rat model of experimental stroke. J Neurosci Res 76(4):519–527. https://doi.org/10.1002/jnr.20087

Kim JH, Lee SS, Jung MH, Yeo HD, Kim HJ, Yang JI, Roh GS, Chang SH, Park DJ (2010) N-acetylcysteine attenuates glycerol-induced acute kidney injury by regulating MAPKs and Bcl-2 family proteins. Nephrol Dial Transplant 25(5):1435–1443. https://doi.org/10.1093/ndt/gfp659

Kin H, Wang NP, Halkos ME, Kerendi F, Guyton RA, Zhao ZQ (2006) Neutrophil depletion reduces myocardial apoptosis and attenuates NFkappaB activation/TNFalpha release after ischemia and reperfusion. J Surg Res 135(1):170–178. https://doi.org/10.1016/j.jss.2006.02.019

Kin H, Wang NP, Mykytenko J, Reeves J, Deneve J, Jiang R, Zatta AJ, Guyton RA, Vinten-Johansen J, Zhao ZQ (2008) Inhibition of myocardial apoptosis by postconditioning is associated with attenuation of oxidative stress-mediated nuclear factor-kappa B translocation and TNF alpha release. Shock 29(6):761–768. https://doi.org/10.1097/SHK.0b013e31815cfd5a

Klass O, Fischer UM, Antonyan A, Bosse M, Fischer JH, Bloch W, Mehlhorn U (2007) Pneumocyte apoptosis induction during cardiopulmonary bypass: effective prevention by radical scavenging using N-acetylcysteine. J Investig Surg 20(6):349–356. https://doi.org/10.1080/08941930701772165

Laouar A, Glesne D, Huberman E (1999) Involvement of protein kinase C-beta and ceramide in tumor necrosis factor-alpha-induced but not Fas-induced apoptosis of human myeloid leukemia cells. J Biol Chem 274(33):23526–23534

Lau ST, Lin ZX, Leung PS (2010) Role of reactive oxygen species in brucein D-mediated p38-mitogen-activated protein kinase and nuclear factor-kappaB signalling pathways in human pancreatic adenocarcinoma cells. Br J Cancer 102(3):583–593. https://doi.org/10.1038/sj.bjc.6605487

Lee BS, Kang SU, Hwang HS, Kim YS, Sung ES, Shin YS, Lim YC, Kim CH (2012) An agonistic antibody to human death receptor 4 induces apoptotic cell death in head and neck cancer cells through mitochondrial ROS generation. Cancer Lett 322(1):45–57. https://doi.org/10.1016/j.canlet.2012.02.007

Lesiak K, Koprowska K, Zalesna I, Nejc D, Duchler M, Czyz M (2010) Parthenolide, a sesquiterpene lactone from the medical herb feverfew, shows anticancer activity against human melanoma cells in vitro. Melanoma Res 20(1):21–34. https://doi.org/10.1097/CMR.0b013e328333bbe4

Li L, Yue GG, Pu JX, Sun HD, Fung KP, Leung PC, Han QB, Lau CB, Leung PS (2014) Eriocalyxin B-induced apoptosis in pancreatic adenocarcinoma cells through thiol-containing antioxidant systems and downstream signalling pathways. Curr Mol Med 14(5):673–689

Liao YJ, Bai HY, Li ZH, Zou J, Chen JW, Zheng F, Zhang JX, Mai SJ, Zeng MS, Sun HD, Pu JX, Xie D (2014) Longikaurin A, a natural ent-kaurane, induces G2/M phase arrest via downregulation of Skp2 and apoptosis induction through ROS/JNK/c-Jun pathway in hepatocellular carcinoma cells. Cell Death Dis 5:e1137. https://doi.org/10.1038/cddis.2014.66

Lin H, Sue YM, Chou Y, Cheng CF, Chang CC, Li HF, Chen CC, Juan SH (2010) Activation of a nuclear factor of activated T-lymphocyte-3 (NFAT3) by oxidative stress in carboplatin-mediated renal apoptosis. Br J Pharmacol 161(7):1661–1676. https://doi.org/10.1111/j.1476-5381.2010.00989.x

Liu HN, Giasson BI, Mushynski WE, Almazan G (2002) AMPA receptor-mediated toxicity in oligodendrocyte progenitors involves free radical generation and activation of JNK, calpain and caspase 3. J Neurochem 82(2):398–409

Liu JQ, Lee TF, Chen C, Bagim DL, Cheung PY (2010) N-acetylcysteine improves hemodynamics and reduces oxidative stress in the brains of newborn piglets with hypoxia-reoxygenation injury. J Neurotrauma 27(10):1865–1873. https://doi.org/10.1089/neu.2010.1325

Liu H, Zhou BH, Qiu X, Wang HS, Zhang F, Fang R, Wang XF, Cai SH, Du J, Bu XZ (2012) T63, a new 4-arylidene curcumin analogue, induces cell cycle arrest and apoptosis through activation of the reactive oxygen species-FOXO3a pathway in lung cancer cells. Free Radic Biol Med 53(12):2204–2217. https://doi.org/10.1016/j.freeradbiomed.2012.10.537

Liu C, Wan X, Ye T, Fang F, Chen X, Chen Y, Dong Y (2014) Matrix metalloproteinase 2 contributes to pancreatic Beta cell injury induced by oxidative stress. PLoS One 9(10):e110227. https://doi.org/10.1371/journal.pone.0110227

Luo J, Tsuji T, Yasuda H, Sun Y, Fujigaki Y, Hishida A (2008) The molecular mechanisms of the attenuation of cisplatin-induced acute renal failure by N-acetylcysteine in rats. Nephrol Dial Transplant 23(7):2198–2205. https://doi.org/10.1093/ndt/gfn090

Ma T, Zhu J, Chen X, Zha D, Singhal PC, Ding G (2013) High glucose induces autophagy in podocytes. Exp Cell Res 319(6):779–789. https://doi.org/10.1016/j.yexcr.2013.01.018

Mao X, Wang T, Liu Y, Irwin MG, Ou JS, Liao XL, Gao X, Xu Y, Ng KF, Vanhoutte PM, Xia Z (2013) N-acetylcysteine and allopurinol confer synergy in attenuating myocardial ischemia injury via restoring HIF-1alpha/HO-1 signaling in diabetic rats. PLoS One 8(7):e68949. https://doi.org/10.1371/journal.pone.0068949

Martin H, Abadie C, Heyd B, Mantion G, Richert L, Berthelot A (2006) N-acetylcysteine partially reverses oxidative stress and apoptosis exacerbated by Mg-deficiency culturing conditions in primary cultures of rat and human hepatocytes. J Am Coll Nutr 25(5):363–369

Messier EM, Day BJ, Bahmed K, Kleeberger SR, Tuder RM, Bowler RP, Chu HW, Mason RJ, Kosmider B (2013) N-acetylcysteine protects murine alveolar type II cells from cigarette smoke injury in a nuclear erythroid 2-related factor-2-independent manner. Am J Respir Cell Mol Biol 48(5):559–567. https://doi.org/10.1165/rcmb.2012-0295OC

Milacic V, Chen D, Ronconi L, Landis-Piwowar KR, Fregona D, Dou QP (2006) A novel anticancer gold(III) dithiocarbamate compound inhibits the activity of a purified 20S proteasome and 26S proteasome in human breast cancer cell cultures and xenografts. Cancer Res 66(21):10478–10486. https://doi.org/10.1158/0008-5472.can-06-3017

Moon C, Lee YJ, Park HJ, Chong YH, Kang JL (2010) N-acetylcysteine inhibits RhoA and promotes apoptotic cell clearance during intense lung inflammation. Am J Respir Crit Care Med 181(4):374–387. https://doi.org/10.1164/rccm.200907-1061OC

Naziroglu M, Senol N, Ghazizadeh V, Yuruker V (2014) Neuroprotection induced by N-acetylcysteine and selenium against traumatic brain injury-induced apoptosis and calcium entry in hippocampus of rat. Cell Mol Neurobiol 34(6):895–903. https://doi.org/10.1007/s10571-014-0069-2

Nitobe J, Yamaguchi S, Okuyama M, Nozaki N, Sata M, Miyamoto T, Takeishi Y, Kubota I, Tomoike H (2003) Reactive oxygen species regulate FLICE inhibitory protein (FLIP) and susceptibility to Fas-mediated apoptosis in cardiac myocytes. Cardiovasc Res 57(1):119–128

Ozdulger A, Cinel I, Koksel O, Cinel L, Avlan D, Unlu A, Okcu H, Dikmengil M, Oral U (2003) The protective effect of N-acetylcysteine on apoptotic lung injury in cecal ligation and puncture-induced sepsis model. Shock 19(4):366–372

Panda PK, Mukhopadhyay S, Behera B, Bhol CS, Dey S, Das DN, Sinha N, Bissoyi A, Pramanik K, Maiti TK, Bhutia SK (2014) Antitumor effect of soybean lectin mediated through reactive oxygen species-dependent pathway. Life Sci 111(1-2):27–35. https://doi.org/10.1016/j.lfs.2014.07.004

Park SA, Choi KS, Bang JH, Huh K, Kim SU (2000) Cisplatin-induced apoptotic cell death in mouse hybrid neurons is blocked by antioxidants through suppression of cisplatin-mediated accumulation of p53 but not of Fas/Fas ligand. J Neurochem 75(3):946–953

Park MH, Jo M, Won D, Song HS, Song MJ, Hong JT (2012) Snake venom toxin from Vipera lebetina turanica sensitizes cancer cells to TRAIL through ROS- and JNK-mediated upregulation of death receptors and downregulation of survival proteins. Apoptosis 17(12):1316–1326. https://doi.org/10.1007/s10495-012-0759-5

Pathania D, Kuang Y, Sechi M, Neamati N (2015) Mechanisms underlying the cytotoxicity of a novel quinazolinedione-based redox modulator, QD232, in pancreatic cancer cells. Br J Pharmacol 172(1):50–63. https://doi.org/10.1111/bph.12855

Pawlas N, Malecki A (2009) Neuroprotective effect of N-acetylcysteine in neurons exposed to arachidonic acid during simulated ischemia in vitro. Pharmacol Rep 61(4):743–750

Peng YW, Buller CL, Charpie JR (2011) Impact of N-acetylcysteine on neonatal cardiomyocyte ischemia-reperfusion injury. Pediatr Res 70(1):61–66. https://doi.org/10.1203/PDR.0b013e31821b1a92

Prehn JH, Jordan J, Ghadge GD, Preis E, Galindo MF, Roos RP, Krieglstein J, Miller RJ (1997) Ca2+ and reactive oxygen species in staurosporine-induced neuronal apoptosis. J Neurochem 68(4):1679–1685

Qu X, Li Q, Wang X, Yang X, Wang D (2013) N-acetylcysteine attenuates cardiopulmonary bypass-induced lung injury in dogs. J Cardiothorac Surg 8:107. https://doi.org/10.1186/1749-8090-8-107

Reid AJ, Shawcross SG, Hamilton AE, Wiberg M, Terenghi G (2009) N-acetylcysteine alters apoptotic gene expression in axotomised primary sensory afferent subpopulations. Neurosci Res 65(2):148–155. https://doi.org/10.1016/j.neures.2009.06.008

Risso PS, Koike MK, Abrahao Mde S, Ferreira NC, Montero EF (2014) The effect of n-acetylcysteine on hepatic histomorphology during hypothermic preservation. Acta Cir Bras 29(Suppl 3):28–32

Roh JL, Kim EH, Park JY, Kim JW, Kwon M, Lee BH (2014) Piperlongumine selectively kills cancer cells and increases cisplatin antitumor activity in head and neck cancer. Oncotarget 5(19):9227–9238. https://doi.org/10.18632/oncotarget.2402

Romano G, Briguori C, Quintavalle C, Zanca C, Rivera NV, Colombo A, Condorelli G (2008) Contrast agents and renal cell apoptosis. Eur Heart J 29(20):2569–2576. https://doi.org/10.1093/eurheartj/ehn197

Rudiger HA, Graf R, Clavien PA (2003) Sub-lethal oxidative stress triggers the protective effects of ischemic preconditioning in the mouse liver. J Hepatol 39(6):972–977

Seril DN, Liao J, Ho KL, Yang CS, Yang GY (2002) Inhibition of chronic ulcerative colitis-associated colorectal adenocarcinoma development in a murine model by N-acetylcysteine. Carcinogenesis 23(6):993–1001

Shen WH, Zhang CY, Zhang GY (2003) Antioxidants attenuate reperfusion injury after global brain ischemia through inhibiting nuclear factor-kappa B activity in rats. Acta Pharmacol Sin 24(11):1125–1130

Shi Y, Sahu RP, Srivastava SK (2008) Triphala inhibits both in vitro and in vivo xenograft growth of pancreatic tumor cells by inducing apoptosis. BMC Cancer 8:294. https://doi.org/10.1186/1471-2407-8-294

Singh I, Pahan K, Khan M, Singh AK (1998) Cytokine-mediated induction of ceramide production is redox-sensitive. Implications to proinflammatory cytokine-mediated apoptosis in demyelinating diseases. J Biol Chem 273(32):20354–20362

Sun L, Gu L, Wang S, Yuan J, Yang H, Zhu J, Zhang H (2012) N-acetylcysteine protects against apoptosis through modulation of group I metabotropic glutamate receptor activity. PLoS One 7(3):e32503. https://doi.org/10.1371/journal.pone.0032503

Sun Y, Pu LY, Lu L, Wang XH, Zhang F, Rao JH (2014) N-acetylcysteine attenuates reactive-oxygen-species-mediated endoplasmic reticulum stress during liver ischemia-reperfusion injury. World J Gastroenterol 20(41):15289–15298. https://doi.org/10.3748/wjg.v20.i41.15289

Syrkina O, Jafari B, Hales CA, Quinn DA (2008) Oxidant stress mediates inflammation and apoptosis in ventilator-induced lung injury. Respirology 13(3):333–340. https://doi.org/10.1111/j.1440-1843.2008.01279.x

Tang Y, Chen R, Huang Y, Li G, Huang Y, Chen J, Duan L, Zhu BT, Thrasher JB, Zhang X, Li B (2014) Natural compound Alternol induces oxidative stress-dependent apoptotic cell death preferentially in prostate cancer cells. Mol Cancer Ther 13(6):1526–1536. https://doi.org/10.1158/1535-7163.mct-13-0981

Tayman C, Tonbul A, Kosus A, Hirfanoglu IM, Uysal S, Haltas H, Tatli MM, Andiran F (2012) N-acetylcysteine may prevent severe intestinal damage in necrotizing enterocolitis. J Pediatr Surg 47(3):540–550. https://doi.org/10.1016/j.jpedsurg.2011.09.051

Wang H, Xu DX, Lu JW, Zhao L, Zhang C, Wei W (2007a) N-acetylcysteine attenuates lipopolysaccharide-induced apoptotic liver damage in D-galactosamine-sensitized mice. Acta Pharmacol Sin 28(11):1803–1809

Wang X, Svedin P, Nie C, Lapatto R, Zhu C, Gustavsson M, Sandberg M, Karlsson JO, Romero R, Hagberg H, Mallard C (2007b) N-acetylcysteine reduces lipopolysaccharide-sensitized hypoxic-ischemic brain injury. Ann Neurol 61(3):263–271. https://doi.org/10.1002/ana.21066

Wang Q, Zhang X, Ding Q, Hu B, Xie Y, Li X, Yang Q, Xiong L (2011) Limb remote postconditioning alleviates cerebral reperfusion injury through reactive oxygen species-mediated inhibition of delta protein kinase C in rats. Anesth Analg 113(5):1180–1187. https://doi.org/10.1213/ANE.0b013e31822b885f

Wang R, Liang S, Yue H, Chen L (2012) Using a novel in vivo model to study the function of nuclear factor kappa B in cerebral ischemic injury. Med Sci Monit 18(11):BR461–BR467

Wang HW, Yang W, Lu JY, Li F, Sun JZ, Zhang W, Guo NN, Gao L, Kang JR (2013a) N-acetylcysteine administration is associated with reduced activation of NF-kB and preserves lung dendritic cells function in a zymosan-induced generalized inflammation model. J Clin Immunol 33(3):649–660. https://doi.org/10.1007/s10875-012-9852-3

Wang Q, Hou Y, Yi D, Wang L, Ding B, Chen X, Long M, Liu Y, Wu G (2013b) Protective effects of N-acetylcysteine on acetic acid-induced colitis in a porcine model. BMC Gastroenterol 13:133. https://doi.org/10.1186/1471-230x-13-133

Wang Y, Tang Q, Jiang S, Li M, Wang X (2013c) Anti-colorectal cancer activity of macrostemonoside A mediated by reactive oxygen species. Biochem Biophys Res Commun 441(4):825–830. https://doi.org/10.1016/j.bbrc.2013.10.148

Wang C, Chen K, Xia Y, Dai W, Wang F, Shen M, Cheng P, Wang J, Lu J, Zhang Y, Yang J, Zhu R, Zhang H, Li J, Zheng Y, Zhou Y, Guo C (2014) N-acetylcysteine attenuates ischemia-reperfusion-induced apoptosis and autophagy in mouse liver via regulation of the ROS/JNK/Bcl-2 pathway. PLoS One 9(9):e108855. https://doi.org/10.1371/journal.pone.0108855

Wu CT, Sheu ML, Tsai KS, Chiang CK, Liu SH (2011) Salubrinal, an eIF2alpha dephosphorylation inhibitor, enhances cisplatin-induced oxidative stress and nephrotoxicity in a mouse model. Free Radic Biol Med 51(3):671–680. https://doi.org/10.1016/j.freeradbiomed.2011.04.038

Wu XY, Luo AY, Zhou YR, Ren JH (2014) N-acetylcysteine reduces oxidative stress, nuclear factorkappaB activity and cardiomyocyte apoptosis in heart failure. Mol Med Rep 10(2):615–624. https://doi.org/10.3892/mmr.2014.2292

Xiao T, Choudhary S, Zhang W, Ansari NH, Salahudeen A (2003) Possible involvement of oxidative stress in cisplatin-induced apoptosis in LLC-PK1 cells. J Toxicol Environ Health A 66(5):469–479. https://doi.org/10.1080/15287390306449

Xie SQ, Wang JH, Ma HX, Cheng PF, Zhao J, Wang CJ (2009) Polyamine transporter recognition and antitumor effects of anthracenymethyl homospermidine. Toxicology 263(2-3):127–133. https://doi.org/10.1016/j.tox.2009.07.001

Xie J, Zhou X, Hu X, Jiang H (2014) H2O2 evokes injury of cardiomyocytes through upregulating HMGB1. Hell J Cardiol 55(2):101–106

Yang Y, Yang D, Yang D, Jia R, Ding G (2014) Role of reactive oxygen species-mediated endoplasmic reticulum stress in contrast-induced renal tubular cell apoptosis. Nephron Exp Nephrol 128(1-2):30–36. https://doi.org/10.1159/000366063

Zhang L, Sharma S, Zhu LX, Kogai T, Hershman JM, Brent GA, Dubinett SM, Huang M (2003) Nonradioactive iodide effectively induces apoptosis in genetically modified lung cancer cells. Cancer Res 63(16):5065–5072

Zhang LH, Jia YL, Lin XX, Zhang HQ, Dong XW, Zhao JM, Shen J, Shen HJ, Li FF, Yan XF, Li W, Zhao YQ, Xie QM (2013) AD-1, a novel ginsenoside derivative, shows anti-lung cancer activity via activation of p38 MAPK pathway and generation of reactive oxygen species. Biochim Biophys Acta 1830(8):4148–4159. https://doi.org/10.1016/j.bbagen.2013.04.008

Zhang L, Zhu Z, Liu J, Zhu Z, Hu Z (2014) Protective effect of N-acetylcysteine (NAC) on renal ischemia/reperfusion injury through Nrf2 signaling pathway. J Recept Signal Transduct Res 34(5):396–400. https://doi.org/10.3109/10799893.2014.908916

Inflammation

Rabindra Tirouvanziam

7.1 Inflammation: Working Definition and Organizing Principles

The term "inflammation" can have various meanings. For patients and clinicians, inflammation designates organ-level or systemic responses associated with acute or chronic symptoms in diseases as varied as asthma, rheumatoid arthritis, inflammatory bowel disease, or autism. For basic researchers, inflammation relates to the induction of specific genes in structural components of tissues, and the recruitment and activation of immune cells mediating a reaction to self-injury or infection, leading to the symptoms noted above. Seminal work redefined the signals that induce inflammation in living organisms, introducing the concept of danger signaling (Gallucci and Matzinger 2001). Danger signaling is mediated by pathogen-associated molecular patterns (PAMPs) and/or damage-associated molecular patterns (DAMPs), for which tissue and immune cells have evolved pattern recognition receptors (PRRs) that trigger relevant responses upon PAMP/DAMP ligation (Vajjhala et al. 2017).

Downstream of PRR activation, multiple pathways are induced that regulate cellular and organismal defense and reparative responses to the perceived danger. Pro-inflammatory pathways mediate feed-forward and amplifying signals in activated cells and organs involved in an inflammatory reaction. Resilience pathways counterbalance the effect of the former, enabling the use of resources for adaptive and reparative mechanisms. Both pro-inflammatory and resilience pathways are enabled by changes in metabolic pathways, which modulate use of energy resources to

R. Tirouvanziam
Center for CF and Airways Disease Research, Children's Healthcare of Atlanta, Atlanta, GA, USA

Department of Pediatrics, Emory University School of Medicine, Atlanta, GA, USA
e-mail: tirouvanziam@emory.edu

© Springer Nature Singapore Pte Ltd. 2019
R. E. Frye, M. Berk (eds.), *The Therapeutic Use of N-Acetylcysteine (NAC) in Medicine*, https://doi.org/10.1007/978-981-10-5311-5_7

enable proper amplification of signaling and downstream effector functions. Regulation of pro-inflammatory, resilience, and metabolic pathways in inflammation depends on posttranslational modification (PTM) of proteins, of which phosphorylation of tyrosine, serine, and threonine residues has been the most studied (Liu et al. 2016). Besides phosphorylation, oxidation/reduction of cysteine, selenocysteine, and methionine residues is also an essential regulatory mechanism (Rahman et al. 2005). Consequently, basic and clinical researchers for more than three decades have attempted to modulate inflammation through redox agents, including, but not limited to, N-Acetylcysteine (NAC).

7.2 NAC: Cysteine/Glutathione Prodrug and "Suicide Antioxidant"

NAC is an intermediate of cysteine metabolism and a popular prodrug used to rapidly ramp up cysteine levels in the body and thereby increase the antioxidant shield (Atkuri et al. 2007; Rushworth and Megson 2014). Cysteine bears a reactive SH group that can participate in redox reactions. Oxidation of cysteine gives rise to its disulfide bond-bearing counterpart, cystine. The cysteine/cystine redox couple is the most abundant in human plasma. In cells, however, the most abundant redox couple is formed by glutathione (GSH) and glutathione disulfide (GSSG). GSH is a tripeptide formed by glutamate, cysteine, and glycine, in which the central cysteine is relatively protected from spontaneous oxidation. Cells have evolved a whole array of enzymes to synthesize, oxidize, and conjugate GSH to provide reparative and detoxifying power to cells and reduce GSSG back into GSH (Couto et al. 2016). GSSG reduction into GSH uses NADPH as an electron donor (Kojer and Riemer 2014). Interestingly, NADPH is also used as an electron donor by the major inflammatory enzyme NADPH oxidase, which uses NAPDH to reduce molecular oxygen into superoxide, the first step in the production of reactive oxygen species (ROS) such as hydrogen peroxide, hydroxyl radical, and hypohalous acids (Winterbourn et al. 2016). Thus, NADPH can be used either to reduce oxidation by maintaining GSH levels or reduce oxygen to produce ROS, thereby shifting the redox balance toward oxidation and the oxygen balance toward hypoxia, causing cells to effectively pivot from a homeostatic/reparative state to an oxidative/destructive state and *vice versa.*

GSH synthesis occurs in all cells, but the liver in humans is essential to maintaining appropriate circulating GSH levels (Lu 1999). Since cysteine is relatively rare in the diet, it is the rate-limiting amino acid for GSH synthesis (Yin et al. 2016). Dietary cysteine is taken up in the intestine and shuttled via the portal route from the intestine to the liver. While dietary cysteine needs to be actively taken up by ATP-dependent processes through the intestinal epithelium, oral NAC passively diffuses through the plasma membrane of intestinal epithelial cells thanks to its *N*-acetyl moiety, making it an efficient cysteine and GSH prodrug (Fig. 7.1). Once in the cytosol of intestinal epithelial cells, NAC loses its *N*-acetyl group under cytosolic esterase activity, and the resulting cysteine is then transported to the liver and integrated into GSH or circulates in blood. The surface area in the human intestine is

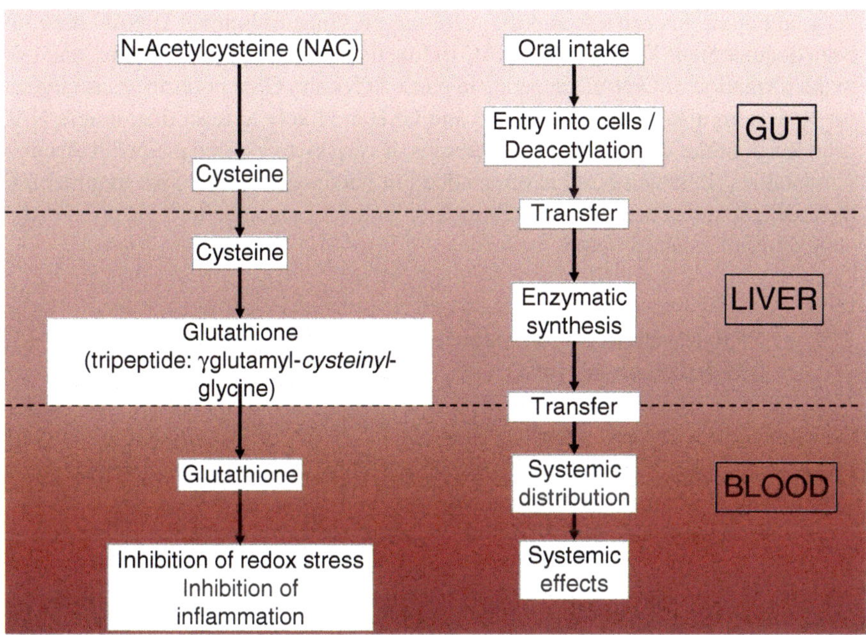

Fig. 7.1 **Mechanism of action of oral NAC.** Oral NAC is passively absorbed through the intestinal epithelium and deacetylated intracellularly, yielding cysteine. Cysteine is then transported to the liver via first-pass metabolism (portal route) and used to synthesize GSH. The liver serves as a source for systemic GSH, which is made available for other tissues in the body for redox metabolism

very high, such that high doses of NAC (hundreds of mg per day) can be administered orally with little risk (Greene et al. 2016). Consequently, plasma NAC remains low to undetectable after oral NAC administration (Pendyala and Creaven 1995). NAC can also be delivered intravenously, notably for acetaminophen overdose and contrast agent-induced nephrotoxicity, or as a mucolytic through oral or inhalation routes for acute and chronic obstructive airway diseases (Rushworth and Megson 2014). NAC skin creams are also available over the counter and have been tested in some animal models (Tsai et al. 2014). As an intravenous drug, NAC serves partially as a cysteine/GSH prodrug during its passage in the liver and partially as an electron donor to directly reduce oxidized molecules (e.g., antagonizing toxic acetaminophen adducts). The resulting oxidation of NAC leads to the formation of its disulfide form, N,N'-diacetyl-cystine (DiNAC). As a topical drug, NAC functions almost exclusively as an electron donor to reduce oxidized and/or cross-linked proteins, such as airway mucins. Unlike GSSG, DiNAC is not easily reduced, essentially making a large fraction of NAC delivered through topical routes a "suicide antioxidant," available for only one redox reaction. DiNAC itself has chemical properties that make it a potent mediator in its own right (Pettersson et al. 2008).

Theoretically, a portion of NAC delivered through the oral route may directly react with intestinal mucins, bacteria, and the apical surface of intestinal epithelial cells, although this process and the resulting presence of luminal DiNAC have not been documented. The ability of NAC to function as a suicide antioxidant, and lead to the formation of DiNAC, depends in part on Cys and GSH pools in areas targeted for NAC administration. Indeed, Cys and GSH are likely to react first, unless NAC is added in molar excess. For these reasons, it is risky to extrapolate results from *in vitro* studies (in which NAC is often added in wide excess) to *in vivo* treatment, as the mechanisms of action of NAC can widely differ among them. This point is discussed in more details below.

7.3   PRR-Medicated Induction of Inflammation and Its Modulation by NAC

Inflammation is controlled by the ligation of PRRs by PAMPs and/or DAMPs (Vajjhala et al. 2017). PAMPs are generated by both commensal and newly acquired (and potentially harmful) bacteria, fungi, and sometimes more complex life-forms (e.g., protozoans or nematodes) and inform hosts on their density and activity (Rana et al. 2015). Prototypical PAMPs are lipopolysaccharide (LPS) and flagellin (both expressed by gram-negative bacteria) and lipoteichoic acid (expressed by fungi). PAMP signaling often requires dual or multiple, rather than single, stimuli (Odendall and Kagan 2017). Interestingly, PAMPs do not only signal the presence of pathogenic microorganisms but also that of commensals, thereby promoting the maintenance of adequate passive or active shielding mechanisms against invasion (Sharma et al. 2010). Therefore, modulating PAMP signaling can affect both homeostatic and inflammatory responses.

DAMPs, also designated as "alarmins," include various molecules derived from host cells that, when released into the extracellular milieu, signal the abnormal breakdown of cells, and thus significant stress, thereby calling for an organized, reparative response (Rider et al. 2017). Interestingly, some DAMPs can also tune down shielding mechanisms during a short period of postnatal colonization to enable establishment of commensalism without triggering septic reactions (Ulas et al. 2017). Examples of DAMPs include interleukin (IL)-1, IL-33, cytosolic calcium-binding proteins of the S100A family, and the nuclear factor high-mobility group box protein 1 (HMGB1) (Bertheloot and Latz 2017). Often, DAMPs are modified through redox chemistry by ROS produced during cell activation and can accumulate both inside and outside stressed cells (Li et al. 2013). HMGB1 exemplifies the importance of redox chemistry in DAMP signaling, since its roles as a chemoattractant for inflammatory cells and an activator of the receptor for advanced glycation end product (RAGE) pathway shift depending on it being present in its reduced form, partially oxidized and disulfide bond-bearing form, or fully oxidized, denatured form (Janko et al. 2014). Extracellular release of HMGB1 depends on the cell's redox balance, which can potentially be impacted by NAC (Gabryel et al. 2011).

Toll-like receptor 4 (TLR4) is a member of the TLR family of surface and endosomal PRRs and a prototypical example of how PRRs function. TLR4 is the main PRR for LPS, aided by the co-receptor CD14 and the adaptor molecules lipid-binding protein and MD2 (Ryu et al. 2017). However, TLR4 has also emerged recently as a promiscuous receptor for multiple DAMPs, following either direct ligation or indirect activation by a co-receptor. For example, TLR4 can be ligated by S100A8/S100A9 (Pruenster et al. 2016), as well as HMGB1 (Sims et al. 2010). Of relevance here, TLRs bear critical cysteine residues that regulate their activation, and NAC treatment has been described, depending on models and specific TLRs, to either preserve TLR activity in the face of denaturation by specific oxidants (Kim et al. 2009) or conversely prevent TLR hyperactivity in response to ROS signaling (Yoshino and Kashiwakura 2017). Extracellular ATP, a DAMP linked to host cell demise, is a strong inducer of another PRR family, that of the inflammasome, which also responds to PAMPs (de Torre-Minguela et al. 2017). Inflammasomes are formed upon ligand-induced aggregation of intracellular protein complexes leading to activation of cysteine aspartate proteases (caspases) and subsequent processing of the inflammatory mediators pro-IL-1 and pro-IL-18 into their mature forms. Signaling through the NLRP3 inflammasome, for example, can be promoted by intracellular ROS (Han et al. 2015) and antagonized by NAC (Liu et al. 2015). As another example of PRRs, recent literature has highlighted the role of scavenger receptors, of which several families are recognized (PrabhuDas et al. 2017). A key functional role is fulfilled by redox-sensitive C-terminal cysteine-rich domains in these scavenger receptors (Novakowski et al. 2016). Among these, CD36 has been studied in detail for its modulation by NAC. At the mRNA and protein levels, increased intracellular ROS levels increase CD36 expression, an effect antagonized by NAC treatment (Mimche et al. 2012). However, the exofacial domain of CD36 is regulated very precisely by the extracellular redox balance (itself modulated by NAC), with significant changes in conformation and binding mediated by oxidoreduction of critical cysteine residues (Gruarin et al. 2001). Interestingly, HMGB1 itself can also be recognized and taken up via scavenger receptors (in addition to RAGE and TLRs), triggering downstream signaling in macrophages (Komai et al. 2017). As illustrated by the above examples of TLR4, NLRP3 inflammasome, and CD36, it appears that PRRs are sensitive to redox signaling both intracellularly and extracellularly and therefore can be modulated by NAC treatment *in vitro* and in animal models.

7.4 Molecular Pathways of Inflammation and Their Modulation by NAC

Downstream of TLR4 ligation, a cascade of phosphorylation ensues involving multiple kinases and adaptor proteins, leading to the translocation of the nuclear factor kappa B (NFkB) family of transcription factors to the nucleus and subsequent transcription of response genes. These include, but are not limited to, pro-inflammatory cytokines and oxidative enzymes such as the proteins assembling into the NOX complex (Anrather et al. 2006). Intracellular ROS, generated by NOX activity [or alternatively by dual oxidase (Duox) activity or mitochondrial leak (O'Neill et al. 2015)], also converge onto mitogen-activated protein kinase (MAPK) pathways, which lead to the activation of the transcription factor activator protein-1 (AP-1) (Youn et al. 2016) and production of downstream mediators and effector proteins. In turn, newly formed mediators such as cytokines can trigger signaling through the Janus kinase (JAK)/signal transducer and activator of transcription (STAT) family of proteins (Majoros et al. 2017). NFkB, MAPK/AP-1, and JAK/STAT pathways collectively form a core of generally pro-inflammatory, feed-forward cascades that further increase inflammatory cell recruitment to a damaged tissue (Fig. 7.2). They also promote ROS production while depending on ROS to induce specific PTMs to some of their signaling components. Consistent with the central role of ROS and redox PTMs in the regulation and function of NFkB, MAPK/AP-1, and JAK/STAT pathways, NAC treatment has been used in numerous studies as a ROS-scavenging and down-modulating strategy to tune down signaling through these pathways (Amore et al. 2013; Park et al. 2012; Zafarullah et al. 2003).

As a set of coordinated measures to counteract potential damaging effects of pro-inflammatory pathways, cells and tissues undergoing inflammatory reactions also activate resilience pathways (Fig. 7.2). These include the heme oxygenase-1 (HO-1), hypoxia-inducible factor (HIF), aryl hydrocarbon receptor (AhR), and reverse strand of Erb (REV-ERB) signaling cascades (Kojetin and Burris 2014; Soares et al.

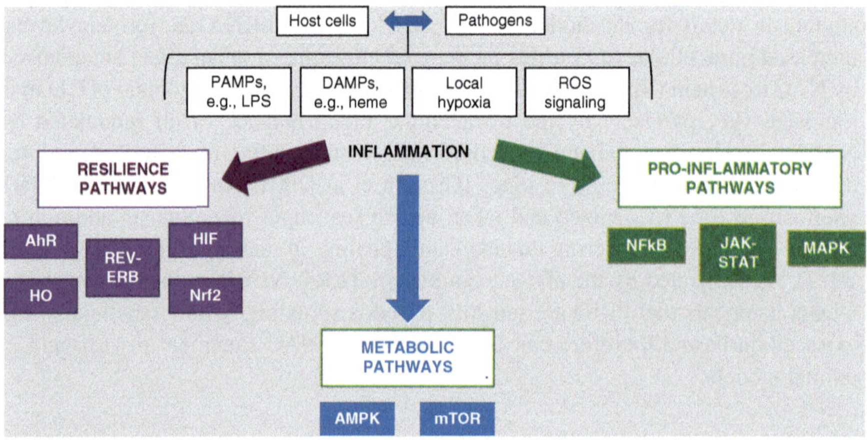

Fig. 7.2 Pro-inflammatory, resilience, and metabolism pathways involved in inflammation. Inflammation is triggered in response to insults involving host cells alone or in interaction with pathogens. Resulting changes in the presence of PAMPs and DAMPs as well as changes in oxygen levels (local hypoxia) and ROS signaling engage three sets of signaling pathways. Pro-inflammatory pathways (green, right) include the NFkB, JAK/STAT, and MAPK signaling cascades. Pro-inflammatory pathways promote leukocyte recruitment to tissues, increased ROS production, and deployment of effector functions such as phagocytosis and killing. Resilience pathways (purple, left) include the AhR, HIF, HO, Nrf2, and REV-ERB signaling cascades. Resilience pathways promote adaptive and reparative responses that guard against tissue damage and counteract potential negative effects of pro-inflammatory pathways. Finally, metabolic pathways (blue, center) include the AMPK and mTOR signaling cascades. Metabolic pathways license cells and tissues to use energy resources for mRNA translation, protein production, and various cellular activities (cell movement, uptake and secretion, mitosis) required during inflammatory reactions

2017). Typically, these pathways promote anti-inflammatory, tolerance, and repair responses when triggered by danger signals. For example, ROS directly trigger the translocation of the master regulator of antioxidant responses in cells, the transcription factor nuclear factor-erythroid 2-related factor 2 (Nrf2). Nrf2 controls numerous genes with antioxidant function, by binding on a consensus sequence in their promoter dubbed the antioxidant response element (ARE). Nrf2-/ARE-regulated genes include GSH synthase subunits, and GSH reductases, which regulate GSH turnover, as well as superoxide dismutase, and catalase, which controls the degradation of superoxide and hydrogen peroxide, respectively (Sies et al. 2017). As another example, extracellular heme released by damaged red blood cells in the context of hemorrhage or malaria infection can trigger HO-1 signaling, which in turn leads to the production of heme and iron-chelating factors to limit damage exerted by heme (Soares et al. 2017). Extracellular heme can also trigger REV-ERB signaling, with profound effects on circadian regulation, behavior, and metabolism (Kojetin and Burris 2014).

Low oxygen levels resulting from anemia or abnormal lung function, or from rapid oxygen depletion in tissues following NOX activation, can trigger HIF signaling, which in turn increases angiogenesis, and erythropoiesis, leading to increased oxygenation (Devraj et al. 2017). Environmental toxicants such as benzopyrenes, bacterial metabolites such as indoles, as well as kynurenine produced by host immune regulatory cells endowed with the tryptophan-metabolizing enzyme indoleamine dioxygenase (IDO) can lead to AhR pathway activation (Jaronen and Quintana 2014). In turn, AhR pathway activation leads to an increase in levels of IDO itself, as well as of enzymes of the cytochrome p450 (CYP) family (Go et al. 2015). After xenobiotics are modified by CYP enzymes, they are conjugated to GSH by GSH-S-transferases (GST) and made to exit cells as GS-X conjugates (Gundert-Remy et al. 2014). As a direct antioxidant and GSH prodrug, NAC can counter the effects of heme and iron, themselves potent activators of ROS signaling (Dutra and Bozza 2014). NAC can also provide the necessary fuel to support detoxifying activities via the CYP/GST families of enzymes (Lash 2007). Finally, NAC treatment was shown to stabilize Hsp90, a HIF cofactor, thereby promoting HIF signaling (Zhang et al. 2014). On the flipside, activation of resilience pathways by ROS can be stunted, or even inhibited by NAC treatment, if timed improperly. This is particularly true of the Nrf2 (Romanque et al. 2011) and HO-1 (Zhao et al. 2016) pathways. Thus, NAC can act both as a potentiator and inhibitor of resilience pathways.

The activation of pro-inflammatory and resilience responses requires the mobilization of energy resources for cell signaling, *de novo* mRNA transcription, protein translation, mediator release, cell movement, etc. These responses are under the control of core metabolic pathways, which license cells and tissues to use extracellular nutrient and intracellular reserves to fuel the increase in cellular activity, itself predicated on the maintenance of adequate ATP levels (Gleeson and Sheedy 2016). The major route for tryptophan catabolism, the kynurenine pathway evoked earlier, is also the main source for *de novo* synthesis of NAD (Gonzalez Esquivel et al. 2017). Carbohydrate, protein, and fatty acid degradation lead, from NAD, to the formation of the redox intermediate NADH. NADH is in turn consumed to generate the mitochondrial proton gradient required to produce ATP and sustain cellular activities in homeostasis and in inflammation. Another important catabolic pathway in inflammation is that of glucose degradation via glucose-6-phosphate dehydrogenase, a rate-limiting enzyme in the pentose phosphate pathway (Park et al. 2017). This leads to the generation of NADPH, which is the electron donor for ROS production by NOX and for GSSG reduction into GSH by GSH reductase.

The two key switches controlling cell metabolism in homeostasis and during inflammation are the AMP kinase (AMPK) and Akt/mechanistic target of rapamycin (mTOR) pathways (Zhao et al. 2017). Most often, AMPK and Akt/mTOR pathways are mutualistically inhibitory and together regulate the balance between catabolism (resource breakdown to fuel activity) and anabolism (buildup of new proteins, organelles, and cells for adaptive and reparative responses). In recent years, modulation of the AMPK and mTOR pathways as a way to regulate the timing and amplitude of inflammatory reactions has been the focus of much research (Antonioli et al. 2016; Weichhart et al. 2015). Considering that redox reactions are central to metabolism, with NADH and NAPDH as the main holders and distributors of reducing power in cells, with GSH being directly linked to both of these critical redox intermediates, it is clear that NAC, as a potent GSH prodrug, can affect metabolism in significant ways. Independent of its role as a GSH prodrug, NAC can inhibit AMPK and autophagy (Rahman et al. 2014), and activate mTOR and anabolic activities (Yi et al. 2016), directly affecting the balance between these two pathways and between catabolism and anabolism. Thus, NAC can potentially regulate proinflammatory, resilience, and metabolic pathways involved in inflammation.

7.5 Guiding Principles for Interpreting Studies of NAC in Inflammation

The difference in biological activities and fate of the cysteine group borne by NAC depending upon its mode of administration is a critical factor to take into account in basic and translational studies of inflammation. For example, substantial NAC administration to cells *in vitro* may simultaneously (1) change the redox status of surface receptors, (2) leave DiNAC in the extracellular fluid to carry out other effects, (3) penetrate in cells and crowd out normal esterase substrates, (4) acutely increase cysteine levels in the cytosol and cause cysteinylation of proteins, and (5) boost GSH synthetic pathway and thereby impact protein glutathionylation, GSH-dependent detoxification, redox potential in the cytosol and organelles, and NADPH use as an electron donor to reduce GSSG into GSH. By contrast, NAC administration in animals and patients will impact specific cell types differentially: oral or intravenous delivery may affect leukocytes, depending on the dosing and underlying level of oxidation in the gut or liver, which may require NAC to react as a direct antioxidant, rather than a GSH prodrug, while airway or skin topical delivery is unlikely to affect leukocytes systemically. Because of these issues, *in vitro* and *in vivo* studies on the effects of NAC are often discrepant.

In addition, there can be significant discrepancies between animal models and humans, which diverge significantly with regard to physiological properties governing NAC pharmacokinetics and pharmacodynamics. For example, high-dose oral NAC may face differential saturation of gut absorption and subsequent NAC leakage into the plasma, which is rarely, if ever, a concern in humans (Pendyala and Creaven 1995). In a mouse model, excess plasma NAC was shown to react with nitric oxide to form the *S*-nitroso-NAC adduct, with damaging side effects (Palmer et al. 2007). It is also worth noting that despite their primary role in mediating oxidative stress and feed-forward pro-inflammatory signaling, ROS also play a homeostatic role and are required to mediate local changes in redox potential and PTMs of critical proteins during normal development and function (Cortese-Krott et al. 2017). Therefore, excessive intake of reducing equivalents may cause reductive stress, leading to inability of cells and organs to mount proper adaptive responses (Handy and Loscalzo 2016).

Among human subjects, there may be differences in NAC absorption and GSH metabolism, notably related to genetic mutations and underlying inflammatory or metabolic conditions, which can in turn impact the clinical efficacy and outcomes of NAC treatment. It is beyond our scope here to provide an exhaustive digest of all clinical trials of NAC, in various modes of administration, doses, and formulations, for conditions associated with inflammation. The clinical role of NAC as an anti-inflammatory agent in cystic fibrosis (Tam et al. 2013), liver damage linked to acetaminophen overdose (Brok et al. 2006), sepsis and other systemic inflammatory disorders (Szakmany et al. 2012), drug-induced kidney damage (Jun et al. 2012), and neurological disorders (Deepmala et al. 2015) is reviewed elsewhere and is outlined in the specific clinical chapters in the next section of the book. Taken together, the current body of basic and clinical knowledge on NAC suggests that, although much is known about its activity *in vitro*, one has to use caution when extrapolating it to specific cohorts of patients to treat redox imbalance and/or inflammation, as many factors can influence outcomes. Stringent design and randomization are critical to ensure appropriate clinical assessment of this multifunctional compound.

References

Amore A, Formica M, Giacchino F, Gigliola G, Bonello F, Conti G, Camilla R, Coppo R (2013) N-Acetylcysteine in hemodialysis diabetic patients resets the activation of NF-kB in lymphomonocytes to normal values. J Nephrol 26(4):778–786. https://doi.org/10.5301/jn.5000167

Anrather J, Racchumi G, Iadecola C (2006) NF-kappaB regulates phagocytic NADPH oxidase by inducing the expression of gp91phox. J Biol Chem 281(9):5657–5667. https://doi.org/10.1074/jbc.M506172200

Antonioli L, Colucci R, Pellegrini C, Giustarini G, Sacco D, Tirotta E, Caputi V, Marsilio I, Giron MC, Nemeth ZH, Blandizzi C, Fornai M (2016) The AMPK enzyme-complex: from the regulation of cellular energy homeostasis to a possible new molecular target in the management of chronic inflammatory disorders. Expert Opin Ther Targets 20(2):179–191. https://doi.org/10.1517/14728222.2016.1086752

Atkuri KR, Mantovani JJ, Herzenberg LA, Herzenberg LA (2007) N-Acetylcysteine--a safe antidote for cysteine/glutathione deficiency. Curr Opin Pharmacol 7(4):355–359. https://doi.org/10.1016/j.coph.2007.04.005

Bertheloot D, Latz E (2017) HMGB1, IL-1alpha, IL-33 and S100 proteins: dual-function alarmins. Cell Mol Immunol 14(1):43–64. https://doi.org/10.1038/cmi.2016.34

Brok J, Buckley N, Gluud C (2006) Interventions for paracetamol (acetaminophen) overdose. Cochrane Database Syst Rev 2:Cd003328. https://doi.org/10.1002/14651858.CD003328.pub2

Cortese-Krott MM, Koning A, Kuhnle GG, Nagy P, Bianco C, Pasch A, Wink DA, Fukuto J, Jackson AA, van Goor H, Olson KR, Feelisch M (2017) The reactive species interactome: evolutionary emergence, biological significance, and opportunities for redox metabolomics and personalized medicine. Antioxid Redox Signal 27:684–712. https://doi.org/10.1089/ars.2017.7083

Couto N, Wood J, Barber J (2016) The role of glutathione reductase and related enzymes on cellular redox homoeostasis network. Free Radic Biol Med 95:27–42. https://doi.org/10.1016/j.freeradbiomed.2016.02.028

Deepmala SJ, Kumar N, Delhey L, Berk M, Dean O, Spielholz C, Frye R (2015) Clinical trials of N-acetylcysteine in psychiatry and neurology: a systematic review. Neurosci Biobehav Rev 55:294–321. https://doi.org/10.1016/j.neubiorev.2015.04.015

Devraj G, Beerlage C, Brune B, Kempf VA (2017) Hypoxia and HIF-1 activation in bacterial infections. Microbes Infect 19(3):144–156. https://doi.org/10.1016/j.micinf.2016.11.003

Dutra FF, Bozza MT (2014) Heme on innate immunity and inflammation. Front Pharmacol 5:115. https://doi.org/10.3389/fphar.2014.00115

Gabryel B, Bielecka A, Bernacki J, Labuzek K, Herman ZS (2011) Immunosuppressant cytoprotection correlates with HMGB1 suppression in primary astrocyte cultures exposed to combined oxygen-glucose deprivation. Pharmacol Rep 63(2):392–402

Gallucci S, Matzinger P (2001) Danger signals: SOS to the immune system. Curr Opin Immunol 13(1):114–119

Gleeson LE, Sheedy FJ (2016) Metabolic reprogramming & inflammation: fuelling the host response to pathogens. Semin Immunol 28(5):450–468. https://doi.org/10.1016/j.smim.2016.10.007

Go RE, Hwang KA, Choi KC (2015) Cytochrome P450 1 family and cancers. J Steroid Biochem Mol Biol 147:24–30. https://doi.org/10.1016/j.jsbmb.2014.11.003

Gonzalez Esquivel D, Ramirez-Ortega D, Pineda B, Castro N, Rios C, Perez de la Cruz V (2017) Kynurenine pathway metabolites and enzymes involved in redox reactions. Neuropharmacology 112(Pt B):331–345. https://doi.org/10.1016/j.neuropharm.2016.03.013

Greene SC, Noonan PK, Sanabria C, Peacock WF (2016) Effervescent N-acetylcysteine tablets versus oral solution N-acetylcysteine in fasting healthy adults: an open-label, randomized, single-dose, crossover, relative bioavailability study. Curr Ther Res Clin Exp 83:1–7. https://doi.org/10.1016/j.curtheres.2016.06.001

Gruarin P, Primo L, Ferrandi C, Bussolino F, Tandon NN, Arese P, Ulliers D, Alessio M (2001) Cytoadherence of Plasmodium falciparum-infected erythrocytes is mediated by a redox-dependent conformational fraction of CD36. J Immunol 167(11):6510–6517

Gundert-Remy U, Bernauer U, Blomeke B, Doring B, Fabian E, Goebel C, Hessel S, Jackh C, Lampen A, Oesch F, Petzinger E, Volkel W, Roos PH (2014) Extrahepatic metabolism at the body's internal-external interfaces. Drug Metab Rev 46(3):291–324. https://doi.org/10.3109/03602532.2014.900565

Han S, Cai W, Yang X, Jia Y, Zheng Z, Wang H, Li J, Li Y, Gao J, Fan L, Hu D (2015) ROS-mediated NLRP3 inflammasome activity is essential for burn-induced acute lung injury. Mediat Inflamm 2015:720457. https://doi.org/10.1155/2015/720457

Handy DE, Loscalzo J (2016) Responses to reductive stress in the cardiovascular system. Free Radic Biol Med 109:114–124. https://doi.org/10.1016/j.freeradbiomed.2016.12.006

Janko C, Filipovic M, Munoz LE, Schorn C, Schett G, Ivanovic-Burmazovic I, Herrmann M (2014) Redox modulation of HMGB1-related signaling. Antioxid Redox Signal 20(7):1075–1085. https://doi.org/10.1089/ars.2013.5179

Jaronen M, Quintana FJ (2014) Immunological relevance of the coevolution of IDO1 and AHR. Front Immunol 5:521. https://doi.org/10.3389/fimmu.2014.00521

Jun M, Venkataraman V, Razavian M, Cooper B, Zoungas S, Ninomiya T, Webster AC, Perkovic V (2012) Antioxidants for chronic kidney disease. Cochrane Database Syst Rev 10:Cd008176. https://doi.org/10.1002/14651858.CD008176.pub2

Kim YS, Park ZY, Kim SY, Jeong E, Lee JY (2009) Alteration of Toll-like receptor 4 activation by 4-hydroxy-2-nonenal mediated by the suppression of receptor homodimerization. Chem Biol Interact 182(1):59–66. https://doi.org/10.1016/j.cbi.2009.07.009

Kojer K, Riemer J (2014) Balancing oxidative protein folding: the influences of reducing pathways on disulfide bond formation. Biochim Biophys Acta 1844(8):1383–1390. https://doi.org/10.1016/j.bbapap.2014.02.004

Kojetin DJ, Burris TP (2014) REV-ERB and ROR nuclear receptors as drug targets. Nat Rev Drug Discov 13(3):197–216. https://doi.org/10.1038/nrd4100

Komai K, Shichita T, Ito M, Kanamori M, Chikuma S, Yoshimura A (2017) Role of scavenger receptors as damage-associated molecular pattern receptors in Toll-like receptor activation. Int Immunol 29(2):59–70. https://doi.org/10.1093/intimm/dxx010

Lash LH (2007) Glutathione-dependent bioactivation. Curr Protoc Toxicol 6:12. https://doi.org/10.1002/0471140856.tx0612s34

Li G, Tang D, Lotze MT (2013) Menage a Trois in stress: DAMPs, redox and autophagy. Semin Cancer Biol 23(5):380–390. https://doi.org/10.1016/j.semcancer.2013.08.002

Liu Y, Yao W, Xu J, Qiu Y, Cao F, Li S, Yang S, Yang H, Wu Z, Hou Y (2015) The anti-inflammatory effects of acetaminophen and N-acetylcysteine through suppression of the NLRP3 inflammasome pathway in LPS-challenged piglet mononuclear phagocytes. Innate Immun 21(6):587–597. https://doi.org/10.1177/1753425914566205

Liu J, Qian C, Cao X (2016) Post-translational modification control of innate immunity. Immunity 45(1):15–30. https://doi.org/10.1016/j.immuni.2016.06.020

Lu SC (1999) Regulation of hepatic glutathione synthesis: current concepts and controversies. FASEB J 13(10):1169–1183

Majoros A, Platanitis E, Kernbauer-Holzl E, Rosebrock F, Muller M, Decker T (2017) Canonical and non-canonical aspects of JAK-STAT signaling: lessons from interferons for cytokine responses. Front Immunol 8:29. https://doi.org/10.3389/fimmu.2017.00029

Mimche PN, Thompson E, Taramelli D, Vivas L (2012) Curcumin enhances non-opsonic phagocytosis of plasmodium falciparum through up-regulation of CD36 surface expression on monocytes/macrophages. J Antimicrob Chemother 67(8):1895–1904. https://doi.org/10.1093/jac/dks132

Novakowski KE, Huynh A, Han S, Dorrington MG, Yin C, Tu Z, Pelka P, Whyte P, Guarne A, Sakamoto K, Bowdish DM (2016) A naturally occurring transcript variant of MARCO reveals the SRCR domain is critical for function. Immunol Cell Biol 94(7):646–655. https://doi.org/10.1038/icb.2016.20

O'Neill S, Brault J, Stasia MJ, Knaus UG (2015) Genetic disorders coupled to ROS deficiency. Redox Biol 6:135–156. https://doi.org/10.1016/j.redox.2015.07.009

Odendall C, Kagan JC (2017) Activation and pathogenic manipulation of the sensors of the innate immune system. Microbes Infect 19(4-5):229–237. https://doi.org/10.1016/j.micinf.2017.01.003

Palmer LA, Doctor A, Chhabra P, Sheram ML, Laubach VE, Karlinsey MZ, Forbes MS, Macdonald T, Gaston B (2007) S-nitrosothiols signal hypoxia-mimetic vascular pathology. J Clin Invest 117(9):2592–2601. https://doi.org/10.1172/JCI29444

Park SK, Dahmer MK, Quasney MW (2012) MAPK and JAK-STAT signaling pathways are involved in the oxidative stress-induced decrease in expression of surfactant protein genes. Cell Physiol Biochem 30(2):334–346. https://doi.org/10.1159/000339068

Park YJ, Choe SS, Sohn JH, Kim JB (2017) The role of glucose-6-phosphate dehydrogenase in adipose tissue inflammation in obesity. Adipocytes 6:147–153. https://doi.org/10.1080/21623945.2017.1288321

Pendyala L, Creaven PJ (1995) Pharmacokinetic and pharmacodynamic studies of N-acetylcysteine, a potential chemopreventive agent during a phase I trial. Cancer Epidemiol Biomark Prev 4(3):245–251

Pettersson K, Kjerrulf M, Jungersten L, Johansson K, Langstrom G, Kalies I, Lenkei R, Walldius G, Lind L (2008) The new oral immunomodulating drug DiNAC induces brachial artery vasodilatation at rest and during hyperemia in hypercholesterolemic subjects, likely by a nitric oxide-dependent mechanism. Atherosclerosis 196(1):275–282. https://doi.org/10.1016/j.atherosclerosis.2006.10.031

PrabhuDas MR, Baldwin CL, Bollyky PL, Bowdish DME, Drickamer K, Febbraio M, Herz J, Kobzik L, Krieger M, Loike J, McVicker B, Means TK, Moestrup SK, Post SR, Sawamura T, Silverstein S, Speth RC, Telfer JC, Thiele GM, Wang XY, Wright SD, El Khoury J (2017) A consensus definitive classification of scavenger receptors and their roles in health and disease. J Immunol 198(10):3775–3789. https://doi.org/10.4049/jimmunol.1700373

Pruenster M, Vogl T, Roth J, Sperandio M (2016) S100A8/A9: from basic science to clinical application. Pharmacol Ther 167:120–131. https://doi.org/10.1016/j.pharmthera.2016.07.015

Rahman I, Biswas SK, Jimenez LA, Torres M, Forman HJ (2005) Glutathione, stress responses, and redox signaling in lung inflammation. Antioxid Redox Signal 7(1-2):42–59. https://doi.org/10.1089/ars.2005.7.42

Rahman M, Mofarrahi M, Kristof AS, Nkengfac B, Harel S, Hussain SN (2014) Reactive oxygen species regulation of autophagy in skeletal muscles. Antioxid Redox Signal 20(3):443–459. https://doi.org/10.1089/ars.2013.5410

Rana A, Ahmed M, Rub A, Akhter Y (2015) A tug-of-war between the host and the pathogen generates strategic hotspots for the development of novel therapeutic interventions against infectious diseases. Virulence 6(6):566–580. https://doi.org/10.1080/21505594.2015.1062211

Rider P, Voronov E, Dinarello CA, Apte RN, Cohen I (2017) Alarmins: feel the stress. J Immunol 198(4):1395–1402. https://doi.org/10.4049/jimmunol.1601342

Romanque P, Cornejo P, Valdes S, Videla LA (2011) Thyroid hormone administration induces rat liver Nrf2 activation: suppression by N-acetylcysteine pretreatment. Thyroid 21(6):655–662. https://doi.org/10.1089/thy.2010.0322

Rushworth GF, Megson IL (2014) Existing and potential therapeutic uses for N-acetylcysteine: the need for conversion to intracellular glutathione for antioxidant benefits. Pharmacol Ther 141(2):150–159. https://doi.org/10.1016/j.pharmthera.2013.09.006

Ryu JK, Kim SJ, Rah SH, Kang JI, Jung HE, Lee D, Lee HK, Lee JO, Park BS, Yoon TY, Kim HM (2017) Reconstruction of LPS transfer cascade reveals structural determinants within LBP, CD14, and TLR4-MD2 for efficient LPS recognition and transfer. Immunity 46(1):38–50. https://doi.org/10.1016/j.immuni.2016.11.007

Sharma R, Young C, Neu J (2010) Molecular modulation of intestinal epithelial barrier: contribution of microbiota. J Biomed Biotechnol 2010:305879. https://doi.org/10.1155/2010/305879

Sies H, Berndt C, Jones DP (2017) Oxidative stress. Annu Rev Biochem 86:715–748. https://doi.org/10.1146/annurev-biochem-061516-045037

Sims GP, Rowe DC, Rietdijk ST, Herbst R, Coyle AJ (2010) HMGB1 and RAGE in inflammation and cancer. Annu Rev Immunol 28:367–388. https://doi.org/10.1146/annurev.immunol.021908.132603

Soares MP, Teixeira L, Moita LF (2017) Disease tolerance and immunity in host protection against infection. Nat Rev Immunol 17(2):83–96. https://doi.org/10.1038/nri.2016.136

Szakmany T, Hauser B, Radermacher P (2012) N-acetylcysteine for sepsis and systemic inflammatory response in adults. Cochrane Database Syst Rev 9:Cd006616. https://doi.org/10.1002/14651858.CD006616.pub2

Tam J, Nash EF, Ratjen F, Tullis E, Stephenson A (2013) Nebulized and oral thiol derivatives for pulmonary disease in cystic fibrosis. Cochrane Database Syst Rev 7:Cd007168. https://doi.org/10.1002/14651858.CD007168.pub3

de Torre-Minguela C, Mesa Del Castillo P, Pelegrin P (2017) The NLRP3 and pyrin inflammasomes: implications in the pathophysiology of autoinflammatory diseases. Front Immunol 8:43. https://doi.org/10.3389/fimmu.2017.00043

Tsai ML, Huang HP, Hsu JD, Lai YR, Hsiao YP, Lu FJ, Chang HR (2014) Topical N-acetylcysteine accelerates wound healing in vitro and in vivo via the PKC/Stat3 pathway. Int J Mol Sci 15(5):7563–7578. https://doi.org/10.3390/ijms15057563

Ulas T, Pirr S, Fehlhaber B, Bickes MS, Loof TG, Vogl T, Mellinger L, Heinemann AS, Burgmann J, Schoning J, Schreek S, Pfeifer S, Reuner F, Vollger L, Stanulla M, von Kockritz-Blickwede M, Glander S, Barczyk-Kahlert K, von Kaisenberg CS, Friesenhagen J, Fischer-Riepe L, Zenker S, Schultze JL, Roth J, Viemann D (2017) S100-alarmin-induced innate immune programming protects newborn infants from sepsis. Nat Immunol 18(6):622–632. https://doi.org/10.1038/ni.3745

Vajjhala PR, Ve T, Bentham A, Stacey KJ, Kobe B (2017) The molecular mechanisms of signaling by cooperative assembly formation in innate immunity pathways. Mol Immunol 86:23. https://doi.org/10.1016/j.molimm.2017.02.012

Weichhart T, Hengstschlager M, Linke M (2015) Regulation of innate immune cell function by mTOR. Nat Rev Immunol 15(10):599–614. https://doi.org/10.1038/nri3901

Winterbourn CC, Kettle AJ, Hampton MB (2016) Reactive oxygen species and neutrophil function. Annu Rev Biochem 85:765–792. https://doi.org/10.1146/annurev-biochem-060815-014442

Yi D, Hou Y, Wang L, Long M, Hu S, Mei H, Yan L, Hu CA, Wu G (2016) N-acetylcysteine stimulates protein synthesis in enterocytes independently of glutathione synthesis. Amino Acids 48(2):523–533. https://doi.org/10.1007/s00726-015-2105-z

Yin J, Ren W, Yang G, Duan J, Huang X, Fang R, Li C, Li T, Yin Y, Hou Y, Kim SW, Wu G (2016) L-Cysteine metabolism and its nutritional implications. Mol Nutr Food Res 60(1):134–146. https://doi.org/10.1002/mnfr.201500031

Yoshino H, Kashiwakura I (2017) Involvement of reactive oxygen species in ionizing radiation-induced upregulation of cell surface Toll-like receptor 2 and 4 expression in human monocytic cells. J Radiat Res 58:626–635. https://doi.org/10.1093/jrr/rrx011

Youn GS, Lee KW, Choi SY, Park J (2016) Overexpression of HDAC6 induces pro-inflammatory responses by regulating ROS-MAPK-NF-kappaB/AP-1 signaling pathways in macrophages. Free Radic Biol Med 97:14–23. https://doi.org/10.1016/j.freeradbiomed.2016.05.014

Zafarullah M, Li WQ, Sylvester J, Ahmad M (2003) Molecular mechanisms of N-acetylcysteine actions. Cell Mol Life Sci 60(1):6–20

Zhang Z, Yan J, Taheri S, Liu KJ, Shi H (2014) Hypoxia-inducible factor 1 contributes to N-acetylcysteine's protection in stroke. Free Radic Biol Med 68:8–21. https://doi.org/10.1016/j.freeradbiomed.2013.11.007

Zhao Z, Zhao J, Xue J, Zhao X, Liu P (2016) Autophagy inhibition promotes epithelial-mesenchymal transition through ROS/HO-1 pathway in ovarian cancer cells. Am J Cancer Res 6(10):2162–2177

Zhao Y, Hu X, Liu Y, Dong S, Wen Z, He W, Zhang S, Huang Q, Shi M (2017) ROS signaling under metabolic stress: cross-talk between AMPK and AKT pathway. Mol Cancer 16(1):79. https://doi.org/10.1186/s12943-017-0648-1

Part III

The Clinical Use of N-Acetylcysteine (NAC)

Clinical Trials on N-Acetylcysteine

Richard Eugene Frye

8.1 Introduction

Clinical trials using N-Acetylcysteine (NAC) started in the late 1960s and have grown ever since with a rapid growth started in the 1990s. The number of studies hits a relative peak within the last decade at about 125 clinical trials per year (see Fig. 8.1).

8.2 History of Clinical Trials Investigating N-Acetylcysteine (NAC)

NAC has been studied in clinical trials in many different medical disorders, most likely due to multiple pathways it modulates and its favorable safety profile. Figure 8.2 outlines the number of studies broken down by medical specialty. NAC has been studied in several renal and pulmonary diseases as well as in cardiology, particularly cardiac surgery. While well-known for its use for acetaminophen toxicity, the number of clinical studies is not extensive. Other emerging areas of study of NAC include exercise physiology, psychiatry, and neurology. Below we discuss the details of some of the more well-studied areas of medicine.

Clinical trials studying the use of NAC in protecting the kidney from radiological contrast agents started relatively recently, in the year 2000, and have grown considerably. Many such studies have focused on high-risk patients with either preexisting kidney disease or those undergoing cardiac procedures (Fig. 8.3). Additionally, a small number of studies have investigated the use of NAC in chronic kidney disease and acute kidney injury.

R. E. Frye
Barrow Neurological Institute, Phoenix Children's Hospital, University of Arizona College of Medicine – Phoenix, Phoenix, AZ, USA
e-mail: rfrye@phoenixchildrens.com

© Springer Nature Singapore Pte Ltd. 2019
R. E. Frye, M. Berk (eds.), *The Therapeutic Use of N-Acetylcysteine (NAC) in Medicine*, https://doi.org/10.1007/978-981-10-5311-5_8

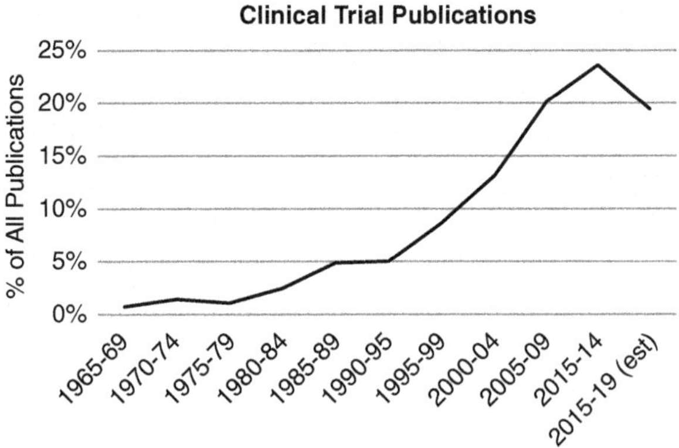

Fig. 8.1 Percent of total clinical trials performed in 5-year blocks starting in 1965. The years 2017–2019 are estimated from 2015–2016

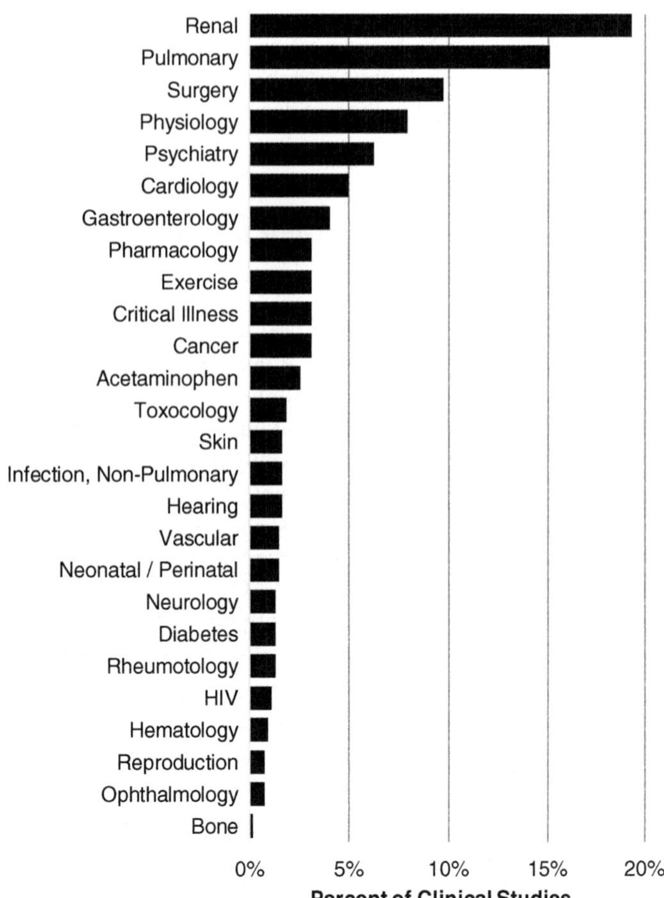

Fig. 8.2 Percent of clinical trials on NAC by medical specialty

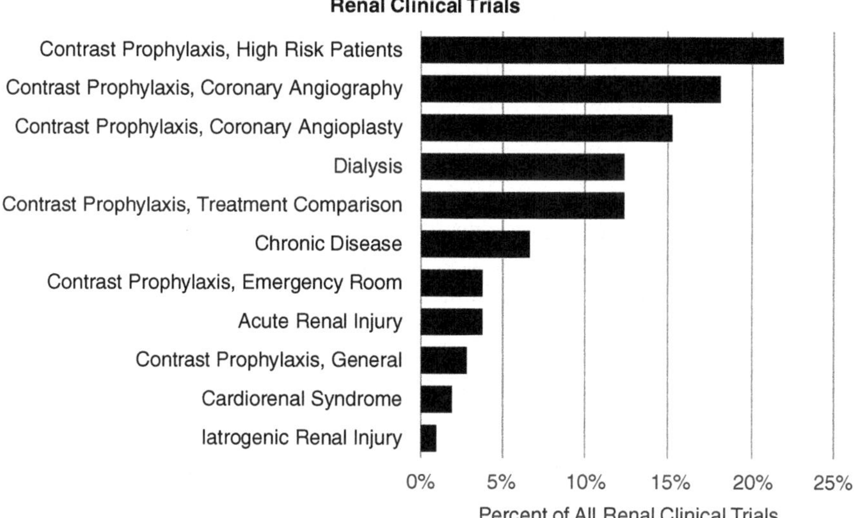

Fig. 8.3 Renal clinical trials on NAC

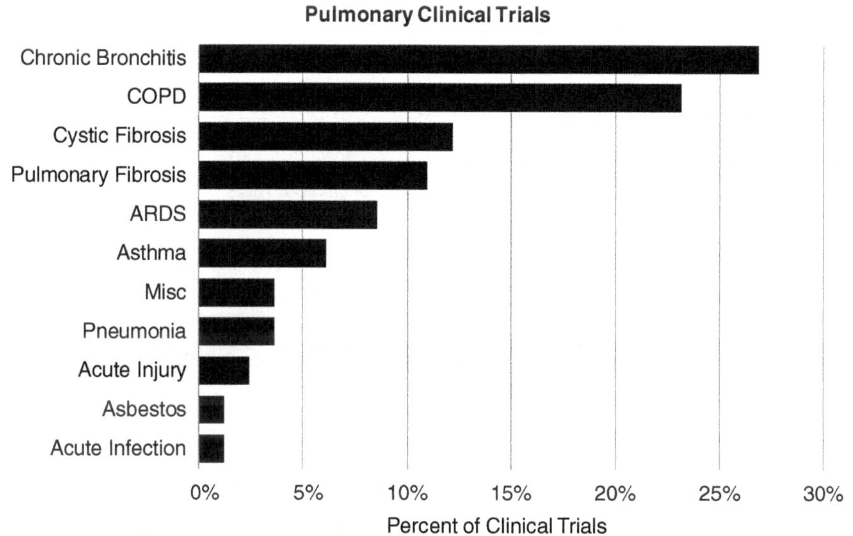

Fig. 8.4 Pulmonary clinical trials on NAC

Pulmonary clinical trials studying the use of NAC are the second most numerous and some of the earliest clinical trials studying NAC (Fig. 8.4). The great majority of the clinical trials have focused on chronic obstructive conditions including chronic bronchitis and chronic obstructive pulmonary disease (COPD). The second most numerous pulmonary studies are on chronic restrictive lung diseases such as cystic fibrosis and pulmonary fibrosis. Given the large number of studies on these chronic lung diseases, other studies on acute pulmonary conditions that have emerged.

Clinical trials to prevent surgical complications using NAC date back to the 1960–1970 where the prevention of pulmonary complications was investigated (Fig. 8.5). In the late 1980s and early 1990s, there was interest in the use of NAC during abdominal surgery, and in the 1990s there was a growth in the investigation of its use in liver transplantation. In the 2000s, interest grew in its use for cardiac surgery.

The clinical use of NAC in psychiatry (Fig. 8.6) is a relatively recent development with most studies being conducted within the last 5–7 years. Over half of the

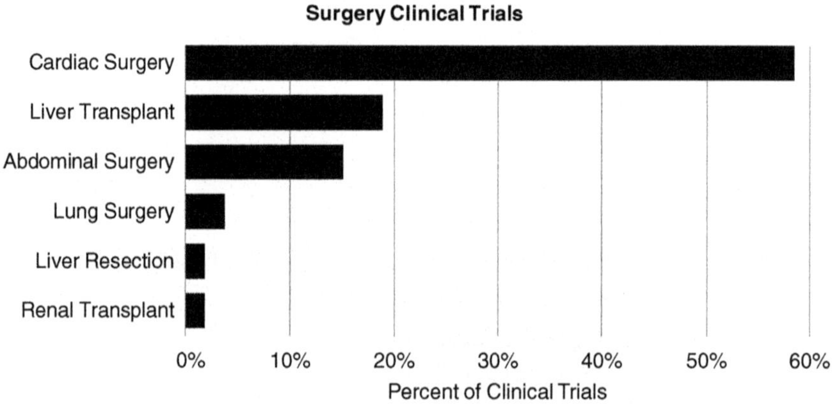

Fig. 8.5 Surgical clinical trials on NAC

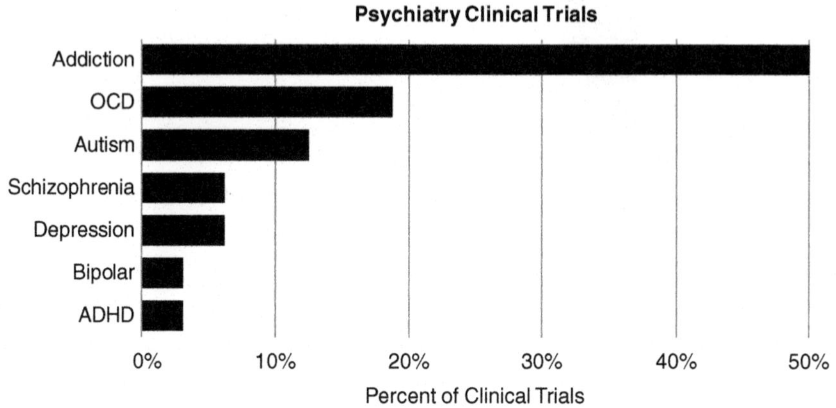

Fig. 8.6 Psychiatric clinical trials on NAC

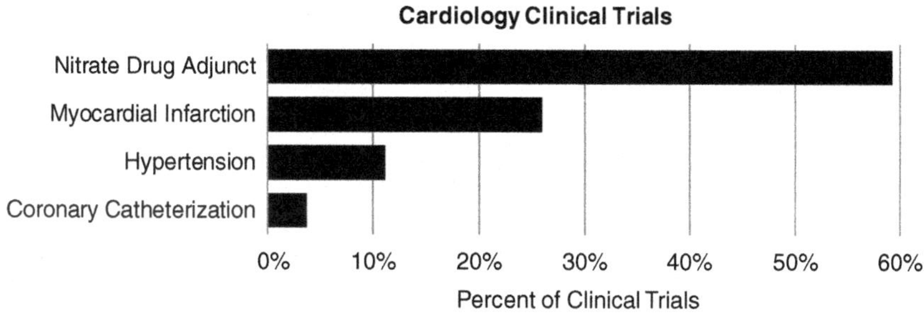

Fig. 8.7 Cardiology clinical trials on NAC

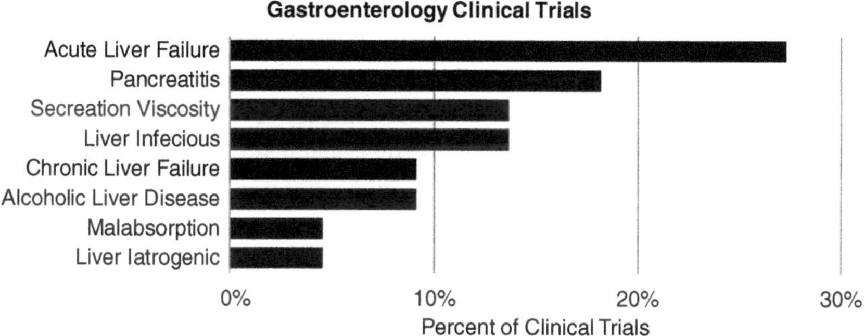

Fig. 8.8 Gastroenterology clinical trials on NAC

studies in psychiatry have explored the use of NAC in various addictions. Investigation of NAC in other areas of psychiatry is growing.

The investigation of NAC in cardiology is one of the largest areas when trials that have examined cardiac surgery and coronary angioplasty and angiography are included (Fig. 8.7). Excluding these latter areas, a large number of studies have examined the effect of NAC as an adjunct to common nitrate drugs such as nitroglycerin. Other areas include its use in reducing the size of myocardial infarction, reducing hypertension, and its use in coronary catheterization not related to angioplasty and angiography specifically.

Aside from liver surgery, NAC has been studied for many indications, including both chronic and acute conditions, in gastroenterology (Fig. 8.8).

8.3   Organization of the Clinical Section of the Book

The clinical section of the book aims to provide the most comprehensive analysis of the use of NAC in medicine. Since NAC has been used in a wide variety of medical condition, this section is divided into the major medical applications with separate chapters dedicated to the areas where there are the most trials or the more interesting emerging fields where its use appears promising.

Each chapter systematically reviews the clinical trials in the specific area of medicine and rates the level of evidence for each study reviewed and then generates a grade of recommendation based on this level of evidence using an objective criteria system that is outlined below. In addition to these grades, a recommendation is made for the use of NAC for specific disorders or conditions.

The section starts with clinical trials in the area where NAC is most well-known, toxicology, which is reviewed in two chapters, one on poisoning, including acetaminophen poisoning, and another on metal toxicity, an emerging field in which NAC may be helpful. Next the use of NAC in the fields of neurology and psychiatry is reviewed with psychiatry divided into two chapters, with one chapter dedicated to addiction. Additional chapters review the use of NAC in other fields where it is commonly used. A chapter is also dedicated to those areas with only a handful of clinical trials, to ensure the book is comprehensive. A chapter is also dedicated to clinical studies that have examined the physiological effects of NAC in humans. Further, a chapter that proposes that NAC may be a treatment for disease characterized by glutathione deficiency is provided. Finally, a chapter reviews the adverse effects associated with NAC as well as the formulations and pharmacology of NAC.

8.4   Methods for Selecting Clinical Trials

Each chapter reviews the evidence for the use of NAC for specific medical conditions using a systematic approach. Systematic reviews use the PICO (Problem-Intervention-Comparison-Outcomes) framework (Richardson and Detsky 1995). The problem specifically addressed treatment or prevention of the conditions within the medical areas being reviewed, and the intervention was NAC as compared to placebo or other standard treatments (although this was uncommon). The goal was to consider all outcomes reported as well as determine the common adverse effects.

8.4.1   Search Strategy

A systematic review uses the common medical literature databases such as PubMed, Ovid MEDLINE, Google Scholar, CINAHL, Embase, Scopus, Cochrane, and ERIC databases, usually from inception through the date of writing the review. To identify studies using NAC, terms such as "N-Acetylcysteine," "acetylcysteine," or "NAC" are used. These terms are combined with specific diseases that are part of the specific medical areas being investigated. Other filter terms such as "human" or "clinical trials" are not uncommonly used. Also it is customary to review the references in publications identified by the search to determine if any relevant publications may have been missed.

8.4.2   Study Selection

Commonly, one or more of the authors of the chapter review the titles and abstracts of all potentially relevant publications. Studies are usually included if they meet specific criteria such as (a) human randomized controlled trials, nonrandomized trials, case studies, and/or case series and (b) report of a direct clinical effect of NAC as an outcome. Studies are commonly excluded if they (a) do not involve humans, (b) do not provide new or unique data (review articles, letter to the editor, duplicate article), and (c) do not measure a clinical outcome or do not report a clinical measure (this is an exception in the physiological studies reviewed in one chapter in this section).

8.5 Methods for Developing Recommendations

8.5.1 Level of Evidence Ratings

A grade of recommendation (GOR) is given for each medical condition studied based on the level of evidence (LOE) for each study. Using a well-established scale (Howick et al. 2011), each clinical trial is individually assessed to determine the LOE, ranging from level 1 to 5 (see Table 8.1). After assessing all identified studies for each disorder, a GOR ranging from A (solid evidence) to D (limited, inconsistent, or inconclusive evidence) is assigned (see Table 8.2). Since a condition can be given a GOR of D for several reasons, a modifier is used if the evidence represents a single case report or series (SC), demonstrated a neutral effect (NE), or was found to be possibly detrimental (DE).

8.5.2 Data Analysis and Synthesis

The information about each medical condition is summarized and synthesized in several ways. A GOR for each medical condition is summarized based on the LOE for each study identified. Since the GOR is based on the quality of the clinical study

Table 8.1 Levels of evidence

Level	Description
1a	SR or meta-analysis of RCTs with homogeneity or Cochrane review with favorable findings
1b	Prospective high-quality RCT (medium sized with N between 50 and 100 or large sized with N over 100 and/or higher validity trials based on adequate follow-up, intent to treat analysis, randomization, baseline similarity, equal treatment, and dropout rate)
2a	SR of cohort (prospective, nonrandomized) studies with homogeneity
2b	Individual cohort (prospective, nonrandomized) study or low-quality RCT (small sized with N less than 50 and/or lower validity trials based on adequate follow-up, intent to treat analysis, randomization, baseline similarity, equal treatment, and dropout rate)
3a	SR of case-control (retrospective) studies with homogeneity
3b	Individual case-control (retrospective) study
4	Open-label trials, case series, or reports
5	Expert opinion without critical appraisal or based on physiology or bench research

RCT randomized controlled trial, *SR* systematic review

Table 8.2 Grade of recommendation

Grade	Description
A	At least one level 1a study *or* two level 1b studies
B	At least one level 1b, 2a, or 3a study *or* two level 2b or 3b studies
C	At least one level 2b or 3b study *or* two level 4 studies
D	Level 5 evidence *or* troublingly inconsistent or inconclusive studies of any level *or* studies reporting no improvements
N	No studies identified

and not necessarily the outcome, the recommendation on whether NAC should be utilized for the specific medical condition is based on both the strength of the evidence and the outcome of the studies. A study is given 1 point for positive on primary outcome measures and 0 for negative outcomes on all measures. Studies are given 0.5 point if the study is positive for few but not all outcomes or positive in subgroup analysis only. Based on points, the percentage positive of total studies is calculated. If 100% of the studies are positive and GOR was either A or B, then the recommendation for treatment is "Yes" to use NAC for that specific disorder. For percentage positive between 50 and 100%, the recommendation for treatment was "Mixed." If there was only one study or a few small studies on a disorder, the recommendation for clinical treatment is "None" as it is not advisable to base treatment recommendations on one study, and treatment must be based on the specific characteristics of the patient as well as the expert judgment of the treating physician. If the GOR was either C or D, the recommendation could be "Mixed" or "None" depending on the quality and the individual studies. If the overall percentage was less than 50%, independent of the GOR, usually a recommendation for treatment of "No" was highly considered based on the quality of the individual studies. The number of studies is based on actual trial conducted and not on the number of articles to avoid duplication. For each medical condition, a table provides the details of each study along with the LOE grading and point based on outcomes for most chapters. In addition, the text discusses the summary of all the studies for each disorder. Finally, the discussion in each chapter synthesizes this information to summarize the potential clinical use of NAC and comments on the mechanisms of action.

References

Howick J, Chalmers I, Glasziou P, Greenhalgh T, Heneghan C, Liberati A, Moschetti I, Phillips B, Thornton H, Goddard O, Hodgkinson M (2011) The Oxford 2011 Levels of Evidence. http://www.cebm.net/index.aspx?o=5653
Richardson WS, Detsky AS (1995) Users' guides to the medical literature. VII. How to use a clinical decision analysis. A. Are the results of the study valid? Evidence-based Medicine Working Group. JAMA 273(16):1292–1295

N-Acetylcysteine in the Poisoned Patient

9

Angela L. Chiew and Geoffrey K. Isbister

9.1 Introduction

N-Acetylcysteine (NAC) has been used as an antidote for a variety of different poisonings (Table 9.1). Most commonly it is used in paracetamol poisoning where it is the mainstay of treatment. Its use has led to a substantial reduction in mortality following paracetamol overdose. NAC is effective in paracetamol overdose because it replenishes glutathione, which is required to breakdown the toxic metabolite of paracetamol (Olsson et al. 1988).

NAC has been proposed for poisonings other than paracetamol, such as paraquat, amanita, essential oils and hydrocarbons. However, there is very limited evidence for its use in these poisonings with only case reports or series or animal studies to support its effectiveness.

NAC has been well established as the treatment for paracetamol poisoning for over 30 years. In this chapter, we review the use of NAC in paracetamol poisoning, the randomised controlled trials (RCT) supporting its effectiveness, NAC regimens and studies of its adverse effects. We systematically analyse the RCT's for NAC in

Electronic supplementary material The online version of this article (https://doi.org/10.1007/978-981-10-5311-5_9) contains supplementary material, which is available to authorized users.

A. L. Chiew (✉)
Clinical Toxicology Unit, Department of Emergency Medicine, Prince of Wales Hospital, Randwick, NSW, Australia

Department of Pharmacology, School of Medical Sciences, University of Sydney, Sydney, NSW, Australia
e-mail: angela.chiew@health.nsw.gov.au

G. K. Isbister
Clinical Toxicology Research Group, University of Newcastle, Callaghan, NSW, Australia

Department of Clinical Toxicology and Pharmacology, Calvary Mater, Newcastle, NSW, Australia

© Springer Nature Singapore Pte Ltd. 2019
R. E. Frye, M. Berk (eds.), *The Therapeutic Use of N-Acetylcysteine (NAC) in Medicine*, https://doi.org/10.1007/978-981-10-5311-5_9

Table 9.1 Summary of the proposed uses in toxicology for NAC, toxic effect of the ingestion and mechanism of action of NAC for that toxin

Toxin	Toxic effect	Mechanism of NAC
Paracetamol	Acute liver injury, hepatotoxicity, fulminant liver failure and renal injury	Replenishes glutathione which is essential in the metabolism of NAPQI (Olsson et al. 1988, Jones 1998). Supplies thiol groups, which can directly bind with NAPQI in hepatocytes (Jones 1998) and enhances non-toxic sulphate conjugation (Buckpitt et al. 1979)
Paraquat (herbicide)	Multisystem organ failure, in particular pulmonary and renal toxicity	Beneficial effects may be through scavenging of reactive oxygen species, increasing glutathione and reducing inflammation, lipid peroxidation and apoptosis (Hoffer et al. 1997; Cappelletti et al. 1998; Yeh et al. 2006). NAC reduces paraquat-induced apoptosis (Cappelletti et al. 1998) and inflammatory response (Yeh et al. 2006) in human lung cultures
Amatoxin (predominately *Amanita phalloides* mushroom)	Gastrointestinal symptoms, hepatorenal toxicity, fulminant hepatic failure	NAC replenishes glutathione and scavenges free radicals (Smith and Davis 2016)
Orellanine toxin (*Cortinarius* species mushroom)	Gastrointestinal symptoms, acute kidney injury can result in chronic renal disease, acute liver injury	Antioxidant effect
Clove oil (essential oil)	Respiratory symptoms, seizures, coma and hepatic injury	Animal data suggest that eugenol is metabolised by hepatic cytochrome P450 enzymes to a quinone intermediate that causes hepatotoxicity (Mizutani et al. 1991). NAC replenishes glutathione
Pennyroyal (hydrocarbon)	Gastrointestinal symptoms, coma, hepatic injury, hepatotoxicity	Pulegone is converted by the cytochrome P450 system (CYP 1A2 and 2E1) to other hepatotoxins (Gordon et al. 1987; Thomassen et al. 1988). Similar to clove oil, pulegone and its metabolites deplete glutathione levels; hence, NAC is used to replenish glutathione
Chloroform (hydrocarbon)	CNS depression, respiratory depression and delayed hepatotoxicity	Chloroform is metabolised by cytochrome P450 to phosgene and free radicals, which cause mitochondrial damage and hepatocellular death (Pohl et al. 1977; Pandit et al. 2012). NAC replenishes glutathione and antioxidant effect
Carbon tetrachloride (hydrocarbon)	Coma, hypotension, respiratory depression and hepatorenal toxicity	The mechanism of toxicity is due to its toxic metabolite trichloromethyl that may covalently bind to macromolecules or react further (Recknagel et al. 1989). NAC has an antioxidant effect

NAPQI N-acetyl-p-benzoquinone imine

paracetamol poisoning and systematically analyse clinical case reports and studies of NAC used in the management of other poisons.

9.2   Methods

We aimed to identify research studies that reported NAC as a treatment to improve all toxic ingestions/poisonings. A systematic online literature search was conducted using broad search terms like "overdose", "poisoning", "toxin" or "antidote". We also looked at specific toxins—"paracetamol", "acetaminophen", "paraquat", "amanita", "essential oils" and "hydrocarbons". We also searched the references cited in the identified publications for additional studies. We only looked at NAC as a treatment for poisoning or overdose, not as a treatment of adverse effects of drugs given in therapeutic doses. For paracetamol (i.e. acetaminophen), we only looked at RCTs as it is an accepted treatment.

Much of the evidence for the use of NAC in non-paracetamol toxic ingestion is from case reports and small case series. Furthermore, NAC was often used in combination with other treatments, hence making any recommendations difficult. Instead we have summarised the findings of these in a table of results, and we provided a grade of recommendation (GOR) for each toxin based on the level of evidence for each study.

9.3   Paracetamol (Acetaminophen)

Paracetamol is one of the most common medications taken in both deliberate self-poisoning and unintentional overdose worldwide. Furthermore, it is the most common cause of acute liver failure in North America, Europe and Australia (Larson et al. 2005; Lancaster et al. 2015). The main toxicity following paracetamol poisoning is acute liver injury that results from the formation of a toxic metabolite of paracetamol, N-acetyl-p-benzoquinone imine (NAPQI). NAPQI is responsible for the hepatocellular injury that occurs with paracetamol toxicity.

In adults taking therapeutic doses, paracetamol is metabolised into two major non-toxic metabolites—sulphate and glucuronide conjugates—which account for 30 and 55% of paracetamol metabolism (Mitchell et al. 1974). NAPQI is formed in small amounts following a therapeutic dose of paracetamol. It is a highly reactive toxic metabolite formed by cytochrome P450 2E1 and is responsible for the hepatocellular injury that occurs with paracetamol toxicity. The small amounts of NAPQI produced after therapeutic doses are detoxified by irreversible glutathione-dependent conjugation reactions to two non-toxic metabolites, mercapturic acid and cysteine conjugates (Mitchell et al. 1974). In therapeutic paracetamol doses, these two metabolites are excreted at 4% (as a fraction of the parent dose) each, with over 80% excreted in the urine in the first 12 h following ingestion (Mitchell et al. 1974; Prescott 1980). In overdose, the increased formation of NAPQI depletes glutathione, and once glutathione is depleted by more than two-thirds, it covalently binds to critical cellular proteins (Mitchell et al. 1973). It is hypothesised that this results in loss of activity of critical proteins and eventually hepatic cell death.

Before there was an effective antidote for paracetamol poisoning, the morbidity was high. Prescott et al. reported 89% of patients developing severe liver damage if they had an initial concentration above 300 mg/L at 4 h or a concentration above a line decreasing from this point with a half-life of 4 h and 28% if the concentration was between 200 and 300 mg/L at 4 h (Prescott et al. 1977).

9.3.1   How N-Acetylcysteine Works in Paracetamol Poisoning

Glutathione consists of three amino acids, glycine, cysteine and glutamic acid. It has many important physiological roles such as forming conjugates with various molecules and acting as a potent free radical and reactive oxygen species scavenger (Forman et al. 2009). It is also an essential cofactor for many enzymes and is involved in several metabolic and signalling pathways. Glutathione is essential in the metabolism of NAPQI and covalently binds to the toxic paracetamol metabolite NAPQI in a 1:1 ratio (Jones 1998). The amino acid cysteine is the main factor limiting the synthesis of glutathione. NAC is a cysteine precursor; it is hydrolysed intracellularly to cysteine, which replenishes glutathione (Olsson et al. 1988). Its efficacy as a specific antidote for paracetamol poisoning relies mainly on its ability to stimulate glutathione synthesis (Prescott et al. 1989). NAC also supplies thiol groups, which can directly bind with NAPQI in hepatocytes (Jones 1998) and enhance nontoxic sulphate conjugation (Buckpitt et al. 1979; Table 9.1).

9.3.2   Evidence of Effectiveness of N-Acetylcysteine in the Treatment of Paracetamol Poisoning and Review of Randomised Controlled Trials

In the late 1960s, it was recognised that paracetamol overdose could result in acute liver injury and death (Davidson and Eastham 1966). It was not until the 1970s that several antidotes that replenish glutathione and detoxify NAPQI were developed; these included methionine, cysteine, cysteamine and dimercaprol (Prescott et al. 1976). Before NAC was available as a treatment for paracetamol poisoning, the morbidity following paracetamol overdose was significant, with a mortality rate reported by Prescott et al. of 5% in untreated patients with an initial paracetamol concentration above the probable risk nomogram line (Prescott et al. 1979). After the introduction of NAC in the 1980s, the mortality rate fell to 0.4% (Gunnell et al. 1997).

Cysteamine and methionine were shown to decrease the risk of developing hepatotoxicity in three small randomised controlled trials (RCTs; Douglas et al. 1976; Hamlyn et al. 1981; Hughes et al. 1977). However, their use was limited as cysteamine was associated with severe headache, nausea and vomiting in nearly all patients, while methionine only came in an oral preparation (Hamlyn et al. 1981; Douglas et al. 1976; Hughes et al. 1977).

Prescott et al. (1979), in an observational study of 200 participants, showed that first-line intravenous (IV) NAC was more effective than cysteamine and methionine and had noticeably less adverse effects (Prescott et al. 1979). This study compared IV NAC versus supportive treatment or comparison antidotes (cysteamine and methionine). All participants had a paracetamol concentration above the 200 mg/L at 4 h nomogram treatment line. IV NAC was given as three infusions, with an initial dose of 150 mg/kg over 15 m followed by 50 mg/kg over 4 h and 100 mg/kg over the next 16 h (total dose 300 mg/kg in 20.25 h). The comparison antidote and supportive groups were historical control groups, treated 3 and 10 years earlier, respectively. In this study, 1 out of 62 patients treated within 10 h with IV NAC developed severe liver damage compared with 33 out of 57 (58%) control patients. However, the rate of severe liver injury in the historical control methionine group in this study was 20%, compared to 4–10% in other studies (Prescott et al. 1979; Meredith et al. 1978; Crome et al. 1976).

Since this time, NAC has been accepted as an antidote for paracetamol overdose, in the IV dosing regimen proposed by Prescott et al. or a longer 72 h oral regimen, used mainly in the United States (Williamson et al. 2013; Woo et al. 2000). Smilkstein et al. reported the results of a large multicentre observational study in the United States of 2540 patients receiving oral NAC for the treatment of paracetamol poisoning. In this study, there were only 11 deaths with a mortality rate of 0.43%. Rates of hepatotoxicity increased with increasing treatment delay from time of ingestion beyond 8 h. They showed that the 72 h oral regimen is at least as effective as the IV 20 h protocol and possibly superior in those treated beyond 10 h (Smilkstein et al. 1988).

The current recommendations for the treatment of paracetamol poisoning vary between countries. Treatment with NAC is usually based on the patients' paracetamol concentration. Nomograms define risk lines for hepatotoxicity by graphs plotting concentration versus time. Risk lines define high risk (300 mg/L at 4 h line), probable risk (200 mg/L at 4 h line) and possible risk (150 mg/L at 4 h line; Rumack and Matthew 1975; Prescott et al. 1979; Smilkstein et al. 1991). In the United Kingdom, a lower risk line is defined at 100 mg/L at 4 h (MHRA 2012).

There are few RCTs investigating interventions in patients who are poisoned by paracetamol (Park et al. 2015), but we identified five RCTs (Online Table 9.1). Only one had survival as their primary outcome, and this was conducted in patients with paracetamol-induced fulminant hepatic failure (Keays et al. 1991). In this trial of 50 participants, Keays et al. (1991) found that IV NAC compared with placebo for paracetamol-induced fulminant hepatic failure appeared to reduce mortality, with a significant difference in survival rates between the two groups of 28% (95% CI for the difference: 3 to 53%, $P = 0.04$). The survival rates was 48% (12/25 patients) in the NAC group compared with 20% (5/25) in the control group (Keays et al. 1991).

More recent RCTs of IV NAC have investigated the optimal way to administer NAC, in order to minimise adverse events (AEs). However, none of these were powered to look at efficacy. There are four RCTs looking at alternative IV NAC regimens compared with the standard three-bag regimen (150 mg/kg of NAC over 15 m followed by 50 mg/kg over 4 h and 100 mg/kg over the next 16 h, total dose

300 mg/kg in 20.25 h; Bateman et al. 2014; Kerr et al. 2005; Eizadi-Mood et al. 2013; Arefi et al. 2013). Kerr et al. looked at the effect of slowing the loading dose from 15 m to 1 h. In this trial of 180 participants, an infusion time of 15 m did not significantly increase the risk of specific AEs (e.g. anaphylactoid reactions, gastro-intestinal disorders, etc.) or drug-related AEs within 2 h, compared to administration over 60 m. The frequency of drug-related AEs was 45% in the 15 m group and 38% in the 60 m group (absolute difference, 7%; 95% CI for the difference, −8 to 22%; $P = 0.36$ (Kerr et al. 2005)).

Bateman et al. compared two different IV NAC regimens, a modified 12 h regimen that has an initial lower loading dose given over 2 h (100 mg/kg) followed by 200 mg/kg over 10 h versus the standard 20.25 h schedule (Bateman et al. 2014). They showed that the modified 12 h regimen resulted in a significant reduction in the incidence of vomiting, retching or need for anti-emetics at 2 h (39/108 versus 79/109; adjusted odds ratio 0.26; 97.5% CI, 0.13–0.52; $p < 0.0001$). A reduced rate of severe anaphylactoid reactions was seen in the shorter modified regimen ($n = 5$) versus the standard regimen ($n = 31$) (adjusted common odds ratio 0.23, 97.5% CI, 0.12–0.43; $p < 0.0001$). There was no significant difference in efficacy detected between the two regimens, with an adjusted odds ratio of 0.60 (95% CI: 0.2–1.83), for an ALT increase of 50%. However, the trial was under-powered for this outcome (Bateman et al. 2014).

Arefi et al. (2013) investigated oral NAC versus the standard 20.25 h IV NAC (Arefi et al. 2013). This was a small study of 66 patients published originally in Farsi (Persian). It reported no statistically significant difference in AST, ALT, bilirubin and prothrombin time in the oral versus the IV group at 24, 48 and 72 h. However, the numbers were small in both groups ($n = 33$), and the trial was not powered to show a difference in efficacy. Nausea and hypotension were significantly more prevalent in the oral compared with the IV NAC treatment group. Nausea occurred in 19/33 (57.6%) in the oral group versus 11/33 (33.3%) in the IV group ($p = 0.04$). This trial had a high risk of bias and did not report the method of randomisation, outcome measures, power calculations or numbers excluded. Patients were "excluded" from the IV arm if anaphylactoid reactions were unresponsive to decreasing the administration rate and given oral NAC, and it was unclear if these participants were included in the intention to treat analysis (Arefi et al. 2013).

Eizadi-Mood et al. (2013) looked at a combination of IV and oral NAC versus a standard 20.25 h IV NAC regimen in 50 participants (Eizadi-Mood et al. 2013). Again, this study was not powered for efficacy, and the main outcome was the rate of anaphylactoid reactions defined as nausea and vomiting, dyspnoea and flushing. This study was at high risk of bias and had a methodological flaw in that the investigators post hoc excluded those who vomited twice after oral NAC and did not analyse them as intention to treat. The authors found that 13.3% of those who had a combination of oral and IV NAC vomited versus 28.5% in the IV NAC group. Adding the excluded 10 patients with vomiting increases this rate to 48% and reverses the conclusions of the study (Eizadi-Mood et al. 2013).

Hence the management of paracetamol poisoning is based on observational studies, case series and animal data (Park et al. 2015). A controlled trial comparing NAC to no treatment would be unethical, because the use of IV and oral NAC for paracetamol poisoning has coincided with a marked decrease in morbidity. Future trials are therefore likely to focus on the optimum NAC regimen and NAC route or compare NAC to other antidotes such as methionine.

9.3.3 Dosage Regimens

Two different NAC regimens were initially developed, a 20.25 h IV regimen in the United Kingdom and a 3-day oral regimen in the United States (US) due to a lack of licensing for IV NAC in the USA (Rumack and Bateman 2012; Smilkstein et al. 1988). The dosing regimen for IV NAC was developed in Edinburgh and chosen to give a large loading dose as patients were thought to be glutathione depleted on presentation (Prescott et al. 1977). The IV regimen was 20.25 h based on five times a theoretical 4-hour half-life of paracetamol (Prescott et al. 1977; Rumack and Bateman 2012). The traditional IV three-bag infusion delivers 300 mg/kg of NAC over 20.25 h with an initial 150 mg/kg of NAC over 15 m followed by 50 mg/kg over 4 h and 100 mg/kg over the next 16 h. The 16 h infusion was based on providing 6.25 mg/kg/h of NAC, theorised to be sufficient based on liver glutathione turnover to maintain glutathione concentrations (Rumack and Bateman 2012; Rumack 2002). In the USA and Australia, this loading dose is given over 1 h.

In the USA there were concerns about the prolonged paracetamol half-life seen in overdose in some patients. Based on a 12 h paracetamol half-life that can occur in overdose, a 72 h oral regimen was developed (Rumack and Bateman 2012). The oral NAC regimen is given as a loading dose of 140 mg/kg, with maintenance doses of 70 mg/kg that is repeated every 4 h for a total of 17 doses (Smilkstein et al. 1991). Figure 9.1 shows the infusion rate and accumulated NAC dose of the oral versus the IV regimen.

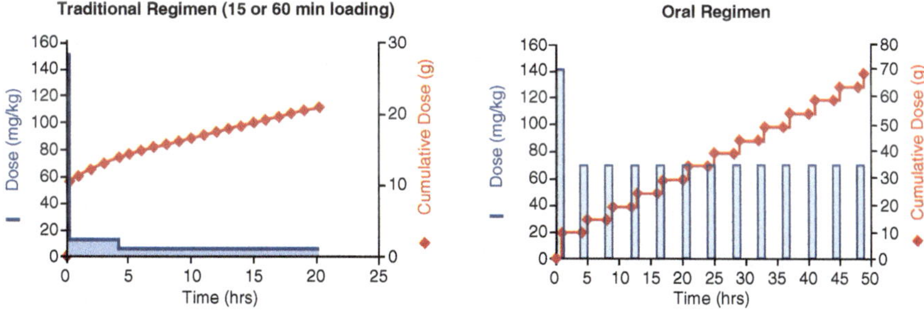

Fig. 9.1 N-Acetylcysteine infusion (mg/kg) and cumulative N-Acetylcysteine dose (g) in a 70 kg patient versus time. Blue line (left y-axis) shows the infusion rate in mg/kg. Red line (right y-axis) shows the cumulative dose of acetylcysteine (g) for a 70 kg person. Note different scale right y-axis between the two graphs as larger cumulative dose of acetylcysteine administered with the oral regimen

There are various observational studies that have looked at differing NAC regimens to decrease the rate of AEs or decrease drug administration errors. To decrease rates of AEs, these regimens lengthen the loading dose to 4 h, most commonly 200 mg/kg of NAC over 4 h (Isbister et al. 2016; Wong and Graudins 2016). Observational studies of these two regimens reported fewer systemic hypersensitivity (4–8%) and severe non-IgE anaphylactic (0–0.5%) reactions, but rates of gastrointestinal reactions remained high (27–39%; Isbister et al. 2016; Wong and Graudins 2016).

While Oakley et al. (2011) and Johnson et al. (2011) have looked at regimens to simplify NAC administration and reduce administration errors by either using a two-bag regimen (Oakley) or a single-bag method and altering the rate of the infusion (Johnson), Johnson et al. reviewed their protocol retrospectively and still found 13.5 errors per 100 administration interventions (Johnson et al. 2011; Oakley et al. 2011).

Questions have also been raised as to whether the dose of NAC is adequate in those who take large paracetamol overdoses. The current IV NAC regimen is adequate to detoxify an ingested paracetamol dose of 15.9 g (Rumack and Bateman 2012). With debate over whether the third infusion 100 mg/kg over 16 h (6.25 mg/kg/h) is adequate for larger overdoses and whether higher doses are required, NAC regimens have been proposed that increase the 16 h infusion in those who ingest large paracetamol overdoses or who have high paracetamol concentrations. Rumack and Bateman theoretically proposed that a patient who ingested 47.7 g of paracetamol would require this third infusion to be increased to 17.5 mg/kg/h (Rumack and Bateman 2012). However, there are few studies investigating increased NAC doses and whether this reduces risk of hepatotoxicity. The most commonly proposed modification to the standard IV NAC regimen is doubling the dose of NAC in the 16 h infusion (from 100 to 200 mg/kg), in those with high paracetamol concentrations. A recent survey of international clinical toxicologists and poison centres found that 61% of the 164 respondents would increase the dose of NAC in the 100 mg/kg over 16 h infusion in patients with a high paracetamol concentration. However, the paracetamol concentration at which the dose should be increased varied widely between respondents (Juma et al. 2015).

Indeed, further research is required to determine what the optimum dose of NAC is and what regimen results in the least AEs. The current IV NAC regimen of 300 mg/kg over 20 h is adequate in most overdoses. Administering this as a two-bag regimen, 200 mg/kg over 4 h and then 100 mg/kg over 16 h appears to be more practical, associated with less AEs and with similar effectiveness. However its efficacy compared to the standard regimen still requires further studies. Table 9.2

Table 9.2 Common indications for NAC following paracetamol ingestion

Acute paracetamol ingestion with a paracetamol concentration above the paracetamol nomogram line
Toxic paracetamol ingestion presenting >8 h post ingestion
Acute liver injury as a result of paracetamol ingestion acute or supratherapeutic
Ingestion of a toxic dose of modified release paracetamol

Table 9.3 Recommended intravenous regimens for NAC administration

Standard three-bag IV NAC regimen	Two-bag IV NAC regimen
First infusion: 150 mg/kg in 200 mL of 5% glucose dextrose over 60 min	First infusion: followed by 200 mg/kg in 500 mL of 5% glucose dextrose over 4 h
Second infusion: followed by 50 mg/kg in 500 mL of 5% glucose dextrose over 4 h	Second infusion: followed by 100 mg/kg in 1 L of 5% glucose dextrose over 16 h
Third infusion: followed by 100 mg/kg in 1 L of 5% glucose dextrose over 16 h	

Note: NAC is also compatible in normal saline and ½ normal saline

outlines some of the common indications for NAC following paracetamol poisoning, but note these indications vary depending on local guidelines. Table 9.3 outlines the most commonly administered NAC regimens, the traditional three-bag and the newly proposed two-bag regimen.

9.3.4 Potential Adverse Effects

Both oral and IV NAC are associated with AEs. Since NAC was introduced, there have been reports of AEs, ranging from mild to severe. These include rash, nausea and vomiting, angioedema, flushing, tachycardia, bronchospasm, hypotension and death (Schmidt 2013; Sandilands and Bateman 2009; Mant et al. 1984), with the most common AEs from IV NAC being nausea and vomiting and cutaneous systemic hypersensitivity reactions (Sandilands and Bateman 2009). The rates of AEs vary greatly between observational studies. The difference in reported rates depends on whether they were studied prospectively or retrospectively and which AEs were recorded, total versus gastrointestinal versus systemic hypersensitivity reactions. A review of the larger IV observational NAC studies revealed reported rates of AEs from NAC varied from 8.5 to 77% (Chiew et al. 2015). Oral NAC administration often results in rashes, nausea, vomiting, and abdominal pain and can be unpalatable to some patients.

The main mechanism for AEs is a non-IgE-mediated systemic hypersensitivity (anaphylactic) reaction. In patients having moderate to severe AEs, a 2.5-fold increase in histamine concentrations has been reported, without elevated tryptase concentrations (Pakravan et al. 2008).

AEs most commonly occur within the first hour of treatment and appear to be associated with peak NAC concentrations and so a rate-dependent effect (Sandilands and Bateman 2009). Various risk factors have been identified for developing AEs, with higher rates in females, those with a family history of allergy or past history of asthma (Pakravan et al. 2008; Schmidt and Dalhoff 2001; Waring et al. 2008; Sandilands and Bateman 2009). A lower paracetamol concentration has been associated with both an increased and a decreased risk of AEs in various studies (Schmidt 2013; Carroll et al. 2015).

Various new regimens have been trialled to decrease the rate of AEs. As outlined above in the one RCT and various observational studies, they have shown by decreasing or slowing the initial loading dose there is a decrease in AEs. This is presumably due to a decrease in the peak NAC concentration.

9.4   N-Acetylcysteine in Non-paracetamol Poisonings

NAC has been used as a treatment in a variety of overdoses for its antioxidant effects, particularly in those poisons with a high morbidity where few other treatment options are available. NAC has been proposed to be effective in the treatment of many drugs, chemicals and toxins including paraquat, amanita, clove oil, pennyroyal oil, carbon tetrachloride and chloroform toxicity. The proposed mechanisms for the effectiveness of NAC in these toxins are outlined in Table 9.1. The evidence for use of NAC in these is limited due to the uncommon and sporadic occurrence of these poisonings and is usually limited to case reports, occasional case series and animal studies.

9.4.1   Paraquat

Paraquat is a herbicide that is highly toxic in overdose with an overall mortality rate of greater than 50%. As little as one mouthful (15–30 mL) of 20% concentrate may produce multisystem organ failure, pulmonary toxicity and death (Gawarammana and Buckley 2011). In Asia it is a significant cause of morbidity and in many countries, such as Sri Lanka, is the leading single agent causing death from poisoning (Dawson et al. 2010). Paraquat generates highly reactive oxygen and nitrite species that result in toxicity in most organs. Paraquat toxicity is most severe in the lungs and results in acute alveolitis, pneumonitis and lung fibrosis (Gawarammana and Buckley 2011). Furthermore, paraquat poisoning can also cause severe renal and liver injury.

There are no widely accepted treatment guidelines for paraquat poisoning, with management varying from supportive care alone to various combinations of immune modulation, antioxidant therapy, haemoperfusion and haemodialysis (Gawarammana and Buckley 2011). Initial management typically consists of decreasing absorption with gastric lavage and activated charcoal (Vale and Kulig 2004). Following decontamination other treatments trialled include immunosuppressive agents (such as cyclophosphamide, MESNA, methylprednisolone and dexamethasone), haemodialysis and antioxidants (such as NAC, vitamin C, vitamin E, deferoxamine and salicylic acid; Gawarammana and Buckley 2011).

NAC is a potential treatment for paraquat toxicity and works via multiple mechanisms including scavenging of reactive oxygen species, increasing glutathione and reducing inflammation, lipid peroxidation and apoptosis. NAC has been shown to reduce paraquat-induced apoptosis and inflammatory response in human lung cultures and improves survival in rats (Yeh et al. 2006; Cappelletti et al. 1998). Despite its potential benefits, there are limited studies in human paraquat poisoning. There are case reports and few case series that treat patients with IV NAC in combination with various other therapies (Davarpanah et al. 2015; Drault et al. 1999; Lheureux et al. 1995; Gil et al. 2008; Raghu et al. 2013; Dinis-Oliveira et al. 2006; Cherukuri et al. 2014). Doses of NAC vary between cases. From this limited data and based on the relative safety of NAC and high toxicity of paraquat, NAC should be commenced in most paraquat poisonings (see Online Table 9.2).

9.4.2   Mushroom Toxins

9.4.2.1 Amatoxin

Amatoxin is the most potent hepatotoxin in cyclopeptide mushrooms and irreversibly binds to RNA polymerase II, causing hepatic necrosis (Berger and Guss 2005). *Amanita phalloides* is a cyclopeptide variety of mushroom containing amatoxin that is responsible for more than 90% of mushroom-related fatalities (Berger and Guss 2005). Ingestions of as little as one mushroom cap can cause fulminant hepatic failure and death (Berger and Guss 2005). The clinical features of amanita poisoning involve three major stages, an asymptomatic latency period, a gastrointestinal phase include vomiting, abdominal pain and watery diarrhoea that can result in severe dehydration and lastly a hepatic-kidney toxicity stage. The final hepatic-kidney stage starts 48–72 h post-ingestion and lasts for 6–16 days and can result in acute hepatic failure, renal failure and death (Poucheret et al. 2010).

Treatment firstly involves gastrointestinal decontamination including multiple-dose activated charcoal, supportive care, various antidotes and as a last resort liver transplant (Enjalbert et al. 2002; Poucheret et al. 2010; Broussard et al. 2001; Roberts et al. 2013). Multiple antidotes have been used to treat patients with *Amanita phalloides* poisoning with limited evidence for all. These include silymarin complex (silibinin); antioxidants such as NAC and vitamins E and C; benzylpenicillin (penicillin G), rifampicin, cimetidine or other beta-lactam antibiotics; thioctic acid; hormones; and steroids. These antidotes have been administered alone or, more commonly, in combination (Roberts et al. 2013; Enjalbert et al. 2002; Poucheret et al. 2010).

NAC is thought to be beneficial as amatoxin results in a decrease in glutathione synthesis and in production of reactive oxygen species that ultimately lead to damage to all components within the cell, resulting in cell death and glutathione depletion. NAC replenishes glutathione and scavenges free radicals (Smith and Davis 2016). NAC has been shown to increase non-transplant survival and is beneficial in grade I–II encephalopathy (Craig et al. 2010). Pourchet et al. retrospectively analysed 2110 cases of amatoxin poisoning from a database built up from Enjalbert et al. over a 20-year period. They found silibinin to be the most effective antidote, administered in 624 cases, alone or in combination with other treatments; it decreased the mortality from 10.7 to 5.6%. NAC was given in 192 treated patients and reduced the mortality rate to 6.8% (Poucheret et al. 2010; Enjalbert et al. 2002). NAC has also been used as an antidote in multiple case series and case reports, often in combination with other treatments such as silibinin (Garcia et al. 2015; Roberts et al. 2013; Karvellas et al. 2016; Montanini et al. 1999; Vanooteghem et al. 2014; Grabhorn et al. 2013; Zevin et al. 1997; Boyer et al. 2001; French et al. 2011; Ahishali et al. 2012; Chen et al. 2012; Ward et al. 2013). From these case reports and series, NAC appears beneficial in the management of amanita toxicity especially when used in combination with other treatments (Online Table 9.3).

9.4.2.2 Orellanine Toxin (*Cortinarius* Species)

Cortinarius mushrooms including *Cortinarius speciosissimus*, *C. orellanus*, and *C. orellanoides* contain the tubulotoxin orellanine that is typically found in Europe and North America. Ingestion of *Cortinarius* species may result in mild early gastrointestinal symptoms and transient liver damage followed by a delayed onset of acute kidney injury, developing over several days to up to 2 weeks (Dinis-Oliveira et al. 2016; Esposito et al. 2015). Renal impairment is due to severe interstitial nephritis, acute focal tubular damage and interstitial fibrosis (Dinis-Oliveira et al. 2016). It is estimated that 30–45% of individuals who ingest nephrotoxic *Cortinarius* mushrooms develop acute renal failure. Of these, half usually recover and half progress to chronic renal failure and require ongoing haemodialysis or kidney transplant (Dinis-Oliveira et al. 2016).

Treatment strategies include symptomatic treatment, haemodialysis, plasmapheresis, steroids and NAC (Kerschbaum et al. 2012) and, in severe cases, renal replacement therapy and renal transplant (Nagaraja et al. 2015). NAC has been reported to be effective in a few case reports (Kerschbaum et al. 2012; Kilner et al. 1999; Wornle et al. 2004; Online Table 9.3) with some authors recommending that early treatment with high-dose antioxidant therapy and steroids may be effective in reducing the risk of chronic renal failure (Kerschbaum et al. 2012). However others have reported no benefit of NAC following *C. orellanus* ingestion (Grebe et al. 2013; Esposito et al. 2015). Grebe et al. (2013) reviewed eight patients who accidentally ingested *C. orellanus*, and NAC and corticosteroids were administered to six patients. However, all patients developed acute renal injury, and after 12 months, seven patients had chronic renal disease of which three required ongoing renal replacement therapy. The author's concluded that NAC and corticosteroid treatment did not seem to have a beneficial effect on either acute or chronic kidney disease in these cases. However, they did note the ineffectiveness of NAC and corticosteroids in this case series may have been due to the long delay between consumption and treatment initiation (Grebe et al. 2013).

9.4.3   Essential Oils

9.4.3.1 Clove Oil

Clove oil is an essential oil that is used as a "remedy" for toothache. It is obtained from the distillation of dried flower buds of the *Eugenia caryophyllata* tree and contains 70–90% eugenol. Eugenol causes hepatotoxicity in a similar way to paracetamol poisoning with eugenol being metabolised by cytochrome P450 to quinone intermediates. In animal studies glutathione-depleted mice develop hepatotoxicity from clove oil (Mizutani et al. 1991). These rat studies have also shown that hepatotoxicity can be prevented by administration of NAC (El Rahi et al. 2015).

Toxic effects from clove oil ingestion include central nervous system (CNS) depression, seizures, aspiration pneumonitis, respiratory depression, renal failure, hypoglycaemia lactic acidosis and liver injury (Eisen et al. 2004; Hartnoll and Douek 1993). Children have developed severe hepatotoxicity after drinking as little as 5–10 mL (Hartnoll and Douek 1993). Treatment includes good supportive care with the use of NAC having a strong theoretical basis (Eisen et al. 2004). There are few case reports of NAC being used successfully in patients with hepatotoxicity secondary to clove oil ingestion in a similar regimen to that used in paracetamol poisoning (see Online Table 9.4; Eisen et al. 2004; Hartnoll and Douek 1993; Janes et al. 2005). In both of these case reports, NAC was commenced only after LFTs became abnormal. Given the biologically plausible effect of NAC in clove oil poisoning, it is indicated in these circumstances. However, the question remains whether if given earlier it could prevent an acute liver injury.

9.4.3.2 Pennyroyal Oil

Pennyroyal is an herbal extract or oil derived from leaves of the plant in the mint genus (*Mentha pulegium*) or *Hedeoma pulegioides*; it was used in the past as an insect repellent and an abortifacient. Gastrointestinal symptoms are noted at doses of pennyroyal oil as low as 10 mL, with cases of centrilobular hepatitis following ingestion of 30 mL or more (Sullivan Jr et al. 1979; Woolf 1999; Bakerink et al. 1996). Pennyroyal extract contains many components; the main toxic competent is pulegone which accounts for 85% of its composition. Pulegone can cause acute multi-organ injury, including acute hepatic necrosis.

There are very few case reports in the literature; Anderson et al. report a case of a child who ingested a life-threatening amount of pennyroyal oil, was administered NAC and did not subsequently develop hepatitis (Anderson et al. 1996; Buechel et al. 1983).

9.4.4   Hydrocarbons

9.4.4.1 Chloroform

Chloroform is a halogenated hydrocarbon and is used as a general anaesthetic agent and general industrial solvent. Chloroform is metabolised by cytochrome P450 to phosgene and free radicals, which cause mitochondrial damage and hepatocellular death (Pandit et al. 2012; Pohl et al. 1977). Most cases of chloroform toxicity are the result of inhalational exposures, with few cases of oral ingestion. Hepatotoxicity has been reported after inhalation and skin exposure (Kang et al. 2014). Cases of oral ingestion of chloroform are rare but have been associated with severe toxicity such as CNS depression, respiratory depression and delayed hepatotoxicity. From these case reports of oral chloroform ingestion, the onset of hepatotoxicity was at approximately 36 h post ingestion, even more delayed than following paracetamol ingestion (Jayaweera et al. 2016).

NAC has been successfully administered in several cases, in the same regimen as used for paracetamol poisoning (Online Table 9.5; Dell'Aglio et al. 2010; Jayaweera et al. 2016). These cases have commenced NAC early aiming to prevent liver injury and late following the onset of liver injury (Dell'Aglio et al. 2010; Boyer and de Roos 1998). There have also been cases in the literature that have survived without NAC (Kim 2008). There is very limited evidence to guide treatment, but given the severity of the toxicity that can result, early NAC treatment may be beneficial with little harm.

9.4.4.2 Carbon Tetrachloride

Carbon tetrachloride is a clear, colourless, volatile and stable chlorinated hydrocarbon that was formerly widely used in fire extinguishers, as a precursor to refrigerants and as a cleaning agent. Due to its ozone-depleting properties, its use is restricted but is still used in laboratories and industry. Carbon tetrachloride is highly toxic with as little as 5–10 mL by ingestion or inhalation causing toxicity (Flanagan and Meredith 1991). The early features of acute carbon tetrachloride poisoning include nausea, vomiting, ataxia and confusion. Severe cases can develop coma, hypotension, respiratory depression and hepatorenal toxicity that can be fatal (Ruprah et al. 1985). The mechanism of toxicity is due to its toxic metabolite trichloromethyl that may covalently bind to macromolecules or react further (Recknagel et al. 1989).

Patients have been managed with antioxidants/free radical scavengers, including vitamin E, sulphhydryl compounds and hyperbaric oxygen (Mathieson et al. 1985). The use of NAC was reported in a case series of 19 patients poisoned with carbon tetrachloride (Online Table 9.5; Ruprah et al. 1985). Thirteen were treated with intravenous NAC of which seven developed mild hepatic injury, one moderate hepatic injury and one (history of chronic alcohol abuse) severe hepatorenal injury requiring haemodialysis. This is in comparison to the six patients (one lost to follow-up) who were not given NAC of which three developed hepatorenal failure requiring dialysis and one died. The authors suggest prompt treatment with NAC may minimise hepatorenal damage following carbon tetrachloride poisoning.

9.4.5 Other

There are numerous case reports where NAC has been trialled for a varying group of toxins either to treat liver injury or for its antioxidant effect (Online Table 9.6; Bhat and Kenchetty 2015; Sheikh-Hamad et al. 1997; El Rahi et al. 2015; Howard et al. 1987). Human volunteer, animal studies case reports and case series have trialled NAC as a potential treatment for a wide variety of adverse drug reactions such as haematological complications of gold therapy and hypersensitivity from co-trimoxazole and phenytoin (Chyka et al. 2000).

NAC has also been used in cases of idiosyncratic drug-induced liver injury (DILI) from a number of causes (Elliott et al. 2016; Mudalel et al. 2015). The mechanism underlying hepatotoxicity in idiosyncratic DILI is not clearly understood; however, it does not involve glutathione depletion. With the proposed benefits of NAC via its antioxidant effects (Chughlay et al. 2015), a systematic review of NAC for the treatment of DILI identified just one RCT of NAC vs. placebo (Chughlay et al. 2016). This RCT was a part of a larger study; there were 45 participants with DILI, of which 19 received NAC and 26 placebo (Lee et al. 2009). The primary outcome was mortality with four deaths in the NAC arm compared with nine deaths in the placebo arm, odds ratio of 0.50 (95% CI = 0.13–1.98, $P = 0.33$). Furthermore, transplant-free survival was higher in the NAC group 58% ($n = 11$) vs. 27% ($n = 7$), odds ratio of 0.27 (95% CI 0.076, 0.942, $P = 0.04$; Lee et al. 2009; Chughlay et al. 2016). This study was not powered for either outcome; hence, the authors of the systematic review concluded that the numbers were too small to draw any firm conclusions (Chughlay et al. 2016).

9.5 Summary

NAC is the mainstay of treatment for paracetamol poisoning, and its use has led to a significant reduction in both the mortality and morbidity following paracetamol overdose, with more recent trials of NAC focusing on optimising the NAC regimen to decrease rates of side effects or shorten treatment time.

NAC use is not just confined to paracetamol and has been utilised for a wide variety of toxins and ingestions, with a proposed mechanism of action in these cases either due to NAC's antioxidant and/or glutathione-replenishing effects. The evidence for its use in many of these toxins is often limited to animal studies, case reports or small case series, due to the uncommon occurrence of these cases. Recommendations for use of NAC for these various toxins are shown in Table 9.4. Due to the relative safety of NAC and the high morbidity associated with many of these ingestions, NAC is often recommended.

Table 9.4 Overall ratings of NAC based on clinical studies presented by toxin

Toxin	Randomised control trials number (number positive)	Grade of recommendation	Recommendation for treatment
Paracetamol	5 (4 RCTs primary outcome rate of adverse events. 1 trial primary outcome was effectiveness which was a positive trial)	B	There are few RCTs investigating NAC in patients who are poisoned by paracetamol, the majority are testing differing NAC regimens. However, multiple large observational studies show the efficacy of NAC. Hence NAC is the mainstay of treatment for paracetamol poisoning
Toxin	Uncontrolled studies number (number positive)	Grade of recommendation	Recommendation for treatment
Paraquat (herbicide)	6 (4) Note 1 case series no recommendation	C	From limited data and based on the relative safety of NAC and high toxicity of paraquat, NAC should be commenced in most paraquat poisonings
Amatoxin (predominately *Amanita phalloides* mushroom)	11 (10) Note 1 case series no recommendation	C	From these case reports and series, NAC appears beneficial and is recommended in the management of amanita toxicity especially when used in combination with other treatments
Orellanine toxin (*Cortinarius* species mushroom)	5 (3)	D	Mixed results, in those studies that showed no benefit patient treatment was delayed due to late presentation. Early treatment with high-dose antioxidant therapy together with steroids may be effective in reducing the risk of chronic renal failure
Clove oil (essential Oil)	2 (2)	C	From limited data and based on the relative safety of NAC and high toxicity of clove oil, NAC is recommended
Pennyroyal (hydrocarbon)	2 (2)	C	From limited data and based on the relative safety of NAC and high toxicity of clove oil, NAC is recommended
Chloroform (hydrocarbon)	4 (4)	C	There is very limited evidence to guide treatment, but given the severity of the toxicity that can result, early NAC treatment may be beneficial with little harm
Carbon tetrachloride (hydrocarbon)	2 (2)	C	From very limited data NAC is recommended

References

Ahishali E, Boynuegri B, Ozpolat E, Surmeli H, Dolapcioglu C, Dabak R, Bahcebasi ZB, Bayramicli OU (2012) Approach to mushroom intoxication and treatment: can we decrease mortality? Clin Res Hepatol Gastroenterol 36(2):139–145. https://doi.org/10.1016/j.clinre.2011.11.004

Anderson IB, Mullen WH, Meeker JE, Khojasteh Bakht SC, Oishi S, Nelson SD, Blanc PD (1996) Pennyroyal toxicity: measurement of toxic metabolite levels in two cases and review of the literature. Ann Intern Med 124(8):726–734

Arefi M, Behnoush B, Pouraziz H, Yousefinejad V (2013) Comparison of oral and intravenous N-acetylcysteine administration in the treatment of acetaminophen poisoning. Scientific Journal of Kurdistan University of Medical. Sciences 18(2):36–43

Bakerink JA, Gospe SM Jr, Dimand RJ, Eldridge MW (1996) Multiple organ failure after ingestion of pennyroyal oil from herbal tea in two infants. Pediatrics 98(5):944–947

Bateman DN, Dear JW, Thanacoody HK, Thomas SH, Eddleston M, Sandilands EA, Coyle J, Cooper JG, Rodriguez A, Butcher I, Lewis SC, Vliegenthart AD, Veiraiah A, Webb DJ, Gray A (2014) Reduction of adverse effects from intravenous acetylcysteine treatment for paracetamol poisoning: a randomised controlled trial. Lancet 383(9918):697–704. https://doi.org/10.1016/S0140-6736(13)62062-0

Berger KJ, Guss DA (2005) Mycotoxins revisited: part I. J Emerg Med 28(1):53–62. https://doi.org/10.1016/j.jemermed.2004.08.013

Bhat S, Kenchetty KP (2015) N-acetyl cysteine in the management of rodenticide consumption - life saving? JCDR 9(1):OC10–OC13. https://doi.org/10.7860/jcdr/2015/11484.5455

Boyer ELSPJ, de Roos F (1998) Limited hepatotoxicity following a massive chloroform ingestion treated with oral N-acetyl-cysteine. J Toxicol Clin Toxicol 36:427–534

Boyer J-C, Hernandez F, Estorc J, De La Coussaye J-E, Bali J-P (2001) Management of maternal amanita phalloïdes poisoning during the first trimester of pregnancy: a case report and review of the literature. Clin Chem 47(5):971

Broussard CN, Aggarwal A, Lacey SR, Post AB, Gramlich T, Henderson JM, Younossi ZM (2001) Mushroom poisoning--from diarrhea to liver transplantation. Am J Gastroenterol 96(11):3195–3198. https://doi.org/10.1111/j.1572-0241.2001.05283.x

Buckpitt AR, Rollins DE, Mitchell JR (1979) Varying effects of sulfhydryl nucleophiles on acetaminophen oxidation and sulfhydryl adduct formation. Biochem Pharmacol 28(19):2941–2946

Buechel DW, Haverlah VC, Gardner ME (1983) Pennyroyal oil ingestion: report of a case. J Am Osteopath Assoc 82(10):793–794

Cappelletti G, Maggioni MG, Maci R (1998) Apoptosis in human lung epithelial cells: triggering by paraquat and modulation by antioxidants. Cell Biol Int 22(9-10):671–678. https://doi.org/10.1006/cbir.1998.0305

Carroll R, Benger J, Bramley K, Williams S, Griffin L, Potokar J, Gunnell D (2015) Epidemiology, management and outcome of paracetamol poisoning in an inner city emergency department. EMJ 32(2):155–160. https://doi.org/10.1136/emermed-2013-202518

Chen WC, Kassi M, Saeed U, Frenette CT (2012) A rare case of amatoxin poisoning in the state of Texas. Case Rep Gastroenterol 6(2):350–357. https://doi.org/10.1159/000339692

Cherukuri H, Pramoda K, Rohini D, Thunga G, Vijaynarayana K, Sreedharan N, Varma M, Pandit V (2014) Demographics, clinical characteristics and management of herbicide poisoning in tertiary care hospital. Toxicol Int 21(2):209–213. https://doi.org/10.4103/0971-6580.139813

Chiew AL, Isbister GK, Duffull SB, Buckley NA (2015) Evidence for the changing regimens of acetylcysteine. Br J Clin Pharmacol 81:471–481. https://doi.org/10.1111/bcp.12789

Chughlay MF, Kramer N, Werfalli M, Spearman W, Engel ME, Cohen K (2015) N-acetylcysteine for non-paracetamol drug-induced liver injury: a systematic review protocol. Syst Rev 4:84. https://doi.org/10.1186/s13643-015-0075-6

Chughlay MF, Kramer N, Spearman CW, Werfalli M, Cohen K (2016) N-acetylcysteine for non-paracetamol drug-induced liver injury: a systematic review. Br J Clin Pharmacol 81(6):1021–1029. https://doi.org/10.1111/bcp.12880

Chyka PA, Butler AY, Holliman BJ, Herman MI (2000) Utility of acetylcysteine in treating poisonings and adverse drug reactions. Drug Saf 22(2):123–148

Craig DG, Lee A, Hayes PC, Simpson KJ (2010) Review article: the current management of acute liver failure. Aliment Pharmacol Ther 31(3):345–358. https://doi.org/10.1111/j.1365-2036.2009.04175.x

Crome P, Vale JA, Volans GN, Widdop B, Goulding R (1976) Oral methionine in the treatment of severe paracetamol (Acetaminophen) overdose. Lancet 2(7990):829–830

Davarpanah MA, Hosseinzadeh F, Mohammadi SS (2015) Treatment following intoxication with lethal dose of paraquat: a case report and review of literature. Iran Red Crescent Med J 17(10):e19373. https://doi.org/10.5812/ircmj.19373

Davidson DG, Eastham WN (1966) Acute liver necrosis following overdose of paracetamol. Br Med J 2(5512):497–499

Dawson AH, Eddleston M, Senarathna L, Mohamed F, Gawarammana I, Bowe SJ, Manuweera G, Buckley NA (2010) Acute human lethal toxicity of agricultural pesticides: a prospective cohort study. PLoS Med 7(10):e1000357. https://doi.org/10.1371/journal.pmed.1000357

Dell'Aglio DM, Sutter ME, Schwartz MD, Koch DD, Algren DA, Morgan BW (2010) Acute chloroform ingestion successfully treated with intravenously administered N-acetylcysteine. J Med Toxicol 6(2):143–146. https://doi.org/10.1007/s13181-010-0071-0

Dinis-Oliveira RJ, Sarmento A, Reis P, Amaro A, Remiao F, Bastos ML, Carvalho F (2006) Acute paraquat poisoning: report of a survival case following intake of a potential lethal dose. Pediatr Emerg Care 22(7):537–540. https://doi.org/10.1097/01.pec.0000223179.07633.8a

Dinis-Oliveira RJ, Soares M, Rocha-Pereira C, Carvalho F (2016) Human and experimental toxicology of orellanine. Hum Exp Toxicol 35(9):1016–1029. https://doi.org/10.1177/0960327115613845

Douglas AP, Hamlyn AN, James O (1976) Controlled trial of cysteamine in treatment of acute paracetamol (acetaminophen) poisoning. Lancet 1(7951):111–115

Drault JN, Baelen E, Mehdaoui H, Delord JM, Flament F (1999) Massive paraquat poisoning. Favorable course after treatment with n-acetylcysteine and early hemodialysis. Ann Fr Anesth Reanim 18(5):534–537

Eisen JS, Koren G, Juurlink DN, Ng VL (2004) N-acetylcysteine for the treatment of clove oil-induced fulminant hepatic failure. J Toxicol 42(1):89–92

Eizadi-Mood N, Sabzghabaee AM, Siadat S, Yaraghi A, Shariati M, Gheshlaghi F et al (2013) Intravenous acetylcysteine versus oral and intravenous acetylcysteine: does a combination therapy decrease side effects of acetylcysteine? Pak J Med Sci 29(1):308–311

El Rahi C, Thompson-Moore N, Mejia P, De Hoyos P (2015) Successful use of N-acetylcysteine to treat severe hepatic injury caused by a dietary fitness supplement. Pharmacotherapy 35(6):e96–e101. https://doi.org/10.1002/phar.1572

Elliott TR, Symes T, Kannourakis G, Angus P (2016) Resolution of norfloxacin-induced acute liver failure after N-acetylcysteine therapy: further support for the use of NAC in drug-induced ALF? BMJ Case Rep 2016:bcr2015213189. https://doi.org/10.1136/bcr-2015-213189

Enjalbert F, Rapior S, Nouguier-Soule J, Guillon S, Amouroux N, Cabot C (2002) Treatment of amatoxin poisoning: 20-year retrospective analysis. J Toxicol Clin Toxicol 40(6):715–757

Esposito P, La Porta E, Calatroni M, Bianzina S, Libetta C, Gregorini M, Rampino T, Dal Canton A (2015) Renal involvement in mushroom poisoning: the case of Orellanus syndrome. Hemodial Int 19(4):E1–E5. https://doi.org/10.1111/hdi.12275

Flanagan RJ, Meredith TJ (1991) Use of N-acetylcysteine in clinical toxicology. Am J Med 91(3C):131S–139S

Forman HJ, Zhang H, Rinna A (2009) Glutathione: overview of its protective roles, measurement, and biosynthesis. Mol Asp Med 30(1-2):1–12. https://doi.org/10.1016/j.mam.2008.08.006

French LK, Hendrickson RG, Horowitz BZ (2011) Amanita phalloides poisoning. Clin Toxicol 49(2):128–129. https://doi.org/10.3109/15563650.2011.557663

Garcia J, Costa VM, Costa AE, Andrade S, Carneiro AC, Conceicao F, Paiva JA, de Pinho PG, Baptista P, de Lourdes Bastos M, Carvalho F (2015) Co-ingestion of amatoxins and isoxazoles-containing mushrooms and successful treatment: a case report. Toxicon 103:55–59. https://doi.org/10.1016/j.toxicon.2015.06.012

Gawarammana IB, Buckley NA (2011) Medical management of paraquat ingestion. Br J Clin Pharmacol 72(5):745–757. https://doi.org/10.1111/j.1365-2125.2011.04026.x

Gil HW, Kang MS, Yang JO, Lee EY, Hong SY (2008) Association between plasma paraquat level and outcome of paraquat poisoning in 375 paraquat poisoning patients. Clin Toxicol 46(6):515–518. https://doi.org/10.1080/15563650701549403

Gordon WP, Huitric AC, Seth CL et al (1987) The metabolism of the abortifacient terpene, (R)-(+)-pulegone, to a proximate toxin, menthofuran. Drug Metab Dispos 15:589–594

Grabhorn E, Nielsen D, Hillebrand G, Brinkert F, Herden U, Fischer L, Ganschow R (2013) Successful outcome of severe Amanita phalloides poisoning in children. Pediatr Transplant 17(6):550–555. https://doi.org/10.1111/petr.12108

Grebe SO, Langenbeck M, Schaper A, Berndt S, Aresmouk D, Herget-Rosenthal S (2013) Antioxidant treatment and outcome of Cortinarius orellanus poisoning: a case series. Ren Fail 35(10):1436–1439. https://doi.org/10.3109/0886022x.2013.826110

Gunnell D, Hawton K, Murray V, Garnier R, Bismuth C, Fagg J, Simkin S (1997) Use of paracetamol for suicide and non-fatal poisoning in the UK and France: are restrictions on availability justified? J Epidemiol Community Health 51(2):175–179

Hamlyn AN, Lesna M, Record CO, Smith PA, Watson AJ, Meredith T, Volans GN, Crome P (1981) Methionine and cysteamine in paracetamol (acetaminophen) overdose, prospective controlled trial of early therapy. J Int Med Res 9(3):226–231

Hartnoll G, Douek D (1993) Near fatal ingestion of oil of cloves. Arch Dis Child 69:392–393

Hoffer E, Shenker L, Baum Y, Tabak A (1997) Paraquat-induced formation of leukotriene B4 in rat lungs: modulation by Nacetylcysteine. Free Radic Biol Med 22:567–572

Howard RJ, Blake DR, Pall H, Williams A, Green ID (1987) Allopurinol/N-acetylcysteine for carbon monoxide poisoning. Lancet 2(8559):628–629

Hughes RD, Gazzard BG, Hanid MA, Trewby PN, Murray-Lyon IM, Davis M, Williams R, Bennet JR (1977) Controlled trial of cysteamine and dimercaprol after paracetamol overdose. Br Med J 2(6099):1395–1395

Isbister GK, Downes MA, McNamara K, Berling I, Whyte IM, Page CB (2016) A prospective observational study of a novel 2-phase infusion protocol for the administration of acetylcysteine in paracetamol poisoning. Clin Toxicol 54(2):120–126. https://doi.org/10.3109/15563650.2015.1115057

Janes SE, Price CS, Thomas D (2005) Essential oil poisoning: N-acetylcysteine for eugenol-induced hepatic failure and analysis of a national database. Eur J Pediatr 164(8):520–522. https://doi.org/10.1007/s00431-005-1692-1

Jayaweera D, Islam S, Gunja N, Cowie C, Broska J, Poojara L, Roberts MS, Isbister GK (2016) Chloroform ingestion causing severe gastrointestinal injury, hepatotoxicity and dermatitis confirmed with plasma chloroform concentrations. Clin Toxicol 55(2):147–150. https://doi.org/10.1080/15563650.2016.1249795

Johnson MT, McCammon CA, Mullins ME, Halcomb SE (2011) Evaluation of a simplified N-acetylcysteine dosing regimen for the treatment of acetaminophen toxicity. Ann Pharmacother 45(6):713–720. https://doi.org/10.1345/aph.1P613

Jones AL (1998) Mechanism of action and value of N-acetylcysteine in the treatment of early and late acetaminophen poisoning: a critical review. J Toxicol Clin Toxicol 36(4):277–285

Juma SA, Villeneuve E, Elliot A, Palmer RB, Gosselin S (2015) Doubling the third dose of intravenous N-acetylcysteine survey: an international practice perspective (abstract). Clin Toxicol 4:233–403. https://doi.org/10.3109/15563650.2015.1024953

Kang YJ, Ahn J, Hwang YI (2014) Acute liver injury in two workers exposed to chloroform in cleanrooms: a case report. Ann Occup Environ Med 26(1):49. https://doi.org/10.1186/s40557-014-0049-5

Karvellas CJ, Tillman H, Leung AA, Lee WM, Schilsky ML, Hameed B, Stravitz RT, McGuire BM, Fix OK (2016) Acute liver injury and acute liver failure from mushroom poisoning in North America. Liver Int 36(7):1043–1050. https://doi.org/10.1111/liv.13080

Keays R, Harrison PM, Wendon JA, Forbes A, Gove C, Alexander GJ, Williams R (1991) Intravenous acetylcysteine in paracetamol induced fulminant hepatic failure: a prospective controlled trial. BMJ 303(6809):1026–1029

Kerr F, Dawson A, Whyte IM, Buckley N, Murray L, Graudins A, Chan B, Trudinger B (2005) The Australasian Clinical Toxicology Investigators Collaboration randomized trial of different loading infusion rates of N-acetylcysteine. Ann Emerg Med 45(4):402–408. https://doi.org/10.1016/j.annemergmed.2004.08.040

Kerschbaum J, Mayer G, Maurer A (2012) High-dose antioxidant therapy and steroids might improve the outcome of acute renal failure from intoxication by Cortinarius rubellus: report of two cases. Clin Kidney J 5(6):576–578. https://doi.org/10.1093/ckj/sfs129

Kilner RG, D'Souza RJ, Oliveira DB, MacPhee IA, Turner DR, Eastwood JB (1999) Acute renal failure from intoxication by Cortinarius orellanus: recovery using anti-oxidant therapy and steroids. Nephrol Dial Transplant 14(11):2779–2780

Kim H (2008) A case of acute toxic hepatitis after suicidal chloroform and dichloromethane ingestion. Am J Emerg Med 26(9):1073.e3–1073.e6. https://doi.org/10.1016/j.ajem.2008.03.050

Lancaster EM, Hiatt JR, Zarrinpar A (2015) Acetaminophen hepatotoxicity: an updated review. Arch Toxicol 89(2):193–199. https://doi.org/10.1007/s00204-014-1432-2

Larson AM, Polson J, Fontana RJ, Davern TJ, Lalani E, Hynan LS, Reisch JS, Schiodt FV, Ostapowicz G, Shakil AO, Lee WM (2005) Acetaminophen-induced acute liver failure: results of a United States multicenter, prospective study. Hepatology 42(6):1364–1372. https://doi.org/10.1002/hep.20948

Lee WM, Hynan LS, Rossaro L, Fontana RJ, Stravitz RT, Larson AM, Davern TJ, Murray NG, McCashland T, Reisch JS, Robuck PR (2009) Intravenous N-acetylcysteine improves transplant-free survival in early stage non-acetaminophen acute liver failure. Gastroenterology 137(3):856–864., 864.e851. https://doi.org/10.1053/j.gastro.2009.06.006

Lheureux P, Leduc D, Vanbinst R, Askenasi R (1995) Survival in a case of massive paraquat ingestion. Chest 107(1):285–289

Mant TG, Tempowski JH, Volans GN, Talbot JC (1984) Adverse reactions to acetylcysteine and effects of overdose. Br Med J 289(6439):217–219

Mathieson PW, Williams G, MacSweeney JE (1985) Survival after massive ingestion of carbon tetrachloride treated by intravenous infusion of acetylcysteine. Hum Toxicol 4(6):627–631

Meredith TJ, Crome P, Volans G, Goulding R (1978) Treatment of paracetamol poisoning. Br Med J 1(6121):1215–1216

MHRA (2012) Treating paracetamol overdose with intravenous acetylcysteine: new guidance. Accessed 6 Nov 2016

Mitchell JR, Jollow DJ, Potter WZ, Davis DC, Gillette JR, Brodie BB (1973) Acetaminophen-induced hepatic necrosis. I. Role of drug metabolism. J Pharmacol Exp Ther 187(1):185–194

Mitchell JR, Thorgeirsson SS, Potter WZ, Jollow DJ, Keiser H (1974) Acetaminophen-induced hepatic injury: protective role of glutathione in man and rationale for therapy. Clin Pharmacol Ther 16(4):676–684

Mizutani T, Satoh K, Nomura H (1991) Hepatotoxicity of eugenol and related compounds in mice depleted of glutathione: structural requirements for toxic potency. Res Commun Chem Pathol Pharmacol 73(1):87–95

Montanini S, Sinardi D, Pratico C, Sinardi AU, Trimarchi G (1999) Use of acetylcysteine as the life-saving antidote in Amanita phalloides (death cap) poisoning. Case report on 11 patients. Arzneimittelforschung 49(12):1044–1047

Mudalel ML, Dave KP, Hummel JP, Solga SF (2015) N-acetylcysteine treats intravenous amiodarone induced liver injury. World J Gastroenterol 21(9):2816–2819. https://doi.org/10.3748/wjg.v21.i9.2816

Nagaraja P, Thangavelu A, Nair H, Kumwenda M (2015) Successful living related kidney transplantation for end-stage renal failure caused by orellanine syndrome. QJM 108(5):413–415. https://doi.org/10.1093/qjmed/hcs201

Oakley E, Robinson J, Deasy C (2011) Using 0.45% saline solution and a modified dosing regimen for infusing N-acetylcysteine in children with paracetamol poisoning. Emerg Med Australas 23(1):63–67. https://doi.org/10.1111/j.1742-6723.2010.01376.x

Olsson B, Johansson M, Gabrielsson J, Bolme P (1988) Pharmacokinetics and bioavailability of reduced and oxidized N-acetylcysteine. Eur J Clin Pharmacol 34(1):77–82

Pakravan N, Waring WS, Sharma S, Ludlam C, Megson I, Bateman DN (2008) Risk factors and mechanisms of anaphylactoid reactions to acetylcysteine in acetaminophen overdose. Clin Toxicol 46(8):697–702. https://doi.org/10.1080/15563650802245497

Pandit A, Sachdeva T, Bafna P (2012) Drug-induced hepatotoxicity: a review. J Appl Pharmaceut Sci 2(5):233–243

Park BK, Dear JW, Antoine DJ (2015) Paracetamol (acetaminophen) poisoning. BMJ Clin Evid 2007:2101

Pohl LR, Bhooshan B, Whittaker NF, Krishna G (1977) Phosgene: a metabolite of chloroform. Biochem Biophys Res Commun 79(3):684–691

Poucheret P, Fons F, Dore JC, Michelot D, Rapior S (2010) Amatoxin poisoning treatment decision-making: pharmaco-therapeutic clinical strategy assessment using multidimensional multivariate statistic analysis. Toxicon 55(7):1338–1345. https://doi.org/10.1016/j.toxicon.2010.02.005

Prescott LF (1980) Kinetics and metabolism of paracetamol and phenacetin. Br J Clin Pharmacol 10(Suppl 2):291S–298S

Prescott LF, Sutherland GR, Park J, Smith IJ, Proudfoot AT (1976) Cysteamine, methionine, and penicillamine in the treatment of paracetamol poisoning. Lancet 2(7977):109–113

Prescott LF, Park J, Ballantyne A, Adriaenssens P, Proudfoot AT (1977) Treatment of paracetamol (acetaminophen) poisoning with N-acetylcysteine. Lancet 2(8035):432–434

Prescott LF, Illingworth RN, Critchley JA, Stewart MJ, Adam RD, Proudfoot AT (1979) Intravenous N-acetylcystine: the treatment of choice for paracetamol poisoning. Br Med J 2(6198):1097–1100

Prescott LF, Donovan JW, Jarvie DR, Proudfoot AT (1989) The disposition and kinetics of intravenous N-acetylcysteine in patients with paracetamol overdosage. Eur J Clin Pharmacol 37(5):501–506

Raghu K, Mahesh V, Sasidhar P, Reddy PR, Venkataramaniah V, Agrawal A (2013) Paraquat poisoning: a case report and review of literature. J Fam Commun Med 20(3):198–200. https://doi.org/10.4103/2230-8229.122023

Recknagel RO, Glende EA Jr, Dolak JA, Waller RL (1989) Mechanisms of carbon tetrachloride toxicity. Pharmacol Ther 43(1):139–154

Roberts DM, Hall MJ, Falkland MM, Strasser SI, Buckley NA (2013) Amanita phalloides poisoning and treatment with silibinin in the Australian Capital Territory and New South Wales. Med J Aust 198(1):43–47

Rumack BH (2002) Acetaminophen hepatotoxicity: the first 35 years. J Toxicol Clin Toxicol 40(1):3–20

Rumack BH, Bateman DN (2012) Acetaminophen and acetylcysteine dose and duration: past, present and future. Clin Toxicol 50(2):91–98. https://doi.org/10.3109/15563650.2012.659252

Rumack BH, Matthew H (1975) Acetaminophen poisoning and toxicity. Pediatrics 55(6):871–876

Ruprah M, Mant TG, Flanagan RJ (1985) Acute carbon tetrachloride poisoning in 19 patients: implications for diagnosis and treatment. Lancet 1(8436):1027–1029

Sandilands EA, Bateman DN (2009) Adverse reactions associated with acetylcysteine. Clin Toxicol 47(2):81–88. https://doi.org/10.1080/15563650802665587

Schmidt LE (2013) Identification of patients at risk of anaphylactoid reactions to N-acetylcysteine in the treatment of paracetamol overdose. Clin Toxicol 51(6):467–472. https://doi.org/10.3109/15563650.2013.799677

Schmidt LE, Dalhoff K (2001) Risk factors in the development of adverse reactions to N-acetylcysteine in patients with paracetamol poisoning. Br J Clin Pharmacol 51(1):87–91

Sheikh-Hamad D, Timmins K, Jalali Z (1997) Cisplatin-induced renal toxicity: possible reversal by N-acetylcysteine treatment. JASN 8(10):1640–1644

Smilkstein MJ, Knapp GL, Kulig KW, Rumack BH (1988) Efficacy of oral N-acetylcysteine in the treatment of acetaminophen overdose. Analysis of the national multicenter study (1976 to 1985). N Engl J Med 319(24):1557–1562. https://doi.org/10.1056/nejm198812153192401

Smilkstein MJ, Bronstein AC, Linden C, Augenstein WL, Kulig KW, Rumack BH (1991) Acetaminophen overdose: a 48-hour intravenous N-acetylcysteine treatment protocol. Ann Emerg Med 20(10):1058–1063

Smith MR, Davis RL (2016) Mycetismus: a review. Gastroenterol Rep 4(2):107–112. https://doi. org/10.1093/gastro/gov062

Sullivan JB Jr, Rumack BH, Thomas H Jr, Peterson RG, Bryson P (1979) Pennyroyal oil poisoning and hepatotoxicity. JAMA 242(26):2873–2874

Thomassen D, Slattery JT, Nelson SD (1988) Contribution of menthofuran to the hepatotoxicity of pulegone: assessment based on matched area under the curve and on matched time course. J Pharmacol Exp Ther 244(3):825–829

Vale JA, Kulig K (2004) Position paper: gastric lavage. J Toxicol 42(7):933–943

Vanooteghem S, Arts J, Decock S, Pieraerts P, Meersseman W, Verslype C, Van Hootegem P (2014) Four patients with amanita phalloides poisoning. Acta Gastroenterol Belg 77(3):353–356

Ward J, Kapadia K, Brush E, Salhanick SD (2013) Amatoxin poisoning: case reports and review of current therapies. J Emerg Med 44(1):116–121. https://doi.org/10.1016/j. jemermed.2012.02.020

Waring WS, Stephen AF, Robinson OD, Dow MA, Pettie JM (2008) Lower incidence of anaphylactoid reactions to N-acetylcysteine in patients with high acetaminophen concentrations after overdose. Clin Toxicol 46(6):496–500. https://doi.org/10.1080/15563650701864760

Williamson K, Wahl MS, Mycyk MB (2013) Direct comparison of 20-hour IV, 36-hour oral, and 72-hour oral acetylcysteine for treatment of acute acetaminophen poisoning. Am J Ther 20(1):37–40. https://doi.org/10.1097/MJT.0b013e318250f829

Wong A, Graudins A (2016) Simplification of the standard three-bag intravenous acetylcysteine regimen for paracetamol poisoning results in a lower incidence of adverse drug reactions. Clin Toxicol 54(2):115–119. https://doi.org/10.3109/15563650.2015.1115055

Woo OF, Mueller PD, Olson KR, Anderson IB, Kim SY (2000) Shorter duration of oral N-acetylcysteine therapy for acute acetaminophen overdose. Ann Emerg Med 35(4):363–368

Woolf A (1999) Essential oil poisoning. J Toxicol 37(6):721–727. https://doi.org/10.1081/ CLT-100102450

Wornle M, Angstwurm MW, Sitter T (2004) Treatment of intoxication with Cortinarius speciosissimus using an antioxidant therapy. Am J Kidney Dis 43(4):e3–e6

Yeh ST, Guo HR, Su YS, Lin HJ, Hou CC, Chen HM, Chang MC, Wang YJ (2006) Protective effects of N-acetylcysteine treatment post acute paraquat intoxication in rats and in human lung epithelial cells. Toxicology 223(3):181–190. https://doi.org/10.1016/j.tox.2006.03.019

Zevin S, Dempsey D, Olson K (1997) Amanita phalloides mushroom poisoning– Northern California, January 1997. J Toxicol 35(5):461–463. https://doi.org/ 10.3109/15563659709001230

The Use of N-Acetylcysteine as a Chelator for Metal Toxicity

Daniel A. Rossignol

10.1 Introduction

N-Acetylcysteine (NAC) is a derivative of cysteine, an amino acid. NAC can function as a chelator to remove metals, including mercury, cadmium, chromium, arsenic, and gold (Blanusa et al. 2005). It also has antioxidant properties and functions as a free radical scavenger and has been shown to increase glutathione levels (Kelly 1998). NAC may function to protect against toxicant exposures by limiting damage from the toxicant (by reducing oxidative stress) and also by removing (chelating) toxicants (Kelly 1998). Even though NAC has been shown to remove heavy metals from tissue, NAC does not appear to cause an increase in excretion of essential metals such as iron, zinc, copper, calcium, or magnesium, resulting in advantages and a potential better safety profile than other chelating agents (Hjortso et al. 1990). This chapter is a systematic review that identifies studies using NAC to chelate heavy metals or act as a protectant against heavy metals. Studies were categorized for humans and animals and then sorted by heavy metal.

10.2 Methods

For this chapter the terms, "mercury," "lead," "arsenic," "nickel," "aluminum," "heavy metal," "toxicant," "chelate," and "remove" were used. These search terms were used in combination with "NAC" and "N-Acetylcysteine" to identify papers. Figure 10.1 depicts the publications identified during the search process. For all identified records, the titles and abstracts were screened to identify potentially

Electronic supplementary material The online version of this article (https://doi.org/10.1007/978-981-10-5311-5_10) contains supplementary material, which is available to authorized users.

D. A. Rossignol
Rossignol Medical Center, Aliso Viejo, CA, USA

© Springer Nature Singapore Pte Ltd. 2019
R. E. Frye, M. Berk (eds.), *The Therapeutic Use of N-Acetylcysteine (NAC) in Medicine*, https://doi.org/10.1007/978-981-10-5311-5_10

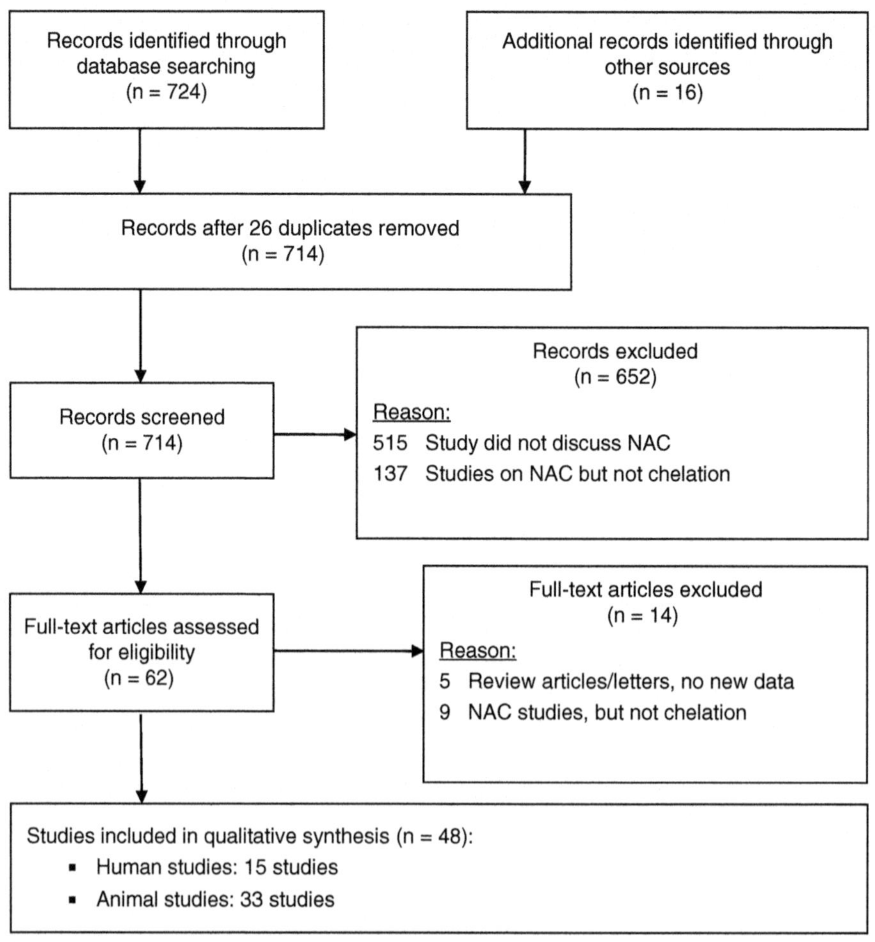

Fig. 10.1 Flow diagram of study selection for review

relevant studies. After screening all records, 62 studies were identified and each paper was then reviewed. After review, 48 studies met inclusion criteria (15 human studies and 33 animal studies; Fig. 10.1).

10.3 Animal Studies

A total of 33 studies (Fig. 10.1) were identified using NAC as a chelator of heavy metals in animals or animal cell lines.

10.3.1 Mercury

Eleven studies examined the use of NAC as a potential chelator of mercury (both organic and inorganic mercury) with eight (73%) studies reporting improvements.

In one study, NAC was given to rats treated with mercuric chloride, and the addition of NAC led to a reduction in the mercury content in the kidney and liver (Girardi and Elias 1991). Rats exposed to mercury vapor were treated with NAC which led to an increase in survival time and a decrease in mercury levels in both blood and lung tissue (Livardjani et al. 1991). Mice exposed to methylmercury had a significant increase in the rate of mercury excretion and a lower tissue mercury level after oral NAC administration (10 mg/ml); excretion of inorganic mercury was not affected by NAC (Ballatori et al. 1998a). NAC injection into rodents led to a dose-dependent increase in methylmercury (MeHg) excretion and a reduction of mercury burden in the fetus, brain, and placenta in pregnant rats (Aremu et al. 2008). Cysteine administration to young rats exposed to inorganic mercury increased the rate of biliary mercury secretion (Ballatori and Clarkson 1984). In another study, NAC in drinking water (10 mg/ml) led to an increase in the urinary excretion of methylmercury in mice exposed to methylmercury (Ballatori et al. 1998b). NAC significantly increased the excretion of methylmercury in the urine of rats exposed to mercury (Madejczyk et al. 2007). Rats exposed to mercury that were treated with zinc and NAC showed that this combination of treatments prevented blood and liver mercury retention (Oliveira et al. 2015).

Three studies reported no improvement using NAC in mercury exposure. Mice injected with mercuric chloride were treated with 2,3-dimercapto-1-propanesulfonic acid (DMPS) or NAC, and then kidney, liver, and blood samples were examined. In combination with mercuric chloride, both DMPS and NAC showed evidence of renal tissue damage due to the formation of complexes that were toxic; further study was recommended (Brandao et al. 2006). In another study, NAC was fed to mice that were exposed to mercury, chromium, or cadmium, and an increase in congenital malformation was found with these metals when NAC was given (Endo and Watanabe 1988). Finally, one study on rats showed no significant chelator effect with NAC (Khandelwal et al. 1988).

10.3.2 Lead

Eight studies examine the effect of NAC on lead exposure in animals with seven (88%) studies reporting some type of improvement. In one study, cells taken from rats which were exposed to lead were treated with NAC, and this led to increased cell survival and improved the GSH/GSSG ratio; this also led to a protection of lead poisoning through antioxidant mechanisms (Aykin-Burns et al. 2005). In rats treated with lead acetate, NAC lowered the blood lead level by 35–38% (not statistically significant) and led to a decrease in oxidative stress markers (malondialdehyde, MDA) in the cerebellum ($p < 0.0001$; Calderon-Cabrera et al. 2008). DMSA and NAC led to a larger reduction in body lead burden compared to DMSA without NAC (Flora et al. 2004). Rats exposed to lead acetate showed a small reduction in blood lead levels with NAC treatment (28.5% reduction) and DMSA treatment (92.9% reduction) (Gurer et al. 1998). In rats exposed to lead, NAC added to DMSA was more effective at reducing lead levels in the blood and liver compared to DMSA alone (Pande et al. 2001). Rats exposed to lead acetate that were then given NAC had a reduction in oxidative stress markers compared to those not given NAC; the improvement with NAC was greater than with GSH (Sharma et al. 2013). In a study of rats exposed to lead, the administration of NAC led to a reduction of oxidative stress (Tandon et al. 2002). Finally, one study of lead exposure in mice reported no significant changes with NAC (Llobet et al. 1990).

10.3.3 Cadmium

Four studies examined the use of NAC in animals with three (75%) reporting an improvement; one additional study examined NAC in porcine cells exposed to cadmium. In one study of rats treated with cadmium, mercury, and lead, the addition of NAC did not lead to an increased excretion of mercury but caused a fourfold increase in the urinary excretion of cadmium and a gradual increase in the excretion of lead (Ottenwalder and Simon 1987). In another study, NAC improved oxidative stress markers in rats exposed to cadmium (Tandon et al. 2003). In mouse cells exposed to cadmium, NAC was shown to lessen oxidative stress (Figueiredo-Pereira et al. 2002). NAC was fed to mice that were exposed to mercury, chromium, or cadmium, and an increase in congenital malformation was found with these metals when NAC was given (Endo and Watanabe 1988).

One study used porcine cell lines (LLC-PK1 cells) that were exposed to cadmium and then treated with NAC. NAC suppressed cadmium toxicity by reducing the uptake of cadmium into cells; NAC also led to an increase in glutathione levels (Wispriyono et al. 1998).

10.3.4 Chromium and Boron

In one study, rats exposed to lead, boric acid, and chromium were treated with NAC, calcium EDTA, and/or dimercaptosuccinic acid (DMSA); the largest excretion of boron and chromium occurred with NAC; DMSA caused the largest increase in excretion of lead, whereas NAC did not affect lead excretion (Banner Jr et al. 1986).

10.3.5 Arsenic

Six studies examined the use of NAC as a chelator in arsenic exposure with all reporting some type of improvement. In mice exposed to arsenic, survival time was longer after NAC exposure; NAC was ineffective in mice exposed to thallium and cadmium (Henderson et al. 1985). NAC combined with atorvastatin help prevent rat erythrocyte apoptosis after chronic exposure to arsenic (Biswas et al. 2011). The administration of NAC after arsenic trioxide exposure in mice reduced the toxic effect of arsenic on the male genital system (da Silva et al. 2016). Rats exposed to sodium arsenite in drinking water were also treated with NAC or DMSA; NAC improved GSH and oxidative stress markers, including oxidative stress markers in the brain; DMSA lowered blood and liver arsenic concentrations (Flora 1999). In guinea pigs exposed to 50 ppm arsenic in drinking water for 8 months, NAC combined with DMSA depleted arsenic from blood and tissue better than DMSA alone (Kannan and Flora 2006). Finally, in an animal study, NAC showed protective effects against arsenic (Shum et al. 1981).

10.3.6 Aluminum

Three studies examined the use of NAC in animals exposed to aluminum with two studies (67%) reporting improvements. After the injection of aluminum phosphide into the stomach of rats, NAC infusion led to increased survival time and decreased myocardial oxidative injury (Azad et al. 2001). In another study of rats exposed to aluminum, survival time was the longest in the rats treated with NAC and vitamin C (Gheshlaghi et al. 2015). Finally, in a study of mice, after intraperitoneal injection of aluminum, NAC was not as effective as other agents (Domingo et al. 1986).

10.3.7 Gold

In one study of rats treated with gold, NAC administration led to an increased excretion of gold after gold exposure (Ottenwalder and Simon 1987).

10.4 Human Studies

A total of 15 studies (Fig. 10.1) were identified using NAC as a chelator of heavy metals in humans or human cells. Five of the human studies were controlled (Kasperczyk et al. 2013, 2014a, b, 2015; Lorber et al. 1973), but four of the studies used the same population (Kasperczyk et al. 2013, 2014a, b, 2015). Two studies used NAC in human cells exposed to lead (Ustundag and Duydu 2007) or arsenic (Ghani et al. 2014).

10.4.1 Effects on Essential Metals

In the human studies, NAC did not appear to cause an increase in excretion of essential metals such as iron, zinc, copper, calcium, or magnesium. For example, in one study NAC (200 mg three times a day) was given to ten healthy volunteers for 2 weeks, and plasma levels of calcium, magnesium, iron, zinc, and copper were measured; no significant changes were found (Hjortso et al. 1990). However, another study of two soldiers injured from inhalation of zinc chloride smoke who then developed adult respiratory distress syndrome (ARDS) reported increased urinary excretion of zinc and a decreased plasma level of zinc in one of the patients (Hjortso et al. 1988).

10.4.2 Mercury

Two uncontrolled case studies reported improvements with the use of NAC in people exposed to mercury (Online Table 10.1). A 20-year-old man who had methylmercury ingestion from a fungicide was treated with hemodialysis with NAC infusion (36 h after ingestion of fungicide), and the urinary organic mercury rate of elimination was about 40 times higher during hemodialysis and 84-fold after hemodialysis—this was a dramatic increase; there was also a 50% reduction in mercury blood levels (Lund et al. 1984). A 36-year-old woman exposed to metallic mercury by oral ingestion 1 week earlier presented to the emergency room with diarrhea, fever, and abdominal pain and showed improvements in symptoms with NAC treatment (Sarikaya et al. 2010).

10.4.3 Lead

Five studies examined the use of NAC in people exposed to lead in the workplace or in human lymphocytes; four of these studies contained a control group, but these four studies evaluated the same 200 individuals; each of the four publications reported on different outcomes (Online Table 10.2). In these four publications, 200 healthy male workers exposed to lead from Poland were divided into four groups: one group was a control group (not treated); one group received NAC 200 mg PO qd (200 mg group); one group received NAC 200 mg PO bid (400 mg group); and the final group received NAC 400 mg PO bid (800 mg group). In the first published study, the groups receiving oral NAC (all three groups, total of 200–800 mg daily dose) had a significant reduction in blood lead levels compared to workers who did not receive NAC; glutathione (GSH) significantly increased in the NAC 400 and 800 mg groups; glucose-6-phosphate dehydrogenase (G6PD) significantly increased in all NAC groups; and lipofuscin (LPS) significantly decreased in all NAC groups (Kasperczyk et al. 2013). In the second publication, workers taking NAC had a normalization of antioxidant enzyme concentrations in blood cells compared to those not treated with NAC; MDA significantly decreased in all NAC groups; superoxide dismutase (SOD), glutathione peroxidase (GPx), and catalase (CAT) levels normalized in the NAC groups (Kasperczyk et al. 2014a). In the third publication, the groups receiving NAC at 400 and 800 mg/day for 12 weeks had a significant reduction in lipid hydroperoxides (a marker of lipid peroxidation) and an increase in alpha-tocopherol levels; the reduction of lipid peroxidation was dose-dependent; lipid hydroperoxides (LHP) significantly decreased in the 400 and 800 mg groups; alpha-tocopherol significantly increased in the 400 and 800 mg groups; and the lipid peroxidation improved in a dose-dependent fashion (Kasperczyk et al. 2014b). Finally, in the fourth publication, the groups receiving NAC had significant reductions in homocysteine levels and protein carbonyl groups; iron and transferrin were unchanged (Kasperczyk et al. 2015). One study examined human lymphocytes taken from a 45-year-old healthy female who was exposed to lead, and the addition of NAC led to less induced genotoxicity as shown by a significant reduction in sister chromatid exchange frequencies (Ustundag and Duydu 2007).

10.4.4 Gold

Four studies examined the use of NAC for gold exposure (Online Table 10.3). In 23 patients with rheumatoid arthritis (RA) receiving gold injections, the use of NAC led to a significant increase in gold excretion compared to 17 patients in a control group (Lorber et al. 1973). Another case report found intravenous (IV) NAC infusion led to increased daily excretion of gold in a 47-year-old female with rheumatoid arthritis who had been treated with gold over a 5-year period; she also had aplastic anemia that resolved (Hansen et al. 1985). One study gave oral NAC (2000 mg orally three times a day for 1 week) to 13 patients with rheumatoid arthritis and reported an increase in the urinary excretion of gold (Vreugdenhil and Swaak 1990). Finally, in another study, 12 patients who were treated with gold salts were given IV NAC, and the urinary excretion of gold was increased (Godfrey et al. 1982).

10.4.5 Arsenic

Two studies examined the use of NAC in humans or human cells exposed to arsenic (Online Table 10.4). A 32-year-old male who was exposed to arsenic from ant poison was given NAC intravenously every 4 h for 18 doses, and the patient "showed remarkable clinical improvement during the following 24 h" (Martin et al. 1990). In another study using a human U937 monocytic leukemia cell line exposed to arsenite, NAC treatment led to a significant reduction in apoptosis through a chelation mechanism (Ghani et al. 2014).

10.5   Discussion

A number of studies examined the use of NAC in conjunction with, or after exposure to, heavy metals in animals. Most of the animal studies investigated NAC in conjunction with exposure to mercury or lead. The majority of the mercury studies (8 out of 11, 73%) reported improvements although two studies reported potential side effects including evidence of renal toxicity (Brandao et al. 2006) and congenital malformation (Endo and Watanabe 1988), and one study reported no significant chelator effect with NAC (Khandelwal et al. 1988). The majority of animal studies investigating lead exposure reported an improvement in metal toxicity with the use of NAC (7 out of 8, 88%) although one study reported no chelator effect (Llobet et al. 1990). Three out of the four (75%) cadmium studies reported an improvement with NAC except for the previously mentioned study reporting evidence of congenital malformation when NAC was given with cadmium (Endo and Watanabe 1988); one study using cadmium in porcine cells also reported an improvement. Improvements were also reported in studies on chromium, boron (1 study), arsenic (6 out of 6 studies, 100%), aluminum (2 out of 3 studies, 67%), and gold (1 study).

Table 10.1 Overall ratings of NAC based on clinical studies presented by metal

Metal	Controlled studies positive% (positive/total)	Uncontrolled studies positive% (positive/total)	Grade of recommendation	Recommendation for treatment
Mercury		100% (2/2)	C	None
Lead	100%(1/1)	100% (1/1)	C	None
Gold	100%(1/1)	100% (3/3)	C	None
Arsenic		100% (2/2)	C	None

Fifteen studies examined the use of NAC in humans or human cells. One study reported that NAC did not deplete essential metals (i.e., iron, zinc, copper, calcium, or magnesium) from the body (Hjortso et al. 1990). Lead was the most commonly examined toxicant (5 out of 15 studies, 33%). Four of the lead studies contained data on the same population of patients but reported multiple improvements in a variety of parameters; these studies were controlled which strengthens the study results. The lead studies reported improvements in oxidative stress markers, inflammatory markers, and glutathione levels, suggesting that NAC has a broad effect on metabolism markers. Two case studies reported improvements with NAC in people poisoned with mercury (Lund et al. 1984; Sarikaya et al. 2010). The remaining studies on gold (4 studies) and arsenic (2 studies) reported improvements or increased excretion of heavy metals.

Table 10.1 provides recommendations as a result of reviewing these studies. Although universally positive, most of the studies were uncontrolled, and four of the controlled studies for lead need to be considered one study for evaluation purposes. Because of the preliminary nature of these studies, the overall rating was C that limits our ability to make a positive recommendation because of the limited evidence. Nevertheless, it should be pointed out that none of these studies reported any significant side effects. We believe this is a promising area of medical research and look forward to further clinical studies to verify these preliminary findings.

The reviewed studies contained some potential limitations. Most of the published studies reported improvements that could be evidence of publication bias (i.e., studies reporting improvements might be more likely to be published), especially for the case reports in humans. Although many of the animal studies had a control group, the only controlled studies of NAC in humans were based off one population of patients. These lead publications were strengthened by the controlled nature. However, the number of human studies is low compared to the number of animal studies. Further human studies would be helpful in examining the use of NAC in humans but overall the use of NAC appears safe.

References

Aremu DA, Madejczyk MS, Ballatori N (2008) N-acetylcysteine as a potential antidote and biomonitoring agent of methylmercury exposure. Environ Health Perspect 116(1):26–31. https://doi.org/10.1289/ehp.10383

Aykin-Burns N, Franklin EA, Ercal N (2005) Effects of N-acetylcysteine on lead-exposed PC-12 cells. Arch Environ Contam Toxicol 49(1):119–123. https://doi.org/10.1007/s00244-004-0025-0

Azad A, Lall SB, Mittra S (2001) Effect of N-acetylcysteine and L-NAME on aluminium phosphide induced cardiovascular toxicity in rats. Acta Pharmacol Sin 22(4):298–304

Ballatori N, Clarkson TW (1984) Dependence of biliary secretion of inorganic mercury on the biliary transport of glutathione. Biochem Pharmacol 33(7):1093–1098

Ballatori N, Lieberman MW, Wang W (1998a) N-acetylcysteine as an antidote in methylmercury poisoning. Environ Health Perspect 106(5):267–271

Ballatori N, Wang W, Lieberman MW (1998b) Accelerated methylmercury elimination in gamma-glutamyl transpeptidase-deficient mice. Am J Pathol 152(4):1049–1055

Banner W Jr, Koch M, Capin DM, Hopf SB, Chang S, Tong TG (1986) Experimental chelation therapy in chromium, lead, and boron intoxication with N-acetylcysteine and other compounds. Toxicol Appl Pharmacol 83(1):142–147

Biswas D, Sen G, Sarkar A, Biswas T (2011) Atorvastatin acts synergistically with N-acetyl cysteine to provide therapeutic advantage against Fas-activated erythrocyte apoptosis during chronic arsenic exposure in rats. Toxicol Appl Pharmacol 250(1):39–53. https://doi.org/10.1016/j.taap.2010.10.002

Blanusa M, Varnai VM, Piasek M, Kostial K (2005) Chelators as antidotes of metal toxicity: therapeutic and experimental aspects. Curr Med Chem 12(23):2771–2794

Brandao R, Santos FW, Zeni G, Rocha JB, Nogueira CW (2006) DMPS and N-acetylcysteine induced renal toxicity in mice exposed to mercury. Biometals 19(4):389–398. https://doi.org/10.1007/s10534-005-4020-3

Calderon-Cabrera L, Duran-Galetta MG, Garcia I, Galetta D, Lacruz L, Naranjo R, Perez B, Ferreira E (2008) Determination of the N-acetylcysteine and methionine effects in the cerebellum of rats intoxicated with lead. Investig Clin 49(1):17–28

Domingo JL, Llobet JM, Gomez M, Corbella J (1986) Acute aluminium intoxication: a study of the efficacy of several antidotal treatments in mice. Res Commun Chem Pathol Pharmacol 53(1):93–104

Endo A, Watanabe T (1988) Analysis of protective activity of N-acetylcysteine against teratogenicity of heavy metals. Reprod Toxicol 2(2):141–144

Figueiredo-Pereira ME, Li Z, Jansen M, Rockwell P (2002) N-acetylcysteine and celecoxib lessen cadmium cytotoxicity which is associated with cyclooxygenase-2 up-regulation in mouse neuronal cells. J Biol Chem 277(28):25283–25289. https://doi.org/10.1074/jbc.M109145200

Flora SJ (1999) Arsenic-induced oxidative stress and its reversibility following combined administration of N-acetylcysteine and meso 2,3-dimercaptosuccinic acid in rats. Clin Exp Pharmacol Physiol 26(11):865–869

Flora SJ, Pande M, Kannan GM, Mehta A (2004) Lead induced oxidative stress and its recovery following co-administration of melatonin or N-acetylcysteine during chelation with succimer in male rats. Cell Mol Biol 50:OL543–OL551

Ghani S, Khan N, Koriyama C, Akiba S, Yamamoto M (2014) N-acetyl-L-cysteine reduces arsenite-induced cytotoxicity through chelation in U937 monocytes and macrophages. Mol Med Rep 10(6):2961–2966. https://doi.org/10.3892/mmr.2014.2612

Gheshlaghi F, Lavasanijou MR, Moghaddam NA, Khazaei M, Behjati M, Farajzadegan Z, Sabzghabaee AM (2015) N-acetylcysteine, ascorbic acid, and methylene blue for the treatment of aluminium phosphide poisoning: still beneficial? Toxicol Int 22(1):40–44. https://doi.org/10.4103/0971-6580.172255

Girardi G, Elias MM (1991) Effectiveness of N-acetylcysteine in protecting against mercuric chloride-induced nephrotoxicity. Toxicology 67(2):155–164

Godfrey NF, Peter A, Simon TM, Lorber A (1982) IV N-acetylcysteine treatment of hematologic reactions to chrysotherapy. J Rheumatol 9(4):519–526

Gurer H, Ozgunes H, Neal R, Spitz DR, Ercal N (1998) Antioxidant effects of N-acetylcysteine and succimer in red blood cells from lead-exposed rats. Toxicology 128(3):181–189

Hansen RM, Csuka ME, McCarty DJ, Saryan LA (1985) Gold induced aplastic anemia. Complete response to corticosteroids, plasmapheresis, and N-acetylcysteine infusion. J Rheumatol 12(4):794–797

Henderson P, Hale TW, Shum S, Habersang RW (1985) N-acetylcysteine therapy of acute heavy metal poisoning in mice. Vet Hum Toxicol 27(6):522–525

Hjortso E, Qvist J, Bud MI, Thomsen JL, Andersen JB, Wiberg-Jorgensen F, Jensen NK, Jones R, Reid LM, Zapol WM (1988) ARDS after accidental inhalation of zinc chloride smoke. Intensive Care Med 14(1):17–24

Hjortso E, Fomsgaard JS, Fogh-Andersen N (1990) Does N-acetylcysteine increase the excretion of trace metals (calcium, magnesium, iron, zinc and copper) when given orally? Eur J Clin Pharmacol 39(1):29–31

Kannan GM, Flora SJ (2006) Combined administration of N-acetylcysteine and monoisoamyl DMSA on tissue oxidative stress during arsenic chelation therapy. Biol Trace Elem Res 110(1):43–59. https://doi.org/10.1385/BTER:110:1:43

Kasperczyk S, Dobrakowski M, Kasperczyk A, Ostalowska A, Birkner E (2013) The administration of N-acetylcysteine reduces oxidative stress and regulates glutathione metabolism in the blood cells of workers exposed to lead. Clin Toxicol 51(6):480–486. https://doi.org/10.3109/1 5563650.2013.802797

Kasperczyk S, Dobrakowski M, Kasperczyk A, Machnik G, Birkner E (2014a) Effect of N-acetylcysteine administration on the expression and activities of antioxidant enzymes and the malondialdehyde level in the blood of lead-exposed workers. Environ Toxicol Pharmacol 37(2):638–647. https://doi.org/10.1016/j.etap.2014.01.024

Kasperczyk S, Dobrakowski M, Kasperczyk A, Zalejska-Fiolka J, Pawlas N, Kapka-Skrzypczak L, Birkner E (2014b) Effect of treatment with N-acetylcysteine on non-enzymatic antioxidant reserves and lipid peroxidation in workers exposed to lead. Ann Agric Environ Med 21(2):272–277. https://doi.org/10.5604/1232-1966.1108590

Kasperczyk S, Dobrakowski M, Kasperczyk A, Romuk E, Rykaczewska-Czerwinska M, Pawlas N, Birkner E (2015) Effect of N-acetylcysteine administration on homocysteine level, oxidative damage to proteins, and levels of iron (Fe) and Fe-related proteins in lead-exposed workers. Toxicol Ind Health 32(9):1607–1618. https://doi.org/10.1177/0748233715571152

Kelly GS (1998) Clinical applications of N-acetylcysteine. Altern Med Rev 3(2):114–127

Khandelwal S, Kachru DN, Tandon SK (1988) Chelation in metal intoxication. XXVIII: effect of thiochelators on mercury (II) toxicity: pre- and post treatment. Biochem Int 16(5):869–878

Livardjani F, Ledig M, Kopp P, Dahlet M, Leroy M, Jaeger A (1991) Lung and blood superoxide dismutase activity in mercury vapor exposed rats: effect of N-acetylcysteine treatment. Toxicology 66(3):289–295

Llobet JM, Domingo JL, Paternain JL, Corbella J (1990) Treatment of acute lead intoxication. A quantitative comparison of a number of chelating agents. Arch Environ Contam Toxicol 19(2):185–189

Lorber A, Baumgartner WA, Bovy RA, Chang CC, Hollcraft R (1973) Clinical application for heavy metal-complexing potential of N-acetylcysteine. J Clin Pharmacol 13(8):332–336

Lund ME, Banner W Jr, Clarkson TW, Berlin M (1984) Treatment of acute methylmercury ingestion by hemodialysis with N-acetylcysteine (Mucomyst) infusion and 2,3-dimercaptopropane sulfonate. J Toxicol Clin Toxicol 22(1):31–49

Madejczyk MS, Aremu DA, Simmons-Willis TA, Clarkson TW, Ballatori N (2007) Accelerated urinary excretion of methylmercury following administration of its antidote N-acetylcysteine requires Mrp2/Abcc2, the apical multidrug resistance-associated protein. J Pharmacol Exp Ther 322(1):378–384. https://doi.org/10.1124/jpet.107.122812

Martin DS, Willis SE, Cline DM (1990) N-acetylcysteine in the treatment of human arsenic poisoning. J Am Board Fam Pract 3(4):293–296

Oliveira VA, Oliveira CS, Mesquita M, Pedroso TF, Costa LM, Fiuza Tda L, Pereira ME (2015) Zinc and N-acetylcysteine modify mercury distribution and promote increase in hepatic metallothionein levels. J Trace Elem Med Biol 32:183–188. https://doi.org/10.1016/j. jtemb.2015.06.006

Ottenwalder H, Simon P (1987) Differential effect of N-acetylcysteine on excretion of the metals Hg, Cd, Pb and Au. Arch Toxicol 60(5):401–402

Pande M, Mehta A, Pant BP, Flora SJ (2001) Combined administration of a chelating agent and an antioxidant in the prevention and treatment of acute lead intoxication in rats. Environ Toxicol Pharmacol 9(4):173–184

Sarikaya S, Karcioglu O, Ay D, Cetin A, Aktas C, Serinken M (2010) Acute mercury poisoning: a case report. BMC Emerg Med 10:7. https://doi.org/10.1186/1471-227X-10-7

Sharma S, Shrivastava S, Shukla S (2013) Reversal of lead-induced toxicity due to the effect of antioxidants. J Environ Pathol Toxicol Oncol 32(2):177–187

Shum S, Skarbovig J, Habersang R (1981) Acute lethal arsenite poisoning in mice: effect of treatment with N-acetylcysteine, D-penicillamine and dimercaprol on survival time. Vet Hum Toxicol 23(Suppl 1):39–42

da Silva RF, dos Borges CS, Villela ESP, Missassi G, Kiguti LR, Pupo AS, Barbosa Junior F, Anselmo-Franci JA, de Kempinas WG (2016) The coadministration of N-acetylcysteine ameliorates the effects of arsenic trioxide on the male mouse genital system. Oxidative Med Cell Longev 2016:4257498. https://doi.org/10.1155/2016/4257498

Tandon SK, Singh S, Prasad S, Srivastava S, Siddiqui MK (2002) Reversal of lead-induced oxidative stress by chelating agent, antioxidant, or their combination in the rat. Environ Res 90(1):61–66

Tandon SK, Singh S, Prasad S, Khandekar K, Dwivedi VK, Chatterjee M, Mathur N (2003) Reversal of cadmium induced oxidative stress by chelating agent, antioxidant or their combination in rat. Toxicol Lett 145(3):211–217

Ustundag A, Duydu Y (2007) The influence of melatonin and N-acetylcysteine in delta-aminolevulinic acid and lead induced genotoxicity in lymphocytes in vitro. Biol Trace Elem Res 117(1-3):53–64. https://doi.org/10.1007/BF02698083

Vreugdenhil G, Swaak AJ (1990) Effects of oral N-acetylcysteine on gold levels in rheumatoid arthritis. Br J Rheumatol 29(5):404–405

Wispriyono B, Matsuoka M, Igisu H, Matsuno K (1998) Protection from cadmium cytotoxicity by N-acetylcysteine in LLC-PK1 cells. J Pharmacol Exp Ther 287(1):344–351

Application of N-Acetylcysteine in Neurological Disorders

11

Reza Bavrsad Shahripour, Ana Hossein Zadeh Maleki, and Andrei V. Alexandrov

11.1 Introduction

Oxidative stress plays a critical role in neuronal dysfunction and death in various neurodegenerative disorders (Arakawa and Ito 2007). Previous studies support the notion that the intrinsic antioxidant glutathione (GSH) and GSH-dependent enzymes have significant role in the protection against neurodegeneration. Additionally, GSH has important role in S-glutathionylation which is important in signal transduction and enzyme regulation (Johnson et al. 2012). Any dysregulation in the GSH-based antioxidant network may promote the initiation and progression of the neurodegenerative diseases (Table 11.1).

The major event in the pathogenesis of Huntington's disease (HD), sporadic Parkinson's disease (PD), focal cerebral ischemia, and traumatic brain injury (TBI) is mitochondrial dysfunction which results in elevated oxidative stress and leads to a decline in GSH level (Arakawa and Ito 2007; Sian et al. 1994). In other neurological disorders such as multiple sclerosis (MS) and amyotrophic lateral sclerosis (ALS), tumor necrosis factor alpha (TNFα) markedly increases followed by increased free radical production (Sharief and Hentges 1991). Specific mutations in the gene encoding superoxide dismutase, decreased activity of glutathione peroxidase (GSHpx), and GSH reductase were reported in the pathogenesis of familial (Bavarsad Shahripour et al. 2014) and sporadic ALS (Wilder et al. 1995). Earlier studies revealed that the pathological production of free radicals and consequent lipid peroxidation have a principal role in the development of vasospasm after subarachnoid hemorrhage (SAH; Sen et al. 2006).

Electronic supplementary material The online version of this article (https://doi.org/10.1007/978-981-10-5311-5_11) contains supplementary material, which is available to authorized users.

R. B. Shahripour · A. H. Z. Maleki · A. V. Alexandrov (✉)
Department of Neurology, University of Tennessee, Memphis, TN, USA
e-mail: Aalexa30@uthsc.edu

Table 11.1 Summary of NAC mechanisms of action across different neurological disorders

Neurological disorder	Mechanism of N-Acetylcysteine (NAC)
Neurodegenerative disorders: Spinocerebellar degeneration, myoclonus epilepsy of Unverricht–Lundborg type	Antioxidant effect by free radical scavenging and increased levels of glutathione (Arakawa and Ito 2007)
Multiple sclerosis	Free radical scavenging and inhibition of TNF-alpha toxicity (Lehmann et al. 1994)
Amyotrophic lateral sclerosis	Increasing the level of glutathione peroxidase and free radical scavenging (Louwerse et al. 1995)
Parkinson's disease	Increasing the level of glutathione and free radical scavenging (Martínez et al. 1999; Schapira a et al. 1990)
Huntington's disease	Free radical trapping and preventing mitochondrial dysfunction (La Fontaine et al. 2000)
Traumatic brain injury	Repair of TBI-induced mitochondrial dysfunction, increasing the reduced antioxidant enzyme and glutathione levels, inhibition of the activation of NF-kB and TNF-alpha (Chen et al. 2008; Hoffer et al. 2002; Hsu et al. 2006)
Focal cerebral ischemia	Nitric oxide synthase (NOS) inhibition, regeneration of endothelium-derived relaxing factor, increasing GSH levels, improving microcirculatory blood flow, and tissue oxygenation (Caplan 2013; Cuzzocrea et al. 2000)
Alzheimer's disease	Blocking the induced oxidative injury, increasing GSH level in cortical and hippocampus areas (Adams Jr et al. 1991)
Subarachnoid hemorrhage	Free radical scavenging, endothelial apoptosis inhibition, lipid peroxidation reduction, increasing glutathione levels, superoxide dismutase (SOD) enzymatic activities, endothelial integrity protection (Sen et al. 2006)
Neuropathy	Increasing the viability of cells through inhibitory reactive oxygen species, attenuation of oxidative stress and apoptosis, inhibition of matrix metallo-proteinase (MMP), blocking the maturation of interleukin-1β (Cameron et al. 2001; Cui et al. 2008; Stevens et al. 2000)
Myopathies	Reducing oxidative stress, improving survival of cultured myotubes, scavenging oxygen free radicals, and repleting low glutathione stores (Ortolani et al. 2000)

N-Acetylcysteine (NAC) is widely known as an antidote for acetaminophen overdose. In the past few decades, it has also been used in several other fields of medicine as well. These diverse clinical applications of NAC are linked to its ability to support the body's antioxidant and nitric oxide (NO) systems against stress, infection, toxic assaults, and inflammatory conditions (Dekhuijzen 2004). Generally any situation that results in a sudden or chronic overconsumption of oxygen in the body can lead to production of the reactive oxygen species (ROS). Several studies report that ROS is detected in (a) mitochondria, (b) inside the capillary system, and (c) as an oxidative burst induced by inflammatory cells (Dekhuijzen 2004; Kerksick and Willoughby 2005).

NAC is an acetylated cysteine residue that is able to magnify protection against oxidative stresses in cell. NAC also performs as an effective free radical scavenger and greatly contributes in maintaining the GSH level in cells. Studies report that NAC can minimize the oxidative effects of ROS through inhibition of GSH depletion (Johnson et al. 2012). By doing so NAC may decrease the inflammatory responses in some diseases such as in chronic obstructive pulmonary disease (COPD), influenza, and idiopathic pulmonary fibrosis. NAC not only can operate as an antioxidant but also can facilitate NO production and vasodilation of the blood vessels. Various applications of NAC in many illnesses such as cancer, cardiovascular diseases, human immunodeficiency virus (HIV) infection, acetaminophen-induced liver toxicity, and metal toxicity have been reviewed in other chapters of this book (Bavarsad Shahripour et al. 2014; Dekhuijzen 2004; Kerksick and Willoughby 2005).

In this chapter we provide a systematic analysis of the recent clinical studies about NAC efficacy in various neurological disorders. Also we mentioned its role in brain function and the pathophysiology of neurological disease as it has been discussed in clinical trials, case series, case reports, and review articles.

11.2 Methods

A systematic online literature search used broad search terms such as "neurologic," "neurology," "neurological disorder," or "specific neurological disorder"—"amyotrophic lateral sclerosis," "ALS," "epilepsy," "seizures," "traumatic brain injury," "TBI," "stroke," "ischemia," "focal cerebral ischemia," "Parkinson's disease," "Huntington's disease," "subarachnoid hemorrhage," "SAH," "multiple sclerosis," "myopathy," "neuropathy," "spinocerebellar ataxia," "hereditary spinocerebellar ataxia," "Freidrich's ataxia," "ataxia–telangiectasia," "olivopontocerebellar atrophy," "progressive myoclonic epilepsy of the Unverricht–Lundborg type (PME–ULD)," and "Alzheimer's disease (AD)." References cited in the identified publications were also reviewed. One reviewer screened titles and abstracts of all potentially relevant publications (Fig. 11.1).

11.3 Evidence of Effectiveness of NAC in the Treatment of Neurological Disorders

11.3.1 Alzheimer's Disease (AD)

Alzheimer's disease (AD) is a progressive degenerative disorder. Previous studies have shown evidence of direct and indirect influence of free radicals in AD. In 1991, Adams Jr et al. (1991) reported an increase in the lipid peroxides level in the temporal and cerebral cortex and a reduction in the GSH level in the cortical and hippocampus areas in patients with AD (Jenner 1994).

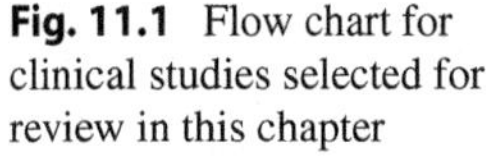

Fig. 11.1 Flow chart for clinical studies selected for review in this chapter

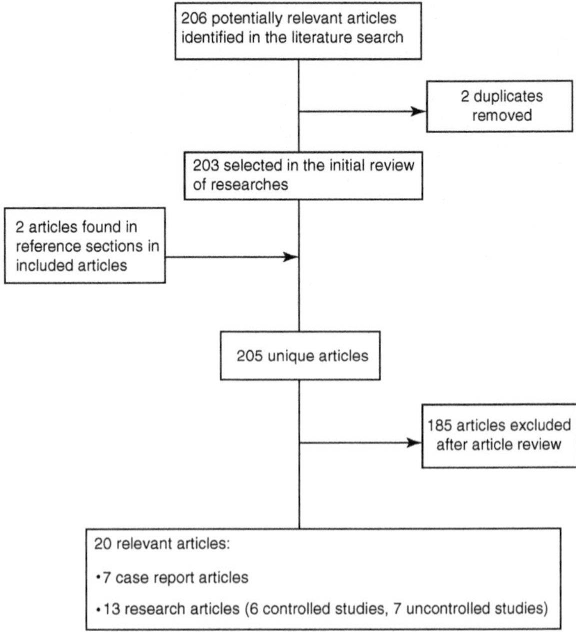

Some clinical trials have evaluated the synergistic effect of combined antioxidants with different chemical compounds such as tocopherol (a compound with vitamin E activity) or selegiline (a selective MAO-B inhibitor) in the treatment of the AD. In 2005, two groups revealed a supportive and protective effect of NAC in some murine models of AD. They documented that NAC administration could block induced oxidative injury in AD models (Tchantchou et al. 2005; Tucker et al. 2005).

Adair et al. (2001) evaluated NAC in a double-blind placebo-controlled (DBPC) trial in patients with AD (Online Table 11.1). All subjects tolerated the drug well and experienced only minor and transient adverse effects (AEs). Although NAC treatment failed to alter the primary outcome measures, it had positive effects on some secondary outcome measures. Their results support future testing of NAC in AD.

McCaddon and Davies (2005) evaluated the co-administration of vitamin B supplements with NAC (600 mg daily) in three patients with dementia and hyperhomocysteinemia. In the first case, a 65-year-old man, with a 3-year history of memory loss and severe cognition impairment (17/30 on the Mini-Mental Status Examination (MMSE)), demonstrated reduced agitation, improved word-finding ability, and increased compliance, although his cognitive score remained unchanged, with NAC treatment. In the second case, a 70-year-old woman with history of short-term memory loss for 3 years (21/30 on the MMSE) demonstrated no change in cognitive function (21/30 on MMSE) with 6-month treatment of monthly injections of hydroxocobalamin and daily oral 5 mg of folic acid. One month after NAC was initiated, her cognitive function improved, her MMSE score markedly improved

(25/30), and she was livelier and happier. The third case was an 81-year-old man with a 5-year history of slowly deteriorating short-term memory loss, verbal aggression, agitation, and unsteady gait who required assistance with most daily activities (68 on the AD Assessment Scale-Cognition Assessment Subscale). Although no changes in cognitive function were observed with monthly hydroxocobalamin injections and oral folate, 1 month after adding 600 mg NAC, he improved 6 points on the AD Assessment Scale-Cognition Assessment Subscale, and he became less agitated and became more content and alert.

Chan et al. (2008) performed a pilot study on a nutriceutical formulation (NF) (folate 400 μg, vitamin B12 6 mg, alpha-tocopherol 30IU, S-adenosylmethionine 400 mg, N-Acetylcysteine 600 mg, and acetyl-L-carnitine 500 mg) on mild-to-moderate AD. They followed 14 cases for about 9 months and demonstrated a clinically markedly delay in the decline in the Dementia Rating Scale (DRS) and clock-drawing test (CDT), about 30% improvement in the Neuropsychiatric Inventory (NPI), and maintenance of performance in the AD Cooperative Study-Activities of Daily Living as reported by their caregivers.

Remington et al. (2009) performed a small 9-month DBPC on 12 institutionalized patients with moderate-to-late-stage probable AD. Unfortunately, all participants in the placebo group dropped out by 6 months, making the study a small-uncontrolled case series. NF delayed the decline in the Dementia Rating Scale-2 (DRS-2) and clock-drawing test (CLOX-1) tests and resulted in improvements in the Neuropsychiatric Inventory and AD Cooperative Study-Activities of Daily Living.

In a phase 2 DBPC multisite clinical trial, 106 AD cases were randomized into the NF or placebo groups for 3 or 6 months (Remington et al. 2015). NF treatment resulted in improvement in the Neuropsychiatric Inventory for the 3-month cohort. According to these findings, this NF formulation may be effective in delaying cognition, mood, and daily function decline in progressive AD cases and may be particularly valuable as a supplement for pharmacological approaches during later stages of this progressive degenerative disease. However, larger trials are warranted (Remington et al. 2015).

Based on two controlled studies with high positive responses and the evidence available, NAC appears to have therapeutic effect in the treatment of Alzheimer's disease (Table 11.2).

11.3.2 Ataxia–Telangiectasia

Ataxia–telangiectasia (AT) is another complex multisystem disorder characterized by ataxia, ocular telangiectasia, and T-cell and B-cell dysfunction with increased susceptibility to cancer and high sensitivity to ionizing radiation (Woods and Taylor 1992). Three siblings aged 7, 11, and 13 years with confirmed AT were treated with NAC in an open-label fashion. After 3 months of treatment, one showed questionable improvements, and the other two patients showed rapid deterioration 2 weeks after NAC cessation (Bavarsad Shahripour et al. 2014; Wilder et al., 1995; Online

Table 11.2 Overall ratings of NAC based on clinical studies presented by condition

Neurological condition	Uncontrolled studies positive % (positive/total)	Controlled studies positive % (positive/total)	Grade of recommendation	Recommendation for treatment
Alzheimer's disease	100 (4/4)	75 (1.5/2)	B	Yes
Ataxia–telangiectasia	50 (0.5/1)		C	None
Freidrich's ataxia	100 (1/1)		C	None
Hereditary spinocerebellar ataxia	100 (2/2)		C	Mixed
Huntington's disease	0 (0/1)		C	None
Motor neuron disease	33 (1/3)	50 (1/2)	B	None
Multiple sclerosis		50 (1/2)	C	None
Neuropathy	100 (1/1)	100 (1/1)	C	Mixed
Olivopontocerebellar atrophy	100 (1/1)		C	None
Progressive myoclonus epilepsy of Unverricht–Lundborg disease	87.5 (3.5/4)		C	Mixed
Subarachnoid hemorrhage	100 (1/1)		C	None
Traumatic brain injury		100 (1/1)	B	None

Table 11.2). Since there are only a few case presentations and a few anecdotal reports on NAC treatment in AT, no recommendations can be made at this point, and more controlled trials are required (Table 11.2).

11.3.3 Focal Cerebral Ischemia

Following cerebral ischemia, the level of ROS increases due to several changes including mitochondria dysfunction. Ischemia also changes different neural and humoral mediator pathways including opioids, NO, adenosine, bradykinin, catecholamines, heat-shock proteins, heme oxygenase, TNFα, angiotensin, and prostaglandins (Caplan 2013). Cuzzocrea et al. (2000) stated that release of excitatory neurotransmitters such as glutamate, which acts on the N-methyl-D-aspartate (NMDA) receptors, has a main role in neural injury after ischemia. The theory of NAC involvement in the microcirculatory blood flow and tissue oxygenation has been supported by animal studies, but studies have also demonstrated that glutamate receptor antagonists reduce neuronal damages following ischemic stroke.

Past studies have shown that NO synthase (NOS) inhibitors and neuronal gene disruption can protect ischemic brain from NMDA neurotoxicity (Bavarsad Shahripour et al. 2014; Cuzzocrea et al. 2000). Harrison et al. (1991) have documented a markedly decrease in the neuronal loss of the pyramidal layer of the cortex in the ischemic animals that received NAC. However, although there are several animal studies demonstrating the protective effect of the NAC treatment after ischemic cascade, no clinical data is available on the use of NAC in acute ischemic stroke patients.

11.3.4 Friedrich's Ataxia

Helveston et al. (1996) presented a 21-year-old female with Friedreich's ataxia. After 13 months of treatment with NAC and other antioxidants, she experienced a significant improvement in her proprioception and, to some extent, her ataxia (Bavarsad Shahripour et al. 2014; Online Table 11.3). Based on a single case presentation on NAC treatment in Friedrich's ataxia, no recommendations can be drawn at this point, and more controlled clinical trials are required (Table 11.2).

11.3.5 Hereditary Spinocerebellar Ataxia (HSCA)

Based on the oxidative role of free radical species in the pathogenesis of cerebellar degeneration disease, NAC may be therapeutically effective. Although there are no published basic research studies or clinical trials about the potential therapeutic role of NAC on HSCA, Wilder et al. presented 18 patients with HSCA who received NAC (Wilder et al. 1995; Online Table 11.4). However, the presentation was never published in a peer-reviewed journal. He reported five siblings with variable

Table 11.3 Ongoing clinical trials on N-Acetylcysteine for neurological disorders

Trial title	NCT no.	Trial status
N-Acetylcysteine for neuroprotection in Parkinson's disease (NAC for PD)	NCT01470027	Recruiting
The role of N-acetyl-L-cysteine (NAC) as an adjuvant to opioid treatment in patients with chronic neuropathic pain	NCT01840345	Recruiting
Overcoming membrane transporters to improve CNS drug delivery—improving brain antioxidants after traumatic brain injury (Pro-NAC)	NCT01322009	Recruiting
Physiological effects of nutritional support in patients with Parkinson's disease	NCT02445651	Recruiting
Repeated-dose oral N-Acetylcysteine for the treatment of Parkinson's disease	NCT02212678	Completed. No results
Antioxidant therapy in RYR1-related congenital myopathy	NCT02362425	Recruiting
N-Acetylcysteine vs placebo to prevent neurotoxicity induced by platinum-containing chemotherapy (NAC-PNP)	NCT00637624	Recruiting
Effect on migraine frequency of combined antioxidant therapy: The MIGRANT study	NCT02629536	Not recruiting yet
Nutrition, neuromuscular electrical stimulation (NMES), and secondary progressive multiple sclerosis (SPMS)	NCT01381354	Ongoing but not recruiting
Acetaminophen in aSAH to inhibit lipid peroxidation and cerebral vasospasm	NCT00585559	Recruiting
Pharmacological treatment of a rare genetic disease: N-Acetylcysteine in myopathy associated selenoprotein N-related myopathy (SEPN1-RM) (SelNac)	NCT02505087	Recruiting

severity of ataxia, dysarthria, and oculomotor disturbances. All of these patients claimed subjective improvement after NAC treatment. The most severely affected sibling (male, age 43) was treated with NAC for 26 months. After NAC treatment, he achieved significantly improved control on his eye movement, and his reading speed increased from 50 to 300 words per minute.

Another reported case was a 67-year-old patient with a 25-year history of progressive HSCA primarily with difficulties in balance and his speech. His deceased father and brother had the same disorder. After a 7-month treatment with NAC, his wife reported no falling, and his speech became comprehensible over the phone (Wilder et al. 1995).

Although all the case reports demonstrate a dramatic response of NAC, a lack of any controlled studies led us to make a mixed recommendation regarding the use of NAC in HSCA (Table 11.2).

11.3.6 Huntington's Disease

Mitochondrial dysfunction has been stated as a major event in the pathogenesis of HD. La Fontaine et al. (2000) successfully created an animal model of HD by intraperitoneally injecting 3-nitropropionic acid (3-NP) to rats. 3-NP worked as an irreversible inhibitor of complex II in the mitochondria (La Fontaine et al. 2000). They found an increase in oxidative stress in both the striatum and cortical synaptosomes in all rats (La Fontaine et al. 2000). Interestingly, pretreatment with NAC (100 mg/kg, daily) 2 h before 3-NP injection protected rats from the oxidative damage and significantly reduced striatal lesion volume (La Fontaine et al. 2000). Sandhir et al. (2012) reported the same protective effect of NAC in the 3-NP-induced HD models and reported an increased generation of ROS and lipid peroxidation in the mitochondria of 3-NP-treated rats (Sandhir et al. 2012). The main histopathologic findings in these rats were increased neural space, neurodegeneration, and gliosis. These findings were accompanied by cognitive and motor deficits (Sandhir et al. 2012). Although several animal studies have shown this beneficial and protective effect of NAC in HD, only two cases have been reported in a conference presentation (Wilder et al., 1995). In their report, treatment with NAC for 3 and 4 months resulted in no obvious improvement in the patient's condition (Online Table 11.5). There is a recent clinical report of a case of Huntington's treated with NAC (Berk 2015).

Based on the evidence available, there is inconsistent evidence of benefit but NAC also appeared to be well tolerated and safe. Thus, until more studies are available, it is difficult to make a recommendation for the use of NAC in HD (Table 11.2).

11.3.7 Motor Neuron Diseases

Rosen et al. (1993) have reported a specific mutation in the gene encoding superoxide dismutase 1 (SOD1) in the familial amyotrophic lateral sclerosis (FALS). This finding supports the role of free radicals in the progression of ALS. Previous studies revealed that the level of SOD1 is reduced in patients with FALS but is often normal in sporadic ALS (Bavarsad Shahripour et al. 2014). However, Wilder et al. (1995) reported normal SOD1 activity in two patients with sporadic ALS but found markedly reduced glutathione peroxidase (GSHpx) and GSH reductase activities. After 12 months of treatment with NAC in one of these patients, not only did his disease stop progressing, but he achieved an increase in grip strength. After 17 months of treatment, the second patient had only mild disease progression. This change in disease progression may have been due to NAC treatment (Online Table 11.6).

de Jong et al. (1987) reported an open-label study of NAC in 40 cases of ALS. After 6 months of treatment with 100 cc of NAC injected subcutaneously, 62% of cases stayed stable, and after 24 months of treatment, 52% had no progression. In another open-label study in 11 patients with ALS reported by Küther and Struppler (1987), all of the patients received 50 cm^3 of 5% NAC injected subcutaneously daily plus vitamin C, as antioxidant, for 1–12 months. According to this report, there was no significant difference in patient survival. Louwerse et al. (1995) reported a DBPC trial of NAC therapy in 111 ALS patients. Their trial did not show any significant increase in 12-month survival (65% vs 54%) or any marked reduction in the disease progression. However, in the subgroup of 81 ALS cases with limb onset of the disease, there was greater survival in the NAC treatment group (28 patients, 74%) as compared to the placebo group (22 patients, 51%) at 12 months (Louwerse et al. 1995).

In a retrospective case–control study by Vyth et al. (1996), the effect of different antioxidants in 36 ALS cases was evaluated. After any new exacerbation of the disease, patients were given a different antioxidant such as vitamins C and E, N-acetylmethionine (NAM), NAC, and dithiothreitol (DTT) or its isomer dithioerythritol (DTE). Antioxidants (such as NAC) did not seem to harm ALS patients, but also they did not seem to prolong their survival either (3.4-month survival before antioxidant use vs 2.8-month survival after use of antioxidants).

At this time there are few controlled clinical trials and no large controlled trial on the therapeutic effect of NAC on motor neuron disease. Based on the evidence available, there is inconsistent evidence of benefit, but NAC also appears to be well tolerated and safe. Thus, until more studies are available, it is difficult to make a recommendation for the use of NAC in motor neuron disease (Table 11.2).

11.3.8 Multiple Sclerosis (MS)

MS disease is associated with a marked increase TNFα, especially in the active phase of the illness. A correlation between TNFα concentration in the cerebrospinal fluid and the severity and progression of the disease has been reported (Sharief and Hentges 1991). An increase in free radical production with cytokine activation has been demonstrated in MS (Glabiński et al. 1993). In animal models NAC inhibited the toxicity of TNFα and the development of MS-like pathology (Lehmann et al. 1994).

For the first time, Wilder et al. (1995) presented ten patients with relapsing-remitting MS (RRMS) treated with NAC for up to 16 months. Two MS patients with long-standing incoherent speech demonstrated a rather dramatic improvement in their speech shortly after starting NAC treatment. However, due to the waxing and waning course of this disease in many patients, it is difficult to determine the efficacy of NAC in a small sample without a control group (Online Table 11.7).

Recently, Schipper et al. (2015) performed an open-label pilot study on seven RRMS cases to evaluate the tolerability and safety of glatiramer acetate (GA) and 2.5 g NAC orally combined. Although none of the MRI changes were statistically significant, there was a significant improvement in the erythrocyte GSSG/GSH ratios after 36 weeks of treatment. Overall, the sustained exposure to high doses of NAC in patients with RRMS was safe and well tolerated and did not show any significant clinical deterioration or neuroimaging abnormality.

At this time there are no controlled clinical trials on the therapeutic effect of NAC in MS. Controlled studies are particularly important in MS as the disease has a waxing and waning course. Based on the evidence available, there is inconsistent evidence of benefit, but NAC appears to be well tolerated and safe. Thus, until more studies are available, it is difficult to make a recommendation for the use of NAC in MS (Table 11.2).

11.3.9 Myopathy

Ryanodine receptor (RYR) has an important role in the skeletal muscle, especially as an essential component of the excitation–contraction coupling process. RYR1-related myopathies refer to a group of congenital myopathies that are the most common non-dystrophic muscle diseases. Currently, for these kinds of congenital myopathies, there is not any curative treatment except for symptomatic therapies and rehabilitation (Dowling et al. 2012). In an effort to discover novel pathogenic mechanisms, Dowling et al. (2012) uncovered a significant abnormality in pathways associated with cellular stress. Their study was based on analyzing two models of RYR1-related myopathies: (a) the relatively relaxed zebra fish and (b) cultured myotubes from patients with RYR1-related myopathies. Expression array analysis in the zebra fish revealed significant abnormalities in pathways associated with cellular stress, including increased oxidant activity, the presence of oxidative stress markers, excessive production of oxidants by mitochondria, and diminished survival under oxidant conditions. Exposure to NAC reduced oxidative stress and improved survival of cultured myotubes from the patient with the RYR1-related myopathy. NAC also led to significant restoration of muscle's function in the relatively relaxed zebra fish. Based on their findings, it appears that oxidative stress is an important pathophysiological mechanism in RYR1-related myopathy, and NAC could be a successful treatment modality for this common myopathy in children (Dowling et al. 2012).

Earlier investigations on muscle biopsy in critically ill patients have focused on the GSH levels in parallel with low glutamine levels (Wernerman et al. 1999; Yu et al. 2002). Ortolani et al. (2000) assessed the effects of either intravenous NAC or GSH in critically ill patients with early septic shock syndrome who were receiving standard therapy. Interestingly, oxidative stress indicators were markedly decreased at day 5 of treatment in the NAC group, especially in the combined GSH and NAC therapy. They hypothesized that potentially glutathione precursors, such as NAC, may improve outcomes in critically ill patients through scavenge oxygen free radicals and replete low glutathione stores. Although NAC therapy in this type of myopathy can be beneficial either in the treatment or prevention, so far there has not been any randomized clinical trial evaluating the efficacy of NAC (Burnham et al. 2005). However, a clinical trial to evaluate the efficacy of antioxidant therapy in RYR1-related congenital myopathy has been registered and is currently recruiting participants (NCT02362425; Table 11.3).

11.3.10 Neuropathy

According to the published preclinical and animal studies, diabetic polyneuropathy (DPN) results from a complex network of interrelated vascular, metabolic, and neurotrophic cascades (Cameron et al. 2001; Calcutt et al. 2004; Stevens et al. 2000; Sima et al. 2000). Studies have shown that metabolic changes are involved in the pathogenesis of DPN, including increased oxidative stress, altered eicosanoid metabolism, activation of nuclear enzyme polymerase (ADP-ribose), and decreased antioxidant defenses (Edwards et al. 2008). Several potential sources of ROS have been suggested such as endothelial NAD(P)H oxidase, xanthine oxidase, nitric oxide synthase, and mitochondrial respiratory chain inefficiency (Cameron et al. 2001). Reduced activity of Cu–Zn superoxide dismutase and glutathione peroxidase as well as decreased levels of glutathione, vitamin E, and L-carnitine has been reported in DPN (Arora et al. 2008; Cui et al. 2008; Ido et al. 1994; Junxian et al. 2006; Nagamatsu et al. 1995). Animal studies have revealed that insulin and antioxidants have significant improvement in nerve function in DPN (Kamboj et al. 2010). Although oxidative stress has been associated with the development of diabetic complications in the preclinical and animal studies, no clinical trial has shown an advantage in using classic antioxidants in diabetes (Ceriello 2006; Shelton et al. 2005).

Rothstein et al. (1994) showed that NAC increased the viability of cells in culture, including spinal motor neurons, through inhibitory reactive oxygen species. The same protective effect has been shown in oligodendrocytes, cortical neurons, and superior cervical ganglion neurons (Ferrari et al. 1995; Mayer and Noble 1994; Ratan et al. 1994; Yan and Greene 1998). Kamboj et al. (2010) documented that the protective effect for NAC was mediated through attenuation of oxidative stress and apoptosis. Based on these findings, he suggested a therapeutic potential of NAC in the attenuation of DPN in rats (Kamboj et al. 2010; Kamboj and Chopra 2008).

Although there are no published clinical trials or case series about the efficacy of NAC in DPN, NAC has been studied in other neuropathies. Lin et al. (2006) reported a pilot study examining the effect of NAC (1200 mg) in 14 patients receiving oxaliplatin as a colorectal cancer treatment. After 12 chemotherapy cycles, 3/5 patients who received NAC developed chemotherapy-induced peripheral neuropathy (CIPN), but only 1/5 had grade 2–4 of toxicity. In the control group, 9/9 patients developed CIPN with 8/9 developing grade 2–4 of toxicity (Online Table 11.8). Another case report showed positive results using a combination of neuroprotectants—NAC, levocarnitine, and pyridoxine—in a 46-day-old male with acute lymphoblastic leukemia who developed severe vincristine- induced peripheral neuropathy (Baker and Lipson 2010).

The mechanisms of neuropathic pain are not clear. Matrix metallo-proteinase (MMP)-9 and MMP-2 have been documented as the key components in neuropathic pain through their facilitation of inflammatory cytokine maturation and induction of neural inflammation (Li and Xu 2016). The inhibitory characteristic of MMPs may represent a new therapeutic approach to neuropathic pain. Based on this theory, Li and Xu (2016) recently stated a markedly reduction in neuropathic pain via a unique inhibitory mechanism of MMP (Li and Xu 2016). This rat study showed that orally administered NAC not only postponed the occurrence of neuropathic pain but also inhibited neuropathic pain induced by maintenance of chronic constrictive injury (CCI). The administration of NAC blocked the maturation of interleukin-1β, which is a critical substrate of MMPs, and also markedly suppressed the neuronal activation induced by CCI, including inhibition of the phosphorylation of protein kinase Cγ, NMDAR1, and mitogen-activated protein kinases. Their results documented an effective treatment for neuropathic pain which is achieved by the MMP activation prevention (Li and Xu 2016). In 2015, a new ongoing clinical trial about NAC impact as an adjuvant therapy in chronic pain has been initiated (NCT01840345; Table 11.3).

Based on the evidence available, there is mixed evidence of benefit, but NAC also appears to be well tolerated and safe. Thus, until more studies are available, it is difficult to make a recommendation for the use of NAC in neuropathy (Table 11.2).

11.3.11 Olivopontocerebellar Atrophy

There is one case report of NAC administration in a known case of olivopontocerebellar atrophy (OPCA) presented by Wilder et al. (1995). The patient had difficulties in balancing and progressive speech disruption with decreased proprioception and pain sensitivity. After 1 month of NAC treatment, marked improvement especially in his speech and balance was seen. After 3 months of treatment with NAC, the patient could discriminate between hot and cold and regained some touch and position sense (Online Table 11.9).

Based on the evidence available, there is inconsistent evidence of benefit, but NAC also appears to be well tolerated and safe. Thus, until more studies are available, it is difficult to make a recommendation for the use of NAC in olivopontocerebellar atrophy (Table 11.2).

11.3.12 Parkinson's Disease (PD)

Multiple neuronal systems are involved in the sporadic PD. The cardinal histopathologies in PD are alpha-synuclein (SCNA) immunopositive, Lewy neurites, and Lewy bodies (Braak et al. 2003). Initially, different areas of the brain including the dorsal part of glossopharyngeal motor nucleus, vagal nerve, anterior part of the olfactory nucleus, and anteromedial part of the temporal mesocortex become affected. Also, increased lipid peroxidation and dramatic decline in GSH level have been reported (Arakawa and Ito 2007). However some published case–control animal studies revealed that GSH concentrations in the substantia nigra (SN) were reduced by 40% in PD animals as compared to controls. On the other hand, since neural degeneration in SN is a common finding in sporadic PD, some investigators believe that the findings from the animal study could be a coincidental finding rather than a casual finding (Dexter et al. 1992; Johnson et al. 2012; Sian et al. 1994). This remarkable decline in GSH level may be related to mitochondrial dysfunction and oxidative stress. Eventually, oxidative stress will increase the accumulation of toxic forms of SNCA (Sian et al. 1994).

Clark et al. (2010) hypothesized a protective role for NAC therapy against SNCA toxicity. They supported this notion based on evidences of temporary increase (less than 1 year) in GSH level in SN in transgenic mice with NAC treatment. After 1 year of treatment with NAC, they reported a reduction in dopaminergic terminal attenuation that was associated with diminished overexpression SNCA. Based on previous animal studies, oxidative stress and GSH depletion eventually result in dopaminergic neuronal loss. This finding has been affirmed in an age-dependent manner in mice specially in pars compacta of the SN (Jiang et al. 2005). Generation of hydrogen peroxide by monoamine oxidase (MAO) and ROS production by catecholamine in the SN are other precipitating factors in PD (Martínez et al. 1999). Furthermore, SN in PD patients is rich in iron and neuromelanin, two other sources that may facilitate the formation of ROS.

According to the animal model studies, Martínez et al. (1999) assumed that new neuroprotective treatments with a sulfur-containing antioxidant such as NAC may be another strategy to approach PD (MAO), and ROS production by catecholamine in the SN is another precipitating factor in PD (Schapira a et al. 1990). Although some clinical trials evaluated the effect of other antioxidants such as vitamins E and C, on PD cases, none of them showed significant effects. This might be because of the poor ability of antioxidants to penetrate the blood–brain barrier (BBB; Pappert et al. 1996; Reilly et al. 1983; Schapira a et al. 1990). On the other hand, other studies demonstrated NAC penetration through BBB which exerted a preventive effect in mice models of PD induced by 1-methyl-4-phenyl-1,2,3,6-tetrahydro-pyridine (MPTP) (Farr et al. 2003; Martínez et al. 1999; Pan et al. 2009).

Holmay et al. (2014) measured brain GSH concentration using 7 tesla magnetic resonance spectroscopy as well as blood redox ratios before and after 150 mg per kg of NAC intravenous infusion in PD patients. NAC was found to increase blood GSH redox ratios in those with PD, which was followed by an increase in brain GSH concentrations. Clinical status of the patients was measured using the disability rating scale during the first month after treatment (6000 mg/day of NAC divided into two equal daily doses for approximately 28 days), but these clinical results have not been published (Holmay et al. 2014). In two ongoing randomized clinical trials, PD patients are being recruited to evaluate the neuroprotective role of NAC (NCT01470027, NCT02445651; Henchcliffe and Shungu 2016; Tuite and Coles 2016; Table 11.3).

NAC appears to be a promising treatment in PD. We believe that additional controlled trials involving administration of NAC or GSH precursors with or without other combined antioxidants are needed (Table 11.2).

11.3.13 Progressive Myoclonic Epilepsy of the Unverricht–Lundborg Type (PME–ULD)

PME–ULD is an autosomal recessive disorder that typically develops between the ages of 6 and 15 years with stimulus-sensitive myoclonus and generalized tonic–clonic (GTC) seizures followed by progressive cerebellar syndrome (Arakawa and

Ito 2007). Based on our search, there is no clinical trial about the efficacy of NAC in PME–ULD, but there are four published case reports.

Selwa (1999) reported a 40-year-old male with a long past medical history of ULD disease. Since the age of 13 years, he had history of unprovoked GTC seizures and morning myoclonus that was unresponsive to phenytoin and phenobarbital. Morning myoclonus became prominent after he left school at the age of 16 years. When phenytoin was tapered, he reported significant improvement in his seizures, but not any slowness or deterioration in cognition or any changes in his ataxia. Seven days after NAC 3 g was prescribed twice daily, the patient's speech improved, his tremor decreased significantly, and he became capable of walking for a whole day. Selwa (1999) reported that the patient had a dramatic response to NAC therapy due to the significant improvements that were observed in his motor function and cognition status (Online Table 11.10).

In 1999, four patients with EPM 1 (Unverricht–Lundborg disease) and one patient with EPM2 (Lafora body disease) were treated with 6 g/day of NAC. Before treatment, GSH peroxidase activity, catalase activity, extracellular superoxide dismutase (SOD), and CuZn–SOD were measured in these patients and compared with controls. Erythrocyte CuZn–SOD was significantly lower in the patients compared to controls. NAC markedly improved and stabilized the neurological symptoms in patients with EPM 1 but not the EPM 2 patient (Ben-Menachem et al. 2000).

Four siblings in Florida with PME–ULD received anticonvulsant treatment for about 20 years without any benefit. All affected siblings had history of GTC seizure with the age onset of 9–11 years old with preceding occurrence of stimulus-sensitive myoclonus between 1 and 3 years of age. Three of four cases had marked mental illness and cognitive deterioration. Treatment with NAC 4–6 g daily resulted in an initial improvement, particularly in mental alertness. The first patient showed a dramatic increase in verbalization and motor function (daily activity) during the 30 months of treatment. The second patient also reported a better motor function during the 30 months of treatment. Before the 26 months of treatment with NAC, the third and fourth patients were in a semicomatose state and weren't able to talk but were only able to respond to gestures. After the treatment, both patients became active enough to change their own position instead of needing to be turned over every 2 h. The third patient started to tell jokes in a primitive manner. In the least affected patient, myoclonus improved to such an extent that she has been able to walk independently for several days at a time after NAC was started (Hurd et al. 1996).

Edwards et al. (2002) reported a variable response in three known cases of ULD with different chronicities of the illness (ages 12, 3, and 9 years). In the first case with a 12-year history of symptoms, dramatic improvement in myoclonus, ataxia, and alertness was reported with this beneficial effect maintained for 2 years. This was associated with an increase in GSH concentrations (from 2.2 to 5.4 μM) in the blood. In the second case with a 3-year history of symptoms, the patient's myoclonus improved after 2 weeks of treatment (3 g/d NAC), but because of developing sensory neuronal deafness after 5 weeks, the patient did not continue treatment. In the third case with 9-year history of symptoms, NAC therapy (3 g/d) showed a good response during the first 2 months, but this response was not maintained after the second month, and the patient withdrew the treatment.

Based on the evidence available, there is mixed evidence of benefit, but NAC also appears to be well tolerated and safe. Thus, until more studies are available, it is difficult to make a recommendation for the use of NAC in PME–ULD (Table 11.2).

11.3.14 Subarachnoid Hemorrhage (SAH)

Vasospasm is one of the major complications after SAH. Earlier studies reveal that the pathological production of free radicals and consequent lipid peroxidation have a principal role in the development of vasospasm after SAH (Sen et al. 2006). Halliwell and Gutteridge (1986) documented that endothelial damage and apoptosis of endothelial cells contribute to cerebral vasospasm after SAH, while Sen et al. (2006) hypothesized that protecting the endothelium from apoptosis might attenuate vasospasm (Guney et al. 2010; Halliwell and Gutteridge 1986; Sen et al. 2006). Later, Guney et al. (2010) demonstrated a significant reduction in the apoptotic index after NAC treatment in animal models with SAH. Their study depicted the protective effect of the intraperitoneal administration of NAC in the rabbits with SAH against cerebral vasospasm development. Also, they discovered that NAC treatment increased the luminal area and reduced the wall thickness of the basilar artery.

Bavarsad Shahripour et al. (2014) reported an experience with a 43-year-old woman with vasospasm after Grade 3 SAH resulting from a ruptured aneurysm. The patient had a dramatic clinical response (improved level of consciousness and headache) to treatment of oral NAC 600 mg twice a day, with vasospasm resolution after 24 h confirmed by computed tomography angiography and transcranial Doppler sonography (Online Table 11.11). They believe that NAC can be part of the preventive therapy of vasospasm after SAH through its antioxidant mechanism. However, there are some human studies that have evaluated the protective function of antioxidants and free radical scavengers in SAH patient, but there is no published study on NAC treatment after SAH. It seems this subject deserves further investigation (Munakata et al. 2009; Saito et al. 1998), and no recommendation is applicable at this point (Table 11.2).

11.3.15 Traumatic Brain Injury

Earlier animal studies have documented the neuroprotective role of NAC treatment after traumatic brain injuries (TBIs). It is believed that NAC repairs the mitochondria and specifically increases reduced antioxidant enzymes (Hicdonmez et al. 2006; Xiong et al. 1999). Previous animal studies have suggested that TBI results in an increase in immune mediators such as interleukin-1b (IL-1b), TNFα, interleukin-6 (IL-6), and intercellular adhesion molecule-1 (ICAM-1). There is evidence regarding the role of inflammation in brain damage after TBI, and the influence of NAC on this inflammation has been reported (Merrill and Benveniste 1996; Morganti-Kossmann et al. 2001). NAC inhibited NF-kB and TNFα activation through augmenting GSH concentrations (Hoffer et al. 2002; Hsu et al. 2006). Based on the animal experiments, NAC treatment may decrease inflammatory responses in injured brain following TBI (Chen et al. 2008).

Hoffer et al. (2013) did the first DBPC study to evaluate the clinical efficacy of NAC treatment in amelioration of acute sequel of mild TBI induced by an improvised explosive blast (n:81). The primary results indicated that NAC treatment was significantly better than placebo (OR = 3.6, p = 0.006). Subjects who received NAC (n:29/41) within 24 hours of the blast had 86% chance of symptom's resolution with no reported side effects versus 42% who received placebo (31/40). This trial demonstrated that NAC has beneficial effects on the severity and resolution of sequel after mild TBI induced by a blast (online Table 11.12).

Based on the evidence available, there is inconsistent evidence of benefit, but NAC also appears to be well tolerated and safe. Thus, until more studies are available, it is difficult to make a recommendation for the use of NAC in TBI (Table 11.2).

11.4 Summary

In our systematic review, we found few clinical trials that tested NAC effects in neurological diseases such as AD, motor neuron diseases, MS, neuropathy, and TBI. There are also ongoing clinical trials (Table 11.3) on the effect of NAC in a variety of neurological disorders.

Of note, two clinical trials in AD reported up to 75% positive response overall, while two open-label studies and one case report showed a 100% positive response. Based on the positive responses and the grade of recommendation, we think NAC can be beneficial in the AD treatment. Unfortunately, NAC applications in ataxia–telangiectasia, Freidrich's ataxia, hereditary spinocerebellar ataxia, and Huntington's disease remain uncertain, and the quality of reports precludes making any recommendation. Considering the nature of the ALS disease and difficulties in its treatment and since there are just few small controlled studies and case reports on NAC treatment, no recommendations could be made at this point. As many as 75% of MS case reports treated with NAC showed either improvement in their disabilities or no new changes in their clinical and imaging status, and it is not possible to make any recommendation at this point since controlled trials are lacking. Based on the grade of recommendation and 100% positive response in patients with neuropathy, we conclude that NAC can be considered as a treatment for neuropathy. Although 87.5% of patients with PME–ULD responded to NAC treatment, the grade of recommendation is C due to the quality of reports. There has been just one case report of NAC application in SAH with vasospasm and clinical symptom resolution. Unfortunately, at this point, no comments can be made and further studies are warranted. Although 100% positive response was observed in patients with mild traumatic brain injury in a DBPC study, it is difficult to give a specific recommendation based on a single study.

As a drug, NAC represents perhaps the ideal xenobiotic, capable of directly entering endogenous biochemical processes as a result of its own metabolism. In addition, NAC may cross the blood–brain barrier (BBB). The use of NAC has been studied in several neurological disorders and seems to be a a novel treatment approach. In our literature reviews, no recommendations could be made for most of the neurological disorders including ataxia–telangiectasia, Freidrich's ataxia, HD, olivopontocerebellar, SAH, and TBI. Studies on hereditary spinocerebellar ataxia, MS, and progressive myoclonus epilepsy of Unverricht–Lundborg diseases demonstrate mixed results, and the evidence for the effectiveness of NAC was negative in motor neuron diseases. NAC showed positive response in anticancer medicine-induced neuropathy in a small controlled trial and a case study potentially making it a favorable treatment option for such neuropathies, but since the sample size of the controlled study was very small, it is hard to give any specific recommendation based on the limited current evidence (Table 11.2).

Thus, the recommendations for use of NAC in the majority of neurological disorders are still limited based on the number and the quality of studies that have been conducted and available for review at this time. While larger controlled trials are needed to establish effectiveness of NAC, available evidence so far and safety profile of NAC support its potential as a novel treatment option for several neurological disorders.

References

Adair JC, Knoefel JE, Morgan N (2001) Controlled trial of *N*-acetylcysteine for patients with probable Alzheimer's disease. Neurology 57(8):1515–1517

Adams JD Jr, Klaidman LK, Odunze IN, Shen HC, Miller CA (1991) Alzheimer's and Parkinson's disease. Brain levels of glutathione, glutathione disulfide, and vitamin E. Mol Chem Neuropathol 14(3):213–226

Arakawa M, Ito Y (2007) *N*-acetylcysteine and neurodegenerative diseases: basic and clinical pharmacology. Cerebellum 6(4):308–314

Arora M, Kumar A, Kaundal RK, Sharma SS (2008) Amelioration of neurological and biochemical deficits by peroxynitrite decomposition catalysts in experimental diabetic neuropathy. Eur J Pharmacol 596(1–3):77–83

Baker SK, Lipson DM (2010) Vincristine-induced peripheral neuropathy in a neonate with congenital acute lymphoblastic leukemia. J Pediatr Hematol Oncol 32(3):e114–e117

Bavarsad Shahripour R, Harrigan MR, Alexandrov AV (2014) *N*-acetylcysteine (NAC) in neurological disorders: mechanisms of action and therapeutic opportunities. Brain Behav 4(2):108–122

Ben-Menachem E, Kyllerman M, Marklund S (2000) Superoxide dismutase and glutathione peroxidase function in progressive myoclonus epilepsies. Epilepsy Res 40(1):33–39

Berk M (2015) *N*-Acetylcysteine for Huntington's? Aust N Z J Psychiatry 49(11):1071–1072

Braak H, Del Tredici K, Rüb U, De Vos RAI, Jansen Steur ENH, Braak E (2003) Staging of brain pathology related to sporadic Parkinson's disease. Neurobiol Aging 24(2):197–211

Burnham EL, Moss M, Ziegler TR (2005) Nutritional consequences of critical illness myopathies myopathies in critical illness: characterization and nutritional aspects 1, 2. J Nutr 135(7):1818–1823

Calcutt NA, Freshwater JD, Mizisin AP (2004) Prevention of sensory disorders in diabetic Sprague-Dawley rats by aldose reductase inhibition or treatment with ciliary neurotrophic factor. Diabetologia 47(4):718–724

Cameron NE, Eaton SE, Cotter MA, Tesfaye S (2001) Vascular factors and metabolic interactions in the pathogenesis of diabetic neuropathy. Diabetologia 44(11):1973–1988

Caplan LR (2013) Creating one problem to try and fix another: the saga of ischemic preconditioning. Brain Behav 3(6):603–605

Ceriello A (2006) Controlling oxidative stress as a novel molecular approach to protecting the vascular wall in diabetes. Curr Opin Lipidol 17(5):510–518

Chan A, Paskavitz J, Remington R, Rasmussen S, Shea TB (2008) Efficacy of a vitamin/nutriceutical formulation for early-stage Alzheimer's disease: a 1-year, open-label pilot study with an 16-month caregiver extension. Am J Alzheimers Dis Other Demen 23(6):571–585

Chen G, Shi J, Hu Z, Hang C (2008) Inhibitory effect on cerebral inflammatory response following traumatic brain injury in rats: a potential neuroprotective mechanism of N-Acetylcysteine. Mediat Inflamm 2008:716458. https://doi.org/10.1155/2008/716458

Clark J, Clore EL, Zheng K, Adame A, Masliah E, Simon DK (2010) Oral N-acetyl-cysteine attenuates loss of dopaminergic terminals in α-synuclein overexpressing mice. PLoS One 5(8):e12333. https://doi.org/10.1371/journal.pone.0012333

Cui X, Li B, Gao H, Wei N, Wang W, Lu M (2008) Effects of grape seed proanthocyanidin extracts on peripheral nerves in streptozocin-induced diabetic rats. J Nutr Sci Vitaminol 54(4): 321–328

Cuzzocrea S, Mazzon E, Costantino G, Serraino I, Dugo L, Calabro G et al (2000) Beneficial effects of n-acetylcysteine on ischaemic brain injury. Br J Pharmacol 130(6):1219–1226

de Jong JM, den Hartog Jager WA, Vyth A, Timmer JG (1987) Attempted treatment of motor neuron disease with N-acetylcysteine and dithiothreitol. Adv Exp Med Biol 209:227–280

Dekhuijzen PNR (2004) Antioxidant properties of N-acetylcysteine: their relevance in relation to chronic obstructive pulmonary disease. Eur Respir J 23(4):629–636

Dexter DT, Jenner P, Schapira AH, Marsden CD (1992) Alterations in levels of iron, ferritin, and other trace metals in neurodegenerative diseases affecting the basal ganglia. Ann Neurol 32:S94–S100

Dowling JJ, Arbogast S, Hur J, Nelson DD, McEvoy A, Waugh T et al (2012) Oxidative stress and successful antioxidant treatment in models of RYR1-related myopathy. Brain 135(4):1115–1127

Edwards MJ, Hargreaves IP, Heales SJ, Jones SJ, Ramachandran V, Bhatia KP et al (2002) N-acetylcysteine and Unverricht-Lundborg disease: variable response and possible side effects. Neurology 59(9):1447–1449

Edwards JL, Vincent AM, Cheng HT, Feldman EL (2008) Diabetic neuropathy: mechanisms to management. Pharmacol Ther 120(1):1–34

Farr SA, Poon HF, Dogrukol-Ak D, Drake J, Banks WA, Eyerman E et al (2003) The antioxidants α-lipoic acid and N-acetylcysteine reverse memory impairment and brain oxidative stress in aged SAMP8 mice. J Neurochem 84(5):1173–1183

Ferrari G, Yan CY, Greene LA (1995) N-acetylcysteine (D- and L-stereoisomers) prevents apoptotic death of neuronal cells. J Neurosci 15(4):2857–2866

Glabiński A, Tawsek NS, Bartosz G (1993) Increased generation of superoxide radicals in the blood of MS patients. Acta Neurol Scand 88(3):174–177

Guney O, Erdi F, Esen H, Kiyici A, Kocaogullar Y (2010) N-acetylcysteine prevents vasospasm after subarachnoid hemorrhage. World Neurosurg 73(1):42–49

Halliwell B, Gutteridge JMC (1986) Oxygen free radicals and iron in relation to biology and medicine: some problems and concepts. Arch Biochem Biophys 246(2):501–514

Harrison PM, Wendon JA, Gimson AE, Alexander GJ, Williams R (1991) Improvement by acetylcysteine of hemodynamics and oxygen transport in fulminant hepatic failure. N Engl J Med 324(26):1852–1857

Helveston W, Cibula JE, Hurd R, Uthman BM, Wilder BJ (1996) Abnormalities of antioxidant metabolism in a case of Friedreich's disease. Clin Neuropharmacol 19(3):271–275

Henchcliffe C, Shungu DC (2016) N-Acetylcysteine for Neuroprotection in Parkinson's disease. https://clinicaltrials.gov/ct2/show/NCT01470027?te

Hicdonmez T, Kanter M, Tiryaki M, Parsak T, Cobanoglu S (2006) Neuroprotective effects of N-acetylcysteine on experimental closed head trauma in rats. Neurochem Res 31(4):473–481

Hoffer E, Baum Y, Nahir a M (2002) *N*-Acetylcysteine enhances the action of anti-inflammatory drugs as suppressors of prostaglandin production in monocytes. Mediat Inflamm 11:321–323

Hoffer ME, Balaban C, Slade MD, Tsao JW, Hoffer B (2013) Amelioration of acute sequelae of blast induced mild traumatic brain injury by *N*-acetyl cysteine: a double-blind, placebo controlled study. PLoS One 8(1):1–10

Holmay MJ, Terpstra M, Coles LD, Tuite J (2014) *N*-acetylcysteine boosts brain and blood glutathione in Gaucher and Parkinson's diseases. Clin Neuropharmacol 36(4):103–106

Hsu BG, Lee RP, Yang FL, Harn HJ, Chen HI (2006) Post-treatment with *N*-acetylcysteine ameliorates endotoxin shock-induced organ damage in conscious rats. Life Sci 79(21):2010–2016

Hurd RW, Wilder BJ, Helveston WR, Uthman BM (1996) Treatment of four siblings with progressive myoclonus epilepsy of the Unverricht-Lundborg type with *N*-acetylcysteine. Neurology 47(5):1264–1268

Ido Y, McHowat J, Chang KC, Arrigoni-Martelli E, Orfalian Z, Kilo C et al (1994) Neural dysfunction and metabolic imbalances in diabetic rats: prevention by acetyl-L-carnitine. Diabetes 43(12):1469–1477

Jenner P (1994) Oxidative damage in neurodegenerative disease. Lancet 344(8925):796–798. https://doi.org/10.1016/S0140-6736(94)92347-7

Jiang C, Wan X, He Y, Pan T, Jankovic J, Le W (2005) Age-dependent dopaminergic dysfunction in Nurr1 knockout mice. Exp Neurol 191(1):154–162

Johnson WM, Wilson-Delfosse AL, Mieyal JJ (2012) Dysregulation of glutathione homeostasis in neurodegenerative diseases. Forum Nutr 4(10):1399–1440

Junxian Y, Zhang Y, Sun S, Shen J, Qiu J, Yin X, Honglin Yin SJ (2006) Inhibitory effects of astragaloside IV on diabetic peripheral neuropathy in rats. Can J Physiol Pharmacol 84:579–587

Kamboj SS, Chopra K (2008) Neuroprotective effect of *N*-acetylcysteine in the development of diabetic encephalopathy in streptozotocin-induced diabetes. Metab Brain Dis 23(4):427–443. https://doi.org/10.1007/s11011-008-9104-7

Kamboj SS, Vasishta RK, Sandhir R (2010) *N*-acetylcysteine inhibits hyperglycemia-induced oxidative stress and apoptosis markers in diabetic neuropathy. J Neurochem 112(1):77–91

Kerksick C, Willoughby D (2005) The antioxidant role of glutathione and *N*-acetyl-cysteine supplements and exercise-induced oxidative stress. J Int Soc Sports Nutr 2(2):38

Küther G, Struppler A (1987) Therapeutic trial with *N*-acetylcysteine in amyotrophic lateral sclerosis. Adv Exp Med Biol 209:281–284

La Fontaine MA, Geddes JW, Banks A, Allan Butterfield D (2000) Effect of exogenous and endogenous antioxidants on 3-nitropropionic acid-induced in vivo oxidative stress and striatal lesions: insights into Huntington's disease. J Neurochem 75(4):1709–1715

Lehmann D, Karussis D, Misrachi-Koll R, Shezen E, Ovadia H, Abramsky O (1994) Oral administration of the oxidant scavenger *N*-acetyl-L-cysteine inhibits acute experimental autoimmune encephalomyelitis. J Neuroimmunol 50:35–42

Li I, Xu L (2016) *N*-acetyl-cysteine attenuates neuropathic pain by suppressing matrix metalloproteinases. Pain 157(8):1711–1723. https://doi.org/10.1097/j.pain.0000000000000575

Lin P-C, Lee M-Y, Wang W-S, Yen C-C, Chao T-C, Hsiao L-T et al (2006) *N*-acetylcysteine has neuroprotective effects against oxaliplatin-based adjuvant chemotherapy in colon cancer patients: preliminary data. Support Care Cancer 14(5):484–487

Louwerse ES, Weverling GJ, Bossuyt PM, Meyjes FE, de Jong JM (1995) Randomized, double-blind, controlled trial of acetylcysteine in amyotrophic lateral sclerosis. Arch Neurol 52(6):559–564

Martínez M, Martínez N, Hernández AI, Ferrándiz ML (1999) Hypothesis: can *N*-acetylcysteine be beneficial in Parkinson's disease? Life Sci 64(15):1253–1257

Mayer M, Noble M (1994) *N*-acetyl-L-cysteine is a pluripotent protector against cell death and enhancer of trophic factor-mediated cell survival in vitro. Proc Natl Acad Sci U S A 91(16):7496–7500

McCaddon A, Davies G (2005) Co-administration of *N*-acetylcysteine, vitamin B12 and folate in cognitively impaired hyperhomocysteinaemic patients. Int J Geriatr Psychiatry 20:99–1000

Merrill JE, Benveniste EN (1996) Cytokines in inflammatory brain lesions: helpful and harmful. Trends Neurosci 19(8):331–338

Morganti-Kossmann MC, Rancan M, Otto VI, Stahel PF, Kossmann T (2001) Role of cerebral inflammation after traumatic brain injury: a revisited concept. Shock 16:165–177

Munakata A, Ohkuma H, Nakano T, Shimamura N, Asano K, Naraoka M (2009) Effect of a free radical scavenger, edaravone, in the treatment of patients with aneurysmal subarachnoid hemorrhage. Neurosurgery 64(3):423–428

Nagamatsu M, Nickander KK, Schmelzer JD, Raya A, Wittrock DA, Tritschler H et al (1995) Lipoic acid improves nerve blood flow, reduces oxidative stress, and improves distal nerve conduction in experimental diabetic neuropathy. Diabetes Care 18(8):1160–1167

Ortolani O, Conti A, De Gaudio AR, Moraldi E, Cantini Q, Novelli G (2000) The effect of glutathione and *N*-acetylcysteine on lipoperoxidative damage in patients with early septic shock. Am J Respir Crit Care Med 161(6):1907–1911

Pan J, Xiao Q, Sheng CY, Hong Z, Yang HQ, Wang G et al (2009) Blockade of the translocation and activation of c-Jun *N*-terminal kinase 3 (JNK3) attenuates dopaminergic neuronal damage in mouse model of Parkinson's disease. Neurochem Int 54(7):418–425

Pappert EJ, Tangney CC, Goetz CG, Ling ZD, Lipton JW, Stebbins GT et al (1996) Alpha-tocopherol in the ventricular cerebrospinal fluid of Parkinson's disease patients: dose-response study and correlations with plasma levels. Neurology 47(4):1037–1042

Ratan RR, Murphy TH, Baraban JM (1994) Oxidative stress induces apoptosis in embryonic cortical neurons. J Neurochem 62(1):376–379

Reilly DK, Hershey L, Rivera-Calimlim L, Shoulson I (1983) On-off effects in Parkinson's disease: a controlled investigation of ascorbic acid therapy. Adv Neurol 37:51–60

Remington R, Chan A, Paskavitz J, Shea TB (2009) Efficacy of a vitamin/nutriceutical formulation for moderate-stage to later-stage Alzheimer's disease: a placebo-controlled pilot study. Am J Alzheimers Dis Other Demen 24(1):27–33

Remington R, Bechtel C, Larsen D, Samar A, Doshanjh L, Fishman P et al (2015) A phase II randomized clinical trial of a nutritional formulation for cognition and mood in Alzheimer's disease. J Alzheimers Dis 45(2):395–405

Rosen DR, Siddique T, Patterson D, Figlewicz DA, Sapp P, Hentati A et al (1993) Mutations in Cu/Zn superoxide dismutase gene are associated with familial amyotrophic lateral sclerosis. Nature 362:59–62

Rothstein JD, Bristol LA, Hosler B, Brown RH, Kuncl RW (1994) Chronic inhibition of superoxide dismutase produces apoptotic death of spinal neurons. Proc Natl Acad Sci U S A 91(10):4155–4159

Saito I, Asano T, Sano K, Takakura K, Abe H, Yoshimoto T et al (1998) Neuroprotective effect of an antioxidant, ebselen, in patients with delayed neurological deficits after aneurysmal subarachnoid hemorrhage. Neurosurgery 42(2):269–278

Sandhir R, Sood A, Mehrotra AKS (2012) *N*-acetylcysteine reverses mitochondrial dysfunctions and behavioral abnormalities in 3-nitropropionic acid-induced Huntington's disease. Neurodegener Dis 9(3):145–157

Schapira a H, Cooper JM, Dexter D, Clark JB, Jenner P, Marsden CD (1990) Mitochondrial complex I deficiency in Parkinson's disease. J Neurochem 54(3):823–827

Schipper HM, Arnold D, Grand'Maison F, Melmed C, Moore F, Levental M et al (2015) Tolerability and safety of combined glatiramer acetate and *N*-acetylcysteine in relapsing-remitting multiple sclerosis. Clin Neuropharmacol 38(4):127–131

Selwa LM (1999) *N*-acetylcysteine therapy for Unverricht-Lundborg disease. Neurology 52(2):426–426

Sen O, Caner H, Aydin MV, Ozen O, Atalay B, Altinors N et al (2006) The effect of mexiletine on the level of lipid peroxidation and apoptosis of endothelium following experimental subarachnoid hemorrhage. Neurol Res 28(8):859–863

Sharief MK, Hentges R (1991) Association between tumor necrosis factor-alpha and disease progression in patients with multiple sclerosis. N Engl J Med 325:467–472

Shelton RJ, Velavan P, Nikitin NP, Coletta AP, Clark AL, Rigby AS et al (2005) Clinical trials update from the American Heart Association meeting: ACORN-CSD, primary care trial of chronic disease management, PEACE, CREATE, SHIELD, A-HeFT, GEMINI, vitamin E meta-analysis, ESCAPE, CARP, and SCD-HeFT cost-effectiveness study. Eur J Heart Fail 7(1):127–135

Sian J, Dexter DT, Lees a J, Daniel S, Agid Y, Javoy-Agid F et al (1994) Alterations in glutathione levels in Parkinson's disease and other neurodegenerative disorders affecting basal ganglia. Ann Neurol 36(3):348–355

Sima AA, Zhang W, Xu G, Sugimoto K, Guberski D, Yorek MA (2000) A comparison of diabetic polyneuropathy in type II diabetic BBZDR/Wor rats and in type I diabetic BB/Wor rats. Diabetologia 43(6):786–793

Stevens MJ, Obrosova I, Cao X, Van Huysen C, Greene DA (2000) Effects of DL-alpha-lipoic acid on peripheral nerve conduction, blood flow, energy metabolism, and oxidative stress in experimental diabetic neuropathy. Diabetes 49(6):1006–1015

Tchantchou F, Graves M, Rogers E, Ortiz D, Shea TB (2005) N-acteyl cysteine alleviates oxidative damage to central nervous system of ApoE-deficient mice following folate and vitamin E-deficiency. J Alzheimers Dis 7(2):135–180

Tucker S, Ahl M, Bush A, Westaway D, Huang X, Rogers JT (2005) Pilot study of the reducing effect on amyloidosis in vivo by three FDA pre-approved drugs via the Alzheimer's APP 5′ untranslated region. Curr Alzheimer Res 2(2):249–254

Tuite P, Coles L (2016) Repeated-dose oral N-acetylcysteine for the treatment of Parkinson's disease. https://clinicaltrials.gov/ct2/show/NCT02212678?te

Vyth A, Timmer JG, Bossuyt PM, Louwerse ES, de Jong JM (1996) Survival in patients with amyotrophic lateral sclerosis, treated with an array of antioxidants. J Neurol Sci 139(Suppl):99–103

Wernerman J, Luo JL, Hammarqvist F (1999) Glutathione status in critically-ill patients: possibility of modulation by antioxidants. Proc Nutr Soc 58(3):677–680

Wilder, B.J, Hurd, R.W., Franzcek, S.C., Helveston, W.R., Uthman, B.M. (1995). Treatment of neurodegenerative disease with N-Acetylcysteine. FIRST ANNUAL HEALTH SCIENCE CENTER RESEARCH WEEK, Gainesville, FL. October 16–20

Woods CG, Taylor AM (1992) Ataxia telangiectasia in the British Isles: the clinical and laboratory features of 70 affected individuals. Q J Med 82(298):169–179

Xiong Y, Peterson PL, Lee CP (1999) Effect of N-acetylcysteine on mitochondrial function following traumatic brain injury in rats. J Neurotrauma 16(11):1067–1082

Yan CY, Greene L (1998) Prevention of PC12 cell death by N-acetylcysteine requires activation of the Ras pathway. J Neurosci 18(11):4042–4049

Yu Y-M, Ryan CM, Fei Z-W, Lu X-M, Castillo L, Schultz JT et al (2002) Plasma L-5-oxoproline kinetics and whole blood glutathione synthesis rates in severely burned adult humans. Am J Physiol Endocrinol Metab 282(2):E247–E258

Application of N-Acetylcysteine in Psychiatric Disorders

12

John Slattery and Richard Eugene Frye

12.1 Introduction

The usage of N-Acetylcysteine (NAC) in psychiatry has gained increased attention over the past decade due to the potential roles of NAC in targeting various physiological systems believe to be disrupted in psychiatric disorders such as glutathione, redox, mitochondrial, glutamate, dopamine, apoptosis, inflammation, and neural plasticity as well as the enteric microbiome (Deepmala et al. 2015; Dean et al. 2011; Samuni et al. 2013; Erny et al. 2015; Dinan and Cryan 2017). Given the safety, tolerability, and broad mechanisms of action targeting putative and associated pathophysiological systems that have been implicated across various psychiatric diseases (see Table 12.1), NAC has been suggested to be a therapy that could potentially ameliorate many psychiatric disease symptoms (Bonvicini et al. 2017; Dimatelis et al. 2015; Verma et al. 2016; Carlsson 2001; Frye et al. 2016a; Rose et al. 2012, 2014; James et al. 2008; Canitano and Pallagrosi 2017; Hardan et al. 2012; Rossignol and Frye 2012a; Mocelin et al. 2015; Kunz et al. 2008; Tuncel et al. 2015; Cikankova et al. 2016; Kim and Andreazza 2012; Dean et al. 2011; Dinan 2009; Brewer and Potenza 2008; Fontenelle et al. 2011; Paydary et al. 2016; Bergman and Ben-Shachar 2016; Morris and Berk 2015). In fact, accumulating evidence suggests that NAC may be effective in treating various psychiatric conditions. In this chapter we will provide a level of evidence for the following conditions: anxiety disorder (AX); attention deficit hyperactivity disorder (ADHD);

Electronic supplementary material The online version of this article (https://doi.org/10.1007/978-981-10-5311-5_12) contains supplementary material, which is available to authorized users.

J. Slattery
BioROSA Technologies Inc, San Francisco, CA, USA

R. E. Frye (✉)
Barrow Neurological Institute, Phoenix Children's Hospital, University of Arizona College of Medicine – Phoenix, Phoenix, AZ, USA
e-mail: rfrye@phoenixchildrens.com

© Springer Nature Singapore Pte Ltd. 2019
R. E. Frye, M. Berk (eds.), *The Therapeutic Use of N-Acetylcysteine (NAC) in Medicine*, https://doi.org/10.1007/978-981-10-5311-5_12

Table 12.1 Summary of NAC mechanisms of action across different psychiatric disorders

Psychiatric disorder	Mechanism of N-Acetylcysteine (NAC)
Anxiety (AX)	Blocks stress response by putatively altering glutamate neurotransmission in zebra fish (Mocelin et al. 2015).
Attention deficit hyperactivity disorder (ADHD)	Related to effect on dopamine projections to the prefrontal cortex and regulation of glutamate neurotransmission. Other mechanisms may be related to regulation of mitochondrial function and/or oxidative stress or a combination of all of the above factors as suggested by various researchers (Bonvicini et al. 2017; Dimatelis et al. 2015; Verma et al. 2016; Carlsson 2001)
Autism spectrum disorder (ASD)	NAC effect in ASD has been attributed to improving glutathione metabolism and modulating glutamate neurotransmission through the glutamate-cystine antiporter system. Since many children with ASD suffer from mitochondrial dysfunction, NAC may also act through supporting mitochondrial metabolism as has been shown in preclinical models (Frye et al. 2016a, b, c; Rose et al. 2012, 2014; James et al. 2008; Canitano and Pallagrosi 2017; Hardan et al. 2012; Rossignol and Frye 2012a, b)
Bipolar disorder (BD)	NAC may promote multiphasic mechanisms of action depending on whether a manic phase (i.e., antioxidant) or depressive state (i.e., anti-inflammatory) is present (Kunz et al. 2008; Tuncel et al. 2015). Markers of mitochondrial dysfunction have also been found in BD, suggesting support for mitochondrial function may be an additional mechanism of NAC (Cikankova et al. 2016). The positive effect of NAC on dopamine neurotransmission and oxidative pathology may be another mechanism of action (Kim and Andreazza 2012)
Depression (DP)	NAC may alter inflammatory mediators IL-6, IL-1β, and TNF that contribute to depressive symptomatology (Dean et al. 2011; Dinan 2009). NAC has also been suggested to alter serotonergic neurotransmission which has long been thought to be disrupted in depression and is a common target for pharmaceutical interventions
Impulse-control disorders (ICD)	NAC may positively modulate glutamate and dopamine systems which are believed to be involved in impulse-control disorders (Brewer and Potenza 2008; Fontenelle et al. 2011)
Obsessive-compulsive disorder (OCD)	NAC may modulate glutamate activity and alter dopamine release and reward-seeking behavior by altering nucleus accumbens dopamine release and glutamate activity, potentially blocking craving and compulsive behavior (Paydary et al. 2016)
Schizophrenia (SZ)	Abnormalities in mitochondrial oxidative phosphorylation have been found in schizophrenia, as well as high levels of oxidative insults and neuroinflammatory along with depressed glutathione. NAC may exert its effects on any and all of these pathological findings (Bergman and Ben-Shachar 2016; Morris and Berk 2015)

IL interleukin, *TNF* tumor necrosis factor

autism spectrum disorder (ASD); bipolar disorder (BD); depression (DP); impulse-control disorders (ICD) including onychophagia, trichotillomania, and excoriation disorder; obsessive-compulsive disorder (OCD); and schizophrenia (SZ). We also discuss the putative mechanisms of action associated with NAC usage that may be involved in response to NAC therapy. This chapter can be considered an update to the systematic review we have recently conducted, where the pathophysiological mechanisms of NAC are considered in-depth (Deepmala et al. 2015).

12.2 Method

All trial designs (both controlled and uncontrolled trials) were considered. A systematic search of PubMed, Ovid MEDLINE, PsycINFO, Google Scholar, CINAHL, Embase, Scopus, Cochrane, and ERIC databases from the inception through April 2017 uses the search terms "N-Acetylcysteine," "acetylcysteine," or "NAC" and "autism," "autistic disorder," "ASD," "Asperger's," "pervasive developmental disorder," "depressive disorder," "major depression," "bipolar disorder," "mania," "hypomania," "psychosis," "schizophrenia," "anxiety," "attention deficit hyperactivity disorder," "ADHD," "obsessive-compulsive disorder," "OCD," "trichotillomania," "nail biting," "skin picking," "impulse control disorder," "onychophagia," "skin picking," and "excoriation disorder." The references cited within the identified publications were also searched for additional studies. One reviewer (JS) screened titles and abstracts of all potentially relevant publications.

12.3 Evidence of Effectiveness of NAC in the Treatment of Psychiatric Disorders

12.3.1 Anxiety

Anxiety is a trait that is associated with many mental disorders such as depression and bipolar and eating disorders, and is also involved in many medical disorders as well. Anxiety disorders occur when excessive fear and anxiety disrupt the ability to function and are persistent lasting for over 6 months or more. Anxiety is believed to involve disruptions in the hypothalamic-pituitary-adrenal (HPA) axis signaling pathway and affects the stress response. Prolonged stress may alter epigenetic regulation (Bartlett et al. 2017) and may be associated with oxidative stress (Boldrini et al. 2017). As such, NAC has been suggested as a possible therapeutic option in anxiety-related disorders. Only a case study (Supplementary Table 12.1) has reported the use of NAC in anxiety (Strawn and Saldana 2012). Thus, the GOR is D and there are insufficient studies to make a recommendation for the use of NAC in anxiety.

12.3.2 Attention Deficit Hyperactivity Disorder (ADHD)

ADHD is one of the most prevalent neurodevelopmental disorders characterized by impulsivity, overactivity, and inattentiveness with an estimated prevalence of 5–7% in childhood (Willcutt 2012). Research suggests that ADHD arises through genetic susceptibility interacting with environmental triggers resulting in disruption of dopamine, norepinephrine, and glutamate systems in the brain (Warton et al. 2009; Perlov et al. 2007; Moore et al. 2006; Sagvolden et al. 2005; Viggiano et al. 2003). More recent studies suggest that oxidative stress and mitochondrial dysfunction may play a role in the etiology and/or pathophysiology of ADHD (Bonvicini et al. 2017; Avcil et al. 2017; Verma et al. 2016). There is only one controlled trial of NAC treatment in ADHD (Supplementary Table 12.2) in a patient population with systemic lupus erythematosus (Garcia et al. 2013). Thus, the GOR is C with no recommendations for treatment because of the lack of research and the fact that the only study published involves an atypical subset of individuals with ADHD.

12.3.3 Autism Spectrum Disorder (ASD)

ASD is a behaviorally defined disorders characterized by deficits in communication and socialization, along with the presence of restricted interests and/or repetitive behaviors (APA 2013). It is currently estimated to affect 1 in 65 children in the United States (CDC 2012). While the etiology of ASD is largely unknown, a growing body of evidence suggests that mitochondrial dysfunction (Rossignol and Frye 2012a, b, 2014; Rose et al. 2017), oxidative stress and abnormalities in redox regulation (Rossignol and Frye 2012b, 2014; Frye and James 2014), immune dysfunction and inflammation (Rossignol and Frye 2012b, 2014), environmental toxicants (Rossignol and Frye 2012b; Rossignol et al. 2014), and disruption in other metabolic processes (Frye and Rossignol 2016; Frye and Rossignol 2014) including folate (Frye et al. 2013b, 2016b, c) and cobalamin (Frye et al. 2013a) may be involved in the pathophysiology of ASD. Attention has focused on interventional strategies that can target these pathophysiological abnormalities, and some of the mechanisms of action of NAC involve the aforementioned pathways.

An overall GOR for NAC in ASD is B (Supplementary Table 12.3). This rating is based on five controlled trials with a total of 3.5 points leading to a 70% positive rating on controlled trials (Hardan et al. 2012; Ghanizadeh and Moghimi-Sarani 2013; Nikoo et al. 2015; Wink et al. 2016; Dean et al. 2017) and four positive uncontrolled trials (Ghanizadeh and Derakhshan 2012; Marler et al. 2014; Stutzman and Dopheide 2015; Celebi 2017) leading to a 100% positive rating on uncontrolled trials. This resulted in a recommendation of "mixed," although the large number of positive trials suggests this is a promising treatment.

Although the most recent controlled trials failed to show improvements on clinical endpoints, the one that measured glutathione metabolism demonstrated NAC improvement in oxidative stress (Wink et al. 2016). While Hardan et al. (2012) found NAC to be safe and effective at addressing irritability in children with ASD, other researchers have looked at NAC to try and improve social abilities in children with ASD (Dean et al. 2017; Wink et al. 2016). Irritability and aggression appear to be symptoms that have repeatedly been shown to improve in many of the controlled (Ghanizadeh and Moghimi-Sarani 2013; Hardan et al. 2012; Nikoo et al. 2015) and open-labeled (Stutzman and Dopheide 2015; Ghanizadeh and Derakhshan 2012; Marler et al. 2014) trials, suggesting that these may be key symptoms to concentration on future high-quality clinical studies. Interestingly, Two controlled study specifically looked at the ability of NAC to complement risperidone, a medication primary used to treat irritability and aggression (Nikoo et al. 2015; Ghanizadeh and Moghimi-Sarani, 2013). One of the negative controlled trials used an unusually low dose of NAC, raising the question of a significant limitation of the study (Dean et al. 2017). Overall, NAC was very well tolerated in most of the studies. The exception is the one case report with mild abdominal pain (Ghanizadeh and Derakhshan 2012) and one controlled study with severe constipation (Hardan et al. 2012). Given that children with ASD commonly have gastrointestinal symptoms (Buie et al. 2010a; Buie et al. 2010b), this may have been unrelated to the treatment.

12.3.4 Bipolar Disorder (BD)

BD, sometimes referred to as manic depression, has a lifetime prevalence of 3% in the general population (Schmitt et al. 2014; Merikangas et al. 2007). Like other psychiatric disorders, oxidative stress, mitochondrial dysfunction, and immune dysregulation have been implicated in BD (Sigitova et al. 2017; Kantrowitz and Javitt 2010; Anderson et al. 2016; de Sousa et al. 2015; Morris and Berk 2015; Callaly et al. 2015; de Sousa et al. 2014). NAC has been investigated as a possible adjunct to standard of care in BD in three high-quality DBPC studies (Berk et al. 2008b; Berk et al. 2012; Dean et al. 2012; Magalhaes et al. 2011a, b, 2012, 2013; Rapado-Castro et al. 2017; Waterdrinker et al. 2015) and one open-label study (Berk et al. 2011a) with the majority of the studies demonstrating that NAC can improve a wide range of symptoms in DB (Supplementary Table 12.4).

12.3.5 Depressive Disorder

Unfortunately few studies have examined the effect of NAC on major depression (Supplementary Table 12.5). One high-quality DBPC study demonstrated positive results on some, but not all, measures (Berk et al. 2014), and NAC has been documented to be beneficial for major depression in an open-label study (Carvalho et al. 2013). This results in a GOR of B with a mixed recommendation for treatment. Clearly more studies are needed with these promising results.

12.3.6 Impulse-Control Disorders

Several controlled and uncontrolled trials have investigated the usage of NAC in impulse-control disorders. These will be outlined below (Supplementary Table 12.6).

12.3.6.1 Nail Biting
There has been one low-quality DBPC study on the effect of NAC treatment on nail biting with positive but inconsistent results (Ghanizadeh et al. 2013) and one case

series (Berk et al. 2009) and case report (Odlaug and Grant 2007) documenting positive response to NAC for nail biting. The GOR is a C with mixed recommendations for treatment. Clearly larger controlled trials are needed to see if NAC is helpful in nail biting.

12.3.6.2 Skin Picking

One high-quality DPBC trial demonstrated significant reductions in skin picking symptoms using NAC at a starting dose of 1200 mg/d and ramping up to 3000 mg/d in a 12-week trial (Grant et al. 2016). In addition, there is a case report (Grant et al. 2012), case series (Silva-Netto et al. 2014), and open-label trial (Miller and Angulo 2014) documenting the effectiveness of NAC in skin picking. Given this evidence the GOR for skin picking is B with a yes recommendation for use given the consistently positive results. Still we believe that replication in larger controlled trials is necessary.

12.3.6.3 Trichotillomania

There is one positive high-quality DBPC study (Grant et al. 2009) as well as one low-quality negative DBPC study (Bloch et al. 2013) on the use of NAC in trichotillomania (Supplementary Table 12.6). There have also been two case reports (Taylor and Bhagwandas 2014; Pinto et al. 2017) and two case series (Rodrigues-Barata et al. 2012; Ozcan and Seckin 2016) documenting the positive effect of NAC treatment on trichotillomania. Thus, the GOR for NAC treatment in trichotillomania is a B with mixed recommendation for use of NAC to treat trichotillomania in the clinic. Larger controlled trials are needed to replicate and extend these promising findings.

12.3.7 Obsessive-Compulsive Disorder (OCD)

OCD is a debilitating disorder characterized by excessive and obtrusive thoughts and/or ritualistic behaviors (Markarian et al. 2010). Patients with OCD often have tics, anxiety, depression, and thoughts of suicidal ideation with an increased risk of suicide (APA 2013). Excessive glutamatergic activity along with altered dopamine reward system signaling is thought to play a role in the pathophysiology of OCD and may result in significant oxidative stress (Wu et al. 2012; Ting and Feng 2008; Chakrabarty et al. 2005; Paydary et al. 2016). Given the significant morbidity that OCD can cause, along with the limited treatment options, finding safe and effective treatments is vital. Due to NAC's roles in oxidative stress, glutamate and dopamine, the therapeutic benefits of NAC have been investigated in OCD. Three low-quality DPBC studies have examined the role of NAC treatment in OCD with two of the studies demonstrating positive outcomes (Afshar et al. 2012; Paydary et al. 2016) and the third DBPC trial showing positive outcomes initially with the effect diminishing later in the trial (Sarris et al. 2015; Supplementary Table 12.7). There has also been a case report (Lafleur et al. 2006) and case series (Yazici and Percinel 2015) documenting the effectiveness of NAC in OCD. The overall GOR for NAC in OCD is B due to multiple positive controlled studies with mixed recommendations for treatment.

12.3.8 Schizophrenia (SZ)

SZ, or schizophrenia spectrum disorders, refers to a group of thought disorders characterized by delusional beliefs, unclear or confused thinking, and auditory and/or visual hallucinations and generally is classified into positive and/or negative symptoms (APA 2013). Generally speaking, the positive symptoms refer to hallucinations, while negative symptoms refer to deficits in social motivation and emotional response/reactivity, anhedonia, cognitive deficits, and deficits in activities of daily living and impaired quality of life. Prevalence rates seem to affect approximately 1.1% of the US adult population (Messias et al. 2007; NIMH 2016). Emerging research is showing that oxidative stress, mitochondrial dysfunction, and immune abnormalities, along with genetic/epigenetic and environmental factors, seem to contribute to the etiopathology of SZ (Monpays et al. 2016; Morris et al. 2016; Nagano et al. 2015; Li et al. 2015; Morris and Berk 2015; Rajasekaran et al. 2015; Faizi et al. 2014; Assies et al. 2014). There has been one high-quality DBPC (Berk et al. 2008a, b) and two low-quality DBPC (Farokhnia et al. 2013; Rapado-Castro et al. 2017) studies on the use of NAC for SZ (Supplementary Table 12.8), all of them demonstrating positive results. However the most recent study examined a wide range of cognitive function but only found a significant improvement in working memory so this is considered a mixed positive result (Rapado-Castro et al. 2017). In addition, there is one case report documenting the beneficial effects of NAC on SZ (Bulut et al. 2009). The GOR for NAC in SZ is a B with mixed recommendation for treatment. Indeed, further high-quality clinical trials need to be conducted.

12.4 Summary

NAC appears to be a safe and potentially effective treatment add-on in many psychiatric disorders. The evidence for the effectiveness of NAC in psychiatric disorders is growing with many clinical trials underway (Table 12.2). Although the recommendation for the clinical use of NAC is stated as mixed for many psychiatric disorders (Table 12.3), most of the psychiatric disorders with high-quality studies did suggest effectiveness of NAC for at least some of the symptoms. Future clinical trials may better focus on the specific symptoms which NAC may address as primarily outcomes and select subpopulations which may optimally respond to NAC as well as optimizing dosing of NAC. Future trials will need to carefully consider these factors when designing and executing trials. However, for now, given the excellent safety profile for NAC in many psychiatric disorders, it may be a prime candidate for a treatment trial for individuals with psychiatric disorders where primary treatments are suboptimal.

Table 12.2 Ongoing clinical trials on N-Acetylcysteine for psychiatric disorders

Trial title	NCT no.	Trial status
N-Acetylcysteine (NAC) for pediatric obsessive-compulsive disorder	NCT01172275	The study is ongoing, but not recruiting participants
The effect of N-Acetylcysteine on cortical erosion in early stage schizophrenia (Breier-Stanley)	NCT01339858	This study is ongoing, but not recruiting participants
Treatment of cognitive and negative symptoms in schizophrenia with N-Acetylcysteine (NAC2)	NCT02505477	This study is currently recruiting participants
N-Acetylcysteine (NAC) for pediatric obsessive-compulsive disorder	NCT01172275	This study is ongoing, but not recruiting participants
A new treatment approach for major depressive disorder based upon targeting monoamine oxidase A (MAO-A)	NCT02269540	This study is currently recruiting participants
"Multimodal prevention of psychosis—a randomized trial investigating the efficacy of N-Acetylcysteine (NAC) and integrated preventive psychological intervention (IPPI) in subjects clinically at high risk for psychosis" (ESPRIT-B1)	NCT03149107	This study is not yet open for participant recruitment
A feasibility study of N-Acetylcysteine (NAC) for self-injurious behavior in children with autism spectrum disorder	NCT03008889	This study is not yet open for participant recruitment
The effect of N-Acetylcysteine (NAC) on inflammatory and oxidative stress biomarkers	NCT02420418	This study is not yet open for participant recruitment
A pilot study investigating the efficacy of minocycline and N-Acetylcysteine for bipolar depression	NCT02719392	This study is currently recruiting participants
Open-label study of N-Acetylcysteine in children and adolescents 5–17 with bipolar spectrum disorders	NCT02357290	This study is currently recruiting participants
N-Acetylcysteine supplementation in therapy refractory major depressive disorders	NCT02972398	This study is currently recruiting participants
N-Acetylcysteine in the treatment of depressive symptoms in bipolar offspring	NCT02865629	This study is currently recruiting participants
N-Acetylcysteine and aspirin as an adjunctive treatment for bipolar disorder (SMRI-bipolar)	NCT01797575	Completed. No results

Table 12.3 Overall ratings of NAC based on clinical studies presented by condition

Psychiatric conditions	Uncontrolled studies positive % (positive/ total)	Controlled studies positive % (positive/ total)	Grade of recommendation	Recommendation for treatment
Anxiety	100% (1/1)		D—SC	None
Attention deficit hyperactivity disorder		100% (1/1)	C	None
Autism	100% (4/4)	70% (3.5/5)	B	Mixed

Table 12.3 (Continued)

Psychiatric conditions	Uncontrolled studies positive % (positive/ total)	Controlled studies positive % (positive/ total)	Grade of recommendation	Recommendation for treatment
Bipolar disorder	100% (1/1)	66% (2/3)	A	Mixed
Depressive disorder	100% (1/1)	50% (0.5/1)	B	Mixed
Impulse-control disorder—overall	100% (12/12)	63% (2.5/4)	B	Mixed
Impulse control—nail biting	100% (2/2)	50% (0.5/1)	C	Mixed
Impulse control—skin picking	100% (4/4)	100% (1/1)	B	Yes
Impulse control—trichotillomania	100% (6/6)	50% (1/2)	B	Mixed
Obsessive-compulsive disorder	75% (1.5/2)	66% (2/3)	B	Mixed
Schizophrenia	100% (1/1)	83% (2.5/3)	B	Mixed

SC single case report

References

Afshar H, Roohafza H, Mohammad-Beigi H, Haghighi M, Jahangard L, Shokouh P, Sadeghi M, Hafezian H (2012) *N*-acetylcysteine add-on treatment in refractory obsessive-compulsive disorder: a randomized, double-blind, placebo-controlled trial. J Clin Psychopharmacol 32(6):797–803. https://doi.org/10.1097/JCP.0b013e318272677d

Anderson G, Jacob A, Bellivier F, Geoffroy PA (2016) Bipolar disorder: the role of the kynurenine and melatonergic pathways. Curr Pharm Des 22(8):987–1012

APA (2013) Diagnostic and statistical manual of mental disorders, 5th edn. American Psychiatric Association, Washington, DC

Assies J, Mocking RJ, Lok A, Ruhe HG, Pouwer F, Schene AH (2014) Effects of oxidative stress on fatty acid- and one-carbon-metabolism in psychiatric and cardiovascular disease comorbidity. Acta Psychiatr Scand 130(3):163–180. https://doi.org/10.1111/acps.12265

Avcil S, Uysal P, Avcil M, Alisik M, Bicer C (2017) Dynamic thiol/disulfide homeostasis in children with attention deficit hyperactivity disorder and its relation with disease subtypes. Compr Psychiatry 73:53–60. https://doi.org/10.1016/j.comppsych.2016.11.003

Bartlett AA, Singh R, Hunter RG (2017) Anxiety and epigenetics. Adv Exp Med Biol 978:145–166. https://doi.org/10.1007/978-3-319-53889-1_8

Bergman O, Ben-Shachar D (2016) Mitochondrial oxidative phosphorylation system (OXPHOS) deficits in schizophrenia: possible interactions with cellular processes. Can J Psychiatr 61(8):457–469. https://doi.org/10.1177/0706743716648290

Berk M, Copolov D, Dean O, Lu K, Jeavons S, Schapkaitz I, Anderson-Hunt M, Judd F, Katz F, Katz P, Ording-Jespersen S, Little J, Conus P, Cuenod M, Do KQ, Bush AI (2008a) *N*-acetyl cysteine as a glutathione precursor for schizophrenia–a double-blind, randomized, placebo-controlled trial. Biol Psychiatry 64(5):361–368. https://doi.org/10.1016/j.biopsych.2008.03.004

Berk M, Copolov DL, Dean O, Lu K, Jeavons S, Schapkaitz I, Anderson-Hunt M, Bush AI (2008b) *N*-acetyl cysteine for depressive symptoms in bipolar disorder–a double-blind randomized placebo-controlled trial. Biol Psychiatry 64(6):468–475. https://doi.org/10.1016/j.biopsych.2008.04.022

Berk M, Jeavons S, Dean OM, Dodd S, Moss K, Gama CS, Malhi GS (2009) Nail-biting stuff? The effect of *N*-acetyl cysteine on nail-biting. CNS Spectr 14(7):357–360

Berk M, Dean O, Cotton SM, Gama CS, Kapczinski F, Fernandes BS, Kohlmann K, Jeavons S, Hewitt K, Allwang C, Cobb H, Bush AI, Schapkaitz I, Dodd S, Malhi GS (2011a) The efficacy of *N*-acetylcysteine as an adjunctive treatment in bipolar depression: an open label trial. J Affect Disord 135(1–3):389–394. https://doi.org/10.1016/j.jad.2011.06.005

Berk M, Munib A, Dean O, Malhi GS, Kohlmann K, Schapkaitz I, Jeavons S, Katz F, Anderson-Hunt M, Conus P, Hanna B, Otmar R, Ng F, Copolov DL, Bush AI (2011b) Qualitative methods in early-phase drug trials: broadening the scope of data and methods from an RCT of *N*-acetylcysteine in schizophrenia. J Clin Psychiatry 72(7):909–913. https://doi.org/10.4088/JCP.09m05741yel

Berk M, Dean OM, Cotton SM, Gama CS, Kapczinski F, Fernandes B, Kohlmann K, Jeavons S, Hewitt K, Moss K, Allwang C, Schapkaitz I, Cobb H, Bush AI, Dodd S, Malhi GS (2012) Maintenance *N*-acetyl cysteine treatment for bipolar disorder: a double-blind randomized placebo controlled trial. BMC Med 10:91. https://doi.org/10.1186/1741-7015-10-91

Berk M, Dean OM, Cotton SM, Jeavons S, Tanious M, Kohlmann K, Hewitt K, Moss K, Allwang C, Schapkaitz I, Robbins J, Cobb H, Ng F, Dodd S, Bush AI, Malhi GS (2014) The efficacy of adjunctive *N*-acetylcysteine in major depressive disorder: a double-blind, randomized, placebo-controlled trial. J Clin Psychiatry 75(6):628–636. https://doi.org/10.4088/JCP.13m08454

Bloch MH, Panza KE, Grant JE, Pittenger C, Leckman JF (2013) *N*-Acetylcysteine in the treatment of pediatric trichotillomania: a randomized, double-blind, placebo-controlled add-on trial. J Am Acad Child Adolesc Psychiatry 52(3):231–240. https://doi.org/10.1016/j.jaac.2012.12.020

Boldrini P, Fusco A, Nicoletti F, Badiani A, Saso L (2017) Potential use of modulators of oxidative stress as add-on therapy in patients with anxiety disorders. Curr Drug Targets 18. https://doi.org/10.2174/1389450118666170425153356

Bonvicini C, Faraone SV, Scassellati C (2017) Common and specific genes and peripheral bio-markers in children and adults with attention-deficit/hyperactivity disorder. World J Biol Psychiatry:1–52. https://doi.org/10.1080/15622975.2017.1282175

Brewer JA, Potenza MN (2008) The neurobiology and genetics of impulse control disorders: relationships to drug addictions. Biochem Pharmacol 75(1):63–75. https://doi.org/10.1016/j.bcp.2007.06.043

Buie T, Campbell DB, Fuchs GJ 3rd, Furuta GT, Levy J, Vandewater J, Whitaker AH, Atkins D, Bauman ML, Beaudet AL, Carr EG, Gershon MD, Hyman SL, Jirapinyo P, Jyonouchi H, Kooros K, Kushak R, Levitt P, Levy SE, Lewis JD, Murray KF, Natowicz MR, Sabra A, Wershil BK, Weston SC, Zeltzer L, Winter H (2010a) Evaluation, diagnosis, and treatment of gastrointestinal disorders in individuals with ASDs: a consensus report. Pediatrics 125(Suppl 1):S1–S18. https://doi.org/10.1542/peds.2009-1878C

Buie T, Fuchs GJ 3rd, Furuta GT, Kooros K, Levy J, Lewis JD, Wershil BK, Winter H (2010b) Recommendations for evaluation and treatment of common gastrointestinal problems in children with ASDs. Pediatrics 125(Suppl 1):S19–S29. https://doi.org/10.1542/peds.2009-1878D

Bulut M, Savas HA, Altindag A, Virit O, Dalkilic A (2009) Beneficial effects of *N*-acetylcysteine in treatment resistant schizophrenia. World J Biol Psychiatry 10(4 Pt 2):626–628. https://doi.org/10.1080/15622970903144004

Callaly E, Walder K, Morris G, Maes M, Debnath M, Berk M (2015) Mitochondrial dysfunction in the pathophysiology of bipolar disorder: effects of pharmacotherapy. Mini Rev Med Chem 15(5):355–365

Canitano R, Pallagrosi M (2017) Autism spectrum disorders and schizophrenia spectrum disorders: excitation/inhibition imbalance and developmental trajectories. Front Psych 8:69. https://doi.org/10.3389/fpsyt.2017.00069

Carlsson ML (2001) On the role of prefrontal cortex glutamate for the antithetical phenomenology of obsessive compulsive disorder and attention deficit hyperactivity disorder. Prog Neuro-Psychopharmacol Biol Psychiatry 25(1):5–26

Carvalho AF, Macedo DS, Goulia P, Hyphantis TN (2013) *N*-acetylcysteine augmentation to tranylcypromine in treatment-resistant major depression. J Clin Psychopharmacol 33(5):719–720. https://doi.org/10.1097/JCP.0b013e31829839c6

CDC (2012) Prevalence of autism spectrum disorders—autism and developmental disabilities monitoring network, 14 Sites, United States, 2008. Morbidity and Mortality Weekly Report

Celebi F (2017) *N*-acetylcysteine may reduce repetitive behaviors in children with autism: a case series. Psychiatry Clin Psychopharmacol:1–4. https://doi.org/10.1080/24750573.2017.1309817

Chakrabarty K, Bhattacharyya S, Christopher R, Khanna S (2005) Glutamatergic dysfunction in OCD. Neuropsychopharmacology 30(9):1735–1740. https://doi.org/10.1038/sj.npp.1300733

Cikankova T, Sigitova E, Zverova M, Fisar Z, Raboch J, Hroudova J (2016) Mitochondrial dysfunctions in bipolar disorder: effect of the disease and pharmacotherapy. CNS Neurol Disord Drug Targets 16(2):176–186

de Sousa RT, Machado-Vieira R, Zarate CA Jr, Manji HK (2014) Targeting mitochondrially mediated plasticity to develop improved therapeutics for bipolar disorder. Expert Opin Ther Targets 18(10):1131–1147. https://doi.org/10.1517/14728222.2014.940893

de Sousa RT, Streck EL, Forlenza OV, Brunoni AR, Zanetti MV, Ferreira GK, Diniz BS, Portela LV, Carvalho AF, Zarate CA Jr, Gattaz WF, Machado-Vieira R (2015) Regulation of leukocyte tricarboxylic acid cycle in drug-naive bipolar disorder. Neurosci Lett 605:65–68. https://doi.org/10.1016/j.neulet.2015.08.022

Dean O, Giorlando F, Berk M (2011) *N*-acetylcysteine in psychiatry: current therapeutic evidence and potential mechanisms of action. J Psychiatry Neurosci 36(2):78–86. https://doi.org/10.1503/jpn.100057

Dean OM, Bush AI, Copolov DL, Kohlmann K, Jeavons S, Schapkaitz I, Anderson-Hunt M, Berk M (2012) Effects of *N*-acetyl cysteine on cognitive function in bipolar disorder. Psychiatry Clin Neurosci 66(6):514–517. https://doi.org/10.1111/j.1440-1819.2012.02392.x

Dean OM, Gray KM, Villagonzalo KA, Dodd S, Mohebbi M, Vick T, Tonge BJ, Berk M (2017) A randomised, double blind, placebo-controlled trial of a fixed dose of *N*-acetyl cysteine in children with autistic disorder. Aust N Z J Psychiatry 51(3):241–249. https://doi.org/10.1177/0004867416652735

Deepmala SJ, Kumar N, Delhey L, Berk M, Dean O, Spielholz C, Frye R (2015) Clinical trials of *N*-acetylcysteine in psychiatry and neurology: a systematic review. Neurosci Biobehav Rev 55:294–321. https://doi.org/10.1016/j.neubiorev.2015.04.015

Dimatelis JJ, Hsieh JH, Sterley TL, Marais L, Womersley JS, Vlok M, Russell VA (2015) Impaired energy metabolism and disturbed dopamine and glutamate signaling in the striatum and prefrontal cortex of the spontaneously hypertensive rat model of attention-deficit hyperactivity disorder. J Mol Neurosci 56(3):696–707. https://doi.org/10.1007/s12031-015-0491-z

Dinan TG (2009) Inflammatory markers in depression. Curr Opin Psychiatry 22(1):32–36. https://doi.org/10.1097/YCO.0b013e328315a561

Dinan TG, Cryan JF (2017) The microbiome-gut-brain axis in health and disease. Gastroenterol Clin N Am 46(1):77–89. https://doi.org/10.1016/j.gtc.2016.09.007

Erny D, Hrabe de Angelis AL, Jaitin D, Wieghofer P, Staszewski O, David E, Keren-Shaul H, Mahlakoiv T, Jakobshagen K, Buch T, Schwierzeck V, Utermohlen O, Chun E, Garrett WS, McCoy KD, Diefenbach A, Staeheli P, Stecher B, Amit I, Prinz M (2015) Host microbiota constantly control maturation and function of microglia in the CNS. Nat Neurosci 18(7):965–977. https://doi.org/10.1038/nn.4030

Faizi M, Salimi A, Rasoulzadeh M, Naserzadeh P, Pourahmad J (2014) Schizophrenia induces oxidative stress and cytochrome C release in isolated rat brain mitochondria: a possible pathway for induction of apoptosis and neurodegeneration. Iran J Pharm Res 13(Suppl):93–100

Farokhnia M, Azarkolah A, Adinehfar F, Khodaie-Ardakani MR, Hosseini SM, Yekehtaz H, Tabrizi M, Rezaei F, Salehi B, Sadeghi SM, Moghadam M, Gharibi F, Mirshafiee O, Akhondzadeh S (2013) *N*-acetylcysteine as an adjunct to risperidone for treatment of negative symptoms in patients with chronic schizophrenia: a randomized, double-blind, placebo-controlled study. Clin Neuropharmacol 36(6):185–192. https://doi.org/10.1097/wnf.0000000000000001

Fontenelle LF, Oostermeijer S, Harrison BJ, Pantelis C, Yucel M (2011) Obsessive-compulsive disorder, impulse control disorders and drug addiction: common features and potential treatments. Drugs 71(7):827–840. https://doi.org/10.2165/11591790-000000000-00000

Frye RE, James SJ (2014) Metabolic pathology of autism in relation to redox metabolism. Biomark Med 8(3):321–330. https://doi.org/10.2217/bmm.13.158

Frye RE, Rossignol DA (2014) Treatments for biomedical abnormalities associated with autism spectrum disorder. Front Pediatry 2:66. https://doi.org/10.3389/fped.2014.00066

Frye RE, Rossignol DA (2016) Identification and treatment of pathophysiological comorbidities of autism spectrum disorder to achieve optimal outcomes. Clin Med Insights Pediatr 10:43–56. https://doi.org/10.4137/CMPed.S38337

Frye RE, Melnyk S, Fuchs G, Reid T, Jernigan S, Pavliv O, Hubanks A, Gaylor DW, Walters L, James SJ (2013a) Effectiveness of methylcobalamin and folinic acid treatment on adaptive behavior in children with autistic disorder is related to glutathione redox status. Autism Res Treat 2013:609705. https://doi.org/10.1155/2013/609705

Frye RE, Sequeira JM, Quadros EV, James SJ, Rossignol DA (2013b) Cerebral folate receptor autoantibodies in autism spectrum disorder. Mol Psychiatry 18(3):369–381. https://doi.org/10.1038/mp.2011.175

Frye RE, Casanova MF, Fatemi SH, Folsom TD, Reutiman TJ, Brown GL, Edelson SM, Slattery JC, Adams JB (2016a) Neuropathological mechanisms of seizures in autism spectrum disorder. Front Neurosci 10:192. https://doi.org/10.3389/fnins.2016.00192

Frye RE, Delhey L, Slattery J, Tippett M, Wynne R, Rose S, Kahler SG, Bennuri SC, Melnyk S, Sequeira JM, Quadros E (2016b) Blocking and binding folate receptor alpha autoantibodies identify novel autism spectrum disorder subgroups. Front Neurosci 10:80. https://doi.org/10.3389/fnins.2016.00080

Frye RE, Slattery J, Delhey L, Furgerson B, Strickland T, Tippett M, Sailey A, Wynne R, Rose S, Melnyk S, Jill James S, Sequeira JM, Quadros EV (2016c) Folinic acid improves verbal communication in children with autism and language impairment: a randomized double-blind placebo-controlled trial. Mol Psychiatry 23(2):247–256. https://doi.org/10.1038/mp.2016.168

Garcia RJ, Francis L, Dawood M, Lai ZW, Faraone SV, Perl A (2013) Attention deficit and hyperactivity disorder scores are elevated and respond to *N*-acetylcysteine treatment in patients with systemic lupus erythematosus. Arthritis Rheum 65(5):1313–1318. https://doi.org/10.1002/art.37893

Ghanizadeh A, Derakhshan N (2012) *N*-acetylcysteine for treatment of autism, a case report. J Res Med Sci 17(10):985–987

Ghanizadeh A, Moghimi-Sarani E (2013) A randomized double blind placebo controlled clinical trial of *N*-Acetylcysteine added to risperidone for treating autistic disorders. BMC Psychiatry 13:196. https://doi.org/10.1186/1471-244x-13-196

Ghanizadeh A, Derakhshan N, Berk M (2013) *N*-acetylcysteine versus placebo for treating nail biting, a double blind randomized placebo controlled clinical trial. Antiinflamm Antiallergy Agents Med Chem 12(3):223–228

Grant JE, Odlaug BL, Kim SW (2009) *N*-acetylcysteine, a glutamate modulator, in the treatment of trichotillomania: a double-blind, placebo-controlled study. Arch Gen Psychiatry 66(7):756–763. https://doi.org/10.1001/archgenpsychiatry.2009.60

Grant JE, Odlaug BL, Chamberlain SR, Keuthen NJ, Lochner C, Stein DJ (2012) Skin picking disorder. Am J Psychiatry 169(11):1143–1149. https://doi.org/10.1176/appi.ajp.2012.12040508

Grant JE, Chamberlain SR, Redden SA, Leppink EW, Odlaug BL, Kim SW (2016) *N*-acetylcysteine in the treatment of excoriation disorder: a randomized clinical trial. JAMA Psychiat 73(5):490–496. https://doi.org/10.1001/jamapsychiatry.2016.0060

Hardan AY, Fung LK, Libove RA, Obukhanych TV, Nair S, Herzenberg LA, Frazier TW, Tirouvanziam R (2012) A randomized controlled pilot trial of oral *N*-acetylcysteine in children with autism. Biol Psychiatry 71(11):956–961. https://doi.org/10.1016/j.biopsych.2012.01.014

James SJ, Melnyk S, Jernigan S, Hubanks A, Rose S, Gaylor DW (2008) Abnormal transmethylation/transsulfuration metabolism and DNA hypomethylation among parents of children with autism. J Autism Dev Disord 38(10):1976. https://doi.org/10.1007/s10803-008-0614-2

Kantrowitz JT, Javitt DC (2010) *N*-methyl-d-aspartate (NMDA) receptor dysfunction or dysregulation: the final common pathway on the road to schizophrenia? Brain Res Bull 83(3–4):108–121. https://doi.org/10.1016/j.brainresbull.2010.04.006

Kim HK, Andreazza AC (2012) The relationship between oxidative stress and post-translational modification of the dopamine transporter in bipolar disorder. Expert Rev Neurother 12(7):849–859. https://doi.org/10.1586/ern.12.64

Kunz M, Gama CS, Andreazza AC, Salvador M, Cereser KM, Gomes FA, Belmonte-de-Abreu PS, Berk M, Kapczinski F (2008) Elevated serum superoxide dismutase and thiobarbituric acid reactive substances in different phases of bipolar disorder and in schizophrenia. Prog Neuro-Psychopharmacol Biol Psychiatry 32(7):1677–1681. https://doi.org/10.1016/j.pnpbp.2008.07.001

Lafleur DL, Pittenger C, Kelmendi B, Gardner T, Wasylink S, Malison RT, Sanacora G, Krystal JH, Coric V (2006) *N*-acetylcysteine augmentation in serotonin reuptake inhibitor refractory obsessive-compulsive disorder. Psychopharmacology 184(2):254–256. https://doi.org/10.1007/s00213-005-0246-6

Li X, Zhang W, Tang J, Tan L, Luo XJ, Chen X, Yao YG (2015) Do nuclear-encoded core subunits of mitochondrial complex I confer genetic susceptibility to schizophrenia in Han Chinese populations? Sci Rep 5:11076. https://doi.org/10.1038/srep11076

Magalhaes PV, Dean OM, Bush AI, Copolov DL, Malhi GS, Kohlmann K, Jeavons S, Schapkaitz I, Anderson-Hunt M, Berk M (2011a) *N*-acetyl cysteine add-on treatment for bipolar II disorder: a subgroup analysis of a randomized placebo-controlled trial. J Affect Disord 129(1–3):317–320. https://doi.org/10.1016/j.jad.2010.08.001

Magalhaes PV, Dean OM, Bush AI, Copolov DL, Malhi GS, Kohlmann K, Jeavons S, Schapkaitz I, Anderson-Hunt M, Berk M (2011b) *N*-acetylcysteine for major depressive episodes in bipolar disorder. Rev Bras Psiquiatr 33(4):374–378

Magalhaes PV, Dean OM, Bush AI, Copolov DL, Weisinger D, Malhi GS, Kohlmann K, Jeavons S, Schapkaitz I, Anderson-Hunt M, Berk M (2012) Systemic illness moderates the impact of *N*-acetyl cysteine in bipolar disorder. Prog Neuro-Psychopharmacol Biol Psychiatry 37(1):132–135. https://doi.org/10.1016/j.pnpbp.2011.11.011

Magalhaes PV, Dean OM, Bush AI, Copolov DL, Malhi GS, Kohlmann K, Jeavons S, Schapkaitz I, Anderson-Hunt M, Berk M (2013) A preliminary investigation on the efficacy of *N*-acetyl cysteine for mania or hypomania. Aust N Z J Psychiatry 47(6):564–568. https://doi.org/10.1177/0004867413481631

Markarian Y, Larson MJ, Aldea MA, Baldwin SA, Good D, Berkeljon A, Murphy TK, Storch EA, McKay D (2010) Multiple pathways to functional impairment in obsessive-compulsive disorder. Clin Psychol Rev 30(1):78–88. https://doi.org/10.1016/j.cpr.2009.09.005

Marler S, Sanders KB, Veenstra-VanderWeele J (2014) *N*-acetylcysteine as treatment for self-injurious behavior in a child with autism. J Child Adolesc Psychopharmacol 24(4):231–234. https://doi.org/10.1089/cap.2013.0137

Merikangas KR, Akiskal HS, Angst J, Greenberg PE, Hirschfeld RM, Petukhova M, Kessler RC (2007) Lifetime and 12-month prevalence of bipolar spectrum disorder in the National Comorbidity Survey replication. Arch Gen Psychiatry 64(5):543–552. https://doi.org/10.1001/archpsyc.64.5.543

Messias E, Chen CY, Eaton WW (2007) Epidemiology of schizophrenia: review of findings and myths. Psychiatr Clin North Am 30(3):323–338

Miller JL, Angulo M (2014) An open-label pilot study of *N*-acetylcysteine for skin-picking in Prader-Willi syndrome. Am J Med Genet A 164a(2):421–424. https://doi.org/10.1002/ajmg.a.36306

Mocelin R, Herrmann AP, Marcon M, Rambo CL, Rohden A, Bevilaqua F, de Abreu MS, Zanatta L, Elisabetsky E, Barcellos LJ, Lara DR, Piato AL (2015) N-acetylcysteine prevents stress-induced anxiety behavior in zebrafish. Pharmacol Biochem Behav 139 Pt B:121–126. https://doi.org/10.1016/j.pbb.2015.08.006

Monpays C, Deslauriers J, Sarret P, Grignon S (2016) Mitochondrial dysfunction in schizophrenia: determination of mitochondrial respiratory activity in a two-hit mouse model. J Mol Neurosci 59(4):440–451. https://doi.org/10.1007/s12031-016-0746-3

Moore CM, Biederman J, Wozniak J, Mick E, Aleardi M, Wardrop M, Dougherty M, Harpold T, Hammerness P, Randall E, Renshaw PF (2006) Differences in brain chemistry in children and adolescents with attention deficit hyperactivity disorder with and without comorbid bipolar disorder: a proton magnetic resonance spectroscopy study. Am J Psychiatry 163(2):316–318. https://doi.org/10.1176/appi.ajp.163.2.316

Morris G, Berk M (2015) The many roads to mitochondrial dysfunction in neuroimmune and neuropsychiatric disorders. BMC Med 13:68. https://doi.org/10.1186/s12916-015-0310-y

Morris G, Carvalho AF, Anderson G, Galecki P, Maes M (2016) The many neuroprogressive actions of tryptophan catabolites (TRYCATs) that may be associated with the pathophysiology of neuro-immune disorders. Curr Pharm Des 22(8):963–977

Nagano T, Mizuno M, Morita K, Nawa H (2015) Pathological implications of oxidative stress in patients and animal models with schizophrenia: the role of epidermal growth factor receptor signaling. Curr Top Behav Neurosci 29:429–446. https://doi.org/10.1007/7854_2015_399

Nikoo M, Radnia H, Farokhnia M, Mohammadi MR, Akhondzadeh S (2015) N-acetylcysteine as an adjunctive therapy to risperidone for treatment of irritability in autism: a randomized, double-blind, placebo-controlled clinical trial of efficacy and safety. Clin Neuropharmacol 38(1):11–17. https://doi.org/10.1097/wnf.0000000000000063

NIMH (2016) Schizophrenia

Odlaug BL, Grant JE (2007) N-acetyl cysteine in the treatment of grooming disorders. J Clin Psychopharmacol 27(2):227–229. https://doi.org/10.1097/01.jcp.0000264976.86990.00

Ozcan D, Seckin D (2016) N-Acetylcysteine in the treatment of trichotillomania: remarkable results in two patients. J Eur Acad Dermatol Venereol 30(9):1606–1608. https://doi.org/10.1111/jdv.13690

Paydary K, Akamaloo A, Ahmadipour A, Pishgar F, Emamzadehfard S, Akhondzadeh S (2016) N-acetylcysteine augmentation therapy for moderate-to-severe obsessive-compulsive disorder: randomized, double-blind, placebo-controlled trial. J Clin Pharm Ther 41(2):214–219. https://doi.org/10.1111/jcpt.12370

Perlov E, Philipsen A, Hesslinger B, Buechert M, Ahrendts J, Feige B, Bubl E, Hennig J, Ebert D, Tebartz van Elst L (2007) Reduced cingulate glutamate/glutamine-to-creatine ratios in adult patients with attention deficit/hyperactivity disorder–a magnet resonance spectroscopy study. J Psychiatr Res 41(11):934–941. https://doi.org/10.1016/j.jpsychires.2006.12.007

Pinto AC, Andrade TC, Brito FF, Silva GV, Cavalcante ML, Martelli AC (2017) Trichotillomania: a case report with clinical and dermatoscopic differential diagnosis with alopecia areata. An Bras Dermatol 92(1):118–120. https://doi.org/10.1590/abd1806-4841.20175136

Rajasekaran A, Venkatasubramanian G, Berk M, Debnath M (2015) Mitochondrial dysfunction in schizophrenia: pathways, mechanisms and implications. Neurosci Biobehav Rev 48:10–21. https://doi.org/10.1016/j.neubiorev.2014.11.005

Rapado-Castro M, Dodd S, Bush AI, Malhi GS, Skvarc DR, On ZX, Berk M, Dean OM (2017) Cognitive effects of adjunctive N-acetyl cysteine in psychosis. Psychol Med 47(5):866–876. https://doi.org/10.1017/s0033291716002932

Rodrigues-Barata AR, Tosti A, Rodriguez-Pichardo A, Camacho-Martinez F (2012) N-acetylcysteine in the treatment of trichotillomania. Int J Trichol 4(3):176–178. https://doi.org/10.4103/0974-7753.100090

Rose S, Melnyk S, Pavliv O, Bai S, Nick TG, Frye RE, James SJ (2012) Evidence of oxidative damage and inflammation associated with low glutathione redox status in the autism brain. Transl Psychiatry 2:e134. https://doi.org/10.1038/tp.2012.61

Rose S, Frye RE, Slattery J, Wynne R, Tippett M, Melnyk S, James SJ (2014) Oxidative stress induces mitochondrial dysfunction in a subset of autistic lymphoblastoid cell lines. Transl Psychiatry 4:e377. https://doi.org/10.1038/tp.2014.15

Rose S, Bennuri SC, Wynne R, Melnyk S, James SJ, Frye RE (2017) Mitochondrial and redox abnormalities in autism lymphoblastoid cells: a sibling control study. FASEB J 31(3):904–909. https://doi.org/10.1096/fj.201601004R

Rossignol DA, Frye RE (2012a) Mitochondrial dysfunction in autism spectrum disorders: a systematic review and meta-analysis. Mol Psychiatry 17(3):290–314. https://doi.org/10.1038/mp.2010.136

Rossignol DA, Frye RE (2012b) A review of research trends in physiological abnormalities in autism spectrum disorders: immune dysregulation, inflammation, oxidative stress, mitochondrial dysfunction and environmental toxicant exposures. Mol Psychiatry 17(4):389–401. https://doi.org/10.1038/mp.2011.165

Rossignol DA, Frye RE (2014) Evidence linking oxidative stress, mitochondrial dysfunction, and inflammation in the brain of individuals with autism. Front Physiol 5:150. https://doi.org/10.3389/fphys.2014.00150

Rossignol DA, Genuis SJ, Frye RE (2014) Environmental toxicants and autism spectrum disorders: a systematic review. Transl Psychiatry 4:e360. https://doi.org/10.1038/tp.2014.4

Sagvolden T, Johansen EB, Aase H, Russell VA (2005) A dynamic developmental theory of attention-deficit/hyperactivity disorder (ADHD) predominantly hyperactive/impulsive and combined subtypes. Behav Brain Sci 28(3):397–419. https://doi.org/10.1017/s0140525x05000075

Samuni Y, Goldstein S, Dean OM, Berk M (2013) The chemistry and biological activities of N-acetylcysteine. Biochim Biophys Acta 1830(8):4117–4129. https://doi.org/10.1016/j.bbagen.2013.04.016

Sarris J, Oliver G, Camfield DA, Dean OM, Dowling N, Smith DJ, Murphy J, Menon R, Berk M, Blair-West S, Ng CH (2015) N-acetyl cysteine (NAC) in the treatment of obsessive-compulsive disorder: a 16-week, double-blind, randomised, placebo-controlled study. CNS Drugs 29(9):801–809. https://doi.org/10.1007/s40263-015-0272-9

Schmitt A, Malchow B, Hasan A, Falkai P (2014) The impact of environmental factors in severe psychiatric disorders. Front Neurosci 8:19

Sigitova E, Fisar Z, Hroudova J, Cikankova T, Raboch J (2017) Biological hypotheses and biomarkers of bipolar disorder. Psychiatry Clin Neurosci 71(2):77–103. https://doi.org/10.1111/pcn.12476

Silva-Netto R, Jesus G, Nogueira M, Tavares H (2014) N-acetylcysteine in the treatment of skin-picking disorder. Rev Bras Psiquiatr 36(1):101. https://doi.org/10.1590/1516-4446-2013-1154

Strawn JR, Saldana SN (2012) Treatment with adjunctive N-acetylcysteine in an adolescent with selective serotonin reuptake inhibitor-resistant anxiety. J Child Adolesc Psychopharmacol 22(6):472–473. https://doi.org/10.1089/cap.2012.0066

Stutzman D, Dopheide J (2015) Acetylcysteine for treatment of autism spectrum disorder symptoms. Am J Health Syst Pharm 72(22):1956–1959. https://doi.org/10.2146/ajhp150072

Taylor M, Bhagwandas K (2014) N-acetylcysteine in trichotillomania: a panacea for compulsive skin disorders? Br J Dermatol 171(5):1253–1255. https://doi.org/10.1111/bjd.13080

Ting JT, Feng G (2008) Glutamatergic synaptic dysfunction and obsessive-compulsive disorder. Curr Chem Genomics 2:62–75. https://doi.org/10.2174/1875397300802010062

Tuncel OK, Sarisoy G, Bilgici B, Pazvantoglu O, Cetin E, Unverdi E, Avci B, Boke O (2015) Oxidative stress in bipolar and schizophrenia patients. Psychiatry Res 228(3):688–694. https://doi.org/10.1016/j.psychres.2015.04.046

Verma P, Singh A, Nthenge-Ngumbau DN, Rajamma U, Sinha S, Mukhopadhyay K, Mohanakumar KP (2016) Attention deficit-hyperactivity disorder suffers from mitochondrial dysfunction. BBA Clin 6:153–158. https://doi.org/10.1016/j.bbacli.2016.10.003

Viggiano D, Vallone D, Ruocco LA, Sadile AG (2003) Behavioural, pharmacological, morpho-functional molecular studies reveal a hyperfunctioning mesocortical dopamine system in an animal model of attention deficit and hyperactivity disorder. Neurosci Biobehav Rev 27(7):683–689

Warton FL, Howells FM, Russell VA (2009) Increased glutamate-stimulated release of dopamine in substantia nigra of a rat model for attention-deficit/hyperactivity disorder--lack of effect of methylphenidate. Metab Brain Dis 24(4):599–613. https://doi.org/10.1007/s11011-009-9166-1

Waterdrinker A, Berk M, Venugopal K, Rapado-Castro M, Turner A, Dean OM (2015) Effects of N-acetyl cysteine on suicidal ideation in bipolar depression. J Clin Psychiatry 76(5):665. https://doi.org/10.4088/JCP.14l09378

Willcutt EG (2012) The prevalence of DSM-IV attention-deficit/hyperactivity disorder: a meta-analytic review. Neurotherapeutics 9(3):490–499. https://doi.org/10.1007/s13311-012-0135-8

Wink LK, Adams R, Wang Z, Klaunig JE, Plawecki MH, Posey DJ, McDougle CJ, Erickson CA (2016) A randomized placebo-controlled pilot study of N-acetylcysteine in youth with autism spectrum disorder. Mol Autism 7:26. https://doi.org/10.1186/s13229-016-0088-6

Wu K, Hanna GL, Rosenberg DR, Arnold PD (2012) The role of glutamate signaling in the pathogenesis and treatment of obsessive-compulsive disorder. Pharmacol Biochem BehavPharmacology, Biochemistry, and Behavior 100(4):726–735. https://doi.org/10.1016/j.pbb.2011.10.007

Yazici KU, Percinel I (2015) N-acetylcysteine augmentation in children and adolescents diagnosed with treatment-resistant obsessive-compulsive disorder: case series. J Clinical Psychopharmacology 35(4):486–489. https://doi.org/10.1097/jcp.0000000000000362

Clinical Treatment of Addictive Disorders with N-Acetylcysteine

Gregory Powell, Erin A. McClure, M. Foster Olive, and Cassandra D. Gipson

13.1 Introduction

Substance use disorders (SUDs) and addictive behaviors constitute a global health concern, with significant societal costs in health care, crime, and productivity. Recent estimates totaled by the United States (US) National Institute on Drug Abuse (NIDA) for the total costs of SUDs in the USA alone surpassed $700 billion (Centers for Disease Control and Prevention 2016; National Institute on Drug Abuse 2017; National Drug Intelligence Center 2011; US Department of Health and Human Services 2014). It is therefore overwhelmingly beneficial to examine the ability of pharmacotherapies to reduce the use of drugs of abuse and addictive behaviors.

13.2 N-Acetylcysteine as a Potential Treatment for Addiction

There are several advantages for the potential use of NAC to treat SUDs and addictive behaviors. NAC is cost-effective and readily available and has a favorable safety profile. NAC received approval from the Food and Drug Administration (FDA) in 1963 as a mucolytic and still is used clinically as a mucolytic agent for bronchopulmonary disorders (Grandjean et al. 2000) and in the treatment of chronic obstructive pulmonary disease (COPD) (Repine et al. 1997). It is also used as an oral or

Electronic supplementary material The online version of this article (https://doi.org/10.1007/978-981-10-5311-5_13) contains supplementary material, which is available to authorized users.

G. Powell (✉) · M. Foster Olive · C. D. Gipson
Department of Psychology, Arizona State University, Tempe, AZ, USA
e-mail: gregory.powell.1@asu.edu; gpowell6@asu.edu

E. A. McClure
Department of Psychiatry and Behavioral Sciences, Medical University of South Carolina, Charleston, SC, USA

© Springer Nature Singapore Pte Ltd. 2019
R. E. Frye, M. Berk (eds.), *The Therapeutic Use of N-Acetylcysteine (NAC) in Medicine*, https://doi.org/10.1007/978-981-10-5311-5_13

intravenous antidote to treat acetaminophen poisoning (Smilkstein et al. 1988). NAC has a long history of safe use in both adults and children and is commonly available at retail nutritional supplement stores. However, while supplies are readily available, bioavailability is low, ranging from 4% to 10% with oral dosing (Borgström et al. 1986; Olsson et al. 1988; McClure et al. 2014), and thus large doses must be taken when delivered orally.

13.3 Modulation of Glutamate Neurotransmission by N-Acetylcysteine

Preclinical and clinical works have become increasingly focused in recent years on a glutamatergic cystine prodrug, NAC, and its potential therapeutic use against addiction has been extensively reviewed (Gass and Olive 2008; Olive et al. 2012; Asevedo et al. 2014; McClure et al. 2014; Deepmala et al. 2015; Roberts-Wolfe and Kalivas 2015; Minarini et al. 2016; Sherman and McRae-Clark 2016). This chapter will provide a brief background on NAC's potential as a pharmacotherapeutic treatment and examine the clinical literature on NAC in the treatment of addiction.

NAC's hypothesized mechanism of action as an addiction pharmacotherapy is tied to the glutamate homeostasis hypothesis of addiction (Kalivas 2009), where glutamate signaling within the mesocorticolimbic reward system has been disrupted. For a detailed discussion of the glutamate neurotransmitter system and the effect of NAC on glutamate neurotransmission, see Chap. 2 "Neurotransmitter Systems: Glutamate". However, the involvement of the glutamate system in addiction will be reviewed here.

In a drug naïve state, glutamate is released by corticostriatal fibers onto medium spiny neurons of the nucleus accumbens where it binds to postsynaptic receptors (reviewed by Scofield and Kalivas (2014)). Nearby glia are responsible for absorption of glutamate surrounding the synapse, clearing excess excitatory neurotransmitter, primarily through the glutamate transporter GLT-1 (Williams et al. 2005). Glutamate is also released from glia via the cystine-glutamate exchanger system Xc- (containing the catalytic subunit xCT, a potential pharmacotherapeutic target), which transports cystine into glial cells in exchange for outward transport of glutamate (Malarkey and Parpura 2008). After outward transport, glutamate can bind to presynaptic metabotropic glutamate receptors (mGluRs) (Moussawi and Kalivas 2010). These 2/3 subunit mGluRs provide inhibitory feedback on the presynaptic terminal, limiting synaptic glutamate release.

In the dysregulated synaptic environment of the nucleus accumbens in the addicted brain, there are multitudes of drug-induced alterations that potentially influence glutamate transmission. Most notable among them are reductions in levels of GLT-1 (Knackstedt et al. 2009, 2010; Rao and Sari 2012; Gipson et al. 2013) and the catalytic subunit of Xc- (Pierce et al. 1996; Baker et al. 2003a; Berglind et al. 2009). These reductions in glial-mediated glutamate uptake lead to an increase of extrasynaptic glutamate, which activates N-methyl-D-aspartate (NMDA) receptors on postsynaptic dendritic spines resulting in an increase in relapse vulnerability

(Gipson et al. 2013, 2014; Shen et al. 2014) and decreases presynaptic inhibitory mGluR2/3 tone. Without normal inhibitory feedback, excess glutamate is released from the presynaptic terminal, further derailing normal glutamate homeostasis (Knackstedt et al. 2010).

NAC has seen significant preclinical investigation as a potential addiction pharmacotherapy based on its interaction with the Xc- system. NAC is de-acetylated to form the amino acid cysteine and then oxidized to cystine, whereupon it is transported into glia in exchange for glutamate. It is this glia-released glutamate that provides inhibitory feedback on mGluR2/3 presynaptic receptors (Kalivas et al. 2005), thereby limiting the synaptic release of glutamate into the synapse. In slice electrophysiology studies, it has been shown that introducing NAC at low concentrations reduces postsynaptic glutamatergic currents through the presynaptic mGluR2/3 mechanism. However, at higher concentrations of NAC, these same currents are potentiated through the mGluR5 pathway (Kupchik et al. 2012). In addition to increased activation of xCT and GLT-1, NAC has been shown to increase expression of both transporters (Baker et al. 2003b), helping to restore glutamatergic homeostasis.

13.4 Methods

Exhaustive online literature searches of broad search terms include "clinical," "addiction," or specific substance use disorder—"cocaine," "cannabis," "marijuana," "methamphetamine," "nicotine," "tobacco," and "gambling." Where possible, filters were set on the search to limit to studies in humans and only clinical trials. We also searched the references cited in the identified publications for additional studies. One reviewer screened titles and abstracts of all potentially relevant publications.

13.5 Treatment Studies of Addiction with N-Acetylcysteine

This section will review the clinical treatment studies of addiction to cannabis, cocaine, methamphetamine, nicotine, and gambling disorder using NAC (Table 13.1) (See Online Tables 13.1, 13.2, 13.3, 13.4, and 13.5 for summary of studies).

13.5.1 NAC and Cocaine Use Disorder

Preclinical research using rodent self-administration of cocaine has yielded promising results for the ability of NAC to reduce cocaine-seeking behavior, cocaine intake, and cocaine-induced behavioral sensitization (Baker et al. 2003b; Madayag et al. 2007; Moussawi et al. 2009; Amen et al. 2011; Moussawi et al. 2011; Reichel et al. 2011; Murray et al. 2012; Reissner et al. 2015). Importantly, these preclinical works have supported the underlying hypothesis of imbalances in glutamatergic signaling within the nucleus accumbens as a driver of addictive behaviors.

The majority of clinical research thus far examining NAC's therapeutic effects on addictive behaviors has been conducted with cocaine (Online Table 13.1). Initial clinical work on the treatment of cocaine use disorder with NAC was published in 2006 and utilized a double-blind, placebo-controlled, within-subject, inpatient study design to assess the safety and tolerability of NAC in adults with cocaine dependence confirmed by the *Diagnostic and Statistical Manual of Mental Disorders*, Fourth Edition (DSM-IV; First et al. 1994). Thirteen subjects reported significant decreases in cocaine-related withdrawal symptoms, reduced cravings, and less cocaine use for 1 week following the inpatient phase and NAC dosing (LaRowe et al. 2006). A follow-up study containing a portion of LaRowe et al. (2006) subjects investigated NAC's effectiveness on cue-induced craving and demonstrated a reduced desire in adults to use cocaine when in the presence of cocaine-related cues, a reduced interest evoked by viewing cues, and a decrease in time the cues were viewed (LaRowe et al. 2007). NAC also significantly decreased reported craving following cocaine injection in a single-blind study but had no effects on the euphoric components (sensations of the "rush" and "high") of cocaine use (Amen et al. 2011). An open-label trial of NAC among cocaine users showed a reduction in biochemically confirmed cocaine use (Mardikian et al. 2007). Lastly, a large double-blind, placebo-controlled, randomized clinical trial study of NAC intervention failed to show a reduction in active cocaine use (LaRowe et al. 2013). Interestingly in this study, when examining only subjects abstinent from cocaine at the start of the trial, NAC seemed to increase the time to relapse and reduced craving, consistent with previous studies, though this study was not powered to find that effect. This finding suggests that NAC may be more effective at preventing psychostimulant relapse than promoting initial cessation, but that has yet to be directly tested.

There has been one clinical study to image glutamate concentration in the dorsal anterior cingulate cortex (dACC) of 22 human subjects (8 cocaine-dependent, 14 healthy) using proton magnetic resonance spectroscopy after a single dose of NAC (Schmaal et al. 2012). This open-label, randomized, crossover study demonstrated significantly higher baseline levels of glutamate in the dACC of the cocaine-dependent subjects. Administration of NAC reduced glutamate levels of the cocaine-dependent subjects, while no effect was seen in healthy controls. Impulsivity was recorded using the Barratt Impulsiveness Scale and compared to glutamate levels: higher baseline levels of glutamate were associated with exhibited higher impulsivity. Furthermore, both higher impulsivity and higher glutamate levels were predictive of a reduction in glutamate levels in response to NAC treatment. This study is therefore illustrative of NAC's capabilities to address imbalance in glutamate homeostasis and clinical potential.

13.5.2 NAC and Cannabis Use Disorder

Similar to cocaine, there are no FDA-approved pharmacotherapies for cannabis use disorder, though clinical work has also explored NAC as a candidate pharmacotherapeutic agent (Online Table 13.2). There is a notable dearth of preclinical work specifically investigating the effects of NAC on cannabis administration. However, due to NAC's hypothesized mechanism of action and considerable preclinical success for other drugs of abuse, NAC has been investigated clinically for cannabis use disorders.

An open-label study by Gray and colleagues tested NAC's efficacy among adolescents and young adults, reporting a decrease in self-reported cannabis use throughout the duration of the study and a significant reduction in certain constructs of cannabis craving, but no difference was seen in urine cannabinoid tests (Gray et al. 2010). Gray and colleagues (Gray et al. 2012) conducted a double-blind, randomized, placebo-controlled trial of NAC, in addition to a behavioral platform to promote abstinence, in cannabis-dependent adolescents, and found that participants receiving NAC had more than twice the odds of a negative urine cannabinoid test compared to those who received placebo. In a secondary analysis from that clinical trial, Roten and colleagues (Roten et al. 2013) examined cannabis craving changes among participants treated with NAC and found no treatment effect compared to placebo using the Marijuana Craving Questionnaire (MCQ; Heishman et al. 2001), though a decrease in craving was seen over time for both groups. This is potentially indicative of NAC's cessation effects being due to another mechanism and not through craving as initially hypothesized.

13.5.3 NAC and Methamphetamine Use Disorder

As with cannabis, there has been no published preclinical research on the effectiveness of NAC in reducing methamphetamine administration or reinstatement. Regardless, NAC has been explored in clinical research for methamphetamine use (Online Table 13.3), which also currently lacks any FDA-approved pharmacotherapies. Grant and colleagues (Grant et al. 2010) examined a combination of NAC and naltrexone on methamphetamine cravings. Adult men and women were tested in a double-blind, placebo-controlled study where NAC treatment also included a minimum of 50 mg/day of naltrexone. Cravings were measured using a modified Penn Craving Scale (PCS) (Flannery et al. 1999), with additional measurement of self-reported methamphetamine use, urine tests, and tests for illness severity, depression, anxiety, disability, and quality of life at various study time points. Participants on treatment showed no significant difference in cravings or drug use frequency nor any differences in other measured clinical characteristics as compared to placebo. A second study on methamphetamine use disorder utilized a double-blind, crossover design to examine craving (through a cocaine craving scale) (Mousavi et al. 2015). NAC treatment significantly reduced methamphetamine craving, counter to the study discussed previously.

13.5.4 NAC and Tobacco Use Disorder

NAC as a treatment for tobacco use disorder has seen considerable increase over the last decade for both preclinical and clinical research (Online Table 13.4). Preclinical research using rodent models of nicotine self-administration has shown that chronic NAC administration inhibits nicotine-seeking and transient increases in synaptic plasticity within the nucleus accumbens (Gipson et al. 2015). Additionally, acute NAC administration has proven effective at reducing nicotine self-administration without altering motivation for food responding (Ramirez-Niño et al. 2013). NAC therefore has a high potential of effectiveness at treating nicotine addiction in a clinical setting.

A study of 33 healthy individuals attempting to quit smoking measured cigarette craving, withdrawal, and biochemical verification of smoking (through breath carbon monoxide [CO]). Daily oral treatment with 2400 mg NAC yielded no differences in any measurements, though a trend toward fewer cigarettes smoked per day did occur (Knackstedt et al. 2009). In a study of 23 young adults asked to refrain from smoking during a 4-day double-blind, placebo-controlled study, 3600 mg/day NAC produced no difference in nicotine craving but did reduce withdrawal scores and measures of the rewarding properties of the first cigarette posttreatment (Schmaal et al. 2011). Another study tested open-label NAC in combination with the α4β2 nicotinic receptor antagonist varenicline (Chantix®) in daily cigarette smokers and found a reduction in cigarettes smoked per day and decreases in craving and smoking reward, as well as safety and tolerability of this combination pharmacotherapy (McClure et al. 2015). A study from Prado and colleagues (Prado et al. 2015) investigated smoking cessation in 34 tobacco-dependent patients, analyzing the number of cigarettes smoked, exhaled CO, depression severity, and occupational, social, and familial disability according to the Sheehan Disability Scale (Leon et al. 1997). All ratings were made at baseline and 4, 8, and 12 weeks postbaseline. All treatment administration was double-blinded and placebo-controlled and simultaneous with monthly group behavioral therapy. NAC patients received 3000 mg/day in two daily doses. NAC treatment resulted in a significant reduction in cigarette consumption at 12 weeks. Furthermore, at 12 weeks NAC significantly decreased exhaled CO, depression severity, and all disability scores on the Sheehan Disability Scale. Finally, a study investigating the effects of NAC on cannabis smoking also examined NAC's effects on the subset of the study population who smoked cigarettes (McClure et al. 2014). NAC did not alter the number of cigarettes smoked per day in this subpopulation, and co-consumption of nicotine had no apparent effects on cannabis abstinence, though there was a reported trend toward poorer cannabis outcomes for cigarette smokers vs. non-smokers.

There has been one clinical imaging study using functional magnetic resonance imaging (fMRI) to investigate NAC's effects on the frontostriatal resting-state functional connectivity (rsFC) on nicotine withdrawal symptoms (Froeliger et al. 2015). As chronic drug use is thought to produce alterations in synaptic plasticity, the investigation of systems-level functional connectivity between the prefrontal cortex and the striatum could provide significant evidence for NAC's ability to treat disruptions in glutamate homeostasis. In a double-blind, randomized, placebo-controlled study of 16 adult nicotine-dependent subjects, 2400 mg/day NAC increased rates of abstinence, reduced reported craving, and demonstrated increased rsFC compared to placebo. These results are similar to the previous imaging study reported for

NAC's treatment effects on cocaine dependence (Schmaal et al. 2012), suggesting NAC does indeed help to restore regular glutamate homeostasis and signaling.

Studies of NAC for tobacco use disorder have also been conducted with patient populations with co-occurring psychiatric disorders. In one study assessing tobacco use and gambling, NAC augmented behavioral therapy after 6 weeks of treatment in a double-blind, placebo-controlled study of 28 adults. Nicotine dependence scores reduced during the treatment period but returned to baseline at the 3-month follow-up (Grant et al. 2014). Another study on the efficacy of NAC on tobacco, alcohol, and caffeine use in patients with bipolar disorder demonstrated significant decreases in caffeine consumption at one time point, but no effect on tobacco use (Bernardo et al. 2009).

13.5.5 NAC and Gambling Disorder

In addition to SUDs, the DSM-5 lists gambling disorder as similar to drugs of abuse in regard to the activation of the brain reward system and symptom overlap (American Psychiatric Association 2013). NAC, which has been shown to influence intake of other drugs of abuse, therefore has potential as a treatment option for gambling disorder (Online Table 13.5). Grant and colleagues (Grant et al. 2007) utilized NAC in an 8–12-week open-label trial, after which subjects transitioned to a 6-week double-blind, placebo-controlled study. The Yale-Brown Obsessive Compulsive Scale Modified for Pathological Gambling (PG-YBOCS; Grant et al. 2004), Gambling Symptom Assessment Scale (G-SAS; Kim et al. 2001), Clinical Global Impression—Improvement and Severity scales (Guy 1976), Sheehan Disability Scores (Sheehan 1983), and Hamilton Depression and Anxiety Rating Scales (Hamilton 1959, 1960) were utilized as reporters. At the end of the open-label phase of the trials, NAC treatment reduced PG-YBOCS scores, greater than half of subjects listed CGI-improvement scores of "much" to "very much improved," and level of functioning, quality of life, depressive symptoms, and anxiety symptoms all improved, though not to significant levels. The double-blinded portion of the trials showed a statistical trend toward a prolonged response to NAC, indicative of NAC's effectiveness compared to placebo. In a study reported previously for nicotine treatment, double-blind, placebo-controlled administration of 1200–3000 mg/day NAC concurrent with psychosocial intervention showed significant benefits on measures of problem gambling severity after 3 months post-treatment (Grant et al. 2014).

13.6 Tolerability and Safety of NAC

Across multiple studies for several different addictive pathologies, little to no serious adverse events have been reported for NAC. A total of 8 of the 20 studies discussed here report no adverse events. Of the remaining 12, the most commonly reported adverse events include pruritus, headache, gastrointestinal issues including flatulence, diarrhea, and abdominal cramps, dizziness, and elevated blood pressure. One study reported vivid dreams, while another reported insomnia. Dosing for the studies discussed here ranged from 1000 to 3600 mg NAC per day, with consistent use for up to 24 weeks for one study (Bernardo et al. 2009). Most studies were 4 and 12 weeks in duration. This prolonged duration of use also speaks to tolerability profile of NAC. Additionally, NAC does not require a dose induction period to reach the goal dose of medication, which can be started immediately with little issue. In sum, NAC profiles as safe and tolerable for the treatment of addiction and general use, consistent with its availability at many health-focused retail stores.

13.7 Limitations and Future Directions of NAC in the Clinic

In summary, NAC has seen considerable use as a clinical treatment for substance use disorders across several different substances and addiction behaviors with some important successes. NAC has had mixed efficacy in terms of cessation outcomes. Based on preclinical work, NAC may be successful as a relapse prevention pharmacotherapeutic, as it is able to restore balance to the glutamatergic system that is targeted by drugs of abuse. Limited success as a cessation treatment may indicate that its effectiveness is potentially limited to those who have already achieved some initial measure of success to stop drug use.

In addition to NAC's use to treat addiction and addictive-like behaviors, NAC has also seen use for a variety of other psychiatric disorders, as reviewed by Deepmala and colleagues and Berk and colleagues (Berk et al. 2013; Deepmala et al. 2015). These include Alzheimer's disease, amyotrophic lateral sclerosis (ALS), autism spectrum disorders, epilepsy, neuropathy, and schizophrenia, among others. Results from these psychiatric and neurological disorder studies have been mixed, though it is speculated that NAC's effects on multiple metabolic pathways could explain why some clinical results are positive and some negative (Deepmala et al. 2015). Additional investigation is necessary to acquire a better understanding of NAC's viability as a treatment option for a broad spectrum of disease and disorder. Further preclinical investigation of NAC is necessary and ongoing as well, with emphasis on translating NAC's preclinical effectiveness for both alcohol and opioid addiction to the clinic. Efforts should be made to better understand the mixed results from the clinical literature to determine the populations for which NAC will serve as an efficacious pharmacotherapy. NAC has been shown to produce positive outcomes in rodents for both alcohol (Ozaras et al. 2003; Seiva et al. 2009, 2009) and opioids (Zhou and Kalivas 2008), but neither has been tested in clinical populations. The promise of NAC seen with other drugs of abuse highlights the need to expand testing in these instances and has been promoted as such in a review by Holmes et al. (Holmes et al. 2013). Recently, a study investigating NAC's effects on short- and long-term access to cocaine in rodents indicated no effect on either escalation of cocaine self-administration or the overall motivation for cocaine (Ducret et al. 2015). However, treatment with NAC promoted cessation of intake in long-access animals when self-administration was paired with contingent foot shocks, indicative of a reduction in compulsivity, and NAC also reduced consumption and increased latency upon returning to a non-punished schedule. Furthermore, Ducret and colleagues utilized a lower, more human-relevant dose of NAC [60 mg/kg] than most preclinical studies employ. This study therefore underscores the importance of treatment regimen with NAC as seen with previous clinical studies, as animals receiving chronic NAC did not fail to elevate cocaine intake upon starting longer access regimens, but did still alter the neurobiology thought to underlie one potential addiction mechanism. Therefore, NAC treatment during non-abstinent periods may be ineffective at promoting long-term abstinence (Gipson 2016).

Further research into other glial modulators has demonstrated promising results similar to NAC (see reviews by Cooper et al. (2012) and Scofield and Kalivas (2014)). For example, propentofylline (PPF), an atypical methylxanthine derivative, is known as a neuroprotective compound (Sweitzer and De Leo 2011) shown to increase expression of GLT-1 following spinal cord injury in mice (Tawfik et al. 2008). In preclinical tests of PPF in cocaine-administering rats, daily treatment reduced reinstatement through a GLT-1-dependent mechanism (Reissner et al. 2014). Furthermore, acute intraperitoneal injection of PPF suppressed conditioned place preference for methamphetamine and morphine in mice, indicative of a potential role for glial cells in the rewarding properties of both drugs (Narita et al. 2006). Another glial modulator, ibudilast [AV411], has been investigated as it shares similar phosphodiesterase inhibitor properties to PPF (see review by Rolan et al. (2009). Ibudilast has also demonstrated significant effects on methamphetamine consumption, locomotion, sensitization, and reinstatement (Beardsley et al. 2010; Snider et al. 2012), ethanol consumption (Bell et al. 2015), and morphine-induced neurobiological alterations and conditioned place preference (Rolan et al. 2009; Schwarz and Bilbo 2013). In sum, glial modulation represents an exciting research avenue to explore for the reduction of substance use disorders in both the preclinical and clinical fields.

In sum, clinical investigation of NAC's potential as a pharmacotherapeutic treatment of SUDs has shown variable success across drugs, and clinical studies are ongoing (Table 13.2). Controlled studies of NAC in cocaine use disorder and cannabis use disorder have had 50% or greater positive outcomes (Table 13.3).

Table 13.1 Summary of NAC mechanisms of action across different substance use and addictive disorders

Substance use or addictive disorder	Mechanism of N-Acetylcysteine (NAC)
Cocaine use disorder	NAC is thought to restore the balance of glutamate within the mesocorticolimbic reward system typically disrupted by drugs of abuse.
Cannabis use disorder	Notably, expression levels of the astroglial glutamate transporter GLT-1 are reduced (Knackstedt et al. 2009, 2010; Rao and Sari 2012; Gipson
Methamphetamine use disorder	et al. 2013) along with reductions in the catalytic subunit of Xc- (Pierce et al. 1996; Baker et al. 2003a; Berglind et al. 2009). It is thought that
Tobacco use disorder	NAC, de-acetylated and oxidized into cystine, will activate Xc- and cause glial glutamate release onto inhibitory mGluRs located on
Gambling disorder	presynaptic terminals (Kalivas et al. 2005), reducing further glutamate release onto postsynaptic receptors

Table 13.2 Ongoing clinical trials on N-Acetylcysteine for addiction

Trial title	NCT #	Trial status
Effects of N-Acetylcysteine on brain chemistry and behavior in cocaine abusers (NAC)	NCT01392092	Recruiting
Glutamate-glutamine cycling (VCYC) during cocaine abstinence using 13C-MRS	NCT02124941	Recruiting
Neurobiological adaptations and pharmacological interventions in cocaine addiction	NCT02626494	Recruiting
N-Acetylcysteine for tobacco use disorder	NCT02737358	Recruiting
Clinical trial for alcohol use disorder and post-traumatic stress disorder (PTSD)	NCT02966873	Recruiting
Efficacy of N-Acetylcysteine in bipolar disorder and tobacco use disorder (NACBD)	NCT02252341	Recruiting
Achieving cannabis cessation-evaluating N-Acetylcysteine treatment (ACCENT)	NCT01675661	Completed. No results posted

Table 13.3 Overall ratings of NAC based on clinical studies presented by condition

Substance use or addictive disorder	Uncontrolled studies positive% (positive/total)	Controlled studies positive% (positive/total)	Grade of recommendation	Recommendation for treatment
Cocaine use disorder	100% (1/1)	62.5% (2.5/4)	B	Mixed
Cannabis use disorder	50% (0.5/1)	50% (0.5/1)	B	None
Methamphetamine use disorder	–	25% (0.5/2)	B	None
Tobacco use disorder	50% (0.5/1)	50% (3/6)	B	Mixed
Gambling disorder	100% (1/1)	25% (0.5/2)	B	None

Controlled studies of methamphetamine use disorder, tobacco use disorder, and gambling disorder have had less than 50% positive outcomes (but no less than 25%), though the literature remains sparse for some drugs. All uncontrolled studies yielded greater than or equal to 50% positive outcomes. It is therefore necessary to continue investigation of NAC's efficacy as a SUD treatment option. Of particular interest is examination of NAC's apparent differential effects in cessation vs. relapse and how administration timing alters NAC's impact.

References

Amen SL, Piacentine LB, Ahmad ME, Li S-J, Mantsch JR, Risinger RC, Baker DA (2011) Repeated N-acetyl cysteine reduces cocaine seeking in rodents and craving in cocaine-dependent humans. Neuropsychopharmacology 36:871–878. https://doi.org/10.1038/npp.2010.226
American Psychiatric Association (2013) Highlights of changes from DSM-IV-TR to DSM-5

Asevedo E, Mendes AC, Berk M, Brietzke E (2014) Systematic review of N-acetylcysteine in the treatment of addictions. Rev Bras Psiquiatr 36:168–175

Baker D, McFarland K, Lake R, Shen H, Toda S, Kalivas P (2003a) N-acetyl cysteine-induced blockade of cocaine-induced reinstatement. Ann N Y Acad Sci 1003:349–351

Baker DA, McFarland K, Lake RW, Shen H, Tang X-C, Toda S, Kalivas PW (2003b) Neuroadaptations in cystine-glutamate exchange underlie cocaine relapse. Nat Neurosci 6:743–749

Beardsley PM, Shelton KL, Hendrick E, Johnson KW (2010) The glial cell modulator and phosphodiesterase inhibitor, AV411 (ibudilast), attenuates prime-and stress-induced methamphetamine relapse. Eur J Pharmacol 637:102–108

Bell RL, Lopez MF, Cui C, Egli M, Johnson KW, Franklin KM, Becker HC (2015) Ibudilast reduces alcohol drinking in multiple animal models of alcohol dependence. Addict Biol 20:38–42

Berglind WJ, Whitfield TW, LaLumiere RT, Kalivas PW, McGinty JF (2009) A single intra-PFC infusion of BDNF prevents cocaine-induced alterations in extracellular glutamate within the nucleus accumbens. J Neurosci 29:3715–3719

Berk M, Malhi GS, Gray LJ, Dean OM (2013) The promise of N-acetylcysteine in neuropsychiatry. Trends Pharmacol Sci 34:167–177

Bernardo M, Dodd S, Gama CS, Copolov DL, Dean O, Kohlmann K, Jeavons S, Schapkaitz I, Anderson-Hunt M, Bush AI, Berk M (2009) Effects of N-acetylcysteine on substance use in bipolar disorder: a randomised placebo-controlled clinical trial. Acta Neuropsychiatr 21:285–291. https://doi.org/10.1111/j.1601-5215.2009.00397.x

Borgström L, Kågedal B, Paulsen O (1986) Pharmacokinetics of N-acetylcysteine in man. Eur J Clin Pharmacol 31:217–222

Centers for Disease Control and Prevention (2016) Excessive drinking costs U.S. $223.5 billion. http://www.cdc.gov/features/alcoholconsumption/

Cooper ZD, Jones JD, Comer SD (2012) Glial modulators: a novel pharmacological approach to altering the behavioral effects of abused substances. Expert Opin Investig Drugs 21:169–178

Deepmala SJ, Kumar N, Delhey L, Berk M, Dean O, Spielholz C, Frye R (2015) Clinical trials of N-acetylcysteine in psychiatry and neurology: a systematic review. Neurosci Biobehav Rev 55:294–321

Ducret E, Puaud M, Lacoste J, Belin-Rauscent A, Fouyssac M, Dugast E, Murray JE, Everitt BJ, Houeto J-L, Belin D (2015) N-acetylcysteine facilitates self-imposed abstinence after escalation of cocaine intake. Biol Psychiatry 80:226

First MB, Gibbon M, Williams J (1994) Structured clinical interview for DSM-IV-TR axis I disorders, research version, patient edition (SCID-I/P)

Flannery BA, Volpicelli JR, Pettinati HM (1999) Psychometric properties of the Penn alcohol craving scale. Alcohol Clin Exp Res 23:1289–1295

Froeliger B, McConnell PA, Stankeviciute N, McClure EA, Kalivas PW, Gray KM (2015) The effects of N-acetylcysteine on frontostriatal resting-state functional connectivity, withdrawal symptoms and smoking abstinence: a double-blind, placebo-controlled fMRI pilot study. Drug Alcohol Depend 156:234–242

Gass JT, Olive MF (2008) Glutamatergic substrates of drug addiction and alcoholism. Biochem Pharmacol 75:218–265

Gipson CD (2016) Treating addiction: unraveling the relationship between N-acetylcysteine, GLT-1, and behavior. Biol Psychiatry 80:e11

Gipson CD, Kupchik YM, Kalivas PW (2014) Rapid, transient synaptic plasticity in addiction. Neuropharmacology 76:276–286

Gipson CD, Kupchik YM, Shen H, Reissner KJ, Thomas CA, Kalivas PW (2013) Relapse induced by cues predicting cocaine depends on rapid, transient synaptic potentiation. Neuron 77:867–872. https://doi.org/10.1016/j.neuron.2013.01.005

Gipson CD, Reissner KJ, Kupchik YM, Smith ACW, Stankeviciute N, Hensley-Simon ME, Kalivas PW (2013) Reinstatent of nicotine seeking is mediated by glutamatergic plasticity. Proc Natl Acad Sci U S A 110:9124–9129. https://doi.org/10.1073/pnas.1220591110

Gipson CD, Spencer S, Stankeviciute N, Allen N, Garcia-Keller C, Kalivas PW (2015) N-acetylcysteine inhibits nicotine relapse-associated synaptic plasticity and restores glial glutamate transport in nicotine-withdrawn animals. Drug Alcohol Depend 156:e80

Grandjean EM, Berthet P, Ruffmann R, Leuenberger P (2000) Efficacy of oral long-term N-acetylcysteine in chronic bronchopulmonary disease: a meta-analysis of published double-blind, placebo-controlled clinical trials. Clin Ther 22:209–221

Grant JE, Kim SW, Odlaug BL (2007) N-acetyl cysteine, a glutamate-modulating agent, in the treatment of pathological gambling: a pilot study. Biol Psychiatry 62:652–657. https://doi.org/10.1016/j.biopsych.2006.11.021

Grant JE, Odlaug BL, Chamberlain SR, Potenza MN, Schreiber LRN, Donahue CB, Kim SW (2014) A randomized, placebo-controlled trial of N-acetylcysteine plus imaginal desensitization for nicotine-dependent pathological gamblers. J Clin Psychiatry 75:39–45. https://doi.org/10.4088/JCP.13m08411

Grant JE, Odlaug BL, Kim SW (2010) A double-blind, placebo-controlled study of N-acetyl cysteine plus naltrexone for methamphetamine dependence. Eur Neuropsychopharmacol 20:823–828. https://doi.org/10.1016/j.euroneuro.2010.06.018

Grant JE, Steinberg MA, Kim SW, Rounsaville BJ, Potenza MN (2004) Preliminary validity and reliability testing of a structured clinical interview for pathological gambling. Psychiatry Res 128:79–88

Gray KM, Carpenter MJ, Baker NL, DeSantis SM, Kryway E, Hartwell KJ, McRae-Clark AL, Brady KT (2012) A double-blind randomized controlled trial of N-acetylcysteine in cannabis-dependent adolescents. Am J Psychiatry 169:805–812. https://doi.org/10.1176/appi.ajp.2012.12010055

Gray KM, Watson NL, Carpenter MJ, Larowe SD (2010) N-acetylcysteine (NAC) in young marijuana users: an open-label pilot study. Am J Addict 19:187–189. https://doi.org/10.1111/j.1521-0391.2009.00027.x

Guy W (1976) ECDEU assessment manual for psychopharmacology. US Department of Health, Education, and Welfare, Public Health Service, Alcohol, Drug Abuse, and Mental Health Administration, National Institute of Mental Health, Psychopharmacology Research Branch, Division of Extramural Research Programs, Rockville

Hamilton M (1960) A rating scale for depression. J Neurol Neurosurg Psychiatry 23:56–62

Hamilton MAX (1959) The assessment of anxiety states by rating. Br J Med Psychol 32:50–55

Heishman SJ, Singleton EG, Liguori A (2001) Marijuana craving questionnaire: development and initial validation of a self-report instrument. Addiction 96:1023–1034

Holmes A, Spanagel R, Krystal JH (2013) Glutamatergic targets for new alcohol medications. Psychopharmacology 229:539–554

Kalivas PW (2009) The glutamate homeostasis hypothesis of addiction. Nat Rev Neurosci 10:561–572. https://doi.org/10.1038/nrn2515

Kalivas PW, Volkow N, Seamans J (2005) Unmanageable motivation in addiction: a pathology in prefrontal-accumbens glutamate transmission. Neuron 45:647–650

Kim SW, Grant JE, Adson DE, Shin YC (2001) Double-blind naltrexone and placebo comparison study in the treatment of pathological gambling. Biol Psychiatry 49:914–921

Knackstedt LA, LaRowe S, Mardikian P, Malcolm R, Upadhyaya H, Hedden S, Markou A, Kalivas PW (2009) The role of cystine-glutamate exchange in nicotine dependence in rats and humans. Biol Psychiatry 65:841–845. https://doi.org/10.1016/j.biopsych.2008.10.040

Knackstedt LA, Melendez RI, Kalivas PW (2010) Ceftriaxone restores glutamate homeostasis and prevents relapse to cocaine seeking. Biol Psychiatry 67:81–84

Knackstedt LA, Moussawi K, Lalumiere R, Schwendt M, Klugmann M, Kalivas PW (2010) Extinction training after cocaine self-administration induces glutamatergic plasticity to inhibit cocaine seeking. J Neurosci 30:7984–7992

Kupchik YM, Moussawi K, Tang X-C, Wang X, Kalivas BC, Kolokithas R, Ogburn KB, Kalivas PW (2012) The effect of N-acetylcysteine in the nucleus accumbens on neurotransmission and relapse to cocaine. Biol Psychiatry 71:978–986

LaRowe SD, Kalivas PW, Nicholas JS, Randall PK, Mardikian PN, Malcolm RJ (2013) A double blind placebo controlled trial of N-acetylcysteine in the treatment of cocaine dependence. Am J Addict 22:443–452. https://doi.org/10.1111/j.1521-0391.2012.12034.x

LaRowe SD, Mardikian P, Malcolm R, Myrick H, Kalivas P, McFarland K, Saladin M, McRae A, Brady K (2006) Safety and tolerability of N-acetylcysteine in cocaine-dependent individuals. Am J Addict 15:105–110. https://doi.org/10.1080/10550490500419169

LaRowe SD, Myrick H, Hedden S, Mardikian P, Saladin M, McRae A, Brady K, Kalivas PW, Malcolm R (2007) Is cocaine desire reduced by N-acetylcysteine? Am J Psychiatry 164:1115–1117. https://doi.org/10.1176/appi.ajp.164.7.1115

Leon AC, Olfson M, Portera L, Farber L, Sheehan DV (1997) Assessing psychiatric impairment in primary care with the Sheehan disability scale. Int J Psychiatry Med 27:93–105

Madayag A, Lobner D, Kau KS, Mantsch JR, Abdulhameed O, Hearing M, Grier MD, Baker DA (2007) Repeated N-acetylcysteine administration alters plasticity-dependent effects of cocaine. J Neurosci 27:13968–13976

Malarkey EB, Parpura V (2008) Mechanisms of glutamate release from astrocytes. Neurochem Int 52:142–154

Mardikian PN, LaRowe SD, Hedden S, Kalivas PW, Malcolm RJ (2007) An open-label trial of N-acetylcysteine for the treatment of cocaine dependence: a pilot study. Prog Neuro-Psychopharmacol Biol Psychiatry 31:389–394

McClure EA, Baker NL, Gipson CD, Carpenter MJ, Roper AP, Froeliger BE, Kalivas PW, Gray KM (2015) An open-label pilot trial of N-acetylcysteine and varenicline in adult cigarette smokers. Am J Drug Alcohol Abuse 41:52–56

McClure EA, Baker NL, Gray KM (2014) Cigarette smoking during an N-acetylcysteine-assisted cannabis cessation trial in adolescents. Am J Drug Alcohol Abuse 40:285–291. https://doi.org/10.3109/00952990.2013.878718

McClure EA, Gipson CD, Malcolm RJ, Kalivas PW, Gray KM (2014) Potential role of N-acetylcysteine in the management of substance use disorders. CNS Drugs 28:95–106

Minarini A, Ferrari S, Galletti M, Giambalvo N, Perrone D, Rioli G, Galeazzi GM (2016) N-acetylcysteine in the treatment of psychiatric disorders: current status and future prospects. Expert Opin Drug Metab Toxicol 13:279–292

Mousavi SG, Sharbafchi MR, Salehi M, Peykanpour M, Sichani NK, Maracy M (2015) The efficacy of N-acetylcysteine in the treatment of methamphetamine dependence: a double-blind controlled, crossover study. Arch Iran Med 18:28–33

Moussawi K, Kalivas PW (2010) Group II metabotropic glutamate receptors (mGlu 2/3) in drug addiction. Eur J Pharmacol 639:115–122

Moussawi K, Pacchioni A, Moran M, Olive MF, Gass JT, Lavin A, Kalivas PW (2009) N-Acetylcysteine reverses cocaine-induced metaplasticity. Nat Neurosci 12:182–189

Moussawi K, Zhou W, Shen H, Reichel CM, See RE, Carr DB, Kalivas PW (2011) Reversing cocaine-induced synaptic potentiation provides enduring protection from relapse. Proc Natl Acad Sci 108:385–390

Murray JE, Everitt BJ, Belin D (2012) N-Acetylcysteine reduces early-and late-stage cocaine seeking without affecting cocaine taking in rats. Addict Biol 17:437–440

Narita M, Miyatake M, Narita M, Shibasaki M, Shindo K, Nakamura A, Kuzumaki N, Nagumo Y, Suzuki T (2006) Direct evidence of astrocytic modulation in the development of rewarding effects induced by drugs of abuse. Neuropsychopharmacology 31:2476–2488

National Drug Intelligence Center (2011) National drug threat assessment 2011. National Drug Intelligence Center, pp 1–72. doi: https://doi.org/10.1037/e618352012-001

National Institute on Drug Abuse (2017) Trends & statistics. National Institute on Drug Abuse. https://www.drugabuse.gov/related-topics/trends-statistics

Olive MF, Cleva RM, Kalivas PW, Malcolm RJ (2012) Glutamatergic medications for the treatment of drug and behavioral addictions. Pharmacol Biochem Behav 100:801–810

Olsson B, Johansson M, Gabrielsson J, Bolme P (1988) Pharmacokinetics and bioavailability of reduced and oxidized N-acetylcysteine. Eur J Clin Pharmacol 34:77–82

Ozaras R, Tahan V, Aydin S, Uzun H, Kaya S, Senturk H (2003) N-acetylcysteine attenuates alcohol-induced oxidative stress in the rat. World J Gastroenterol 9:125–128

Pierce RC, Bell K, Duffy P, Kalivas PW (1996) Repeated cocaine augments excitatory amino acid transmission in the nucleus accumbens only in rats having developed behavioral sensitization. J Neurosci 16:1550–1560

Prado E, Maes M, Piccoli LG, Baracat M, Barbosa DS, Franco O, Dodd S, Berk M, Vargas Nunes SO (2015) N-acetylcysteine for therapy-resistant tobacco use disorder: a pilot study. Redox Rep 20:215–222. https://doi.org/10.1179/1351000215Y.0000000004

Ramirez-Niño AM, D'Souza MS, Markou A (2013) N-acetylcysteine decreased nicotine self-administration and cue-induced reinstatement of nicotine seeking in rats: comparison with the effects of N-acetylcysteine on food responding and food seeking. Psychopharmacology 225:473–482

Rao PSS, Sari Y (2012) Glutamate transporter 1: target for the treatment of alcohol dependence. Curr Med Chem 19:5148–5156

Reichel CM, Moussawi K, Do PH, Kalivas PW, See RE (2011) Chronic N-acetylcysteine during abstinence or extinction after cocaine self-administration produces enduring reductions in drug seeking. J Pharmacol Exp Ther 337:487–493

Reissner KJ, Brown RM, Spencer S, Tran PK, Thomas CA, Kalivas PW (2014) Chronic administration of the methylxanthine propentofylline impairs reinstatement to cocaine by a GLT-1-dependent mechanism. Neuropsychopharmacology 39:499–506

Reissner KJ, Gipson CD, Tran PK, Knackstedt LA, Scofield MD, Kalivas PW (2015) Glutamate transporter GLT-1 mediates N-acetylcysteine inhibition of cocaine reinstatement. Addict Biol 20:316–323

Repine JE, Bast A, Lankhorst IDA (1997) Oxidative stress in chronic obstructive pulmonary disease. Am J Respir Crit Care Med 156:341–357

Roberts-Wolfe DJ, Kalivas PW (2015) Glutamate transporter GLT-1 as a therapeutic target for substance use disorders. CNS Neurol Disord Drug Targets 14:745–756

Rolan P, Hutchinson MR, Johnson KW (2009) Ibudilast: a review of its pharmacology, efficacy and safety in respiratory and neurological disease. Expert Opin Pharmacother 10:2897–2904

Roten AT, Baker NL, Gray KM (2013) Marijuana craving trajectories in an adolescent marijuana cessation pharmacotherapy trial. Addict Behav 38:1788–1791. https://doi.org/10.1016/j.addbeh.2012.11.003

Schmaal L, Berk L, Hulstijn KP, Cousijn J, Wiers RW, Van Den Brink W (2011) Efficacy of N-acetylcysteine in the treatment of nicotine dependence: a double-blind placebo-controlled pilot study. Eur Addict Res 17:211–216. https://doi.org/10.1159/000327682

Schmaal L, Veltman DJ, Nederveen A, van den Brink W, Goudriaan AE (2012) N-acetylcysteine normalizes glutamate levels in cocaine-dependent patients: a randomized crossover magnetic resonance spectroscopy study. Neuropsychopharmacology 37:2143–2152

Schwarz JM, Bilbo SD (2013) Adolescent morphine exposure affects long-term microglial function and later-life relapse liability in a model of addiction. J Neurosci 33:961–971

Scofield MD, Kalivas PW (2014) Astrocytic dysfunction and addiction consequences of impaired glutamate homeostasis. Neuroscientist 20:610. https://doi.org/10.1177/1073858413520347

Seiva FRF, Amauchi JF, Rocha KKR, Ebaid GX, Souza G, Fernandes AAH, Cataneo AC, Novelli ELB (2009) Alcoholism and alcohol abstinence: N-acetylcysteine to improve energy expenditure, myocardial oxidative stress, and energy metabolism in alcoholic heart disease. Alcohol 43:649–656

Seiva FRF, Amauchi JF, Rocha KKR, Souza GA, Ebaid GX, Burneiko RM, Novelli ELB (2009) Effects of N-acetylcysteine on alcohol abstinence and alcohol-induced adverse effects in rats. Alcohol 43:127–135

Sheehan DV (1983) The anxiety disease. Bantam Books, New York, p 151

Shen H, Gipson CD, Huits M, Kalivas PW (2014) Prelimbic cortex and ventral tegmental area modulate synaptic plasticity differentially in nucleus accumbens during cocaine-reinstated drug seeking. Neuropsychopharmacology 39:1169–1177

Sherman BJ, McRae-Clark AL (2016) Treatment of cannabis use disorder: current science and future outlook. J Hum Pharmacol Drug Ther 36:511–535

Smilkstein MJ, Knapp GL, Kulig KW, Rumack BH (1988) Efficacy of oral N-acetylcysteine in the treatment of acetaminophen overdose. N Engl J Med 319:1557–1562

Snider SE, Vunck SA, van den Oord EJCG, Adkins DE, McClay JL, Beardsley PM (2012) The glial cell modulators, ibudilast and its amino analog, AV1013, attenuate methamphetamine locomotor activity and its sensitization in mice. Eur J Pharmacol 679:75–80

Sweitzer S, De Leo J (2011) Propentofylline: glial modulation, neuroprotection, and alleviation of chronic pain. In: Methylxanthines. Springer, Berlin, pp 235–250

Tawfik VL, Regan MR, Haenggeli C, LaCroix-Fralish ML, Nutile-McMenemy N, Perez N, Rothstein JD, DeLeo JA (2008) Propentofylline-induced astrocyte modulation leads to alterations in glial glutamate promoter activation following spinal nerve transection. Neuroscience 152:1086–1092

US Department of Health and Human Services (2014) The health consequences of smoking—50 years of progress: a report of the Surgeon General

Williams SM, Sullivan RKP, Scott HL, Finkelstein DI, Colditz PB, Lingwood BE, Dodd PR, Pow DV (2005) Glial glutamate transporter expression patterns in brains from multiple mammalian species. Glia 49:520–541

Zhou W, Kalivas PW (2008) N-acetylcysteine reduces extinction responding and induces enduring reductions in cue-and heroin-induced drug-seeking. Biol Psychiatry 63:338–340

14

Richard Eugene Frye

14.1 Introduction

Kidney disease is a prevalent and growing medical problem, affecting more than 20 million people in the United States. Early kidney disease can be silent with symptoms arising only many years after disease has started. Many chronic diseases, including diabetes, high blood pressure, autoimmune disease and vascular diseases, just to name a few, can cause secondary injury to the kidney. Alternatively, the kidneys can be acutely damaged from infection, trauma, or iatrogenic causes. The treatments for kidney disease, which include chronic dialysis and kidney transplant, are less than optimal, making the prevention of kidney disease extremely important.

One of the first studies using N-Acetylcysteine (NAC) in kidney disease was using it as an adjunct to dialysis for removing homocysteine (Bostom et al. 1996). This study demonstrated that NAC did lower homocysteine in general but did not augment clinical outcomes of dialysis. It was not until the 2000s that NAC was again seriously investigated in its use in kidney disease. NAC has been extensively investigated as a preventive treatment for iatrogenic kidney injury, particularly when using radiological contrast agents. Other clinical studies have included its utility in both chronic and acute kidney diseases. This chapter will review the evidence for the use of NAC for these indications.

The proposed pathophysiological mechanisms of NAC are discussed in detail in separate chapters. There are several pathophysiological mechanisms that

Electronic supplementary material The online version of this article (https://doi.org/10.1007/978-981-10-5311-5_14) contains supplementary material, which is available to authorized users.

R. E. Frye
Barrow Neurological Institute, Phoenix Children's Hospital, University of Arizona College of Medicine – Phoenix, Phoenix, AZ, USA
e-mail: rfrye@phoenixchildrens.com

© Springer Nature Singapore Pte Ltd. 2019
R. E. Frye, M. Berk (eds.), *The Therapeutic Use of N-Acetylcysteine (NAC) in Medicine*, https://doi.org/10.1007/978-981-10-5311-5_14

have undergone investigation in renal disease. Improvement in oxidative stress has been studied in the context of radiological contrast exposure (Saitoh et al. 2011; Thiele et al. 2010; Buyukhatipoglu et al. 2010; Sandhu et al. 2006; Drager et al. 2004; Efrati et al. 2003), hemodialysis (HD) (Swarnalatha et al. 2010; Trimarchi et al. 2003; Thaha et al. 2008; Hsu et al. 2010; Shahbazian et al. 2016), and peritoneal dialysis (PD) (Nascimento et al. 2010). The ability of NAC to prevent tubular injury has been studied in radiological contrast exposure (Drager et al. 2004; Levin et al. 2007) and to improve tubular function has been studied in patient with end-stage renal disease (ESRD) (Moist et al. 2010). The ability of NAC to improve endothelial function has been studied in ESRD (Scholze et al. 2004; Wittstock et al. 2009; Renke et al. 2010), HD patients (Sahin et al. 2007; Swarnalatha et al. 2010), and patients exposed to radiological contrast (Efrati et al. 2003). Lastly, modulation of immune system function has been studied in PD (Purwanto and Prasetyo 2012; Nascimento et al. 2010) and HD (Swarnalatha et al. 2010; Saddadi et al. 2014). Table 14.1 outlined the conditions in which NAC has been investigated and the proposed mechanism of action for each condition.

Table 14.1 Summary of proposed NAC mechanisms of action across different renal disorders

Renal disorder	Proposed mechanism of N-Acetylcysteine (NAC)
Protection against kidney injury from radiological contrast	Antioxidant effect by free-radical scavenging and increased levels of glutathione (Saitoh et al. 2011) Preventing tubular injury (Drager et al. 2004) Increase nitric oxide (Efrati et al. 2003)
Protection against kidney injury from amphotericin B	Prevention of renal tubular damage (Adderson et al. 1991)
Kidney transplant	Prevention of ischemia-reperfusion injury (Orban et al. 2015)
Aortic aneurysm repair	Prevention of ischemia-reperfusion injury (Orban et al. 2015)
Prolonged hypotension	Antioxidant and anti-inflammatory effects counteract pathophysiology of shock states (Komisarof et al. 2007)
Hematopoietic stem cell transplantation	Antioxidant and anti-inflammatory effect (Ataei et al. 2015)
Cardiorenal syndrome	Preventing oxidative stress and endothelial dysfunction (Camuglia et al. 2013)
Acute pyelonephritis	Decreased inflammation (Allameh et al. 2015)
Dialysis	Reduction in oxidative stress (Trimarchi et al. 2003) Inflammation (Saddadi et al. 2014) Improving endothelial function (Scholze et al. 2004)
Homocysteine reduction	Increase the acid-soluble homocysteine fraction (Bostom et al. 1996)
End stage renal disease	Improving endothelial function (Sahin et al. 2007) Improving tubular function (Moist et al. 2010)

14.2   Methods

A systematic online literature search to identify all clinical trials using NAC using the filters "human" and "clinical trials." From these the author screened titles and abstracts of all potentially relevant publications.

14.3   NAC in the Prevention of Iatrogenic Induced Renal Disorders

14.3.1   Protection Against Kidney Injury from Radiological Contrast Agents

Contrast-induced nephropathy (CIN), defined as an acute decline in renal function after the administration of intravenous contrast in the absence of other causes, is the third leading cause of acute renal failure in hospitalized patients behind hypotension and surgery complications. Radiological contrast is used in many settings and NAC is provided through several routes (oral, intravenous, combined) and at various doses. This chapter is divided into several parts, including the use of NAC with Computed Tomography (CT) imaging and during angiography. Most of the studies concentrate on patient at risk for developing CIN while a few studies have included patient without risk factors in order to systematically examine risk factors on CIN.

14.3.1.1   Contrast Agents Using Computed Tomography

Seven studies have looked at NAC for the prevention of CIN in older adults at risk for CIN because of medical conditions undergoing CT (Online Table 14.1). Four of the studies were done in the emergency department (ED) setting while the other three studies were in non-emergent settings.

The earliest first two studies in the ED were promising. In one of the first studies Poletti et al. (2007) measured serum creatinine (Cr) and cystatin C (CyC) before and 2 and 4 days after iodine contrast media- enhanced CT imaging in 87 patients with renal insufficiency (RI) (Poletti et al. 2007). CIN was defined as a 25% or greater increase in Cr or CyC. 900 mg of intravenous (IV) NAC given 1 h before and immediately following contrast injection as compared to only IV fluids (IVF) reduced the percentage of patients with Cr defined CIN (hydration 21% vs NAC 5%) but not CyC defined CIN. In the next study, Hsu et al. (2012) prospectively studied ED patients undergoing abdominal or chest contrast-enhanced CT (Hsu et al. 2012). Many patients had risk factors including hypertension, diabetes mellitus (DM), or RI. Patients who agreed to participate in the study received NAC and those who did not agree to be in the study received treatment as usual (TAU) and were considered a control group. Those who received NAC were matched to randomly selected controls based on age and their pre-contrast Cr. 600 mg IV NAC before CT imaging was found to decrease the odds of CIN but not all-cause mortality or the need for temporary hemodialysis.

Following these first two promising studies, two additional studies were conducted with much higher doses of NAC and with populations that had relatively more women. Poletti et al. (2013) studied patient with RI undergoing a contrast-enhanced CT (Poletti et al. 2013). 6 g IV NAC 1 h prior to CT in addition to IVF did not decrease the incidence of CIN as indexes by change in CyC and/or Cr. Traub et al. (2013) enrolled adults with risk factors undergoing contrast-enhanced chest, abdominal, or pelvic CT in the ED. NAC was given as 3 g IV 30 min before the CT and 200 mg/h IV for a minimum of 2 h but up to 15 h (Traub et al. 2013). Placebo patients received analogous treatment of normal saline. The data safety and monitoring board terminated the study early because of futility. NAC treatment did not decrease the incidence of CIN but there were no adverse effects (AEs) of NAC either. This study found that a greater volume of IVF significantly decreased the risk of CIN. Thus, overall it is not clear whether these later studies were negative because of the much higher dose of NAC used, the relatively greater number of women, or the non-standard fluid regime used. Clearly, further research is needed.

Three studies examined the ability of NAC to protect against renal injury in non-emergent CT setting. Kitzler et al. (2012) conducted a three-arm relatively small double-blind placebo-controlled (DBPC) study that found no difference between the NAC, vitamin E, and placebo treatments with respect to the incidence of CIN or the change in Cr or Creatinine Clearance (CCl) (Kitzler et al. 2012). However, in a larger study, Tepel et al. (2000) found that NAC significantly reduced the incidence of CIN (NAC 2% vs 21%) in 83 patients with RI (Tepel et al. 2000), while Sar et al. (2010) demonstrated that NAC resulted in a more favorable change in Cr in 45 type 2 DM patients without RI (Sar et al. 2010). Since the one study that was negative was rather small, given the positive evidence of the other two studies the recommendations for NAC are positive for non-emergent CT imaging with contrast.

Thus, overall, there is clearly some high-quality studies that have examined whether NAC is protective for CIN but the findings remain mixed when considering the results of the various clinical trials. Clearly more research is needed to help clarify the optimal protocol for using NAC during CT imaging with contrast. Thus, the recommendations remain overall mixed for CT imaging with contrast as it appears the efficacy of NAC may depend on the protocol used.

14.3.1.2 Contrast Agents in Angiography

Studies investigating the renal protective effect of NAC during angiography have used various protocols, including oral (Online Table 14.2) and IV (Online Table 14.3) administration routes. In addition, NAC protocols have been compared (Online Table 14.4) and NAC treatment has been compared to other treatments for the prevention of CIN (Online Table 14.5). Each of these various approaches to studying NAC will be discussed separately.

Oral NAC

Based on the physiological data and successful clinical trial of NAC in contrast CT (Tepel et al. 2000), a small clinical trial was conducted to determine if NAC may be helpful during angiography in patient with RI (Diaz-Sandoval et al. 2002). Owing to the success of this pilot study, many other clinical trials were conducted particular on patients believed to at high risk of CIN due to RI. Early follow-up studies were encouraging. Several studies demonstrated that oral NAC reduced the incidence of CIN in patients with RI undergoing coronary angiography (CAG) with or without percutaneous intervention (PCI) (Shyu et al. 2002; Kay et al. 2003; Ochoa et al. 2004; Miner et al. 2004; Briguori et al. 2004; Marenzi et al. 2006). Briguori et al. (2002) found that NAC decreased the overall incidence of CIN in patients with RI in which a low volume of contrast was used but not those in which a high contrast volume was used (Briguori et al. 2002).

Several of these studies that examined the change in renal function indices, including Cr and/or CCl, demonstrated that NAC improved renal function while renal function worsened in the control group, with this difference significant between groups. Two other studies that examined indices of renal function rather than CIN also demonstrated this positive effect of NAC (Efrati et al. 2003; Drager et al. 2004). One study demonstrated the positive effect of NAC on renal indices but did not show a significant change in the incidence of CIN (Balderramo et al. 2004). However, at least 15 other studies during this early phase of investigation did not show any benefit of NAC (Durham et al. 2002; Vallero et al. 2002; El Mahmoud et al. 2003; Oldemeyer et al. 2003; Boccalandro et al. 2003; Fung et al. 2004; Goldenberg et al. 2004; Gulel et al. 2005; Azmus et al. 2005; Gomes et al. 2005; Sandhu et al. 2006; Seyon et al. 2007; Heng et al. 2008; Amini et al. 2009; Ferrario et al. 2009).

In 2011 a large trial of 2308 patients with at least one risk factor for CIN using adequate NAC doses (ACT Trial Investigators 2009) failed to find a significant effect in the overall (ACT Trial Investigators 2011) study or in the DM subgroup (Berwanger et al. 2013). Other contemporary trials have also failed to find an effect (Tanaka et al. 2011; Saitoh et al. 2011; Aslanger et al. 2012), whereas other small (Sadat et al. 2011; Kinbara et al. 2010) and larger (Kim et al. 2010; Awal et al. 2011; Chong et al. 2015; Habib et al. 2016) more contemporary trials have documented the efficacy of NAC in high-risk (Awal et al. 2011; Chong et al. 2015; Habib et al. 2016) and low-risk (Kim et al. 2010; Sadat et al. 2011; Kinbara et al. 2010) patients.

Given that there is many high-quality studies the GOR is A, but given the incredibly mixed findings of the studies it is difficult to make a recommendation for the exact protocol for providing NAC. One great advantage of NAC is the low incidence of AEs especially serious AEs. Given the great potential to prevent a very serious medical complication, the potential for NAC to prevent CIN is still great and further research is indeed needed.

IV NAC

There are eight clinical trials which compare a single dose of IV NAC to placebo with two clinical trials having two publications, one outlining different outcome measures and one concentrating on a high risk subgroup of individuals with RI. Two studies demonstrated positive outcomes. A small pilot study demonstrated that IV NAC at a dose of 100 mg/kg prevented the usual contrast-induced increase in Cr in individuals with RI undergoing CAG and decreased Cr in individuals with RI not receiving contrast at 3 and 24 h after treatment (Sochman and Krizova 2006). The second positive study was a subpopulation of a larger clinical trial which did not demonstrate a protective effect of NAC overall (Carbonell et al. 2007). Carbonell et al. (2010) demonstrated that the subpopulation of individuals with RI undergoing CAG benefited from 600 mg of IV NAC given every 12 h starting at least 6 h before the procedure (Carbonell et al. 2010). Six clinical trials, all of them high quality with very reasonable sample sizes, using both high (Rashid et al. 2004; Kefer et al. 2003; Droppa et al. 2011; Thiele et al. 2010; Jaffery et al. 2012) and low (Webb et al. 2004; Baranska-Kosakowska et al. 2007) dose regimes did not demonstrate a significant benefit of NAC on protecting kidney impairment during angiography. On the other hand, no study reported any AEs of NAC and several specifically stated that no AEs were observed, highlighting the safety of NAC.

Two of three other studies described below compared multiple NAC regimes (Recio-Mayoral et al. 2007; Marenzi et al. 2006; Aslanger et al. 2012) and demonstrated significant effects of IV NAC, particularly at high doses, while another study described below which compared IV NAC to ascorbic acid did not find an effect (Brueck et al. 2013). The potential benefit for NAC is great and the safety is excellent, suggesting that continued research into this treatment may be very beneficial to patients. Caveats to these clinical trials, particularly with regard to primary outcome measures, are discussed below, but clearly IV NAC needs to be compared carefully with oral NAC regimes and the optimal treatment populations considered in future clinical trials.

Comparison of NAC Protocols

Five clinical trials have compared NAC protocols head-to-head. Four of these studies compared low and high NAC doses with all four studies using non-ionic, low-osmolality contrast and demonstrating evidence that high dose NAC was superior to either placebo and/or low dose NAC (Briguori et al. 2004; Recio-Mayoral et al. 2007; Marenzi et al. 2006; Habib et al. 2016). Briguori et al. (2004) demonstrated that a double dose of oral NAC improved outcomes in 224 individuals with RI undergoing coronary and/or peripheral angiography and/or PCI with this effect being driven by individuals who received high doses (≥ 140 ml) of contrast (Briguori et al. 2004). Recio-Mayoral et al. (2007) demonstrated an improvement in CIN incidence and acute anuric renal failure when NAC was given before as well as after emergency PCI in 111 patients (Recio-Mayoral et al. 2007). Marenzi et al. (2006) found that NAC decreased the CIN incidence with a higher dose NAC decreasing incidence to a greater extent than low dose NAC and both low and high dose NAC resulted in significantly better rates of death and composite end-points in 354 patients undergoing PCI (Marenzi et al. 2006). Habib et al. (2016) found that high dose NAC reduced the incidence of CIN to a greater extent than low dose NAC with ascorbic acid or IVF only in 105 high-risk patients with ischemic heart or peripheral vascular disease undergoing CAG (Habib et al. 2016). The only study that did not have positive findings was Aslanger et al. (2012) who compared IV and intrarenal NAC to placebo in patients with acute myocardial infarction undergoing PCI (Aslanger et al. 2012). This latter study is one of the only studies to use an ionic rather than a non-ionic contrast agent, so the results of this study are not completely comparable to other studies and given that most centers now use non-ionic contrast agents, the applicability of this latter study is questionable. However, overall the above studies suggest that high doses of NAC may afford better protection than lower doses during CAG and PCI.

Comparison of NAC vs Other Treatments During Angiography

Four clinical trials compared NAC to other treatments for preventing kidney injury from contrast agents during CAG with or without PCI. In a multicenter DBPC trial in Korea, patients with RI taking statins undergoing CAG with or without PCI were randomized to receive either NAC or ascorbic acid orally (Jo et al. 2009). Maximum increase of Cr level was significantly lower in the NAC group than in the ascorbic acid group, with this effect significant in the DM and high-dose contrast media subgroups but not the severe RI, low ejection fraction or older (>70 years) subgroups. The incidence of CIN favored NAC but was not significant overall except in the DM subgroup. However, in a larger DBPC study of adults with RI undergoing CAG with or without PCI randomized to receive a lower dose of NAC or ascorbic acid IV, there was no difference in CIN incidence, although, as the authors note, the incidence of CIN was higher than expected in this study (Brueck et al. 2013). One small study ($N = 45$) on patients undergoing CAG with or without PCI examined the difference between oral NAC and IV aminophylline as compared to placebo (Kinbara et al. 2010). NAC treatment resulted in a lower incidence of CIN and significantly improved the Cr, CCl, and blood beta-2 microglobulin as compared to placebo; aminophylline also demonstrated favorable effects as compared to placebo. Lastly, a small ($N = 21$) clinical trial of patients with RI undergoing CAG compared NAC and glutathione to IVF only treatment (Saitoh et al. 2011). CIN occurred in one patient in the NAC and control group but the small sample size for this three-arm study makes interpretation of CIN difficult. However, this study did measure biomarkers of oxidative stress.

Critique of Angiograph Studies

Studies examining the protective effect of NAC in angiography with or without percutaneous procedures are very variable with some studies showing clearly promising findings and others failing to find any effect. There is a pattern to studies that are positive. In such studies CIN in the control group is somewhere near 20% and the NAC treatment groups clearly shows a lower incidence of CIN. However, in some studies the background CIN rate may be several times lower (Gomes et al. 2005; Heng et al. 2008) or higher (Droppa et al. 2011; Brueck et al. 2013; Diaz-Sandoval et al. 2002) than usual. Also the standard TAU used in the placebo group can be variable. The most obvious variation in TAU is the type and amount of IVF as some studies have demonstrated that larger amounts of IVF are protective against CIN (Poletti et al. 2013). However, the amount of IVF is often limited on a case-by-case basis if the patient has RI or heart failure. Other factors that significantly predict CIN but may not be well controlled in many studies include contrast volume (Briguori et al. 2002; Azmus et al. 2005; El Mahmoud et al. 2003; Oldemeyer et al.

2003; Chong et al. 2015), baseline RI (Azmus et al. 2005; Oldemeyer et al. 2003; Gulel et al. 2005; Chong et al. 2015; Rashid et al. 2004; Aslanger et al. 2012), gender (Chong et al. 2015), ejection fraction (Azmus et al. 2005; Aslanger et al. 2012), and NAC dose (Habib et al. 2016).

One of the most obvious limitations of the clinical studies is the outcome measure used. The CIN is a predefined measure that might not be sensitive to the protective effect of NAC on the kidney. Indeed, CIN is defined by a significant deterioration in kidney function. However, several studies demonstrate that NAC improves kidney function despite contrast injections (Sar et al. 2010; Shyu et al. 2002; Efrati et al. 2003; Kay et al. 2003; Drager et al. 2004; Awal et al. 2011; Ochoa et al. 2004). Many studies show that this difference was statistically significantly different than controls in which kidney function either didn't improve or, more commonly, worsened (Sar et al. 2010; Shyu et al. 2002; Efrati et al. 2003; Kay et al. 2003; Drager et al. 2004; Awal et al. 2011; Ochoa et al. 2004; Diaz-Sandoval et al. 2002) with some of these studies demonstrating no significant decrease in CIN incidence (Balderramo et al. 2004; Jo et al. 2009). Thus, the CIN based outcome measure may not be sensitive enough to detect the effect of NAC on the kidney.

Further to considering outcome measures, it must be appreciated that medically serious outcome measures such as the need for dialysis and mortality have been found not to be affected despite decreasing the incidence of CIN (Miner et al. 2004), although in other studies such serious outcomes were improved by NAC along with decreasing the incidence of CIN (Poletti et al. 2007; Carbonell et al. 2010; Marenzi et al. 2006). Thus, both the sensitivity of outcome measures and the clinical significance of outcome measures need to be considered in future studies. Indeed, although it may be possible that current studies thus far may have been insensitive to the effect of NAC on kidney function by concentrating on CIN incidence, it is of course important to consider the clinical long-term significance and reversibility of CIN, especially in vulnerable populations.

Perhaps the most interesting findings were in the studies that examined NAC dosing head to head. Several of these trials, all high quality, clearly demonstrated that higher doses of NAC were associated with more favorable outcomes in the context of CAG and/or PCI (Briguori et al. 2004; Marenzi et al. 2006; Habib et al. 2016; Recio-Mayoral et al. 2007). However, this was not true for the studies examining the protective effect of higher doses of NAC during contrast-enhanced CT and some studies examining high dose NAC as compared to placebo (Balderramo et al. 2004; ACT Trial Investigators 2011; Durham et al. 2002; Oldemeyer et al. 2003; Heng et al. 2008). This data suggests that higher doses may be helpful but it may be dependent on the procedure and other factors yet to be elucidated. Given the low percentages of positive trials it is not possible to make recommendations for the use of NAC for renal protection during angiography. Clearly more studies are needed to determine the optimal dose and the optimal patient population. Until consistent data is available, expert medical opinion must be used to guide the use of NAC during angiography.

14.3.2 Protection Against Kidney Injury from Amphotericin B

One study has examined the ability of NAC to prevent amphotericin B-induced nephrotoxicity (Adderson et al. 1991). In a medium-sized DBPC study (level 2b), 40 patients were given either oral NAC 600 mg or placebo twice daily during amphotericin B treatment. NAC was found to significantly decrease Cr/CCl defined nephrotoxicity (OR = 0.29, 95% CI: 0.082–0.993; $p = 0.05$), although an increase in AEs, particularly unpleasant taste, nausea and/or vomiting, was noted in the NAC group. Since there is only one study we cannot make a recommendation at this time but this is a promising area of clinical research.

14.3.3 Kidney Transplant

In a single-blind controlled study, 160 donors (level 2b) received 600 mg IV NAC 1 h before and 2 h after cerebral angiography performed to confirm brain death or TAU (Orban et al. 2015). In the recipients, neither delayed graft function, need for dialysis, Cr, GFR nor daily urine output was affected by NAC treatment. As there is only one study that examined this question, there can be no recommendation made at this time.

14.3.4 Aortic Aneurysm Repair

In a DBPC study (level 2b), 42 patients undergoing elective aortic aneurysm repair received oral NAC 1200 mg twice a day the day before the procedure and IV NAC 600 mg every 12 h for 48 h after the procedure (Macedo et al. 2006). The incidence of acute renal failure, mortality, length of ICU stay did not differ between groups. As there is only one study that examined this question, there can be no recommendation made at this time.

14.3.5 Prolonged Hypotension

A prospective, randomized, DBPC study (level 1b) determined whether NAC could prevent acute renal failure in 142 ICU patients with at least 30 min of hypotension (Komisarof et al. 2007). NAC or placebo was started within 12 h of hypotensive event and was continued for 7 days. NAC did not decrease the incidence of acute renal failure nor did it significantly change the indices of renal function, mortality, or hospital care, although there were trend toward a decreased incidence of acute renal failure in some subgroups. As there is only one study that examined this question, there can be no recommendation made at this time.

14.3.6 Hematopoietic Stem Cell Transplantation

One DBPC study (level 1b) examined the effect of NAC on acute renal injury in 80 patients undergoing hematopoietic stem cell transplantation (Ataei et al. 2015). Patients received placebo or IV NAC 100 mg/kg/day from 6 days prior to 15 days after transplantation. NAC did not decrease the incidence of acute kidney injury, nor did it affect the urine neutrophil gelatinase-associated lipocalin or transplant-related outcomes. Although the frequency of AEs were not different between groups, three patients had to be dropped from the NAC treatment group because of AEs, including abdominal pain, shortness of breath, and rash with pruritus. As there is only one study that examined this question, there can be no recommendation made at this time.

14.4   Treatment of Renal Disease

14.4.1 Cardiorenal Syndrome

In a small DBPC crossover study (level 2b) with 7-day washout, 9 patients with both heart and renal failure were randomized to receive orally either placebo or 500 mg NAC (Camuglia et al. 2013). NAC improved forearm blood flow but not B-type natriuretic peptide nor renal or heart function. The authors suggested that this effect was due to improvement in systemic oxidative stress and endothelial dysfunction. Given that there is only one study we cannot make a recommendation at this time but the positive pilot study suggests that this is a promising area of clinical research.

14.4.2 Acute Pyelonephritis

In a medium-sized DBPC trial (level 2b) the effect of a 5-day weight-based NAC treatment was tested on 70 children with acute pyelonephritis with respect to inflammatory biomarkers (Allameh et al. 2015). NAC did not significantly affect any of the inflammatory or clinical outcome measures, including procalcitonin or C-reactive protein levels, leukocyte or neutrophil counts. Given that there is only one study we cannot make a recommendation at this time.

14.4.3 Dialysis

Several studies have examined the effect of NAC on patients undergoing hemodialysis (HD; 3 studies) and peritoneal dialysis (PD; 1 study).

A prospective randomized placebo-controlled study of 134 patients (level 1b) with end-stage renal disease (ESRD) undergoing HD found that oral NAC 600 mg twice a day significantly reduced the incidence of cardiovascular events, from 47% to 28%, within 2 years of treatment as compared to placebo (Tepel et al. 2003). In another study of 60 patients (level 2b) with ESRD, IV NAC during HD decreased pulse pressure as compared to placebo (Thaha et al. 2006). In a third study (level 2b), 38 HD patients treated with oral NAC 200 mg three times a day were found to have a higher hematocrit as compared to 276 HD patients not receiving NAC (Hsu et al. 2010). Given that there is one level 1b and two level 2b studies, the grade of recommendation is B. With 100% positive outcomes, the recommendation is yes for use of NAC in HD.

Only one study has examined the effect of NAC in PD. In a prospective study of 20 patients treated with chronic PD (level 2b), oral NAC 1200 mg twice daily for 2 weeks was found to improve residual renal function (Feldman et al. 2012). Because of the limited number of studies the grade of recommendation is C. We cannot make a recommendation for use of NAC in PD because of the few studies but with 100% positive outcomes for both HD and PD studies, this is a promising area of clinical research.

14.4.4 Homocysteine

Homocysteine (HC) is particularly important in kidney disease as abnormally high levels commonly persist in dialysis patients, increasing their risk for vascular events. Thus, several studies have examined the effect of NAC on HC levels (Online Table 14.6). In 11 patients undergoing HD (level 2b), NAC given before dialysis lowered HC levels but did not augment the effect of HD on removal of HC (Bostom et al. 1996). In a small DBPC cross-over (level 2b) trial (Scholze et al. 2004) and a larger randomized parallel (level 2b) trial (Thaha et al. 2006), IV NAC during HD was found to significantly lower HC levels. However, two studies did not confirm a HC lower effect of NAC. 1.2 g of oral NAC twice a day did not lower HC levels when given for 4 weeks in a small (level 2b) placebo controlled study (Friedman et al. 2003) or when given with a renin-angiotensin system blocker (level 2b) for 8 weeks (Renke et al. 2010). Thus, the overall grade of recommendation for using NAC for HD patients in order to lower HC levels is B, with a mixed recommendation for treatment. From the studies it seems like providing oral or IV NAC with diagnosis is a yes recommendation as all of the studies are positive, whereas prolonged daily administration of oral NAC is a no recommendation as none of the studies have demonstrated an effect.

14.4.5 End Stage Renal Disease

In an open-label study (level 2b) oral NAC 1200 mg twice a day for four doses did not alter Cr or CyC in 29 ESRD patients (Rehman et al. 2008). Given that there is only one study we cannot make a recommendation at this time.

14.4.6 Proteinuria

In a placebo-controlled, randomized, open-label cross-over study, adding oral NAC 1200 mg/day to a renin-angiotensin-aldosterone system blocker did not improve measures of renal function (Renke et al. 2008) or ambulatory blood pressure (Renke et al. 2010) in 20 non-diabetic patients with proteinuria. Given that there is only one study we cannot make a recommendation at this time.

14.5   Summary

In our systematic review we found many clinical trials that examined the effect of NAC in protecting the kidney from iatrogenic injury, specifically from exposure to radiological contrast, Amphotericin B, kidney transplant, aortic aneurysm repair, prolonged hypotension and hematopoietic stem cell transplantation, and somewhat fewer studies on the treatment of kidney disease, specifically cardiorenal syndrome, acute pyelonephritis, dialysis, chronic renal disease and proteinuria.

Overall there are very variable outcomes with regard to the effects of NAC on renal function. While there are many studies that showed positive effects of NAC on renal function, there are many studies that did not demonstrate significant effects. Importantly, no study found NAC to be detrimental on renal function and very few studies reported any AEs as a result of NAC. Thus, there is little downside to the use of NAC in areas where it appears it might be helpful and there are several biomarker studies that demonstrate improvement in oxidative stress, immune system, and endothelial function. Importantly, because NAC is readily oxidized to di-NAC, which can have oxidative rather than reductive effects, the source and form of NAC administered in these clinical trials is a significant source of variation. For example, in a very large recent clinical trial the importance of protecting the NAC from oxidation was not addressed (Weisbord et al. 2018). Clearly more studies are needed using formulations of NAC that are not oxidized. However, there currently are no active registered clinical trials examining the effect of NAC on renal function.

Thus, the recommendations for use of NAC in the majority of renal disorders are still limited based on the number and the quality of studies (Table 14.2). For prophylactic use of NAC, it use only with radiological contrast in the emergency department at low-dose and non-emergently can be recommended. There are many studies with regard to its use in angiography, but the results are very mixed. Its use as a prophylactic agent has been investigated in other areas but there are very few studies to make any conclusion. For the treatment of kidney disease, NAC seems to be useful in conjunction with hemodialysis, particularly for the purpose of lowering homocysteine. Its use in conjunction with peritoneal dialysis is promising but there are very few studies to make any recommendation. While larger controlled trials are needed to establish effectiveness of NAC, available evidence so far and safety profile of NAC support its potential as a novel treatment option for renal disorders.

Table 14.2 Summary of clinical trials and recommendations

Renal condition	Studies positive % (positive/total)	Grade of recommendation	Recommendation for treatment
Prophylactic treatment			
Contrast for CT in ED: low dose	75% (1.5/2)	A	Yes
Contrast for CT in ED: high dose	0% (0/2)	A	No
Contrast for CT: non-emergent	67% (2/3)	B	Yes
Contrast for CT: overall	50% (3.5/7)	A	Mixed
Angiography: oral route	39% (14/36)	A	None
Angiography: IV route	29% (3.5/12)	A	None
Amphotericin B	100% (1/1)	C	None
Kidney transplant	0% (0/1)	C	None
Aortic aneurysm repair	0% (0/1)	C	None
Prolonged hypotension	0% (0/1)	B	None
Hematopoietic stem cell transplantation	0% (0/1)	B	None
Treatment for renal disease			
Cardiorenal syndrome	50% (0.5/1)	C	None
Acute pyelonephritis	0% (0/1)	C	None
Hemodialysis	100% (3/3)	B	Yes
Homocysteine lowering with hemodialysis	100% (3/3)	B	Yes
Homocysteine lowering given daily	0% (0/2)	B	No
Homocysteine overall	60% (3/5)	B	Mixed
Peritoneal dialysis	100% (1/1)	C	None
End-stage renal disease	0% (0/1)	C	None
Proteinurea	0% (0/1)	C	None

References

ACT Trial Investigators (2009) Rationale, design, and baseline characteristics of the acetylcystein for contrast-induced nephropathy (ACT) trial: a pragmatic randomized controlled trial to evaluate the efficacy of acetylcysteine for the prevention of contrast-induced nephropathy. Trials 10:38. https://doi.org/10.1186/1745-6215-10-38

ACT Trial Investigators (2011) Acetylcysteine for prevention of renal outcomes in patients undergoing coronary and peripheral vascular angiography: main results from the randomized acetylcysteine for contrast-induced nephropathy trial (ACT). Circulation 124(11):1250–1259. https://doi.org/10.1161/circulationaha.111.038943

Adderson EE, Shackelford PG, Quinn A, Carroll WL (1991) Restricted IgH chain V gene usage in the human antibody response to Haemophilus influenzae type b capsular polysaccharide. J Immunol 147:1667–1674

Allameh Z, Karimi A, Rafiei Tabatabaei S, Sharifian M, Salamzadeh J (2015) Effect of N-acetylcysteine on inflammation biomarkers in pediatric acute pyelonephritis: a randomized controlled trial. Iran J Kidney Dis 9(6):454–462

Amini M, Salarifar M, Amirbaigloo A, Masoudkabir F, Esfahani F (2009) N-acetylcysteine does not prevent contrast-induced nephropathy after cardiac catheterization in patients with diabetes mellitus and chronic kidney disease: a randomized clinical trial. Trials 10:45. https://doi.org/10.1186/1745-6215-10-45

Aslanger E, Uslu B, Akdeniz C, Polat N, Cizgici Y, Oflaz H (2012) Intrarenal application of N-acetylcysteine for the prevention of contrast medium-induced nephropathy in primary angioplasty. Coron Artery Dis 23(4):265–270. https://doi.org/10.1097/MCA.0b013e328351aacc

Ataei S, Hadjibabaie M, Moslehi A, Taghizadeh-Ghehi M, Ashouri A, Amini E, Gholami K, Hayatshahi A, Vaezi M, Ghavamzadeh A (2015) A double-blind, randomized, controlled trial on N-acetylcysteine for the prevention of acute kidney injury in patients undergoing allogeneic hematopoietic stem cell transplantation. Hematol Oncol 33(2):67–74. https://doi.org/10.1002/hon.2141

Awal A, Ahsan SA, Siddique MA, Banerjee S, Hasan MI, Zaman SM, Arzu J, Subedi B (2011) Effect of hydration with or without n-acetylcysteine on contrast induced nephropathy in patients undergoing coronary angiography and percutaneous coronary intervention. Mymensingh Med J 20(2):264–269

Azmus AD, Gottschall C, Manica A, Manica J, Duro K, Frey M, Bulcao L, Lima C (2005) Effectiveness of acetylcysteine in prevention of contrast nephropathy. J Invasive Cardiol 17(2):80–84

Balderramo DC, Verdu MB, Ramacciotti CF, Cremona LS, Lemos PA, Orias M, Eduardo M Jr (2004) Renoprotective effect of high periprocedural doses of oral N-acetylcysteine in patients scheduled to undergo a same-day angiography. Rev Fac Cienc Med 61(2):13–19

Baranska-Kosakowska A, Zakliczynski M, Przybylski R, Zembala M (2007) Role of N-acetylcysteine on renal function in patients after orthotopic heart transplantation undergoing coronary angiography. Transplant Proc 39(9):2853–2855. https://doi.org/10.1016/j.transproceed.2007.08.057

Berwanger O, Cavalcanti AB, Sousa AM, Buehler A, Castello-Junior HJ, Cantarelli MJ, Mangione JA, Bergo RR, Sao Thiago LE, Nunes PM, da Motta PA, Kodama A, Victor E, Carvalho VO, Sousa JE (2013) Acetylcysteine for the prevention of renal outcomes in patients with diabetes mellitus undergoing coronary and peripheral vascular angiography: a substudy of the acetylcysteine for contrast-induced nephropathy trial. Circ Cardiovasc Interv 6(2):139–145. https://doi.org/10.1161/circinterventions.112.000149

Boccalandro F, Amhad M, Smalling RW, Sdringola S (2003) Oral acetylcysteine does not protect renal function from moderate to high doses of intravenous radiographic contrast. Catheter Cardiovasc Interv 58(3):336–341. https://doi.org/10.1002/ccd.10389

Bostom AG, Shemin D, Yoburn D, Fisher DH, Nadeau MR, Selhub J (1996) Lack of effect of oral N-acetylcysteine on the acute dialysis-related lowering of total plasma homocysteine in hemodialysis patients. Atherosclerosis 120(1-2):241–244

Briguori C, Colombo A, Violante A, Balestrieri P, Manganelli F, Paolo Elia P, Golia B, Lepore S, Riviezzo G, Scarpato P, Focaccio A, Librera M, Bonizzoni E, Ricciardelli B (2004) Standard vs double dose of N-acetylcysteine to prevent contrast agent associated nephrotoxicity. Eur Heart J 25(3):206–211. https://doi.org/10.1016/j.ehj.2003.11.016

Briguori C, Manganelli F, Scarpato P, Elia PP, Golia B, Riviezzo G, Lepore S, Librera M, Villari B, Colombo A, Ricciardelli B (2002) Acetylcysteine and contrast agent-associated nephrotoxicity. J Am Coll Cardiol 40(2):298–303

Brueck M, Cengiz H, Hoeltgen R, Wieczorek M, Boedeker RH, Scheibelhut C, Boening A (2013) Usefulness of N-acetylcysteine or ascorbic acid versus placebo to prevent contrast-induced acute kidney injury in patients undergoing elective cardiac catheterization: a single-center, prospective, randomized, double-blind, placebo-controlled trial. J Invasive Cardiol 25(6):276–283

Buyukhatipoglu H, Sezen Y, Yildiz A, Bas M, Kirhan I, Ulas T, Turan MN, Taskin A, Aksoy N (2010) N-acetylcysteine fails to prevent renal dysfunction and oxidative stress after noniodine contrast media administration during percutaneous coronary interventions. Pol Arch Med Wewn 120(10):383–389

Camuglia AC, Maeder MT, Starr J, Farrington C, Kaye DM (2013) Impact of N-acetylcysteine on endothelial function, B-type natriuretic peptide and renal function in patients with the cardio-renal syndrome: a pilot cross over randomised controlled trial. Heart Lung Circ 22(4):256–259. https://doi.org/10.1016/j.hlc.2012.10.012

Carbonell N, Blasco M, Sanjuan R, Perez-Sancho E, Sanchis J, Insa L, Bodi V, Nunez J, Garcia-Ramon R, Miguel A (2007) Intravenous N-acetylcysteine for preventing contrast-induced nephropathy: a randomised trial. Int J Cardiol 115(1):57–62. https://doi.org/10.1016/j.ijcard.2006.04.023

Carbonell N, Sanjuan R, Blasco M, Jorda A, Miguel A (2010) N-acetylcysteine: short-term clinical benefits after coronary angiography in high-risk renal patients. Rev Esp Cardiol 63(1):12–19

Chong E, Poh KK, Lu Q, Zhang JJ, Tan N, Hou XM, Ong HY, Azan A, Chen SL, Chen JY, Ali RM, Fang WY, Lau TW, Tan HC (2015) Comparison of combination therapy of high-dose oral N-acetylcysteine and intravenous sodium bicarbonate hydration with individual therapies in the reduction of contrast-induced nephropathy during cardiac catheterisation and percutaneous coronary intervention (CONTRAST): a multi-Centre, randomised, controlled trial. Int J Cardiol 201:237–242. https://doi.org/10.1016/j.ijcard.2015.07.108

Diaz-Sandoval LJ, Kosowsky BD, Losordo DW (2002) Acetylcysteine to prevent angiography-related renal tissue injury (the APART trial). Am J Cardiol 89(3):356–358

Drager LF, Andrade L, Barros de Toledo JF, Laurindo FR, Machado Cesar LA, Seguro AC (2004) Renal effects of N-acetylcysteine in patients at risk for contrast nephropathy: decrease in oxidant stress-mediated renal tubular injury. Nephrol Dial Transplant 19(7):1803–1807. https://doi.org/10.1093/ndt/gfh261

Droppa M, Desch S, Blase P, Eitel I, Fuernau G, Schuler G, Adams V, Thiele H (2011) Impact of N-acetylcysteine on contrast-induced nephropathy defined by cystatin C in patients with ST-elevation myocardial infarction undergoing primary angioplasty. Clin Res Cardiol 100(11):1037–1043. https://doi.org/10.1007/s00392-011-0338-8

Durham JD, Caputo C, Dokko J, Zaharakis T, Pahlavan M, Keltz J, Dutka P, Marzo K, Maesaka JK, Fishbane S (2002) A randomized controlled trial of N-acetylcysteine to prevent contrast nephropathy in cardiac angiography. Kidney Int 62(6):2202–2207. https://doi.org/10.1046/j.1523-1755.2002.00673.x

Efrati S, Dishy V, Averbukh M, Blatt A, Krakover R, Weisgarten J, Morrow JD, Stein MC, Golik A (2003) The effect of N-acetylcysteine on renal function, nitric oxide, and oxidative stress after angiography. Kidney Int 64(6):2182–2187. https://doi.org/10.1046/j.1523-1755.2003.00322.x

El Mahmoud R, Le Feuvre C, Le Quan Sang KH, Helft G, Beygui F, Batisse JP, Metzger JP (2003) Absence of nephro-protective effect of acetylcysteine in patients with chronic renal failure investigated by coronary angiography. Arch Mal Coeur Vaiss 96(12):1157–1161

Feldman L, Shani M, Sinuani I, Beberashvili I, Weissgarten J (2012) N-acetylcysteine may improve residual renal function in hemodialysis patients: a pilot study. Hemodial Int 16(4):512–516. https://doi.org/10.1111/j.1542-4758.2012.00702.x

Ferrario F, Barone MT, Landoni G, Genderini A, Heidemperger M, Trezzi M, Piccaluga E, Danna P, Scorza D (2009) Acetylcysteine and non-ionic isosmolar contrast-induced nephropathy—a randomized controlled study. Nephrol Dial Transplant 24(10):3103–3107. https://doi.org/10.1093/ndt/gfp306

Friedman AN, Bostom AG, Laliberty P, Selhub J, Shemin D (2003) The effect of N-acetylcysteine on plasma total homocysteine levels in hemodialysis: a randomized, controlled study. Am J Kidney Dis 41(2):442–446. https://doi.org/10.1053/ajkd.2003.50054

Fung JW, Szeto CC, Chan WW, Kum LC, Chan AK, Wong JT, Wu EB, Yip GW, Chan JY, Yu CM, Woo KS, Sanderson JE (2004) Effect of N-acetylcysteine for prevention of contrast nephropathy in patients with moderate to severe renal insufficiency: a randomized trial. Am J Kidney Dis 43(5):801–808

Goldenberg I, Shechter M, Matetzky S, Jonas M, Adam M, Pres H, Elian D, Agranat O, Schwammenthal E, Guetta V (2004) Oral acetylcysteine as an adjunct to saline hydration for the prevention of contrast-induced nephropathy following coronary angiography. A randomized controlled trial and review of the current literature. Eur Heart J 25(3):212–218. https://doi.org/10.1016/j.ehj.2003.11.011

Gomes VO, Poli de Figueredo CE, Caramori P, Lasevitch R, Bodanese LC, Araujo A, Roedel AP, Caramori AP, Brito FS Jr, Bezerra HG, Nery P, Brizolara A (2005) N-acetylcysteine does not prevent contrast induced nephropathy after cardiac catheterisation with an ionic low osmolality contrast medium: a multicentre clinical trial. Heart 91(6):774–778. https://doi.org/10.1136/hrt.2004.039636

Gulel O, Keles T, Eraslan H, Aydogdu S, Diker E, Ulusoy V (2005) Prophylactic acetylcysteine usage for prevention of contrast nephropathy after coronary angiography. J Cardiovasc Pharmacol 46(4):464–467

Habib M, Hillis A, Hammad A (2016) N-acetylcysteine and/or ascorbic acid versus placebo to prevent contrast-induced nephropathy in patients undergoing elective cardiac catheterization: the NAPCIN trial; a single-center, prospective, randomized trial. Saudi J Kidney Dis Transpl 27(1):55–61. https://doi.org/10.4103/1319-2442.174072

Heng AE, Cellarier E, Aublet-Cuvelier B, Decalf V, Motreff P, Marcaggi X, Deteix P, Souweine B (2008) Is treatment with N-acetylcysteine to prevent contrast-induced nephropathy when using bicarbonate hydration out of date? Clin Nephrol 70(6):475–484

Hsu SP, Chiang CK, Yang SY, Chien CT (2010) N-acetylcysteine for the management of anemia and oxidative stress in hemodialysis patients. Nephron Clin Pract 116(3):c207–c216. https://doi.org/10.1159/000317201

Hsu TF, Huang MK, Yu SH, Yen DH, Kao WF, Chen YC, Huang MS (2012) N-acetylcysteine for the prevention of contrast-induced nephropathy in the emergency department. Intern Med 51(19):2709–2714

Jaffery Z, Verma A, White CJ, Grant AG, Collins TJ, Grise MA, Jenkins JS, McMullan PW, Patel RA, Reilly JP, Thornton SN, Ramee SR (2012) A randomized trial of intravenous n-acetylcysteine to prevent contrast induced nephropathy in acute coronary syndromes. Catheter Cardiovasc Interv 79(6):921–926. https://doi.org/10.1002/ccd.23157

Jo SH, Koo BK, Park JS, Kang HJ, Kim YJ, Kim HL, Chae IH, Choi DJ, Sohn DW, Oh BH, Park YB, Choi YS, Kim HS (2009) N-acetylcysteine versus AScorbic acid for preventing contrast-induced nephropathy in patients with renal insufficiency undergoing coronary angiography NASPI study-a prospective randomized controlled trial. Am Heart J 157(3):576–583. https://doi.org/10.1016/j.ahj.2008.11.010

Kay J, Chow WH, Chan TM, Lo SK, Kwok OH, Yip A, Fan K, Lee CH, Lam WF (2003) Acetylcysteine for prevention of acute deterioration of renal function following elective coronary angiography and intervention: a randomized controlled trial. JAMA 289(5):553–558

Kefer JM, Hanet CE, Boitte S, Wilmotte L, De Kock M (2003) Acetylcysteine, coronary procedure and prevention of contrast-induced worsening of renal function: which benefit for which patient? Acta Cardiol 58(6):555–560. https://doi.org/10.2143/ac.58.6.2005321

Kim BJ, Sung KC, Kim BS, Kang JH, Lee KB, Kim H, Lee MH (2010) Effect of N-acetylcysteine on cystatin C-based renal function after elective coronary angiography (ENABLE study): a prospective, randomized trial. Int J Cardiol 138(3):239–245. https://doi.org/10.1016/j.ijcard.2008.08.013

Kinbara T, Hayano T, Ohtani N, Furutani Y, Moritani K, Matsuzaki M (2010) Efficacy of N-acetylcysteine and aminophylline in preventing contrast-induced nephropathy. J Cardiol 55(2):174–179. https://doi.org/10.1016/j.jjcc.2009.10.006

Kitzler TM, Jaberi A, Sendlhofer G, Rehak P, Binder C, Petnehazy E, Stacher R, Kotanko P (2012) Efficacy of vitamin E and N-acetylcysteine in the prevention of contrast induced kidney injury in patients with chronic kidney disease: a double blind, randomized controlled trial. Wien Klin Wochenschr 124(9-10):312–319. https://doi.org/10.1007/s00508-012-0169-2

Komisarof JA, Gilkey GM, Peters DM, Koudelka CW, Meyer MM, Smith SM (2007) N-acetylcysteine for patients with prolonged hypotension as prophylaxis for acute renal failure (NEPHRON). Crit Care Med 35(2):435–441. https://doi.org/10.1097/01.ccm.0000253816.83011.db

Levin A, Pate GE, Shalansky S, Al-Shamari A, Webb JG, Buller CE, Humphries KH (2007) N-acetylcysteine reduces urinary albumin excretion following contrast administration: evidence of biological effect. Nephrol Dial Transplant 22(9):2520–2524. https://doi.org/10.1093/ndt/gfl707

Macedo E, Abdulkader R, Castro I, Sobrinho AC, Yu L, Vieira JM Jr (2006) Lack of protection of N-acetylcysteine (NAC) in acute renal failure related to elective aortic aneurysm repair-a randomized controlled trial. Nephrol Dial Transplant 21(7):1863–1869. https://doi.org/10.1093/ndt/gfl079

Marenzi G, Assanelli E, Marana I, Lauri G, Campodonico J, Grazi M, De Metrio M, Galli S, Fabbiocchi F, Montorsi P, Veglia F, Bartorelli AL (2006) N-acetylcysteine and contrast-induced nephropathy in primary angioplasty. N Engl J Med 354(26):2773–2782. https://doi.org/10.1056/NEJMoa054209

Miner SE, Dzavik V, Nguyen-Ho P, Richardson R, Mitchell J, Atchison D, Seidelin P, Daly P, Ross J, McLaughlin PR, Ing D, Lewycky P, Barolet A, Schwartz L (2004) N-acetylcysteine reduces contrast-associated nephropathy but not clinical events during long-term follow-up. Am Heart J 148(4):690–695. https://doi.org/10.1016/j.ahj.2004.05.015

Moist L, Sontrop JM, Gallo K, Mainra R, Cutler M, Freeman D, House AA (2010) Effect of N-acetylcysteine on serum creatinine and kidney function: results of a randomized controlled trial. Am J Kidney Dis 56(4):643–650. https://doi.org/10.1053/j.ajkd.2010.03.028

Nascimento MM, Suliman ME, Silva M, Chinaglia T, Marchioro J, Hayashi SY, Riella MC, Lindholm B, Anderstam B (2010) Effect of oral N-acetylcysteine treatment on plasma inflammatory and oxidative stress markers in peritoneal dialysis patients: a placebo-controlled study. Perit Dial Int 30(3):336–342. https://doi.org/10.3747/pdi.2009.00073

Ochoa A, Pellizzon G, Addala S, Grines C, Isayenko Y, Boura J, Rempinski D, O'Neill W, Kahn J (2004) Abbreviated dosing of N-acetylcysteine prevents contrast-induced nephropathy after elective and urgent coronary angiography and intervention. J Interv Cardiol 17(3):159–165. https://doi.org/10.1111/j.1540-8183.2004.09880.x

Oldemeyer JB, Biddle WP, Wurdeman RL, Mooss AN, Cichowski E, Hilleman DE (2003) Acetylcysteine in the prevention of contrast-induced nephropathy after coronary angiography. Am Heart J 146(6):E23. https://doi.org/10.1016/s0002-8703(03)00511-8

Orban JC, Quintard H, Cassuto E, Jambou P, Samat-Long C, Ichai C (2015) Effect of N-acetylcysteine pretreatment of deceased organ donors on renal allograft function: a randomized controlled trial. Transplantation 99(4):746–753. https://doi.org/10.1097/tp.0000000000000395

Poletti PA, Platon A, De Seigneux S, Dupuis-Lozeron E, Sarasin F, Becker CD, Perneger T, Saudan P, Martin PY (2013) N-acetylcysteine does not prevent contrast nephropathy in patients with renal impairment undergoing emergency CT: a randomized study. BMC Nephrol 14:119. https://doi.org/10.1186/1471-2369-14-119

Poletti PA, Saudan P, Platon A, Mermillod B, Sautter AM, Vermeulen B, Sarasin FP, Becker CD, Martin PY (2007) IV N-acetylcysteine and emergency CT: use of serum creatinine and cystatin C as markers of radiocontrast nephrotoxicity. AJR Am J Roentgenol 189(3):687–692. https://doi.org/10.2214/ajr.07.2356

Purwanto B, Prasetyo DH (2012) Effect of oral N-acetylcysteine treatment on immune system in continuous ambulatory peritoneal dialysis patients. Acta Med Indones 44(2):140–144

Rashid ST, Salman M, Myint F, Baker DM, Agarwal S, Sweny P, Hamilton G (2004) Prevention of contrast-induced nephropathy in vascular patients undergoing angiography: a randomized controlled trial of intravenous N-acetylcysteine. J Vasc Surg 40(6):1136–1141. https://doi.org/10.1016/j.jvs.2004.09.026

Recio-Mayoral A, Chaparro M, Prado B, Cozar R, Mendez I, Banerjee D, Kaski JC, Cubero J, Cruz JM (2007) The Reno-protective effect of hydration with sodium bicarbonate plus N-acetylcysteine in patients undergoing emergency percutaneous coronary intervention: the RENO study. J Am Coll Cardiol 49(12):1283–1288. https://doi.org/10.1016/j.jacc.2006.11.034

Rehman T, Fought J, Solomon R (2008) N-acetylcysteine effect on serum creatinine and cystatin C levels in CKD patients. Clin J Am Soc Nephrol 3(6):1610–1614. https://doi.org/10.2215/cjn.01560408

Renke M, Tylicki L, Rutkowski P, Larczynski W, Aleksandrowicz E, Lysiak-Szydlowska W, Rutkowski B (2008) The effect of N-acetylcysteine on proteinuria and markers of tubular injury in non-diabetic patients with chronic kidney disease. A placebo-controlled, randomized, open, cross-over study. Kidney Blood Press Res 31(6):404–410. https://doi.org/10.1159/000185828

Renke M, Tylicki L, Rutkowski P, Larczynski W, Neuwelt A, Aleksandrowicz E, Lysiak-Szydlowska W, Rutkowski B (2010) The effect of N-acetylcysteine on blood pressure and markers of cardiovascular risk in non-diabetic patients with chronic kidney disease: a placebo-controlled, randomized, cross-over study. Med Sci Monit 16(7):Pi13–Pi18

Sadat U, Walsh SR, Norden AG, Gillard JH, Boyle JR (2011) Does oral N-acetylcysteine reduce contrast-induced renal injury in patients with peripheral arterial disease undergoing peripheral angiography? A randomized-controlled study. Angiology 62(3):225–230. https://doi.org/10.1177/0003319710377078

Saddadi F, Alatab S, Pasha F, Ganji MR, Soleimanian T (2014) The effect of treatment with N-acetylcysteine on the serum levels of C-reactive protein and interleukin-6 in patients on hemodialysis. Saudi J Kidney Dis Transpl 25(1):66–72

Sahin G, Yalcin AU, Akcar N (2007) Effect of N-acetylcysteine on endothelial dysfunction in dialysis patients. Blood Purif 25(4):309–315. https://doi.org/10.1159/000106103

Saitoh T, Satoh H, Nobuhara M, Machii M, Tanaka T, Ohtani H, Saotome M, Urushida T, Katoh H, Hayashi H (2011) Intravenous glutathione prevents renal oxidative stress after coronary angiography more effectively than oral N-acetylcysteine. Heart Vessel 26(5):465–472. https://doi.org/10.1007/s00380-010-0078-0

Sandhu C, Belli AM, Oliveira DB (2006) The role of N-acetylcysteine in the prevention of contrast-induced nephrotoxicity. Cardiovasc Intervent Radiol 29(3):344–347. https://doi.org/10.1007/s00270-005-0127-8

Sar F, Saler T, Ecebay A, Saglam ZA, Ozturk S, Kazancioglu R (2010) The efficacy of n-acetylcysteine in preventing contrast-induced nephropathy in type 2 diabetic patients without nephropathy. J Nephrol 23(4):478–482

Scholze A, Rinder C, Beige J, Riezler R, Zidek W, Tepel M (2004) Acetylcysteine reduces plasma homocysteine concentration and improves pulse pressure and endothelial function in patients with end-stage renal failure. Circulation 109(3):369–374. https://doi.org/10.1161/01.cir.0000109492.65802.ad

Seyon RA, Jensen LA, Ferguson IA, Williams RG (2007) Efficacy of N-acetylcysteine and hydration versus placebo and hydration in decreasing contrast-induced renal dysfunction in patients undergoing coronary angiography with or without concomitant percutaneous coronary intervention. Heart Lung 36(3):195–204. https://doi.org/10.1016/j.hrtlng.2006.08.004

Shahbazian H, Shayanpour S, Ghorbani A (2016) Evaluation of administration of oral N-acetylcysteine to reduce oxidative stress in chronic hemodialysis patients: a double-blind, randomized, controlled clinical trial. Saudi J Kidney Dis Transpl 27(1):88–93. https://doi.org/10.4103/1319-2442.174084

Shyu KG, Cheng JJ, Kuan P (2002) Acetylcysteine protects against acute renal damage in patients with abnormal renal function undergoing a coronary procedure. J Am Coll Cardiol 40(8):1383–1388

Sochman J, Krizova B (2006) Prevention of contrast agent-induced renal impairment in patients with chronic renal insufficiency and heart disease by high-dose intravenous N-acetylcysteine: a pilot-ministudy. Kardiol Pol 64(6):559–564; discussion 565-556

Swarnalatha G, Ram R, Neela P, Naidu MU, Dakshina Murty KV (2010) Oxidative stress in hemodialysis patients receiving intravenous iron therapy and the role of N-acetylcysteine in preventing oxidative stress. Saudi J Kidney Dis Transpl 21(5):852–858

Tanaka A, Suzuki Y, Suzuki N, Hirai T, Yasuda N, Miki K, Fujita M, Tanaka T (2011) Does N-acetylcysteine reduce the incidence of contrast-induced nephropathy and clinical events in patients undergoing primary angioplasty for acute myocardial infarction? Inter Med 50(7):673–677

Tepel M, van der Giet M, Schwarzfeld C, Laufer U, Liermann D, Zidek W (2000) Prevention of radiographic-contrast-agent-induced reductions in renal function by acetylcysteine. N Engl J Med 343(3):180–184. https://doi.org/10.1056/nejm200007203430304

Tepel M, van der Giet M, Statz M, Jankowski J, Zidek W (2003) The antioxidant acetylcysteine reduces cardiovascular events in patients with end-stage renal failure: a randomized, controlled trial. Circulation 107(7):992–995

Thaha M, Widodo, Pranawa W, Yogiantoro M, Tomino Y (2008) Intravenous N-acetylcysteine during hemodialysis reduces asymmetric dimethylarginine level in end-stage renal disease patients. Clin Nephrol 69(1):24–32

Thaha M, Yogiantoro M, Tomino Y (2006) Intravenous N-acetylcysteine during haemodialysis reduces the plasma concentration of homocysteine in patients with end-stage renal disease. Clin Drug Investig 26(4):195–202

Thiele H, Hildebrand L, Schirdewahn C, Eitel I, Adams V, Fuernau G, Erbs S, Linke A, Diederich KW, Nowak M, Desch S, Gutberlet M, Schuler G (2010) Impact of high-dose N-acetylcysteine versus placebo on contrast-induced nephropathy and myocardial reperfusion injury in unselected patients with ST-segment elevation myocardial infarction undergoing primary percutaneous coronary intervention. The LIPSIA-N-ACC (prospective, single-blind, placebo-controlled, randomized Leipzig immediate percutaneous coronary intervention acute myocardial infarction N-ACC) trial. J Am Coll Cardiol 55(20):2201–2209. https://doi.org/10.1016/j.jacc.2009.08.091

Traub SJ, Mitchell AM, Jones AE, Tang A, O'Connor J, Nelson T, Kellum J, Shapiro NI (2013) N-acetylcysteine plus intravenous fluids versus intravenous fluids alone to prevent contrast-induced nephropathy in emergency computed tomography. Ann Emerg Med 62(5):511–520. e525. https://doi.org/10.1016/j.annemergmed.2013.04.012

Trimarchi H, Mongitore MR, Baglioni P, Forrester M, Freixas EA, Schropp M, Pereyra H, Alonso M (2003) N-acetylcysteine reduces malondialdehyde levels in chronic hemodialysis patients—a pilot study. Clin Nephrol 59(6):441–446

Vallero A, Cesano G, Pozzato M, Garbo R, Minelli M, Quarello F, Formica M (2002) [Contrast nephropathy in cardiac procedures: no advantages with prophylactic use of N-acetylcysteine (NAC)]. G Ital Nefrol 19(5):529–533

Webb JG, Pate GE, Humphries KH, Buller CE, Shalansky S, Al Shamari A, Sutander A, Williams T, Fox RS, Levin A (2004) A randomized controlled trial of intravenous N-acetylcysteine for the prevention of contrast-induced nephropathy after cardiac catheterization: lack of effect. Am Heart J 148(3):422–429. https://doi.org/10.1016/j.ahj.2004.03.041

Weisbord SD, Gallagher M, Jneid H, Garcia S, Cass A, Thwin SS, Conner TA, Chertow GM, Bhatt DL, Shunk K, Parikh CR, McFalls EO, Brophy M, Ferguson R, Wu H, Androsenko M, Myles J, Kaufman J, Palevsky PM, PRESERVE Trial Group (2018) Outcomes after angiography with sodium bicarbonate and acetylcysteine. N Engl J Med 378(7):603–614. https://doi.org/10.1056/NEJMoa1710933

Wittstock A, Burkert M, Zidek W, Tepel M, Scholze A (2009) N-acetylcysteine improves arterial vascular reactivity in patients with chronic kidney disease. Nephron Clin Pract 112(3):c184–c189. https://doi.org/10.1159/000218107

Carol Conrad

15.1 Introduction

In this chapter the role of N-Acetylcysteine (NAC) in the treatment of patients with chronic obstructive pulmonary disease (COPD), cystic fibrosis (CF), and idiopathic pulmonary fibrosis (IPF) is discussed and provides the available and most credible evidence that oral NAC treatment may be effective in preventing exacerbations of the inflammatory pulmonary disorders caused by CF and COPD, but not effective and potentially harmful for patients with IPF.

Orally administered NAC is readily absorbed via the intestinal epithelium where it is immediately modified to liberate cysteine, which is transported to the liver, the main site for GSH synthesis. NAC, when taken orally, can reduce oxidative stress in cells. Free NAC in plasma is thought to act as a free radical scavenger, but, as well, it can provide the cysteine molecule that can be metabolized intracellularly to replenish low GSH levels at times of oxidative stress (Atkuri et al. 2007). While NAC can directly scavenge free radicals, the rate constant for its reaction with reactive oxygen species (ROS) such as hydrogen peroxide is several orders of magnitude lower than those of antioxidant enzymes such as superoxide dismutase (SOD), catalase, and glutathione peroxidase (Bonanomi and Gazzaniga 1980).

The airway lumen and the alveolar space of the lung are a unique redox environment unlike other extracellular compartments in other organs. The airway is exposed to higher levels of oxygen than any other mucosal surface in the body. In healthy human airways, the extracellular lung fluid GSH concentration is far higher than that of plasma. Generally, total GSH concentrations in the airway surface liquid (ASL) have been estimated to

Electronic supplementary material The online version of this article (https://doi.org/10.1007/978-981-10-5311-5_15) contains supplementary material, which is available to authorized users.

C. Conrad
Department of Pediatrics, Stanford University, Palo Alto, CA, USA
e-mail: cconrad@stanford.edu

© Springer Nature Singapore Pte Ltd. 2019
R. E. Frye, M. Berk (eds.), *The Therapeutic Use of N-Acetylcysteine (NAC) in Medicine*, https://doi.org/10.1007/978-981-10-5311-5_15

measure 275–500 μM in healthy patients (Roum et al. 1993; Moss et al. 2000; Cantin et al. 1987). GSH is needed to detoxify inhaled pollutants, and in inflammatory diseases, such as CF and COPD, inflammation from the innate and acquired immune defenses leads to significant increase in production of reactive oxygen species. GSH regulates intra- and extracellular oxidative metabolism and inflammatory processes and influences many cellular regulatory functions. It is present at low levels in plasma but can be secreted into certain extracellular compartments, when needed. Thus, GSH levels in the epithelial lining fluid of the lung (ELF) normally are 400 times greater than in plasma. GSH is crucial for balance and control of the inflammatory response in the airway lumen. A deficiency of GSH in the ASL results in injury to airway epithelium, and chronic inflammation compromises the integrity of the airway, causing bronchiectasis, cystic changes in the alveolar space, and eventual respiratory failure and early death.

In CF patients, GSH levels in whole blood, blood neutrophils (Tirouvanziam et al. 2006), and lymphocytes (Lands et al. 1999), and ELF (Tirouvanziam et al. 2002) are markedly decreased. This profound GSH depletion is believed to affect neutrophil recruitment to the lungs of CF patients and may contribute to the exuberant inflammatory response described in these patients.

COPD is a chronic lung disease that is similarly characterized by neutrophilic airway inflammation, leading to the development of chronic bronchitis, fibrosis in the small airways, and/or emphysema. The major risk factor for the development of COPD is chronic exposure to noxious gases and particles, including cigarette smoke (CS; Brusselle et al. 2011). The mechanisms underlying CS-induced airway inflammation in COPD patients are still largely unknown. Airway epithelial cells (AECs) are the first line of defense against inhaled toxicants, and it has been shown that these cells show cellular damage and cell death upon cigarette smoke exposure (Van der Toorn et al. 2013). Thus, to potentially ameliorate the lung dysfunction notable in COPD, NAC has been studied in clinical trials (Table 15.1).

Table 15.1 Summary of NAC mechanisms of action across different pulmonary disorders

Pulmonary disorder	Proposed mechanism of action of NAC after oral administration
Cystic fibrosis	Antioxidant effect by increased levels of glutathione intracellular (Bonanomi and Gazzaniga 1980)
	Anti-inflammatory effect by increased levels of glutathione in airway surface liquid (Stafanger and Koch 1989; Dauletbaev et al. 2009)
	Increase GSH content in neutrophils and lymphocytes (Tirouvanziam et al. 2006)
	Augment total intracellular GSH in deficit states and regulation of whole cell homeostasis (Rushworth and Megson 2014)
	Increase antioxidant capacity of plasma (Skov et al. 2015)
	Reduce airway inflammation by regulating redox signaling (Rahman et al. 2006)
COPD	Resolution of oxidative stress and inflammation (Barnes 2013; Wada and Takizawa 2013)
	Prevent exacerbations (Zheng et al. 2014; Tse et al. 2013)
	Decrease H_2O_2 content in airway surface liquid (De Benedetto et al. 2005)

In IPF, there is evidence that oxidant/antioxidant imbalance and oxidative stress play a role in alveolar epithelial cell injury and fibrogenesis. GSH, which inhibits fibroblast and lymphocyte proliferation and differentiation, is deficient in the epithelial lining fluid as well as intracellularly in bronchoalveolar lavage fluid (BAL) cells of IPF patients (Cantin et al. 1989). Given this evidence, clinicians have considered that an oxidant–antioxidant imbalance may contribute to the disease process in idiopathic pulmonary fibrosis as well.

The ability of NAC to protect isolated cells and animal lung in vivo against oxidant damage could be explained both by its ability to maintain intracellular GSH concentrations and by oxidant scavenging. NAC at low concentrations is a powerful scavenger of the myeloperoxidase-derived oxidant hypochlorous acid (HCIO) and is able to protect α1-antiprotease against damage by this oxidant (Arouma et al. 1989). This HCIO-scavenging action may be of particular importance in the lung, which is susceptible to proteolytic damage if α1-antiprotease is inactivated. It is most likely that the majority of the antioxidant effects attributed to NAC are actually mediated by increased intracellular GSH. This is important because for NAC to confer antioxidant activity, the condition for the therapeutic effect of NAC may require that GSH might have to be depleted intracellularly for NAC to have any beneficial effect.

15.2 Methods

A systematic online literature search using broad search terms was used: N-Acetylcysteine, NAC, COPD, IPF, idiopathic pulmonary fibrosis, cystic fibrosis, clinical trial, efficacy, oxidant, antioxidant, oxidation, oxidative stress, redox, and inflammation.

References cited in the publications were also reviewed. The studies reviewed in this chapter utilized standard methodologies used by Cochrane meta-analysis. Selection criteria for studies reviewed here were randomized, controlled trials comparing oral NAC to placebo in people with CF, COPD, and IPF. The author independently assessed trials for inclusion and analyzed methodological quality. For meta-analysis study reviews, the author independently assessed the studies reviewed for quality of data per the Oxford 2011 Level of Evidence classification (Howick et al. 2011) as outlined in the first chapter of this portion of the book. The level of evidence for efficacy of all studies reviewed is summarized in Online Tables 15.1, 15.2, and 15.3.

Table 15.2 Ongoing clinical trials on N-Acetylcysteine for pulmonary disease

Trial title	NCT #	Trial status
N-Acetylcysteine in early acute respiratory distress syndrome (NARDS)	NCT03346681	Active but not recruiting
Investigating significant health trends in idiopathic pulmonary fibrosis (INSIGHTS-IPF)	NCT01695408	Recruiting
Clinical trial of NAC in asthma (CONA)	NCT02605824	Recruiting

Table 15.3 Summary of clinical trials and recommendations

Pulmonary conditions	Controlled studies % (positive/total)	Grade of recommendation	Recommendation for treatment
Cystic fibrosis	56% (4.5/8)	B	Mixed
Chronic obstructive pulmonary disease	70% (3.5/5)	A	Yes
Idiopathic pulmonary fibrosis	33% (1/3)	A	No

Nine individual clinical studies of oral NAC were reviewed for CF, two meta-analyses and five clinical studies for COPD, and two meta-analyses and five individual clinical studies for IPF.

15.3 The Effectiveness of NAC in the Treatment of Inflammatory Pulmonary Diseases

15.3.1 Cystic Fibrosis (CF)

CF is a lethal autosomal recessive condition caused by mutations in the gene that encodes the transmembrane conductance regulator (CFTR). CFTR plays a key role in cell homeostasis. The primary cause of morbidity and mortality in patients with cystic fibrosis (CF) is lung disease. The pulmonary pathology of CF is characterized by oxidative stress. Symptoms of CF are generally manifest within the first decade of life, and the lungs of CF patients contain excessive amounts of thick, viscous mucus that is difficult to clear. Dysfunctional CFTR impairs the efflux of cell anions such as chloride and bicarbonate as well as reduced glutathione into the airways (Cantin et al. 2006). Due to these and other factors, the patients are susceptible to chronic infection by organisms such as *Staphylococcus aureus* and *Pseudomonas aeruginosa*. Total GSH concentration in CF airway surface liquid (ASL) is greatly decreased, measuring only 92 µM; thus levels are just 20–30% of GSH in healthy pulmonary ASL (Roum et al. 1993). In addition, extensive neutrophilic inflammation in the CF lung is present very early in the course of the disease, due, in part, to elevated levels of interleukin-8 (IL-8) and low levels of IL-10. Neutrophils release oxidants and proteases, particularly elastase. Persistent high-intensity inflammation leads to permanent structural damage of the CF airways. The presence of neutrophil elastase in the CF airway secretions precedes the appearance of bronchiectasis and correlates with lung function deterioration and respiratory exacerbations (Mayer-Hamblett et al. 2007). Both anti-inflammatory and antioxidant therapies are therefore of interest for CF lung disease.

NAC is a drug that was first reported to have clinical benefit in the early 1960s, when it was shown to be an effective mucolytic agent in patients with cystic fibrosis. In 1964, Reas concluded that inhalation of NAC is safe and effective as an inhaled mucolytic agent that increases the clearing of mucus from the lungs of patients with CF (Reas 1964; Hurst et al. 1967). Since those early publications, there have been a few clinical trials completed that assess the efficacy of orally administered NAC to improve lung function, as measured by the forced expiratory volume exhaled in 1 s (FEV$_1$, a measure of obstruction of the airways). Oral antioxidant therapy has been proposed for use in CF since the early 1960s. Until recently, however, substantive evidence that NAC leads to an improvement in airway mechanics or lung function has not been published, though some evidence indicates the potential of NAC to allay deterioration by improving oxidative stress. Figure 15.1 depicts the proposed mechanisms for oxidative imbalance in the airways of CF patients. Mitchell and Elliott (1982) were the first investigators to perform a placebo-controlled study with oral NAC in children with CF. The study was a single-center, randomized, double-blind, placebo-controlled (DBPC), crossover study design in 20 children with CF; mean age was 10.8 years. In the initial 2-week period, all participants took placebo, and then study drug was initiated. The total duration was 6 months (3 months in each limb and a 2-week washout period between the crossover period, when all participants took placebo). Outcomes included clinical assessment, body weight, chest x-ray (CXR) score, daily peak expiratory flow rate (PEF), antibiotic usage, cough frequency (scale of 0–3), and self-assessed sputum viscosity (scale of 0–3). Four subjects withdrew, and final analysis included only 16 participants. No difference was found between the groups, though peak flow as a measure of lung function is not very sensitive, as it measures the function of the larger airways, rather than the small airways, which is the main site of pathology in early CF.

Following that study, Ratjen et al. (1985) performed a placebo-controlled study comparing oral NAC with oral ambroxol (a mucolytic agent with antioxidant and

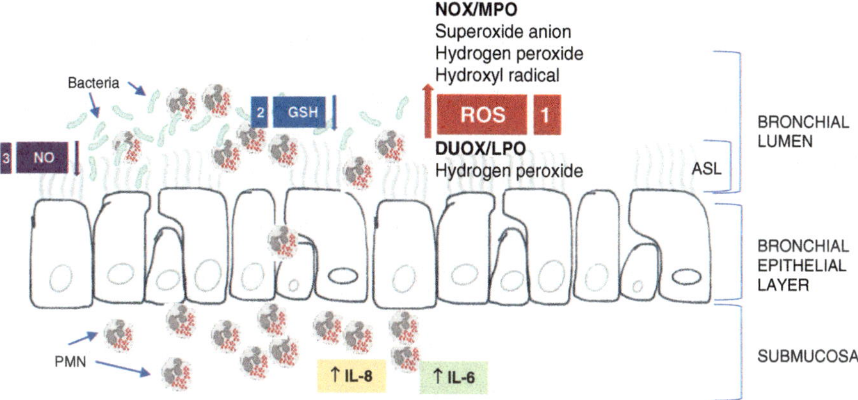

Fig. 15.1 Oxidative imbalance in conductive airways of patients affected by cystic fibrosis. The airway surface liquid (ASL) in CF bronchi is characterized by (1) increased concentration of reactive oxygen species (ROS), (2) lowered levels of glutathione (GSH), and (3) reduced nitric oxide (NO). The net increase of pro-oxidative species in ASL, as a result of derangements of both neutrophils and bronchial epithelial cells, contributes to the progressive lung tissue damage and to the amplification of the inflammatory response in CF airways. This is characterized by the release of chemokines and cytokines (e.g., IL-8 and IL-6, respectively). NOX, NADPH oxidase; MPO, myeloperoxidase; DUOX, dual oxidase; LPO, lactoperoxidase; IL, interleukin (Galli et al. 2012). Used by permission

anti-inflammatory properties). NAC was given orally in a DBPC 12-week trial with 36 CF patients (20 females, 16 males, age range 6–21, mean 13.9 years). The 36 patients were randomly assigned to 3 therapy groups (NAC, ambroxol, and placebo) with the use of a computer program; subjects were matched based on Chrispin-Norman scores and age. After a washout period where patients discontinued routine use of NAC, group 1 received ambroxol (30 mg, three times daily), group 2 received NAC (200 mg, three times daily), and group 3 received placebo. The drugs were indistinguishable with regard to taste, color, or odor. After 12 weeks, the investigators found a significant worsening of FEV_1 for the placebo group, while no changes for either the better or the worse were detected in the NAC and ambroxol groups.

Subsequently, in 1988, a Danish DBPC crossover study of the effects of oral NAC treatment was performed with either 200 mg × 3 daily (patients weighing <30 kg) or 400 mg × 2 daily (>30 kg) for 3 months in 41 CF patients. It was ensured that the subjects' airways were not colonized with *Pseudomonas aeruginosa* by being hospitalized for 14 days for an intravenous (IV) antibiotic "cleanout" (Stafanger et al. 1988). Placebo tablets contained bicarbonate only. The patients were randomized to receive either NAC or placebo for 3 months and were again hospitalized for a 14-day IV antibiotic "cleanout" before the next 3-month period after crossover. The outcome measures included a subjective clinical score, weight, sputum bacteriology, blood leukocyte count, sedimentation rate, titers of specific antimicrobial antibodies, and lung function parameters. The subjects who received NAC were noted to have a mild but statistically significant effect on lung function ($\Delta FEV_1\%$ pred <0.05).

In a follow-up study, the investigators examined the effect of the same dosing regimens in a crossover study alternating treatment with oral placebo or NAC for two 3-month periods (Stafanger and Koch 1989). They studied 52 CF patients with chronic *Pseudomonas aeruginosa* infection and examined clinical measures that included sputum bacteriology and titers of antimicrobial antibodies, as well as changes in lung function. Patients were enrolled immediately after hospitalization for 14-day IV antibiotic treatment directed toward the *Pseudomonas* infection. This IV antibiotic "cleanout" protocol was a routine practice in this CF center at the time. Thirty-one patients completed the study (40% dropout rate), and statistical analysis was performed only on these subjects, thus not on the "intent-to-treat" basis. No significant differences in clinical responses were observed for the entire cohort, but subgroup analysis of CF patients with FEV_1 <70% of predicted who received the NAC in the autumn months rather than summer showed that NAC treatment resulted in a significantly improved FEV_1 versus same subject placebo pretreatment ($p < 0.02$). With this, the authors suggest that NAC benefit might be due to its anti-oxidant/anti-inflammatory properties rather than its mucolytic properties.

The next interventional clinical trials with oral or inhaled NAC were published in 2006. In a phase I dose-ranging/safety study of 18 CF patients and 9 non-CF controls, investigators tested high-dose oral NAC (600–1000 mg three times daily) for 4 weeks to assess for safety and tolerability at the higher doses (Tirouvanziam et al. 2006). Significant increases in blood cell GSH concentrations and decreased sputum neutrophil counts were observed following treatment for all dose levels. No effects were detected on lung function in this short trial. Following the phase I study, the investigators then performed a proof of concept, a DBPC multicenter study in 70 CF subjects. Prior to opening the study to all sites, an early single-center safety study was performed to assure that high doses of NAC were not associated with complications of pulmonary hypertension in humans (Palmer et al. 2007). The subjects were randomly assigned to either 900 mg effervescent tablets of NAC three times daily or matched placebo for 6 months (Conrad et al. 2015). The research participants were randomized by a central pharmacy: 36 to NAC and 34 to placebo. Six participants in the NAC group and two in the placebo group were withdrawn or lost to follow-up. All but one participant in the placebo group were included in the intent-to-treat efficacy analysis. The baseline characteristics and randomization strata were similar between treatment groups. $FEV_1\%$ predicted was <60 in 40% of subjects, 27% of subjects were under 18 years of age, 67% used azithromycin chronically, and none used ibuprofen regularly. The primary outcome measure for the trial was the difference in human neutrophil elastase (HNE) activity levels in sputum measured at the beginning and end of the study. There was no significant change in HNE activity from baseline to week 24 ($p = 0.14$). However, a potentially substantial clinical benefit in the secondary outcome, the FEV_1, was detected. The NAC cohort maintained their baseline FEV_1 and $FEF_{25-75\%}$ throughout the 24-week period, while 4–6% declines in these measures occurred in the placebo cohort ($p = 0.02$; Fig. 15.2). This finding was unexpected, as the study was powered for the primary outcome –change in sputum neutrophil elastase activity. Slightly fewer subjects in the NAC group were treated for pulmonary exacerbations, though the

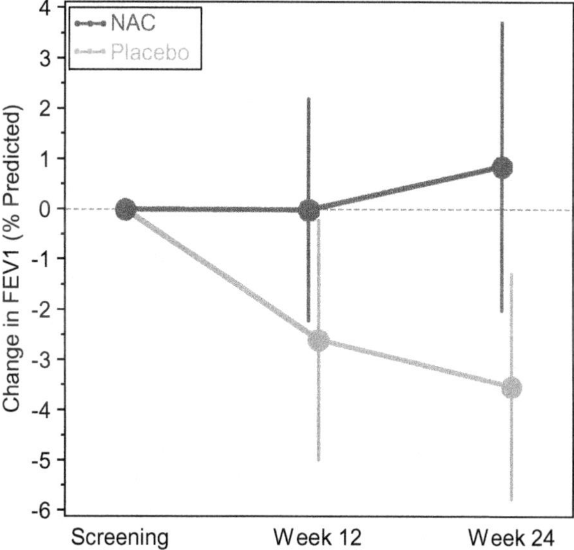

Fig. 15.2 Mean change from baseline in FEV_1 (L) over time by treatment group. The 95% confidence intervals are calculated using one-sample t-tests

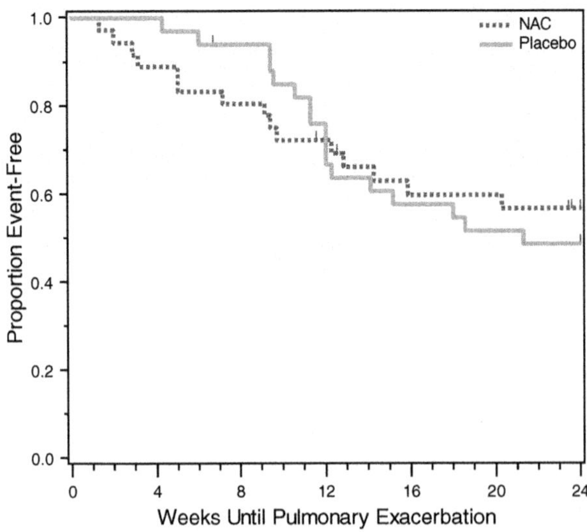

Fig. 15.3 Kaplan–Meier plot of time to pulmonary exacerbation. Censored subjects are denoted with "tick" marks

difference was not significant ($p = 0.48$). However, the Kaplan–Meier plot of time to pulmonary exacerbation did imply a trend toward improvement in this parameter toward the end of the study (Fig. 15.3). Whole blood GSH rather than intracellular levels measured by fluorescence-activated cell sorting (FACS) in neutrophils (as had been measured in the first single-center study) was the measure utilized, primarily due to the lability of neutrophils and the impracticality of transport of sample across centers. The fact that GSH in whole blood tends to be protein-bound or in the intracellular space could explain the lack of significant change in GSH.

Dauletbaev et al. (2009) performed a study to assess the safety and efficacy of high-dose oral NAC in CF patients. The study was a single-center, randomized, DBPC phase II 12-week study comparing low-dose (700 mg/daily) to high-dose (2800 mg/daily) NAC. Twenty-one CF patients with mild-to-moderate lung disease were enrolled. The subjects all underwent a 3-week washout period, followed by a 3-week placebo run-in phase, and then the two groups were randomly assigned to high- or low-dose NAC. The subjects enrolled were comparable in clinical parameters, though the low-dose group $FEV_1\%$ measured 15% higher compared to the higher-dose group at enrolment, though this was not statistically significant in this study ($p = 0.43$). Eleven subjects were randomized to the low-dose NAC and ten to the high-dose NAC. Outcomes included safety and clinical parameters, inflammatory measures (total leukocyte numbers, cell differentials, TNF-α, IL-8) in induced sputum, and concentrations of extracellular GSH in induced sputum and blood. Both doses of NAC were well-tolerated and safe. High-dose NAC did not alter clinical or inflammatory parameters. FEV_1 did not change significantly during medication with either dose of NAC ($p > 0.3$ for both groups). The concentrations of total GSH in induced sputum and blood plasma tended to increase in the high-dose group, but did not reach statistical significance. Inflammatory markers with TNF-α and IL-8 in induced sputum did not decrease. The investigators concluded that high-dose NAC is a well-tolerated and safe medication for a prolonged therapy of patients with CF with a potential to increase extracellular GSH in CF airways.

Pseudomonas aeruginosa lung infection adds an increase to the oxidative burden in CF airways due to increased production of reactive oxygen species as a result of the inflammatory response and impaired inactivation of the antioxidant systems. Skov et al. (2015) conducted an open-label, controlled, randomized trial with high-dose NAC over 4 weeks on 21 patients (11 NAC group and 10 control). Study treatment was 1200 mg of NAC twice daily. The control group maintained usual pulmonary toilet practices, but did not receive a matching placebo. It was hypothesized that high-dose oral NAC, as a source of GSH, would increase the antioxidant capacity of the plasma and subsequently decrease the levels of oxidative burden markers. Biochemical parameters of oxidative burden and plasma levels of antioxidants were measured at the beginning and end of the study. The biomarkers chosen included plasma malondialdehyde (MDA) and 8-isoprostane (8-isoP) and urinary excretion of 8-oxo-7,8-dihydro-2-deoxyguanosine (8-oxodG) and 8-oxo-7,8-dihydroguanosine (8-oxoGuo), as well as total plasma antioxidant levels of vitamin C and oxidized vitamin C (dehydroascorbic acid (DHA)). The secondary efficacy endpoints included lung function (FEV_1) and the oxidative burst in the peripheral blood mononuclear cells (PMNs) as an inflammatory parameter. The investigators detected a significant increase in the total plasma levels of the antioxidant ascorbic acid ($p = 0.037$) and a significant decrease in the levels of the oxidized form of vitamin C (dehydroascorbate; $p = 0.004$) compared to baseline in the NAC group. No significant differences were observed in the control group. The other parameters measuring oxidative burden did not change significantly compared to baseline in either of the groups. Improved lung function ($FEV_1\%$ predicted) was observed in the NAC-treated group, though the changes were not statistically significant.

The sum of these studies implies that long-term, high-dosage use of orally administered NAC can reduce pulmonary oxidative stress and inflammation after an extended time of treatment and can attenuate airway and parenchymal destruction. Growing evidence has suggested that cellular oxidative processes have a fundamental role in inflammation through the activation of stress kinases (c-Jun N-terminal kinases (JNK), mitogen-activated protein kinase (MAPK and p38)) and redox-sensitive transcription factors such as nuclear factor kappa B (NF-kB) and AP-1 (activating protein-1), which differentially regulate the genes for pro-inflammatory mediators and protective antioxidant genes such as gamma-glutamylcysteine synthetase (γ-GCS), manganese-dependent superoxide dismutase (Mn-SOD), and heme oxygenase-1 (HO-1). Oral thiol derivatives may have a mechanism of action in reducing airway inflammation by regulating redox signaling (Fig. 15.4; Rahman et al. 2006). The study by Conrad et al. (2015) is the most definitive study to demonstrate these subtle effects on preserving lung function, which, in CF, predictably deteriorates over a period of 6 months. In the lung, the effects of antioxidant therapy with NAC most likely are related to its

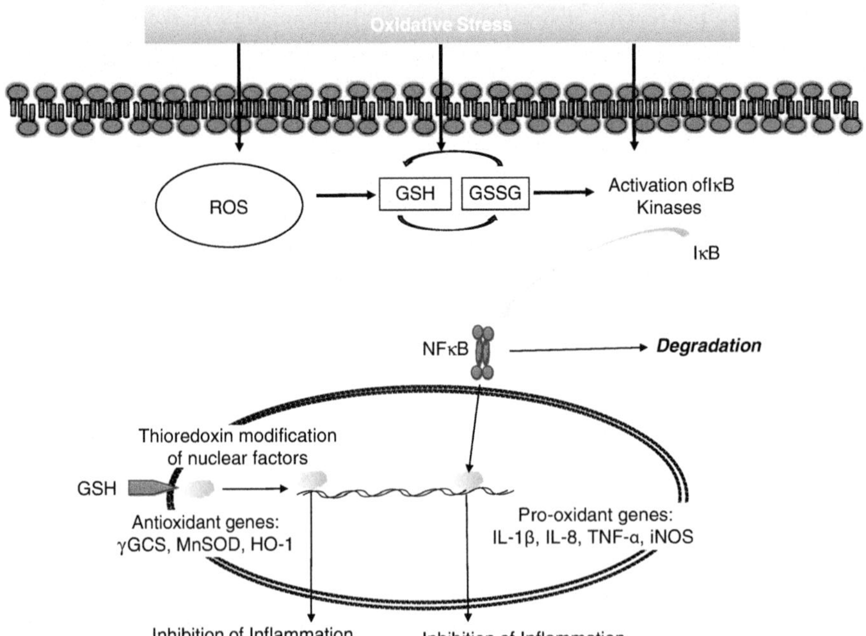

Fig. 15.4 Regulation of inflammatory state in the airway epithelial cell by redox mechanisms. (Modified from Rahman et al. 2006). Inflammatory response is mediated either directly by ROS or by reduced levels of glutathione, which in turn activates NF-kB and p38 MAP kinase. The activation of NF-kB leads to the expression of proinflammatory genes by acetylation of master transcriptional regulator and subunit of NF-kB resulting in inflammation. GSH inhibits oxidative stress-mediated inflammation by suppressing the activity of NF-kB either through Nrf2 (nuclear factor erythroid 2-related factor)-induced phase-2 antioxidant enzymes (GSH), IkB pathway, or decreasing activity of ROS and nuclear activation factors

effect in augmenting total intracellular GSH in deficit states and its contribution to whole cell homeostasis. (Fig. 15.5, Rushworth and Megson 2014).

The summary table at the beginning of the chapter provides information on the studies performed and level of evidence to date of the utility of NAC in treatment of lung disease of CF (Online Table 15.1). This author calculates a level "A" evidence that NAC, taken at high doses, and for at least 6 months can ameliorate deterioration of lung function in CF patients.

15.3.2 Chronic Obstructive Pulmonary Disease (COPD)

COPD is a lung disease associated primarily with cigarette smoking, but inhalation of other noxious agents such as smoke fumes and other injurious particles can also cause sustained lung inflammation in patients who eventually develop COPD. The Global Initiative for Chronic Obstructive Lung Disease (GOLD) is a project initiated by the National Heart, Lung, and Blood Institute (NHLBI) and the World Health

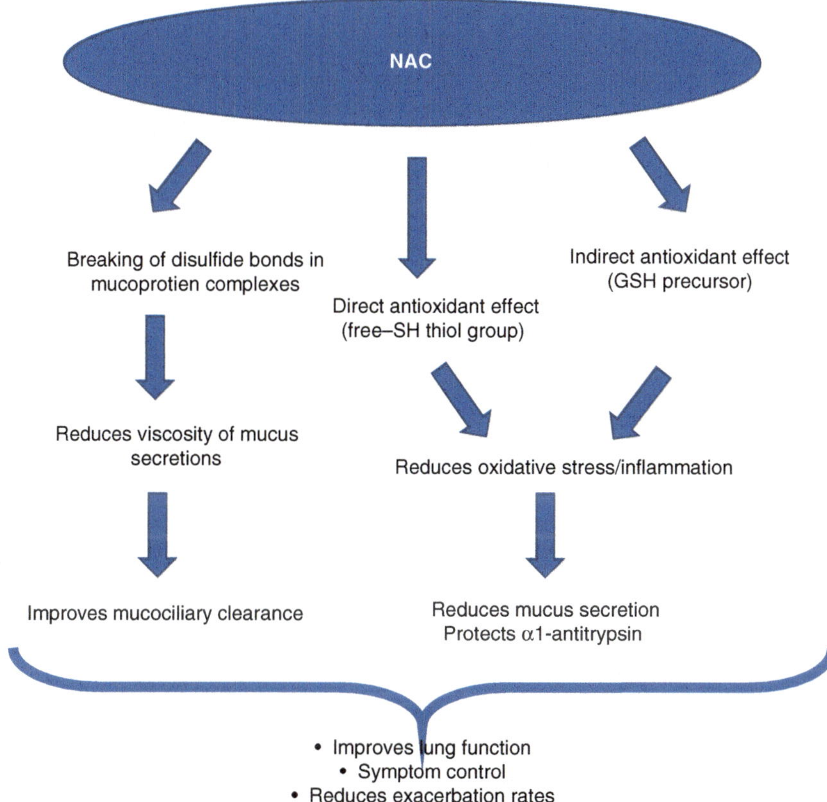

Fig. 15.5 Mechanisms of action of N-Acetylcysteine (NAC). NAC acts as a mucolytic, antioxidant, and anti-inflammatory agent. The free sulfhydryl group confers NAC with the ability to reduce disulfide bonds, thus decreasing mucus viscosity and facilitating mucociliary clearance. The antioxidant activity of NAC may be both direct (the free sulfhydryl group may serve as a ready source of reducing equivalents) and indirect (through replenishment of intracellular GSH levels) antioxidant effects (Modified from Rushworth and Megson 2014)

Organization (WHO). GOLD defines COPD as: "…a common, preventable, and treatable disease that is characterized by persistent respiratory symptoms and airflow limitation that is due to airway and/or alveolar abnormalities usually caused by significant exposure to noxious particles or gases. Chronic airflow limitation characterizes COPD. It is caused by both small airway disease (e.g., obstructive bronchiolitis) and parenchymal destruction (emphysema). Chronic inflammation causes structural changes, small airways narrowing, and destruction of lung parenchyma. A loss of small airways may contribute to airflow imitation and mucociliary dysfunction, a characteristic feature of the disease" (GOLD 2017; www.goldcopd.org).

Oxidative stress plays a key role in driving COPD-related inflammation, even in ex-smokers, and might result in activation of the proinflammatory transcription factor nuclear factor kB (NF-kB), impaired antiprotease defenses, DNA damage, cellular senescence, autoantibody generation, and corticosteroid resistance through inactivation of histone deacetylase 2 (Barnes 2016). Biomarkers such as hydrogen peroxide and 8-isoprostane are increased in sputum and the systemic circulation of COPD patients, and oxidative stress is further increased during exacerbations. Oxidants are released from activated inflammatory cells such as macrophages and neutrophils, and a deficit of endogenous antioxidants may exist in COPD patients. For these reasons, the potential benefit of antioxidant therapy with NAC has been examined in several clinical research trials to assess its efficacy in ameliorating the symptoms of COPD and potential to improve lung function.

Antioxidant therapy has been proposed for use in COPD since the early 1980s, as for CF. There is a large body of evidence that oxidative stress plays an important role in the pathogenesis of COPD (MacNee 2005). Markers of oxidative stress have been demonstrated in the airways, breath condensate, sputum, blood, and urine of smokers and patients with COPD (MacNee 2000; GOLD 2017). There is also evidence that endogenous antioxidants such as reduced GSH and lung GSH biosynthesizing enzymes are significantly decreased in patients with COPD (Malhotra et al. 2008). Furthermore, oxidative stress has been reported to increase concomitantly as GSH levels are depleted during severe COPD exacerbations (Drost et al. 2005). Inhaled bronchodilators and inhaled corticosteroids are the mainstay of treatment for COPD (GOLD 2017; Qaseem et al. 2011). Given their key role in the pathogenesis of COPD, oxidative stress and inflammation could represent promising therapeutic targets for the treatment of this disease (Barnes 2013; Wada and Takizawa 2013).

Cazzola et al. (2015) published the results of a meta-analysis testing the available evidence that NAC treatment may be effective in preventing exacerbations of chronic bronchitis or COPD and evaluating whether there is a substantial difference between the responses induced by low (<600 mg per day) and high ($\geq$600 mg per day) doses of NAC. Thirteen studies were identified for evaluation, and each study was scored utilizing the Jadad scoring system to describe the quality of evidence provided by the design methodology of the trials (Jadad et al. 1996). The Jadad scoring system provides a scale of 0 (worst) to 5 (superior). The major points for scoring include a yes or no answer given to three questions: (1) Was the study described as randomized? (2) Was the study described as double blind? (3) Was there a description of withdrawals and dropouts? Additional points were given if the method of randomization was described in the paper, and was appropriate, or the method of blinding was described and it was appropriate. Points were deducted if the method of randomization was described, but was inappropriate, or the method of blinding was described, but was inappropriate. The point total for the score each study received was not provided. The range of Jadad scores for these 13 studies was 1–4.

From the 13 included studies, performed between the dates of 1976 and 2014, a total of 4155 COPD patients (NAC $n = 1933$; placebo or controls $n = 2222$) were selected. Three studies used high-dose NAC ($\geq$ 600 mg/day), nine used low-dose NAC ($\leq$ 600 mg/day), and one investigated both low- and high-dose NAC. A subgroup analysis was performed on seven studies that were randomized controlled trials (RCTs) in COPD patients (per the American Thoracic Society/European Respiratory Society (ATS/ERS) (Celli and MacNee 2004) or (GOLD 2014) definition) to provide recommendations. The meta-analysis results demonstrate that patients treated with NAC had significantly and consistently fewer exacerbations of chronic bronchitis or COPD (relative risk 0.75, 95% CI 0.66–0.84; $p < 0.01$), although the protective effect was more apparent in chronic bronchitis patients without evidence of airway obstruction. High doses of NAC were also effective in patients suffering from COPD (per GOLD criteria; relative risk 0.75, 95% CI 0.68–0.82; $p = 0.04$).

Fowdar et al. (2017) subsequently performed an updated meta-analysis that included randomized, placebo-controlled trials with oral NAC in COPD. They included 12 studies, ten of which were also included in the Cazzola meta-analysis. Using stricter inclusion criteria, they identified 12 trials that enrolled a total of 2691 patients and occurred between the years 1976 and 2014. The reviewers include studies with the following characteristics: (1) subjects enrolled with stable (per definition) COPD disease status; (2) pulmonary function tests with obstructive characteristics of COPD per GOLD criteria (ten of the studies); (3) the therapeutic intervention with oral NAC for more than 4 weeks, in addition to standard therapy; (4) placebo-controlled; (5) randomized or crossover controlled trial design; (6) and the number of patients with at least one exacerbation as the primary outcome and other effect indexes as the secondary outcomes. Sample sizes ranged from 24 to 1006 participants. Participants were randomly assigned to study drug, NAC ($n = 1339$), or placebo control ($n = 1352$) groups. The baseline characteristics of the two groups did not differ. All studies were randomized. A matching placebo was used to blind both the participants and the investigators in all but one study. Withdrawals and dropouts were described in all but two studies. Overall, the quality of the 12 studies was high per Jadad scoring criteria, which ranged from 2 to 5 (summary of clinical studies in COPD, Online Table 15.2). NAC doses ranged from 257 to 1800 mg/day, and study drug treatment duration ranged from 3 to 36 months. The meta-analysis determined that both high-dose and low-dose NAC treatment with duration of at least 6 months reduced the prevalence of COPD exacerbations. NAC treatment did not affect exacerbation rate, the FEV_1, forced vital capacity (FVC), or inspiratory capacity (IC). The conclusion of the meta-analysis by Fowder et al. was that use of long-term NAC therapy might reduce risk of COPD exacerbation. There was no detectable effect on lung function, and the authors suppose that the reason for that is likely due to previous constriction due to airway remodeling and the development of irreversible airflow constriction.

For both meta-analyses, Zheng et al. (2014) received the highest Jadad score (4 by Cazzola and 5 by Fowder). Zheng et al. performed a DBPC, parallel, multicenter (34 centers) study over 1 year comparing NAC 600 mg or matched placebo taken orally in addition to their usual regimen on the exacerbation rate in 1 year (PANTHEON study). The groups were well-matched in all baseline characteristics, including $FEV_1\%$ of predicted, age, and level of severity of COPD per GOLD criteria. There were no differences noted in baseline therapies prescribed between the two groups. Follow-up visits occurred at 1, 2, 6, 9, and 12 months. Analysis conducted on intent-to-treat (ITT) basis. They did not outline the statistical methods for handling missing data. Four hundred and eighty-two subjects were enrolled into each group (total 964). Seven hundred and sixty-three subjects completed the 1 year study. The primary outcome measure was time to first exacerbation, time to recurrent exacerbation, number of participants requiring systemic corticosteroids or antibiotics or use of short-acting beta-agonist (SABA) rescue medication, St. George's Respiratory Questionnaire (SGRQ – Chinese version), spirometry, and adverse events (including hospitalization or death). After 1 year, 497 acute exacerbations in 482 patients in the NAC group who received at least one dose and had at least one assessment visit (1·16 exacerbations per patient-year) and 641 acute exacerbations in 482 patients in the placebo group (1·49 exacerbations per patient-year; risk ratio 0·78, p = 0·0011). The authors thus concluded that their findings show that in Chinese patients with moderate-to-severe COPD, long-term use of NAC 600 mg twice daily can prevent exacerbations, especially in disease of moderate severity. The report does not supply data regarding assessment of adherence to the medication regimen over the year, though it reports the mean treatment duration of completers was 319·0 days (SD 102·3) in the NAC group and 319·1 days (105·2). Neither do the investigators report the use of concomitant medications such as other antioxidants or alternate therapies, some of which may have efficacy in treatment of lung disease associated with oxidant excess and many of which are likely to be used "off-label" in China where many herbal and homeopathic remedies are utilized in the treatment of disease. Nonetheless, we find the evidence for the use of NAC in COPD to be at a level 1a evidence of efficacy.

Tse et al. (2013) designed a DBPC study to investigate the efficacy of high-dose NAC plus usual therapy in Chinese patients with air trapping and airway resistance of stable COPD, titled the HIACE study. The duration was 1 year in length conducted in Kwong Wah Hospital, Hong Kong. Eligible patients aged 50–80 years of age were randomized to receive NAC 600 mg bid or identical placebo after 4-week run-in. The treating physician and patients were blinded, though a third party was not blinded. The primary outcome was small airways function as assessed via GOLD standard definition of lung function parameters. Other outcome measures included exacerbation and admission rates, and subjects were assessed every 16 weeks for 1 year. One hundred and twenty of 133 patients were eligible for the study. Aside from a predominance of men in each group, baseline characteristics were similar in the two groups. At 1 year, there was a significant improvement in forced expiratory flow ($FEF_{25-75\%}$; p = 0.03) though this measure is not accepted by ATS/ERS as significant. As well, a significant reduction in exacerbation frequency (0.96 times/year vs. 1.71 times/year, p = 0.019) was noted for the NAC group vs. placebo. No major adverse effects were reported. The authors conclude that 1-year treatment with high-dose NAC resulted in significantly improved small airways function and decreased exacerbation frequency in patients with stable COPD, though the sample size in the study was too small to detect an improvement in other lung function parameters such as FEV_1. Therefore, studies with larger sample sizes are warranted to assess the effects of maintenance treatment with high-dose NAC in COPD.

To investigate whether treatment with the inhaled corticosteroid fluticasone propionate (FP) or NAC is effective in primary care patients, Schermer et al. (2009)

performed a 3-year phase IV, randomized, DBPC, double-dummy study comparing the efficacy of inhaled FP 500 mg twice daily, oral NAC 600 mg once daily, or placebo preceded by a 3-month washout and 2-week prednisolone pretreatment. The Cazzola and Fowder meta-analyses awarded this study with a Jadad score of 4 and 5, respectively. Patients were ex-smokers with chronic bronchitis or COPD. Exacerbation rate and quality of life measured with the Chronic Respiratory Questionnaire (CRQ) were the primary outcomes; FEV_1 decline and respiratory symptoms were secondary outcomes. Two hundred and eighty-six patients recruited from 44 general practices were randomized for the study. Results indicate that the exacerbation rate was 1.35 times higher for NAC ($p = 0.054$) and 1.30 times higher for FP ($p = 0.095$) compared with placebo. CRQ total scores did not differ between NAC ($p = 0.306$) or FP ($p = 0.581$) treatment compared to placebo. The authors concluded that in this study comparing low-dose NAC with high-dose fluticasone propionate, no beneficial treatment effects were noted for either study drug compared to placebo.

Decramer et al. (2005) (BRONCUS trial) performed a 3-year, phase III, two-arm, DBPC, parallel-group study of 523 patients from 50 centers with COPD which were randomly assigned to 600 mg daily NAC or placebo. Primary outcomes were yearly reduction in forced expiratory volume in 1 s (FEV_1) and the number of exacerbations per year. Analysis was by intention to treat. The groups were well-matched, blinding was adequate, and those lost to follow up were equal for both groups and accounted for. Both studies received Jadad score of 4 from the meta-analysis reviewers. Overall, yearly exacerbation rates did not differ between patients allocated N-Acetylcysteine and those allocated placebo ($p = 0·85$). In patients who were not taking inhaled corticosteroids ($n = 155$), risk of exacerbation was lower for those assigned NAC than for those assigned placebo ($p = 0.040$). Similarly, patients who were not taking inhaled corticosteroids and were assigned NAC had fewer moderate or severe exacerbations than did those who were assigned placebo ($p = 0.032$). No effect on exacerbation rate was recorded in smokers or non-smokers or in patients in GOLD stage II or III.

A 1-year DBPC study was performed in 2001 to determine the effect of NAC, 600 mg effervescent tablets once a day for 12 months on the concentration of H_2O_2 and thiobarbituric acid reactive substances (TBARs) in expired breath condensate and serum levels of two lipid peroxidation products (TBARs, lipid peroxides) in patients with COPD. Forty-four outpatients with stable COPD (22 in the NAC group and 22 in the placebo group) completed the study. Specimens of expired breath condensate and serum were collected at the randomization visit and then every 3 months over 1 year. The concentration of TBARs and H_2O_2 in expired breath condensate was measured spectrofluorimetrically by the thiobarbituric acid and homovanillic acid methods, respectively. Serum levels of lipid peroxides were determined spectrophotometrically after extraction with butanol and pyridine. Initially, H_2O_2 exhalation did not differ between the placebo and NAC groups up to 6 months of treatment. After this the significant differences were observed. After 9 and 12 months of treatment, NAC group exhaled 2.3-fold ($p < 0.04$) and 2.6-fold ($p < 0.05$) less H_2O_2 than placebo receivers, respectively. No significant effect of

NAC administration on TBARs exhalation and serum levels of TBARs and lipid peroxides was noted over the whole treatment period. Also no significant associations between exhaled H_2O_2 and concentrations of lipid peroxidation products were noted in both treatment groups at any time point. These authors note that their results indicate that long-term oral administration of NAC attenuates H_2O_2 formation in the airways of COPD subjects and prove antioxidant action of drug. However, further studies are necessary to estimate the clinical significance of this finding (Kasielski and Nowak 2001).

Other, less rigorously designed trials have been published. De Benedetto et al. (2005) performed a single blind (to the chemist performing measurements), placebo-controlled study aimed to study the effect of 2 months' treatment with oral NAC compared to placebo on the H_2O_2 content in exhaled air condensate (EAC) of clinically stable COPD patients, mean age 65.93 ± 9.3 years. After clinical examination, pulmonary function tests, and collection of EAC for the basal (T0) assay of H_2O_2, 55 patients were randomly allocated to group A (usual therapy plus oral NAC 600 mg BID for 2 months) or group B (usual therapy plus placebo BID for 2 months). H_2O_2 assay in EAC was repeated at day 15, day 30, and day 60 after the start of therapy in each group. All patients were non-smokers or ex-smokers for at least 5 years, and the two groups were comparable in terms of demographic, respiratory function, and EAC data at baseline. The H_2O_2 level in EAC of group A was significantly decreased at T15 (1.00 ± 0.38 SD mM; $p = 0.003$), T30 (0.91 ± 0.44 mM; $p = 0.007$), and T60 (0.83 ± 0.41 mM; $p = 0.000$) compared to T0 (1.28 ± 0.61 mM). No significant decrease in H_2O_2 of group B was measured at any time point. The investigators conclude that oral NAC 600 mg BID for 2 months rapidly reduces the oxidant burden in airways of stable COPD patients.

Overall, the sum of these studies indicate that NAC may reduce the number of exacerbations in people with COPD by a small amount, but do not appear to cause any harm (Online Table 15.2). The reduction is at most one fewer exacerbation every 3 years. One person in eight may avoid having an exacerbation, provided all take treatment every day for an average of 10 months. Mucolytics have not been shown to slow the decline in lung function in COPD patients, and it is uncertain whether they improve quality of life or hospitalizations (Poole et al. 2015).

In summary, the level of evidence of the benefits of NAC is of an A level recommendation, though overall, the beneficial effects of oral administration of NAC is seen only after treatment periods of at least 6 months for reducing exacerbations and improving symptoms of chronic bronchitis (Stey et al. 2000). A subsequent systematic review of mucolytics in chronic bronchitis or COPD began to stratify where mucolytics might be found to be most cost-effective, advocating their use in patients with severe COPD who are susceptible to repeated exacerbations.

15.3.3 Idiopathic Pulmonary Fibrosis

Idiopathic pulmonary fibrosis (IPF) is a chronic, progressive lung disease of unknown cause that is characterized by the histopathological or radiologic patterns of usual interstitial pneumonia in a typical clinical setting (Raghu et al. 2011; Thannickal et al. 2004). IPF is thought to occur as a consequence of an interaction between multiple risk factors (genetic and environmental) that predispose to an aberrant repair response, particularly by repeated micro-injuries to an aging alveolar epithelium. Abnormalities in multiple pathways involved in wound healing and inflammation lead to the development of IPF. The injury to the lung parenchyma is thought to stimulate epithelial repair mechanisms that, in turn, theoretically initiate aberrant epithelial–fibroblast communication. Rather than leading to resolution, the injury activates myofibroblasts to build a thick collagen matrix in the interstitial compartment of the lung, resulting in extensive remodeling (Richeldi et al. 2017). There is evidence that oxidant/antioxidant imbalance and oxidative stress play a role in alveolar epithelial cell injury and fibrogenesis. The major pulmonary antioxidant, GSH, which inhibits fibroblast and lymphocyte proliferation and differentiation, is lacking in the epithelial lining fluid as well as intracellularly in bronchoalveolar lavage (BAL) fluid cells of IPF patients (Cantin et al. 1989).

The pathology of IPF involves many associated factors, and studies of familial interstitial pneumonia have identified rare genetic variants, including genes associated with surfactant dysfunction (SFTPC, SFTPA2) and telomere biology and maintenance (TERT, TERC, PARN, RTEL, OBFC1; Nogee et al. 2001; Tsakiri et al. 2007; Wang et al. 2009; Stuart et al. 2015; Cogan et al. 2015). Genome-wide association studies (GWAS) have identified common genetic variants that account for about a third of the risk to develop disease. In addition, recent studies indicate the potential importance of alterations in host defense (MUC5B, ATP11A, TOLLIP) and epithelial barrier function (DSP, DPP9; Fingerlin et al. 2013; Noth et al. 2013). Moreover, a common gain-of-function variant in the gene MUC5B promoter region is associated with the greatest relative risk to develop idiopathic pulmonary fibrosis, both familial and sporadic cases. The site of altered MUC5B production has been localized to bronchiolar epithelium, where it might either impede normal lung repair, or, alternatively, enhance injury (Evans et al. 2016).

A number of clinical studies performed to evaluate NAC for the treatment of IPF in combination with "standard therapies" have produced conflicting results. The landmark early trial testing the efficacy of NAC in IPF was performed by Demedts et al. (2005), in the IFIGENIA trial. The results showed that high-dose NAC, added to standard therapy (prednisone and azathioprine), demonstrated a slowing of physiological decline as measured in the FVC and the diffusing capacity for carbon monoxide (D_LCO), as well as an improved lung function in IPF patients compared with standard therapy alone. However, there have been some concerns over the design of the trial due to the relatively small numbers of patients it recruited (Fioret et al. 2011). By contrast, in a DBPC trial, Martinez et al. (2014) studied IPF patients with mild-to-moderate impairment in pulmonary function with a three-drug regimen of prednisone, azathioprine, and NAC; NAC alone; or placebo. The study was interrupted owing to safety concerns associated with the three-drug regimen. The trial continued as a two-group study (acetylcysteine vs. placebo) without other changes; 133 and 131 patients were enrolled in the acetylcysteine and placebo groups, respectively. The primary outcome was the change in forced vital capacity

(FVC) over a 60-week period. At 60 weeks, there was no significant difference in the change in FVC between the NAC group and the placebo group ($p = 0.77$). In addition, there were no significant differences between the NAC group and the placebo group in the rates of death ($p = 0.30$) or acute exacerbation ($p > 0.99$; Raghu et al. 2012). In a 2016 clinical trial, the addition of NAC to pirfenidone unexpectedly increased the rate of decline in FVC (Behr et al. 2016). Based on these conflicting findings, Sun et al. (2016), with a meta-analysis to evaluate the efficacy of NAC for the treatment of IPF, found no beneficial effect of NAC on changes in FVC, carbon monoxide diffusing capacity, rates of adverse events, or death rates.

It has been suggested the perceived benefits of NAC in the initial IFIGENIA trial of 2005 may have been as a result of the protective benefits of NAC with regard to azathioprine toxicity. Interestingly, when the effect of intravenous NAC administration at a range of doses was compared between patients with known IPF and healthy volunteers, there was no difference in the GSH levels noted in the healthy volunteer group (Meyer et al. 1995), reinforcing the concept that NAC only elicits an effect to replenish GSH levels in tissue that is deficient in GSH. Thus, in the final analysis, NAC is not recommended for treatment of IPF.

There are few effective therapies to treat IPF, and the mortality rate is high; thus effective treatments for IPF are urgently needed. Anti-inflammatory therapy with corticosteroids or immunosuppressants does not improve the survival of patients with IPF (Raghu et al. 1991; Pinheiro et al. 2008; Taskar and Coultas 2006). Other pharmacological interventions have included nintedanib, etanercept, warfarin, gleevec, and bosentan, which remain controversial (Canestaro et al. 2016). Pirfenidone was approved by the European Medicines Agency in 2011 for the treatment of IPF (Taniguchi et al. 2011; Behr and Richeldi 2013). Until pirfenidone was approved for the treatment of IPF in 2011, there were not therapeutic trials of any treatment that demonstrated efficacy on the survival of patients with IPF.

15.4 Summary

There have been several investigations into the use of NAC in pulmonary disease, and other studies are ongoing. This chapter reviews some of the major chronic pulmonary diseases, although infectious pulmonary conditions (i.e., bronchiolitis, chronic bronchitis, pneumonia) are reviewed in the chapter on miscellaneous studies. Several clinical trials on the use of NAC in pulmonary disorders are ongoing as outlined in Table 15.2 including two treatment trials on the use of NAC in acute respiratory disease syndrome and asthma and one observation trial on idiopathic pulmonary fibrosis.

There have been very few quality studies investigating the effects of oral NAC in CF. The eight studies included for review in this chapter assessed different doses of NAC through time, and initial studies were 3 months in duration or shorter. The beneficial effects of NAC in CF and COPD appear to be best appreciated after at least 6 months and with higher daily dosing strategies.

Recommendations for the use of NAC in the pulmonary disorders reviewed in this chapter are given in Table 15.3. There is a good grade of recommendation given the quality of the studies performed; however, the outcomes are rather variable. For CF and COPD, the study outcomes are most likely because of different dosing, length of treatment, and subpopulation, with the evidence pointing in a favorable direction for recommendation for the use of oral NAC in people with CF and COPD. However, there is a least one study on IPF in which NAC may have been detrimental, suggesting that, at this time, NAC should not be routinely used in the treatment of IPF until this data is better understood or more studies are available to show benefit (Online Table 15.3). There are few good quality trials investigating the effect of long-term high-dose NAC in patients with CF, and further research is required to investigate the mechanism of its action in CF and in COPD and its role in improving outcomes for these diseases.

References

Aruoma O, Halliwell B, Hoey B et al (1989) The antioxidant action of N-acetylcysteine: its reaction with hydrogen peroxide, hydroxyl radical, superoxide, and hypochlorous acid. Free Radic Biol Med 6:593–597

Atkuri K, Mantovani J, Herzenberg L et al (2007) N-acetylcysteine—a safe antidote for cysteine/glutathione deficiency. Curr Opin Pharmacol 7:355–359

Barnes PJ (2013) New anti-inflammatory targets for chronic obstructive pulmonary disease. Nat Rev Drug Discov 12:543–559

Barnes PJ (2016) Inflammatory mechanisms in patients with chronic obstructive pulmonary disease. J Allergy Clin Immunol 138:16–27

Behr J, Richeldi L (2013) Recommendations on treatment for IPF. Respir Res 14(Suppl 1):S6

Behr J, Bendstrup E, Crestani B et al (2016) Safety and tolerability of acetylcysteine and pirfenidone combination therapy in idiopathic pulmonary fibrosis: a randomised, double-blind, placebo-controlled, phase 2 trial. Lancet Respir Med 4:445–453

Bonanomi L, Gazzaniga A (1980) Toxicological, pharmacokinetic and metabolic studies on acetylcysteine. Eur J Respir Dis Suppl 111:45–51

Brusselle G, Joos G, Bracke K (2011) New insights into the immunology of chronic obstructive pulmonary disease. Lancet 378:1015–1026

Canestaro W, Forrester S, Raghu G et al (2016) Drug treatment of idiopathic pulmonary fibrosis systematic review and network meta-analysis. Chest 149:756–766

Cantin A, North S, Hubbard R et al (1987) Normal alveolar epithelial lining fluid contains high levels of glutathione. J Appl Physiol 63:152–157

Cantin AM, Hubbard RC, Crystal RG (1989) Glutathione defficiency in the epithelial lining fluid of the lower respiratory tract in idiopathic pulmonary fibrosis. Am Rev Respir Dis 139: 370–372

Cantin AM, Bilodeau G, Ouellet C et al (2006) Oxidant stress suppresses CFTR expression. Am J Physiol Cell Physiol 290:C262–C270

Cazzola M, Calzetta L, Page C et al (2015) Influence of N-acetylcysteine on chronic bronchitis or COPD exacerbations: a meta-analysis. Eur Respir Rev 24:451–461

Celli BR, MacNee W (2004) Standards for the diagnosis and treatment of patients with COPD: a summary of the ATS/ERS position paper. Eur Respir J 23:932–946

Cogan JD, Kropski JA, Zhao M et al (2015) Rare variants in RTEL1 are associated with familial interstitial pneumonia. Am J Respir Crit Care Med 191:646–655

Conrad C, Lymp J, Thompson V et al (2015) Long-term treatment with oral N-acetylcysteine: affects lung function but not sputum inflammation in cystic fibrosis subjects. A phase II randomized placebo-controlled trial. J Cyst Fibros 14:219–227

Dauletbaev N, Fischer P, Aulbach B et al (2009) A phase II study on safety and efficacy of high-dose N-acetylcysteine in patients with cystic fibrosis. Eur J Med Res 14:352–358

De Benedetto F, Aceto A, Dragani B et al (2005) Long-term oral n-acetylcysteine reduces exhaled hydrogen peroxide in stable COPD. Pulm Pharmacol Ther 18:41–47

Decramer M, Rutten Van Molken M, Dekhuijzen P et al (2005) Effects of N-acetylcysteine on outcomes in chronic obstructive pulmonary disease (Bronchitis Randomized on NAC Cost-Utility Study, BRONCUS): a randomised placebocontrolled trial. Lancet 365:1552–1560

Demedts M, Behr J, Buhl R et al (2005) High-dose acetylcysteine in idiopathic pulmonary fibrosis. N Engl J Med 353:2229–2242

Drost EM, Skwarski KM, Sauleda J et al (2005) Oxidative stress and airway inflammation in severe exacerbations of COPD. Thorax 60:293–300

Duijvestijn YC, Brand PL (1999) Systematic review of Nacetylcysteine in cystic fibrosis. Acta Paediatr 88:38–41

Evans CM, Fingerlin TE, Schwarz MI et al (2016) Idiopathic pulmonary fibrosis: a genetic disease that involves mucociliary dysfunction of the peripheral airways. Physiol Rev 96:1567–1591

Fingerlin TE, Murphy E, Zhang W et al (2013) Genome-wide association study identifies multiple susceptibility loci for pulmonary fibrosis. Nat Genet 45:613–620

Fioret D, Perez RL, Roman J (2011) Management of idiopathic pulmonary fibrosis. Am J Med Sci 341:450–453

Fowdar K, Chen H, He Z et al (2017) The effect of N-acetylcysteine on exacerbations of chronic obstructive pulmonary disease: a meta-analysis and systematic review. Heart Lung 46:120–128

Galli F, Battistoni A, Gambari R et al (2012) Oxidative stress and antioxidant therapy in cystic fibrosis. Biochim Biophys Acta 1822:690–713

Global Strategy for the Diagnosis, Management and Prevention of COPD, Global Initiative for Chronic Obstructive Lung Disease (GOLD) 2017 report. www.goldcopd.org

GOLD (2014) Updated 2014. Global initiative for chronic obstructive lung disease Inc. Odense, Denmark

Howatt WF, DeMuth GR (1966) A double-blind study of the use of acetylcysteine in patients with cystic fibrosis. Univ Mich Med Cent J 32:82–85

Howick J, Chalmers I, Glasziou P, Greenhalgh T, Heneghan C, Liberati A, Moschetti I, Phillips B, Thornton H, Goddard O, Hodgkinson M (2011) The Oxford 2011 levels of evidence. http://www.cebm.net/index.aspx?o=5653. Accessed 03 Sept 2011

Hurst GA, Shaw PB, LeMaistre CA (1967) Laboratory and clinical evaluation of the mucolytic properties of acetylcysteine. Am Rev Respir Dis 96:962–970

Jadad A, Moore R, Carroll D et al (1996) Assessing the quality of reports of randomized clinical trials: is blinding necessary? Control Clin Trials 17:1–12

Kasielski M, Nowak D (2001) Long-term administration of N-acetylcysteine decreases hydrogen peroxide exhalation in subjects with chronic obstructive pulmonary disease. Respir Med 95:448–456

Lands L, Grey F, Smountas A et al (1999) Lymphocyte glutathione levels in children with cystic fibrosis. Chest 116:201–205

MacNee W (2000) Oxidants/antioxidants and COPD. Chest 117:303S–317S

MacNee W (2005) Pulmonary and systemic oxidant/antioxidant imbalance in chronic obstructive pulmonary disease. Proc Am Thorac Soc 2:50–60

Malhotra D, Th immulappa R, Navas-Acien A et al (2008) Decline in NRF2-regulated antioxidants in chronic obstructive pulmonary disease lungs due to loss of its positive regulator, DJ-1. Am J Respir Crit Care Med 178:592–604

Martinez FJ et al (2014) Randomized trial of Acetylcysteine in idiopathic pulmonary fibrosis. N Engl J Med 370:2093–2101

Mayer-Hamblett N, Aitken M, Accurso F et al (2007) Association between pulmonary function and sputum biomarkers in cystic fibrosis. Am J Respir Crit Care Med 175:822–828

Meyer A, Buhl R, Kampf S, Magnussen H (1995) Intravenous N-acetylcysteine and lung glutathione of patients with pulmonary fibrosis and normals. Am J Respir Crit Care Med 152(3):1055–1060

Mitchell EA, Elliott RB (1982) Controlled trial of oral N-acetylcysteine in cystic fibrosis. Aust Paediatr J 18:40–42

Moss M, Guidot DM, Wong-Lambertina M et al (2000) The effects of chronic alcohol abuse on pulmonary glutathione homeostasis. Am J Respir Crit Care Med 161:414–419

Nogee LM, Dunbar AE, Wert SE et al (2001) A mutation in the surfactant protein C gene associated with familial interstitial lung disease. N Engl J Med 344:573–579

Noth I, Zhang Y, Ma SF et al (2013) Genetic variants associated with idiopathic pulmonary fibrosis susceptibility and mortality: a genome-wide association study. Lancet Respir Med 1:309–317

Palmer LA, Doctor A, Chhabra P et al (2007) S-nitrosothiols signal hypoxia-mimetic vascular pathology. J Clin Invest 117:2592–2601

Pinheiro GA, Antao VC, Wood JM et al (2008) Occupational risks for idiopathic pulmonary fibrosis mortality in the United States. Int J Occup Environ Health 14:117–123

Poole P, Chong J, Cates CJ (2015) Mucolytic agents versus placebo for chronic bronchitis or chronic obstructive pulmonary disease. Cochrane Database Syst Rev 29:CD001287

Qaseem A, Wilt TJ, Weinberger SE et al (2011) Diagnosis and management of stable chronic obstructive pulmonary disease: a clinical practice guideline update from the American College of Physicians, American College of Chest Physicians, American Thoracic Society, and European Respiratory Society. Ann Intern Med 155:179–191

Raghu G, Depaso WJ, Cain K et al (1991) Azathioprine combined with prednisone in the treatment of idiopathic pulmonary fibrosis: a prospective double-blind, randomized, placebo-controlled clinical trial. Am Rev Respir Dis 144:291–296

Raghu G, Collard HR, Egan JJ et al (2011) An official ATS/ERS/JRS/ALAT statement: idiopathic pulmonary fibrosis: evidence based guidelines for diagnosis and management. Am J Respir Crit Care Med 183:788–824

Raghu G, Anstrom K, King T et al (2012) Prednisone, azathioprine, and N-acetylcysteine for pulmonary fibrosis. N Engl J Med 366:1968–1977

Rahman I, Yang SR, Biswas SK (2006) Current concepts of redox signaling in the lungs. Antioxid Redox Signal 8:681–689

Ratjen F, Wonne R, Posselt HG et al (1985) A double-blind placebo controlled trial with oral ambroxol and N-acetylcysteine for mucolytic treatment in cystic fibrosis. Eur J Pediatr 144:374–378

Reas H (1964) The use of N-acetylcysteine in the treatment of cystic fibrosis. J Pediatr 65:542–557

Reas HW (1963) The effect of N-acetylcysteine on the viscosity of tracheobronehial secretions in cystic fibrosis of the pancreas. J Pediatr 62:31

Richeldi L, Collard H, Jones M (2017) Idiopathic pulmonary fibrosis. Lancet 389:1941–1952

Roum JH, Buhl R, McElvaney NG, Borok Z, Crystal RG (1993) Systemic deficiency of glutathione in cystic fibrosis. J Appl Physiol 75:2419–2424

Rushworth GF, Megson IL (2014) Existing and potential therapeutic uses for N-acetylcysteine: the need for conversion to intracellular glutathione for antioxidant benefits. Pharmacol Ther 141(2):150–159. https://doi.org/10.1016/j.pharmthera.2013.09.006

Schermer T, Chavannes N, Dekhuijzen R et al (2009) Fluticasone and N-acetylcysteine in primary care patients with COPD or chronic bronchitis. Respir Med 103:542–551

Sheffner AL (1963) The reduction in vitro in viscosity of mucoprotein solutions by a new mucolytic agent, N-acetyl-l-cysteine. Ann N Y Acad Sci 106:298

Skov M, Pressler T, Lykkesfeldt J et al (2015) The effect of short-term, high-dose oral N-acetylcysteine treatment on oxidative stress markers in cystic fibrosis patients with chronic *P. aeruginosa* infection — a pilot study. J Cyst Fibros 14:211–218

Stafanger G, Koch C (1989) N-acetylcysteine in cystic fibrosis and *Pseudomonas aeruginosa* infection: clinical score, spirometry and ciliary motility. Eur Respir J 2:234–237

Stafanger G, Garne S, Howitz P et al (1988) The clinical effect and the effect on the ciliary motility of oral N-acetylcysteine in patients with cystic fibrosis and primary ciliary dyskinesia. Eur Respir J 1:161–167

Stey C, Steurer J, Bachmann S et al (2000) The effect of oral N-acetylcysteine in chronic bronchitis: a quantitative systematic review. Eur Respir J 16:253–262

Stuart B, Choi J, Zaidi S et al (2015) Exome sequencing links mutations in PARN and RTEL1 with familial pulmonary fibrosis and telomere shortening. Nat Genet 47:512–517

Sun T, Liu J, Zhao DW (2016) Efficacy of N-acetylcysteine in idiopathic pulmonary fibrosis: a systematic review and meta-analysis. Medicine 95:e3629

Taniguchi H, Kondoh Y, Ebina M, Azuma A, Ogura T, Taguchi Y, Suga M, Takahashi H, Nakata K, Sato A, Sugiyama Y, Kudoh S, Nukiwa T, Pirfenidone Clinical Study Group in Japan (2011) The clinical significance of 5% change in vital capacity in patients with idiopathic pulmonary fibrosis: extended analysis of the pirfenidone trial. Respir Res 12:93. https://doi.org/10.1186/1465-9921-12-93

Taskar VS, Coultas DB (2006) Is idiopathic pulmonary fibrosis an environmental disease? Proc Am Thorac Soc 3:293–298

Thannickal VJ, Toews GB, White ES et al (2004) Mechanisms of pulmonary fibrosis. Annu Rev Med 55:395–417

Tirouvanziam R, Khazaal I, Péault B (2002) Primary inflammation in human cystic fibrosis small airways. Am J Physiol Lung Cell Mol Physiol 283:L445–L451

Tirouvanziam R, Conrad CK, Bottiglieri T et al (2006) High-dose oral N-acetylcysteine, a glutathione prodrug, modulates inflammation in cystic fibrosis. Proc Natl Acad Sci U S A 103:4628–4633

Tsakiri KD, Cronkhite JT, Kuan PJ et al (2007) Adult-onset pulmonary fibrosis caused by mutations in telomerase. Proc Natl Acad Sci U S A 104:7552–7557

Tse HN, Raiteri L, Wong KY et al (2013) High-dose N-acetylcysteine in stable COPD: the 1-year, double-blind, randomized, placebo-controlled HIACE study. Chest 144:106–118

Van der Toorn M, Slebos D, de Bruin H et al (2013) Critical role of aldehydes in cigarette smoke-induced acute airway inflammation. Respir Res 14:45

Wada H, Takizawa H (2013) Future treatment for COPD: targeting oxidative stress and its related signal. Recent Patents Inflamm Allergy Drug Discov 7:1–11

Wang Y, Kuan PJ, Xing C et al (2009) Genetic defects in surfactant protein A2 are associated with pulmonary fibrosis and lung cancer. Am J Hum Genet 84:52–59

Zheng JP, Wen FQ, Bai CX et al (2014) Twice daily N-acetylcysteine 600 mg for exacerbations of chronic obstructive pulmonary disease (PANTHEON): a randomised, double-blind placebo-controlled trial. Lancet Respir Med 2:187–194

The Clinical Use of N-Acetylcysteine in Cardiology

16

John P. Marenco and Richard Eugene Frye

16.1 Introduction

Cardiovascular disease is a leading cause of morbidity and mortality for both men and women in the United States. The last 50 years has seen great advancements in our understanding of cardiovascular disease states and has resulted in numerous effective medications and interventional therapies. Treatments are continuing to evolve, and given the number of people affected by cardiac disease, novel and adjunctive treatments continue to be needed to improve outcomes, reduce post-procedural complications, and improve quality of life.

N-Acetylcysteine (NAC) has been shown to be a potent antioxidant and free radical scavenger in part due to its effect on stimulating glutathione (GSH) synthesis and increasing intracellular GSH levels which are decreased in states of increased inflammation and oxidative stress. It has vasodilatory actions that are mediated by its enhancement of nitric oxide and reduction in the development of nitrate tolerance. Some of the first studies using NAC in cardiac disease were in the 1980s with the treatment of angina as an adjunctive treatment to nitrates. It was not until the 1990s that the investigation of NAC into a wider range of cardiac disease states, treatments, and procedures was considered. However, despite a growing number of studies, its clinical utility in treating cardiac disease remains limited. This chapter will review the evidence for the use of NAC for cardiac disorders and procedures and as an adjunct to standard treatments. Table 16.1 outlines the proposed mechanisms of action of NAC for cardiac disorders.

J. P. Marenco
Tufts University School of Medicine, Baystate Medical Center, Springfield, MA, USA

R. E. Frye (✉)
Barrow Neurological Institute, Phoenix Children's Hospital, University of Arizona College of Medicine – Phoenix, Phoenix, AZ, USA
e-mail: rfrye@phoenixchildrens.com

© Springer Nature Singapore Pte Ltd. 2019
R. E. Frye, M. Berk (eds.), *The Therapeutic Use of N-Acetylcysteine (NAC) in Medicine*, https://doi.org/10.1007/978-981-10-5311-5_16

Table 16.1 Summary of NAC mechanisms of action across different cardiac disorders

Cardiac disorder	Mechanism of N-Acetylcysteine (NAC)
Hypertension	Enhancing nitric oxide metabolism by supplying free sulfhydryl groups needed for the activation of guanylate cyclase Inhibition of angiotensin-converting enzyme
Adjunctive to nitrate drug treatments	Enhancing nitric oxide metabolism by supplying free sulfhydryl groups needed for the activation of guanylate cyclase Preventing the oxidation of nitrate compounds
Myocardial infarction	Reducing reactive oxygen species and free radical Antiplatelet effect Reducing activation of inflammatory cascade Inhibition of angiotensin-converting enzyme
Percutaneous coronary intervention	Reducing reactive oxygen species and free radical Antiplatelet effect Reducing activation of inflammatory cascade
Cardiac surgery outcomes	Reducing reactive oxygen species and free radical Antiplatelet effect Reducing activation of inflammatory cascade
Peripheral vascular disease	Antiplatelet effect

16.2   Methods

A systematic online literature search was performed to identify all clinical trials involving cardiovascular disease using NAC using the filters "human" and "clinical trials." From these the author screened titles and abstracts of all potentially relevant publications.

16.3   Evidence of Effectiveness of NAC in the Treatment of Cardiac Disorders

16.3.1 Hypertension

NAC may treat hypertension through enhancing nitric oxide (NO) metabolism and improving endothelial function. In a small open-label randomized crossover study (level 2b), hypertensive smokers already treated with angiotensin-converting enzyme inhibitor therapy received either 600 mg NAC three times a day for 21 days or continued treatment as usual (Barrios et al. 2002). The combination therapy significantly lowered ambulatory systolic and diastolic blood pressure (BP) on 24 h and daytime measurements. In a small double-blind placebo-controlled (DBPC) (level 2b) study, patients with type 2 diabetes and hypertension received placebo or a combination of 600 mg NAC twice a day and 1.2 g L-arginine daily for 6 months (Martina et al. 2008). The combination treatment lowered both systolic and diastolic

BP. Thus, the Grade of Recommendation (GOR) for treatment of hypertension is B with both studies being level 2b. However, given that there are only two small studies, with one being open-label, more studies are needed before a strong recommendation can be made for the use of NAC for hypertension.

16.3.2 NAC for Adjunctive Nitrate Treatments

16.3.2.1 Potentiating the Clinical Effect of Nitrate Drugs

Nitrate drugs like nitroglycerin (NTG) have been a mainstay of therapy for coronary ischemia and for treatment of acute congestive heart failure decompensation for several decades. NAC is believed to augment the hemodynamic and antiplatelet effect of nitrate compounds and limit nitrate tolerance through several mechanisms, including supplying free sulfhydryl groups needed for the activation of guanylate cyclase and preventing the oxidation of nitrate compounds thereby inactivating them and preventing the creation of toxic peroxynitrite.

Several studies have investigated the adjunctive effect of NAC on nitrate treatment for patients with angina. Three studies have examined the effect of NAC on potentiating the clinical effects of nitrates. In patients with severe drug-resistant unstable angina pectoris, 5 g intravenous (IV) NAC reduced the incidence of acute myocardial infarction (AMI) but increased the incidence of symptomatic hypotension when added to IV NTG in a small DBPC study (level 2b) (Horowitz et al. 1988). In a large randomized DBPC (level 1b), the combination of NTG and NAC improved the composite outcome of death, myocardial infarction, or refractory angina requiring revascularization over a 4-month period in 200 patients with unstable angina (Ardissino et al. 1997). Lastly, in a DBPC crossover study (level 2b), 2.4 g oral NAC given twice, combined with 60 mg of the sublingual long-acting nitrate, isosorbide-5-mononitrate, prolonged total exercise time in 10 patients with angina pectoris on beta blockers without nitrate tolerance (Svendsen et al. 1989). Thus, there is a GOR of B for NAC improving clinical endpoints when added to nitrate drugs. There is good potential for using NAC to improve angina treatment, but until the effect of increasing symptomatic hypotension can be studied further, it is difficult to make certain recommendations.

Three studies have examined the effect of NAC potentiating the hemodynamic effect of nitrates. In a small DBPC crossover study (level 2b), 23-h infusion of NTG (0.1 µ/kg/min) combined with NAC (5 mg/kg/h) potentiated the acute venodilatory effect of NTG as estimated by changes in the venous volume and microcirculatory subcutaneous blood flow effects of NTG (Boesgaard et al. 1994). In a small randomized crossover study design (level 2b), IV 100 mg/kg NAC was found to potentiate the effect of isosorbide dinitrate on mean right atrial pressure, mean pulmonary artery wedge pressure, mean pulmonary artery pressure, and cardiac output (Mehra et al. 1994). In a non-blinded study (level 2b) of patients with and without coronary artery disease (CAD), 100 mg/kg of NAC potentiated nitrate-induced large epicardial coronary artery vasodilation in the patients with CAD but not those without

(Nishikawa et al. 1998). NAC also potentiated the increase in coronary blood flow in response to NTG in both those with and without CAD. Thus, this provides a GOR of B for NAC augmenting the hemodynamic effect of nitrates. However, with only a few studies investigating this effect, more research is needed before a definite recommendation regarding its clinical role can be made.

16.3.2.2 Prevention of Nitrate Tolerance

Several studies, most of them small DBPC crossover RCTs with washout periods, have examined the ability of NAC to prevent tolerance to nitrates. Two studies examined transdermal glyceryl trinitrate. NAC 200 mg three times daily failed to prevent tolerance of transdermal glyceryl trinitrate 20 mg on hemodynamic changes following exercise in healthy controls (Hogan et al. 1989) (level 2b), while NAC 400 mg three times daily failed to prevent tolerance of transdermal glyceryl trinitrate 10 mg on hemodynamic changes following exercise in patients with stable angina (Hogan et al. 1990) (level 2b). Thus, these studies do not support an effect of NAC on preventing hemodynamic tolerance of transdermal glyceryl trinitrate (GOR B).

Three studies examined the effect of NAC on isosorbide dinitrate. Controlled released NAC 600 mg four times a day provided a continuing positive effect of isosorbide dinitrate on electrophysiological measurements, including time to 1-mm ST depression and total ST segment depression, during a bicycle exercise test in treated stable angina pectoris patients (level 2b) (Boesgaard et al. 1991). Likewise continuous NAC infusion (5 mg/kg/h) provided a continuing positive effect of IV isosorbide dinitrate, on the aforementioned electrophysiological measurements and time to angina onset in patients with stable angina pectoris during a bicycle exercise tests (level 2b) (Boesgaard et al. 1992). However, a single dose of 100 mg/kg NAC IV did not reverse tolerance to the hemodynamic and antianginal effects of four times a day of 30 mg isosorbide dinitrate during exercise in patients with chronic stable angina (level 2b) (Parker et al. 1987). Although limited in number, these studies suggest that prolonged treatment with NAC may prevent tolerance to the hemodynamic effects of isosorbide dinitrate (GOR B). However, given the small overall sample size of these studies, recommendations for the use of NAC for this indication cannot be made at this time.

Two studies examined the tolerance to NTG following combined infusion of NTG and IV NAC (5 mg/kg/h). In the only non-blinded study (level 2b) in this section, NAC resulted in decreased tolerance to sublingual NTG after 48-h NTG infusion (1.5 μg/kg/min), despite no effect of NAC on counter-regulatory neurohormones (i.e., renin, aldosterone, and norepinephrine) and intravascular volume expansion (Pizzulli et al. 1997). In another small DBPC crossover study (level 2b), NAC added to NTG (0.1 μg/kg/min) prevented NTG tolerance at 23 h (Boesgaard et al. 1994). These studies provide additional support (GOR B) for NAC in the prevention of nitrate tolerance. However, given the small overall sample size of these studies and the fact that there are only two studies, recommendations for the use of NAC for this indication cannot be made at this time.

16.3.2.3 Prevention of Nitrate Adverse Effects

One study investigated whether NAC could prevent nitrite-induced methemoglobinemia. In a randomized placebo-controlled crossover study (level 2b), IV NAC (160 mg/kg) did not change nitrite-induced methemoglobinemia (Tanen et al. 2000).

16.3.3 Acute Myocardial Infarction

NAC is believed to be beneficial during AMI because of several physiological mechanisms that have been studied in animals (Sochman 2002). These potential mechanisms include the amelioration of ischemia-reperfusion injury and adverse remodeling via its antioxidant effects, antiplatelet effects, and enhancement of NO. In a small controlled study (level 2b), 15 g of IV NAC infused over 24 h in combination with NTG and streptokinase resulted in better preservation of left ventricular function and possibly more rapid reperfusion in patients with AMI (Arstall et al. 1995). The infarct size limitation: acute N-Acetylcysteine defense (ISLAND) trial, a controlled randomized three-arm study (level 2b), demonstrated that adding IV NAC (100 mg/kg) to streptokinase-induced recanalization in patients with a first anterior wall myocardial infarction improved global and regional left ventricular ejection fraction and myocardial salvage (Sochman et al. 1995, 1997). In a prospective DBPC study (level 1b), 600 mg NAC twice a day for 3 days lowered serum concentrations of matrix metalloproteinases at 72 h suggesting reduced early remodeling as well as decreased length of hospitalization, major adverse cardiac events at 1-year follow-up, and a decreased incidence of reinfarction (Talasaz et al. 2014). In a small randomized controlled study (level 2b), 15 g of NAC IV over 24 h resulted in higher left ventricular ejection fraction and lower end-systolic and end-diastolic diameters and wall motion score index but no difference in the MB fraction of creatine kinase (Yesilbursa et al. 2006) in AMI patients. Thus, four controlled studies, most of them small, have reported positive effects of NAC during AMI (GOR B), suggesting that this is a very promising area of the therapeutic use of NAC. One limitation of these trials is the paucity of data in patients undergoing early revascularization with percutaneous coronary intervention and stenting as opposed to the use of thrombolytics. Indeed, larger well-designed studies of current era treatment of myocardial infarction are needed to confirm these findings. Several clinical trials are ongoing (Table 16.2).

Table 16.2 Ongoing clinical trials on N-Acetylcysteine for cardiac disease

Trial title	NCT #	Trial status
Effects of N-Acetylcysteine during primary percutaneous coronary intervention (EASE-PRM-PCI)	NCT01878344	Ongoing but not recruiting
Effect of N-Acetylcysteine in myocardial infarction	NCT01741207	Unknown
Effects of N-Acetylcysteine during percutaneous coronary intervention (EASE-PCI)	NCT01878669	Ongoing but not recruiting

One study has examined the effect of NAC of the development of non-thyroidal illness syndrome in patients with AMI. In a multicenter randomized controlled study (level 2b), 1.2 g NAC IV given every 12 h for five doses prevented a decreased in T3 and a normalization of rT3 but did not affect T4 or thyroid-stimulating hormone (Vidart et al. 2014). This study supports the notion that NAC may be useful for patients with AMI but with only one study provides limited evidence for routine use of NAC in patients with AMI for preventing thyroid dysfunction.

16.3.4 Cardiac Surgery

Reactive oxygen species have been shown to be important mediators of myocardial stress associated with ischemia and reperfusion injury in patients undergoing cardioplegia arrest (Mehlhorn et al. 2003). Several studies have investigated whether NAC is helpful during cardiac bypass surgery in general. In a large DBPC (level 1b) of patients undergoing coronary artery bypass surgery with cardiopulmonary bypass, 600 mg NAC oral the day prior to surgery followed by IV NAC (150 mg/kg) just before surgery followed by IV NAC (12.5 mg/kg/h) for 24 h did not change clinical outcomes. In a medium-sized DBPC study (level 2b), IV NAC (300 mg/kg over 24 h) did not improve clinical outcomes in patients at higher risk of postoperative renal failure (Haase et al. 2007). There is one small controlled study of patients undergoing coronary artery bypass surgery (level 2b) NAC (50 mg/kg) infused with cold-blood cardioplegia resulted in lower cardiac troponin I levels following surgery (Koramaz et al. 2006). This later study suggests that delivery and timing of the application of NAC may be important. Lastly, in a large DBPC study (level 1b), IV NAC (100 mg/kg bolus followed by 20 mg/kg/h during bypass until 4 h after bypass surgery) resulted in increased chest tube blood loss and a greater transfusion volume (Wijeysundera et al. 2009). Thus for general use in cardiac surgery, NAC has not been consistently reported to have beneficial effects, and despite its very favorable safety profile, one study seems to suggest that there is increased blood loss with NAC, presumably due to its proposed antiplatelet effects. Thus, until further positive studies are performed, NAC cannot be recommended as an adjunct for cardiac bypass surgery outcomes.

16.3.5 Postoperative Atrial Fibrillation

Postoperative atrial fibrillation (POAF) is the most common arrhythmia occurring after cardiac surgery, being found in 25–40% of such patients (Ommen et al. 1997). While it is generally felt to be benign, it is associated with increased length of stay (LOS), increased cost, and, in some cases, hypotension and mortality. There is evidence that the postoperative state is marked by increased inflammation and oxidative stress as well as alterations in the renin-angiotensin system (Huang et al. 2009; Dilaveris et al. 2005). Based on this evidence, several antioxidant strategies including NAC have been studied for reduction of POAF rates and LOS. Most of the early studies demonstrated a reduction in the rate of POAF with NAC. Ozaydin et al. (Ozaydin et al. 2008) performed a prospective, randomized, placebo-controlled study of 115 patients (level 1b) undergoing cardiac bypass and valve surgery. They received IV NAC 1 h prior to surgery and for 48 h postsurgery. NAC treatment significantly lowered the incidence of POAF lasting longer than 5 min. A subsequent meta-analysis including 8 randomized trials and 578 patients supported the efficacy of NAC in reducing the incidence of POAF (odds ratio = 0.62, 95% CI 0.41–0.93, $P = 0.021$) and showed that NAC was associated with a reduction in all-cause mortality (Liu et al. 2014). Most early trials were small and had variable dosing schedules. In a large DBPC study (level 1b), prophylactic high-dose 1.2 g oral NAC two times a day, begun 2 days before open heart surgery and continued for 5 days after surgery, had no significant effect on the incidence of POAF, in-hospital stay, and postoperative morbidity or mortality (Kazemi et al. 2013). This prompted a second meta-analysis including this new data that still demonstrated that NAC reduced the incidence of POAF (odds ratio = 0.62, 95% CI 0.41–0.93, $P = 0.021$) compared with controls but had no effect on LOS (Gu et al. 2012). Thus, there is good evidence (three level 1b studies; GOR A) that NAC may reduce the incidence of POAF, but the effect on clinical outcomes is inconsistent. Given the fact that one study demonstrated increased blood loss after cardiac surgery with NAC treatment and the lack of a clear clinical outcome, the use of NAC for POAF is probably best decided on a case-by-case basis.

16.3.6 Peripheral Vascular Disease

Two studies have been conducted to determine the utility of inpatients with peripheral vascular disease. In patients undergoing surgical intervention for acute femoral artery occlusion, 300mg NAC before reperfusion, and 8 and 16 h after reperfusion reduced the A-aO2 gradient increase with reperfusion in a controlled study (level 2b) and suggested less severe organ injury in the NAC group (Ege et al. 2006). In a small DBPC crossover study (level 2b), 1.8 g NAC for 4 days plus 2.7 g NAC before the experimental session did not improve walking tolerance or post-occlusive reactive hyperemia in patients with intermittent claudication (da Silva et al. 2015). Given that these two studies examined different populations, it is difficult to combine them to conclude anything certain about the effect of NAC in patients with peripheral vascular disease. Further studies will be needed to examine this population in greater detail.

16.3.7 Cardiac Catheterizations

One study examined the antiplatelet and clinical effect of NAC on outcomes after percutaneous coronary intervention. In a large (level 1b) DBPC intracoronary IV, NAC (100 mg/kg bolus plus 10 mg/kg/h) for 12 h did not reduce the level of platelet activation biomarkers within a 24-h period nor did it reduce a combination endpoint of all-cause death, reinfarction, and target vessel revascularization assessed at 30 days and 2 years following percutaneous coronary intervention (Eshraghi et al. 2016). Major adverse cardiac events at 30 days and 2 years were infrequent in the study, however. This GOR B does not support the use of NAC during percutaneous coronary intervention, but there is only one study at this time to provide any guidance.

16.4 Summary

In our systematic review, we found numerous clinical trials that examined the effect of NAC in treating various cardiac disease states. Although the data for NAC use in several of these conditions such as in the treatment of hypertension and peripheral vascular disease remains limited, clinical trials examining the effect of NAC as an adjunct to nitrate therapy and as a therapy for AMI and during cardiac surgery are more substantial.

We have summarized the evidence and recommendations for the use of NAC for these various conditions in Table 16.3. There is good evidence that NAC may be helpful as an adjunct for nitrate therapy, particularly in the treatment of angina, potentiating the hemodynamic effects of nitrates and preventing nitrate tolerance for certain nitrate formulations. However, one study pointed out that the augmentation of hemodynamic effect of nitrates may also cause symptomatic hypotension, so further studies are needed to determine the optimal combination of nitrate and NAC dosing and to establish its potential benefit in the modern era of early revascularization. There are several positive studies suggesting that NAC may improve outcomes and reduce infarct size after AMI, but more studies are needed to follow up these positive results before NAC can be recommended for routine use in the treatment of AMI. Indeed, several trials are ongoing and should provide greater insight into its potential clinical role (Table 16.2).

Unlike these promising studies, studies examining the use of NAC for cardiac surgery have not demonstrated consistent clinical benefit and must be weighed against limited data suggesting the potential for greater blood loss, presumably due to its antiplatelet effects. However, all of these aforementioned studies provided NAC systematically, whereas the one study that only included it in the cardioplegia demonstrated improvement in biomarkers for myocardial damage. Clearly more research will be needed before NAC can be routinely used in the context of cardiac surgery.

Thus, the recommendations for the use of NAC in the majority of cardiac disorders are still limited based on the number and the quality of studies that have been conducted and available for review at this time. While larger controlled trials are needed to establish efficacy of NAC, available evidence so far and safety profile of NAC support its potential as a novel treatment option for several cardiac disorders.

Table 16.3 Overall ratings of NAC based on clinical studies presented by condition

Reason for treatment	Uncontrolled studies positive% (positive/total)	Controlled studies positive% (positive/total)	Grade of recommendation	Recommendation for treatment
Hypertension		100% (2/2)	B	None
Adjunctive to nitrate drug treatments				None
Angina treatment		100% (3/3)	B	None
Potentiating hemodynamic effect		100% (3/3)	B	None
Preventing nitrate tolerance				None
Transdermal glyceryl trinitrate		0% (0/2)	B	No
Isosorbide dinitrate		67% (2/3)	B	None
Nitroglycerin		100% (2/2)	B	None
Preventing methemoglobinemia		100% (1/1)	C	None
Myocardial infarction		100% (4/4)	B	None
Preventing non-thyroidal illness syndrome		100% (1/1)	C	None
Percutaneous coronary intervention		0% (0/1)	C	None
Improving cardiac surgery outcomes		0% (0/4)	A	No
Post-operative atrial fibrillation		89% (8/9)	A	None
Peripheral vascular disease		0% (0/1)	B	None

References

Ardissino D, Merlini PA, Savonitto S, Demicheli G, Zanini P, Bertocchi F, Falcone C, Ghio S, Marinoni G, Montemartini C, Mussini A (1997) Effect of transdermal nitroglycerin or N-acetylcysteine, or both, in the long-term treatment of unstable angina pectoris. J Am Coll Cardiol 29(5):941–947

Arstall MA, Yang J, Stafford I, Betts WH, Horowitz JD (1995) N-acetylcysteine in combination with nitroglycerin and streptokinase for the treatment of evolving acute myocardial infarction. Safety and biochemical effects. Circulation 92(10):2855–2862

Barrios V, Calderon A, Navarro-Cid J, Lahera V, Ruilope LM (2002) N-acetylcysteine potentiates the antihypertensive effect of ACE inhibitors in hypertensive patients. Blood Press 11(4):235–239

Boesgaard S, Aldershvile J, Pedersen F, Pietersen A, Madsen JK, Grande P (1991) Continuous oral N-acetylcysteine treatment and development of nitrate tolerance in patients with stable angina pectoris. J Cardiovasc Pharmacol 17(6):889–893

Boesgaard S, Aldershvile J, Poulsen HE (1992) Preventive administration of intravenous N-acetylcysteine and development of tolerance to isosorbide dinitrate in patients with angina pectoris. Circulation 85(1):143–149

Boesgaard S, Iversen HK, Wroblewski H, Poulsen HE, Frandsen H, Kastrup J, Aldershvile J (1994) Altered peripheral vasodilator profile of nitroglycerin during long-term infusion of N-acetylcysteine. J Am Coll Cardiol 23(1):163–169

Dilaveris P, Giannopoulos G, Synetos A, Stefanadis C (2005) The role of renin angiotensin system blockade in the treatment of atrial fibrillation. Curr Drug Targets Cardiovasc Haematol Disord 5(5):387–403

Ege T, Eskiocak S, Edis M, Duran E (2006) The role of N-acetylcysteine in lower extremity ischemia/reperfusions. J Cardiovasc Surg 47(5):563–568

Eshraghi A, Talasaz AH, Salamzadeh J, Salarifar M, Pourhosseini H, Nozari Y, Bahremand M, Jalali A, Boroumand MA (2016) Evaluating the effect of intracoronary N-acetylcysteine on platelet activation markers after primary percutaneous coronary intervention in patients with ST-elevation myocardial infarction. Am J Ther 23(1):e44–e51. https://doi.org/10.1097/mjt.0000000000000309

Gu WJ, Wu ZJ, Wang PF, Aung LH, Yin RX (2012) N-acetylcysteine supplementation for the prevention of atrial fibrillation after cardiac surgery: a meta-analysis of eight randomized controlled trials. BMC Cardiovasc Disord 12:10. https://doi.org/10.1186/1471-2261-12-10

Haase M, Haase-Fielitz A, Bagshaw SM, Reade MC, Morgera S, Seevenayagam S, Matalanis G, Buxton B, Doolan L, Bellomo R (2007) Phase II, randomized, controlled trial of high-dose N-acetylcysteine in high-risk cardiac surgery patients. Crit Care Med 35(5):1324–1331. https://doi.org/10.1097/01.ccm.0000261887.69976.12

Hogan JC, Lewis MJ, Henderson AH (1989) N-acetylcysteine fails to attenuate haemodynamic tolerance to glyceryl trinitrate in healthy volunteers. Br J Clin Pharmacol 28(4):421–426

Hogan JC, Lewis MJ, Henderson AH (1990) Chronic administration of N-acetylcysteine fails to prevent nitrate tolerance in patients with stable angina pectoris. Br J Clin Pharmacol 30(4):573–577

Horowitz JD, Henry CA, Syrjanen ML, Louis WJ, Fish RD, Antman EM, Smith TW (1988) Nitroglycerine/N-acetylcysteine in the management of unstable angina pectoris. Eur Heart J 9(Suppl A):95–100

Huang CX, Liu Y, Xia WF, Tang YH, Huang H (2009) Oxidative stress: a possible pathogenesis of atrial fibrillation. Med Hypotheses 72(4):466–467. https://doi.org/10.1016/j.mehy.2008.08.031

Kazemi B, Akbarzadeh F, Safaei N, Yaghoubi A, Shadvar K, Ghasemi K (2013) Prophylactic high-dose oral-N-acetylcysteine does not prevent atrial fibrillation after heart surgery: a prospective double blind placebo-controlled randomized clinical trial. Pacing Clin Electrophysiol 36(10):1211–1219. https://doi.org/10.1111/pace.12190

Koramaz I, Pulathan Z, Usta S, Karahan SC, Alver A, Yaris E, Kalyoncu NI, Ozcan F (2006) Cardioprotective effect of cold-blood cardioplegia enriched with N-acetylcysteine during coronary artery bypass grafting. Ann Thorac Surg 81(2):613–618. https://doi.org/10.1016/j.athoracsur.2005.08.013

Liu XH, Xu CY, Fan GH (2014) Efficacy of N-acetylcysteine in preventing atrial fibrillation after cardiac surgery: a meta-analysis of published randomized controlled trials. BMC Cardiovasc Disord 14:52. https://doi.org/10.1186/1471-2261-14-52

Martina V, Masha A, Gigliardi VR, Brocato L, Manzato E, Berchio A, Massarenti P, Settanni F, Della Casa L, Bergamini S, Iannone A (2008) Long-term N-acetylcysteine and L-arginine administration reduces endothelial activation and systolic blood pressure in hypertensive patients with type 2 diabetes. Diabetes Care 31(5):940–944. https://doi.org/10.2337/dc07-2251

Mehlhorn U, Krahwinkel A, Geissler HJ, LaRosee K, Fischer UM, Klass O, Suedkamp M, Hekmat K, Tossios P, Bloch W (2003) Nitrotyrosine and 8-isoprostane formation indicate free radical-mediated injury in hearts of patients subjected to cardioplegia. J Thorac Cardiovasc Surg 125(1):178–183. https://doi.org/10.1067/mtc.2003.97

Mehra A, Shotan A, Ostrzega E, Hsueh W, Vasquez-Johnson J, Elkayam U (1994) Potentiation of isosorbide dinitrate effects with N-acetylcysteine in patients with chronic heart failure. Circulation 89(6):2595–2600

Nishikawa Y, Kanki H, Ogawa S (1998) Differential effects of N-acetylcysteine on nitroglycerin- and nicorandil-induced vasodilation in human coronary circulation. J Cardiovasc Pharmacol 32(1):21–28

Ommen SR, Odell JA, Stanton MS (1997) Atrial arrhythmias after cardiothoracic surgery. N Engl J Med 336(20):1429–1434. https://doi.org/10.1056/nejm199705153362006

Ozaydin M, Peker O, Erdogan D, Kapan S, Turker Y, Varol E, Ozguner F, Dogan A, Ibrisim E (2008) N-acetylcysteine for the prevention of postoperative atrial fibrillation: a prospective, randomized, placebo-controlled pilot study. Eur Heart J 29(5):625–631. https://doi.org/10.1093/eurheartj/ehn011

Parker JO, Farrell B, Lahey KA, Rose BF (1987) Nitrate tolerance: the lack of effect of N-acetylcysteine. Circulation 76(3):572–576

Pizzulli L, Hagendorff A, Zirbes M, Jung W, Luderitz B (1997) N-acetylcysteine attenuates nitroglycerin tolerance in patients with angina pectoris and normal left ventricular function. Am J Cardiol 79(1):28–33

da Silva ND Jr, Roseguini BT, Chehuen M, Fernandes T, Mota GF, Martin PK, Han SW, Forjaz CL, Wolosker N, de Oliveira EM (2015) Effects of oral N-acetylcysteine on walking capacity, leg reactive hyperemia, and inflammatory and angiogenic mediators in patients with intermittent claudication. Am J Phys Heart Circ Phys 309(5):H897–H905. https://doi.org/10.1152/ajpheart.00158.2015

Sochman J (2002) N-acetylcysteine in acute cardiology: 10 years later: what do we know and what would we like to know?! J Am Coll Cardiol 39(9):1422–1428

Sochman J, Vrbska J, Musilova B, Rocek M (1995) Infarct size limitation: acute N-acetylcysteine defense (ISLAND) trial. Start of the study. Int J Cardiol 49(2):181–182

Sochman J, Vrbska J, Musilova B, Rocek M (1997) Infarct size limitation: acute N-acetylcysteine defense (ISLAND trial): a pilot study. Cor Vasa 39:84–89

Svendsen JH, Klarlund K, Aldershvile J, Waldorff S (1989) N-acetylcysteine modifies the acute effects of isosorbide-5-mononitrate in angina pectoris patients evaluated by exercise testing. J Cardiovasc Pharmacol 13(2):320–323

Talasaz AH, Khalili H, Fahimi F, Jenab Y, Broumand MA, Salarifar M, Darabi F (2014) Effects of N-acetylcysteine on the cardiac remodeling biomarkers and major adverse events following acute myocardial infarction: a randomized clinical trial. American journal of cardiovascular drugs : drugs, devices, and other interventions 14(1):51–61. https://doi.org/10.1007/s40256-013-0048-x

Tanen DA, LoVecchio F, Curry SC (2000) Failure of intravenous N-acetylcysteine to reduce methemoglobin produced by sodium nitrite in human volunteers: a randomized controlled trial. Ann Emerg Med 35(4):369–373

Vidart J, Wajner SM, Leite RS, Manica A, Schaan BD, Larsen PR, Maia AL (2014) N-acetylcysteine administration prevents nonthyroidal illness syndrome in patients with acute myocardial infarction: a randomized clinical trial. J Clin Endocrinol Metab 99(12):4537–4545. https://doi.org/10.1210/jc.2014-2192

Wijeysundera DN, Karkouti K, Rao V, Granton JT, Chan CT, Raban R, Carroll J, Poonawala H, Beattie WS (2009) N-acetylcysteine is associated with increased blood loss and blood product utilization during cardiac surgery. Crit Care Med 37(6):1929–1934. https://doi.org/10.1097/CCM.0b013e31819ffed4

Yesilbursa D, Serdar A, Senturk T, Serdar Z, Sag S, Cordan J (2006) Effect of N-acetylcysteine on oxidative stress and ventricular function in patients with myocardial infarction. Heart Vessel 21(1):33–37. https://doi.org/10.1007/s00380-005-0854-4

The Clinical Use of N-Acetylcysteine in Gastrointestinal Disorders

17

Richard Eugene Frye

17.1 Introduction

The gastrointestinal (GI) system includes the GI tract, from the mouth to the anus, as well as the accessory glands such as the liver, pancreas, and gallbladder. GI disorders include both common ailments that affect a wide range of people, such as constipation and diarrhea, and more uncommon but serious disorders such as liver disease.

Some of the first studies using N-Acetylcysteine (NAC) in GI disorders were in the 1960s with the investigation of cystic fibrosis for abdominal pain and ileus (Snyder et al. 1964; Lillibridge et al. 1967; Gracey et al. 1969). Since it is used as a pulmonary mucolytic in this disorder, it was hypothesized that it might improve malabsorption through a similar mechanism in cystic fibrosis (Mitchell and Elliott 1981). It was not until the 1990s that the investigation of NAC into a wider number of GI diseases, particularly liver disease, lead to its successful use in preventing liver failure in acetaminophen overdose. So far, studies still remain limited for many GI conditions. This chapter will review the evidence for the use of NAC for GI disorders and surgery. Proposed biological mechanisms of action are provided in Table 17.1.

R. E. Frye
Barrow Neurological Institute, Phoenix Children's Hospital, University of Arizona College of Medicine – Phoenix, Phoenix, AZ, USA
e-mail: rfrye@phoenixchildrens.com

© Springer Nature Singapore Pte Ltd. 2019
R. E. Frye, M. Berk (eds.), *The Therapeutic Use of N-Acetylcysteine (NAC) in Medicine*, https://doi.org/10.1007/978-981-10-5311-5_17

Table 17.1 Summary of NAC mechanisms of action across different gastrointestinal disorders

Gastrointestinal disorder	Mechanism of N-Acetylcysteine (NAC)
Cystic fibrosis	Reduce thickened mucous in gastrointestinal tract
Liver disease	Improve hemodynamics, tissue oxygen delivery, and hepatic blood flow Restore glutathione and reduce oxidative stress Restore mitochondrial function Reduce inflammatory mediators, particularly toll-like receptors 2 and 4, TNF-alpha, IL-1β, IL-17, and IL-6
Pancreatitis	Restore glutathione and reduce oxidative stress
Liver surgery	Protective effects on ischemia-reperfusion liver injury Improve hemodynamics
Endoscopy	Reduce thickened mucous in gastrointestinal tract

17.2   Methods

A systematic online literature search was done to identify all clinical trials on GI disorders using NAC using the filters "human" and "clinical trials." From these the author reviewer screened titles and abstracts of all potentially relevant publications.

17.3   Evidence of Effectiveness of NAC in the Treatment of Gastrointestinal Disorders

17.3.1 Cystic Fibrosis

17.3.1.1   Abdominal Pain/Ileus

NAC was first reported to treat ileus in cystic fibrosis in a case series of children with fecal retention (Snyder et al. 1964). In an uncontrolled study of six pediatric patients (one who refused to ingest the NAC), all of the patients who ingested the NAC demonstrated hastened recovery from their abdominal pain without any adverse effects (Gracey et al. 1969). Other case reports (Perman et al. 1975; Lillibridge et al. 1967) and case series that include adult patients that previously required operative treatment (Hanly and Fitzgerald 1983) documented the usefulness of NAC in ileus and abdominal discomfort. Unfortunately, these positive uncontrolled studies have not been followed up with any controlled studies, thereby limiting the grade of recommendation (GOR) possible. Clearly, controlled studies are needed to determine the efficacy of NAC in this important population.

17.3.1.2   Malabsorption

A small double-blind placebo-controlled (DBPC) crossover study (level 2b) determined that 200 mg NAC three times a day for 4 weeks did not significantly affect steatorrhea caused by pancreatic insufficiency associated with cystic fibrosis

(Mitchell and Elliott 1981). As this is the only study in this category (GOR C), no recommendations can be made.

17.3.2 NAC for Liver Disease

Given the effectiveness of NAC for supporting the liver function in the context of acetaminophen toxicity, others have investigated the use of NAC for other types of liver disease, including acute and chronic liver failure from idiopathic, infectious, iatrogenic, and alcohol-related causes.

17.3.2.1 Acute Liver Failure

Two studies, one specifically in children, examined the ability of NAC to improve outcomes in acute liver failure not due to acetaminophen toxicity. In a large prospective DBPC (level 1b) study, IV NAC (loading dose of 150 mg/kg over 1 h, followed by 12.5 mg/kg/h × 4 h, followed by infusion of 6.25 mg/kg/h for 67 h) significantly improved transplant-free survival, particularly in those with grade 1 or 2 hepatic encephalopathy but did not improve survival at 3 weeks (Lee et al. 2009). Although NAC was well-tolerated, nausea and vomiting did occur more frequently in the NAC group. As a follow-up to this large study, others have performed follow-up studies, examining predictors of liver transplant (Singh et al. 2013) and inflammatory markers in patients with grade 1 or 2 hepatic encephalopathy (Stravitz et al. 2013). In a large DBPC study (level 1b) of children, IV NAC (150 mg/kg/day) given up to 7 days improved the 1-year liver transplant-free survival but not the overall 1-year survival, hospital or intensive care stay length, or organ failure (Squires et al. 2013). Thus, two level 1b studies study demonstrated positive outcomes (GOR A) suggesting that NAC is useful for acute liver failure not due to acetaminophen toxicity but in both studies secondary outcome measures but not primary outcome measures per positive. It should be noted that NAC showed limited benefit for patients with high-grade (grade 3 and 4) hepatic encephalopathy, so further research is needed to guide treatment indications.

17.3.2.2 Chronic Liver Failure

In a small controlled (no treatment) study (level 2b) of patients with nonalcoholic steatohepatitis, oral NAC 600 mg daily for 4 weeks improved a subset of transaminases but not a wide number of metabolic measures, resulting in the authors raising doubt that NAC provided a significant therapeutic effect (Pamuk and Sonsuz 2003). This study could be viewed as providing safety information regarding NAC in this population, but these data are not strong enough to provide therapeutic recommendations (GOR C).

17.3.2.3 Iatrogenic Hepatitis

In an open-label controlled (no treatment) trial (level 2b), oral NAC (600 mg twice daily) protected elderly patients receiving first-line antituberculosis drugs, including daily doses of isoniazid, rifampicin, pyrazinamide, and ethambutol, from elevation in transaminases or hepatotoxicity (Baniasadi et al. 2010). Although the results of this small study were promising, further studies will be needed before treatment recommendations (GOR C) can be made.

17.3.2.4 Infectious Hepatitis

Three studies have investigated the role of NAC in infectious hepatitis. One small multicenter DBPC trial (level 2b) on patients infected with hepatitis C found that 600 mg oral NAC three times per day for 6 months did not improve transaminase concentrations or hepatitis C clearance, nor were thiol levels positively affected (Bernhard et al. 1998). Given that only one study was conducted on hepatitis C (GOR C), no recommendations can be made.

Two studies, both conducted in China, examined the effect of NAC on chronic hepatitis B patients. In a large DPBC (level 1b) trial, 8 mcg NAC injected with standard therapy for 45 days reduced total bilirubin, hospitalization length, and the elevation in activated prothrombin time (Shi et al. 2005). In a RCT, 8 g NAC was compared to 1.2 g glutathione injected with standard therapy for chronic hepatitis B patients for 28 days in an open-label non-placebo-controlled study. Both therapies reduced total bilirubin and increased activated prothrombin time (Wang et al. 2008). Although the data for treatment of hepatitis B is promising, the few studies conducted (only one placebo controlled) make conclusion (GOR B) of the data premature at this time.

17.3.2.5 Alcohol-Induced Liver Failure

Two studies have examined the treatment effect of NAC in alcohol-related hepatitis. In a small multicenter, single-blinded, placebo-controlled study (level 2b) in patients with biopsy-proven acute alcoholic hepatitis, 300 mg/kg IV NAC for 14 days did not improve 1- and 6-month survival rates, infection rate at 1 month, or the incidence of hepatorenal syndrome (Moreno et al. 2010). In a large open-label placebo-controlled study (level 2b) of severe acute alcoholic hepatitis, IV NAC (300 mg/kg day 1 and 100 mg/kg days 2–5), added to glucocorticoids, significantly improved mortality at 1 month and the incidence of infections and death due to hepatorenal syndrome. Mortality at 6 months and 1 year was only borderline significant improvement (Nguyen-Khac et al. 2011). With two level 2b studies, the GOR is B. However, given the limited number of studies, it is difficult to make any recommendations. Clearly there is some positive data when adding NAC to glucocorticoids; so further research is needed.

17.3.3 Pancreatitis

Two studies have examined whether NAC can prevent post-endoscopic retrograde cholangiopancreatography (ERCP) pancreatitis. In a large DBPC study (level 1b), IV NAC (70 mg/kg 2 h before ERCP and 35 mg/kg every 4 h × 6 doses post-ERCP) did not improve the incidence of post-ERCP pancreatitis or duration of hospitalization (Katsinelos et al. 2005). In another large RCT placebo-controlled study (level 1b), NAC (oral 600 mg 24 and 12 h before ECRP and IV 600 mg every 12 h × 4 doses) did not prevent post-ERCP pancreatitis or change in serum or urine amylase concentrations (Milewski et al. 2006). Thus, with two large controlled level 1b clinical trials (GOR A) demonstrating no effect, a recommendation of no NAC for post-ERCP pancreatitis is made.

Two studies have examined the effect of combination antioxidant therapy on acute pancreatitis. In an observational study (level 2b), a combination antioxidant therapy including selenium, NAC, ascorbic acid, beta-carotene, and alpha-tocopherol given by nasogastric tube did not improve morbidity and mortality (Virlos et al. 2003). In a multicenter DBPC study (level 2b), IV combination of antioxidants, including NAC, selenium, and vitamin C for 7 days, did not improve the incidence of organ dysfunction or patient outcomes (Siriwardena et al. 2007). Thus, with two studies (GOR B) demonstrating no effect of NAC, in combination with other antioxidants, there can be no recommendations made for acute pancreatitis.

17.3.4 The Use of NAC in Liver Surgery

17.3.4.1   Liver Resection

In a large open-label RCT (level 2b) for patients undergoing liver resection, IV NAC (150 mg/kg over 45 min post-op followed by 50 mg/kg over 4 h followed by 100 mg/kg over 16 h followed by 100 mg/kg/day for 3 days) did not change the incidence of adverse effects or liver failure but was associated with a higher incidence of delirium (2.7% and 9.8%), resulting in early trial termination. A multivariate analysis suggested an association between NAC and postoperative complications, specifically florid perceptual and cognitive symptoms together with hyperactive behaviors that reversed after discontinuing NAC (Grendar et al. 2016). The severe cognitive adverse effects are unusually for studies using NAC. The authors did not find any differences in blood work to explain the effect. Thus, NAC cannot be recommended (GOR C) for liver resection, and careful consideration for the mechanisms and adverse effects of NAC needs to be considered before its use during liver resection.

17.3.4.2   Liver Transplant

Eight studies have been conducted on the use of NAC in orthotopic liver transplantation, with six studies conducted on treating the recipient and two studies treating the donor.

In a DBPC study (level 2b), IV NAC given during orthotopic liver transplantation (150 mg/kg over 15 min followed by 12.5 mg/kg/h for 4 h followed by 6.25 mg/kg/h for the remainder of the surgery) to patients with chronic liver disease induced mild vasodilatation, improved oxygen delivery and consumption, and reduced base deficit, but did not improve mortality, morbidity, or postoperative graft function (Bromley et al. 1995). In another placebo-controlled RCT (level 2b), patients undergoing liver transplant who received NAC (just before reperfusion, 150 mg/kg over 15 min followed by 50 mg/kg NAC over 4 h followed by 100 mg/kg over 16 h) demonstrated a reduction in ischemia-reperfusion injury, improved liver function and macrocirculation (Thies et al. 1998). In a small open-label RCT (level 2b), the combination of IV NAC (following reperfusion, 70 mg/kg over 1 h repeated every 12 h for 6 days) along with prostaglandin E1 (0.4 mg/kg/h continuous infusion for 6 days) resulted in a non-significant lower peak transaminase rise and shorter length of hospital stay as well as less severe graft rejection (Bucuvalas et al. 2001). In a placebo-controlled RCT (level 2b), in patients with chronic end-stage liver disease, IV NAC during the anhepatic phase of liver transplant surgery (150 mg/kg over 30 min followed by 50 mg/kg over 4 h followed by 100 mg/kg over 16 h) did not improve oxygen extraction ratio during hepatic artery revascularization nor postoperative graft function (Steib et al. 1998). In a small placebo-controlled (level 2b) study, NAC (just before reperfusion 150 mg/kg over 15 min followed by 50 mg/kg over 4 h followed by 100 mg/kg over 16 h) did not change peak transaminase concentration (Weigand et al. 2001). In a large DPBC study (level 1b), IV NAC (140 mg/kg over 1 h followed by 70 mg/kg every 4 h × 12 doses) did not affect survival or graft function (Hilmi et al. 2010). Thus, of the six studies, one study was positive, another showed positivity in secondary outcomes, and another demonstrated some nonsignificant positive outcomes, but three other studies did not confirm these positive findings. However, NAC was well-tolerated without significant adverse effects. Given that the studies demonstrate significant heterogeneity in the etiology of the liver disease requiring transplantation, it is very possible that specific underlying diseases may respond better than others to NAC supplementation. Thus, further studies are needed to determine if NAC can be helpful in improving outcomes in orthotopic liver transplantation when given to a liver recipient.

The two studies treating the donor with NAC demonstrated more consistent results. In a large single-blind (level 1b) study, IV NAC (30 mg/kg 1 h before liver procurement and 300 mg through the portal vein just before cross-clamping) significantly improved graft survival at 3 and 12 months and lowered postoperative complications (D'Amico et al. 2013). In another controlled study (level 2b), IV NAC (6 g given to a donor about 1 hr before extraction) improved transaminases, prothrombin time, and bile production in the recipient and lowered graft dysfunction and improved graft rejection (Regueira et al. 1997). Thus, the two studies that examined giving NAC to the donor before procurement both suggested that NAC had several positive effects. Given that both studies were adequate in size and well done (GOR B), it is reasonable to suggest that NAC may be used in this context to improve outcomes in orthotopic liver transplantation.

17.3.5 Endoscopy

Five studies have examined whether pretreatment with oral NAC improved visibility during upper endoscopy. Four studies, some rather large, found positive effects of NAC. In a large blinded placebo-controlled study (level 1b), 400 mg NAC 20 min before upper endoscopy improved the mucosal visibility of the stomach and significantly improved total mucosal visibility (Chang et al. 2007). In a large DBPC (level 1b), oral 300 mg NAC combined with 100 mg dimethicone decreased the water flush used during narrowband imaging upper gastrointestinal endoscopy (Chen et al. 2013). In a DBPC study (level 2b), NAC solution 20 min before gastroscopy was associated with a lower volume of flush required to obtain clear mucosa and a faster overall procedure time (Neale et al. 2013). In a very large controlled blinded study (level 1b), 200 mg NAC added to 100 mg simethicone improved total mucosal visibility scores and reduced the need for flushing during upper endoscopy (Chang et al. 2014). Only one study did not find a positive association with NAC treatment and improved visibility during endoscopy. In a large DBPC study, 600 mg NAC did not improve total mucosal visibility score during upper endoscopy (Asl and Sivandzadeh 2011). Thus, these studies provide a GOR A for the use of NAC prior to endoscopy for improving mucosa visibility.

17.4   Summary

In our systematic review, we found several clinical trials that examined the effect of NAC in treating several GI conditions. We have summarized the evidence and recommendations for the use of NAC for these various conditions in Table 17.2. For some conditions, such as acute liver failure, liver failure in general, post-endoscopic retrograde cholangiopancreatography, orthotopic liver

Table 17.2 Overall ratings of NAC based on clinical studies presented by condition

Reason for treatment	Uncontrolled studies positive% (positive/ total)	Controlled studies positive% (positive/ total)	Grade of recommendation	Recommendation for treatment
Cystic fibrosis	100% (5/5)	0% (0/1)	C	None
Abdominal pain/ileus	100% (5/5)		C	None
Fat malabsorption		0% (0/1)	C	None
Liver failure (overall)		50% (4/8)	A	Mixed
Acute liver failure		50% (1/2)	A	Mixed
Chronic liver failure		50% (0.5/1)	C	None
Iatrogenic liver dysfunction		100% (1/1)	C	None
Hepatitis C		0% (0/1)	C	None
Hepatitis B	100% (1/1)	100% (1/1)	B	None
Alcohol induced liver failure		25% (0.5/2)	B	None
Pancreatitis (overall)	0% (0/1)	0% (3/3)	A	No
Post endoscopic retrograde cholangiopancreatography		0% (2/2)	A	No
Acute pancreatitis	0% (0/1)	0% (0/1)	B	None
Liver surgery (overall)	0% (0/1)	67% (4/6)	A	Mixed
Liver resection	0% (0/1)		C	None
Orthotopic liver transplantation (recipient)		33% (2/6)	A	Mixed
Orthotopic liver transplantation (donor)		100% (2/2)	B	Yes
Endoscopy		80% (4/5)	A	Yes

Table 17.3 Ongoing clinical trials on N-Acetylcysteine for gastrointestinal disorders

Trial title	NCT no.	Trial status
Effectiveness of N-Acetylcysteine on preservation solution during liver transplantation	NCT01866644	Unknown
A trial of intravenous N-Acetylcysteine In The management of antituberculous drug-induced hepatitis (NAC in TB DIH)	NCT02182167	Recruiting
The protective effect for liver organ in patients with anti-TB drugs using of acetylcysteine (NAC)	NCT02889757	Not yet recruiting
Prospective cohort study on drug-induced liver injury in China (DILI-P)	NCT02961413	Recruiting
N-Acetylcysteine to reduce infection and mortality for alcoholic hepatitis (NACAH)	NCT03069300	Recruiting
G-CSF plus NAC in severe alcoholic hepatitis	NCT02971306	Recruiting
Fatty liver disease in obese children	NCT02117700	Not yet recruiting

transplantation, and endoscopy, there are an adequate number of good quality clinical trials to make some recommendations. From these studies, NAC appears to be effective for orthotopic liver transplantation when given to the donor and for endoscopy to improve visualization. Mixed, but promising, results are found for using NAC for orthotopic liver transplantation when given to the recipient, treating acute liver failure and liver failure overall, although the data may suggest that the efficacy of NAC may vary depending on etiology of liver failure—an area that deserves further research. Studies on pancreatitis, including acute pancreatitis and post-endoscopic retrograde cholangiopancreatography, were not positive, suggesting that NAC may not have a therapeutic role in pancreatitis. Studies on patient with cystic fibrosis, for at least abdominal pain and ileus, are promising, but the lack of controlled studies limits the ability to make recommendations.

There are also ongoing clinical trials (Table 17.3) on the effect of NAC in GI disorders. There is one study examining the effect of NAC as a preservation solution for the donor liver, which is a variation on the other liver transplantation studies. This is a very promising area of NAC research that could significantly decrease mortality and morbidity in a high-risk patient group. As an extension to the positive study on the positive effect of NAC for preventing iatrogenic liver injury from antituberculosis drugs, three clinical trials are expanding on this initial study, two specifically on antituberculosis drugs. As an extension of the several clinical trials on the use of NAC for chronic liver failure, two studies are examining the role of NAC in alcoholic hepatitis and one study in obese children with fatty liver disease.

From this review, NAC has therapeutic potential in many GI disorders although the number and quality of the studies are limited in many disorders. Clearly, GI disorders are a promising area for the use of NAC as a therapeutic agent. Thus, more studies are needed in this area to better define the dosing regime and the more precise subpopulation that is optimally responsive to NAC therapy.

References

Asl SM, Sivandzadeh GR (2011) Efficacy of premedication with activated Dimethicone or N-acetylcysteine in improving visibility during upper endoscopy. World J Gastroenterol 17(37):4213–4217. https://doi.org/10.3748/wjg.v17.i37.4213

Baniasadi S, Eftekhari P, Tabarsi P, Fahimi F, Raoufy MR, Masjedi MR, Velayati AA (2010) Protective effect of N-acetylcysteine on antituberculosis drug-induced hepatotoxicity. Eur J Gastroenterol Hepatol 22(10):1235–1238. https://doi.org/10.1097/MEG.0b013e32833aa11b

Bernhard MC, Junker E, Hettinger A, Lauterburg BH (1998) Time course of total cysteine, glutathione and homocysteine in plasma of patients with chronic hepatitis C treated with interferon-alpha with and without supplementation with N-acetylcysteine. J Hepatol 28(5):751–755

Bromley PN, Cottam SJ, Hilmi I, Tan KC, Heaton N, Ginsburg R, Potter DR (1995) Effects of intraoperative N-acetylcysteine in orthotopic liver transplantation. Br J Anaesth 75(3):352–354

Bucuvalas JC, Ryckman FC, Krug S, Alonso MH, Balistreri WF, Kotagal U (2001) Effect of treatment with prostaglandin E1 and N-acetylcysteine on pediatric liver transplant recipients: a single-center study. Pediatr Transplant 5(4):274–278

Chang CC, Chen SH, Lin CP, Hsieh CR, Lou HY, Suk FM, Pan S, Wu MS, Chen JN, Chen YF (2007) Premedication with pronase or N-acetylcysteine improves visibility during gastroendoscopy: an endoscopist-blinded, prospective, randomized study. World J Gastroenterol 13(3):444–447

Chang WK, Yeh MK, Hsu HC, Chen HW, Hu MK (2014) Efficacy of simethicone and N-acetylcysteine as premedication in improving visibility during upper endoscopy. J Gastroenterol Hepatol 29(4):769–774. https://doi.org/10.1111/jgh.12487

Chen MJ, Wang HY, Chang CW, Hu KC, Hung CY, Chen CJ, Shih SC (2013) The add-on N-acetylcysteine is more effective than dimethicone alone to eliminate mucus during narrow-band imaging endoscopy: a double-blind, randomized controlled trial. Scand J Gastroenterol 48(2):241–245. https://doi.org/10.3109/00365521.2012.749509

D'Amico F, Vitale A, Piovan D, Bertacco A, Ramirez Morales R, Chiara Frigo A, Bassi D, Bonsignore P, Gringeri E, Valmasoni M, Garbo G, Lodo E, D'Amico FE, Scopelliti M, Carraro A, Gambato M, Brolese A, Zanus G, Neri D, Cillo U (2013) Use of N-acetylcysteine during liver procurement: a prospective randomized controlled study. Liver Transpl 19(2):135–144. https://doi.org/10.1002/lt.23527

Gracey M, Burke V, Anderson CM (1969) Treatment of abdominal pain in cystic fibrosis by oral administration of n-acetyl cysteine. Arch Dis Child 44(235):404–405

Grendar J, Ouellet JF, McKay A, Sutherland FR, Bathe OF, Ball CG, Dixon E (2016) Effect of N-acetylcysteine on liver recovery after resection: a randomized clinical trial. J Surg Oncol 114(4):446–450. https://doi.org/10.1002/jso.24312

Hanly JG, Fitzgerald MX (1983) Meconium ileus equivalent in older patients with cystic fibrosis. Br Med J (Clin Res Ed) 286(6375):1411–1413

Hilmi IA, Peng Z, Planinsic RM, Damian D, Dai F, Tyurina YY, Kagan VE, Kellum JA (2010) N-acetylcysteine does not prevent hepatorenal ischaemia-reperfusion injury in patients undergoing orthotopic liver transplantation. Nephrol Dial Transplant 25(7):2328–2333. https://doi.org/10.1093/ndt/gfq077

Katsinelos P, Kountouras J, Paroutoglou G, Beltsis A, Mimidis K, Zavos C (2005) Intravenous N-acetylcysteine does not prevent post-ERCP pancreatitis. Gastrointest Endosc 62(1):105–111

Lee WM, Hynan LS, Rossaro L, Fontana RJ, Stravitz RT, Larson AM, Davern TJ 2nd, Murray NG, McCashland T, Reisch JS, Robuck PR (2009) Intravenous N-acetylcysteine improves transplant-free survival in early stage non-acetaminophen acute liver failure. Gastroenterology 137(3):856–864, 864.e851. https://doi.org/10.1053/j.gastro.2009.06.006

Lillibridge CB, Docter JM, Eidelman S (1967) Oral administration of n-acetyl cysteine in the prophylaxis of "meconium ileus equivalent". J Pediatr 71(6):887–889

Milewski J, Rydzewska G, Degowska M, Kierzkiewicz M, Rydzewski A (2006) N-acetylcysteine does not prevent post-endoscopic retrograde cholangiopancreatography hyperamylasemia and acute pancreatitis. World J Gastroenterol 12(23):3751–3755

Mitchell EA, Elliott RB (1981) Failure of oral N-acetylcysteine to improve the malabsorption of cystic fibrosis. Aust Paediatr J 17(3):207–208

Moreno C, Langlet P, Hittelet A, Lasser L, Degre D, Evrard S, Colle I, Lemmers A, Deviere J, Le Moine O (2010) Enteral nutrition with or without N-acetylcysteine in the treatment of severe acute alcoholic hepatitis: a randomized multicenter controlled trial. J Hepatol 53(6):1117–1122. https://doi.org/10.1016/j.jhep.2010.05.030

Neale JR, James S, Callaghan J, Patel P (2013) Premedication with N-acetylcysteine and simethicone improves mucosal visualization during gastroscopy: a randomized, controlled, endoscopist-blinded study. Eur J Gastroenterol Hepatol 25(7):778–783. https://doi.org/10.1097/MEG.0b013e32836076b2

Nguyen-Khac E, Thevenot T, Piquet MA, Benferhat S, Goria O, Chatelain D, Tramier B, Dewaele F, Ghrib S, Rudler M, Carbonell N, Tossou H, Bental A, Bernard-Chabert B, Dupas JL (2011) Glucocorticoids plus N-acetylcysteine in severe alcoholic hepatitis. N Engl J Med 365(19):1781–1789. https://doi.org/10.1056/NEJMoa1101214

Pamuk GE, Sonsuz A (2003) N-acetylcysteine in the treatment of non-alcoholic steatohepatitis. J Gastroenterol Hepatol 18(10):1220–1221

Perman J, Breslow L, Ingal D (1975) Nonoperative treatment of meconium ileus equivalent. Am J Dis Child 129(10):1210–1211

Regueira FM, Cienfuegos JA, Pardo F, Hernandez JL, Diez-Caballero A, Sierra A, Nwose E, Espi A, Baixauli J, Rotellar F (1997) Improvement in early function of the hepatic graft after treatment of the donor with N-acetylcysteine: clinical study. Transplant Proc 29(8):3350–3352

Shi XF, Guo SH, Wu G, Mao Q, Yu YS, Wang JK, Zhang L, Wang ZY, Zhang XQ, Zhang QH, Zhao YR, Zeng WQ (2005) [A multi-center clinical study of N-acetylcysteine on chronic hepatitis B]. Zhonghua Gan Zang Bing Za Zhi 13(1):20–23

Singh S, Hynan LS, Lee WM (2013) Improvements in hepatic serological biomarkers are associated with clinical benefit of intravenous N-acetylcysteine in early stage non-acetaminophen acute liver failure. Dig Dis Sci 58(5):1397–1402. https://doi.org/10.1007/s10620-012-2512-x

Siriwardena AK, Mason JM, Balachandra S, Bagul A, Galloway S, Formela L, Hardman JG, Jamdar S (2007) Randomised, double blind, placebo controlled trial of intravenous antioxidant (n-acetylcysteine, selenium, vitamin C) therapy in severe acute pancreatitis. Gut 56(10):1439–1444. https://doi.org/10.1136/gut.2006.115873

Snyder WH Jr, Gwinn JL, Landing BH, Asay LD (1964) Fecal retention in children with cystic fibrosis. Report of three cases. Pediatrics 34:72–77

Squires RH, Dhawan A, Alonso E, Narkewicz MR, Shneider BL, Rodriguez-Baez N, Olio DD, Karpen S, Bucuvalas J, Lobritto S, Rand E, Rosenthal P, Horslen S, Ng V, Subbarao G, Kerkar N, Rudnick D, Lopez MJ, Schwarz K, Romero R, Elisofon S, Doo E, Robuck PR, Lawlor S, Belle SH (2013) Intravenous N-acetylcysteine in pediatric patients with nonacetaminophen acute liver failure: a placebo-controlled clinical trial. Hepatology 57(4):1542–1549. https://doi.org/10.1002/hep.26001

Steib A, Freys G, Collin F, Launoy A, Mark G, Boudjema K (1998) Does N-acetylcysteine improve hemodynamics and graft function in liver transplantation? Liver Transpl Surg 4(2):152–157

Stravitz RT, Sanyal AJ, Reisch J, Bajaj JS, Mirshahi F, Cheng J, Lee WM (2013) Effects of N-acetylcysteine on cytokines in non-acetaminophen acute liver failure: potential mechanism of improvement in transplant-free survival. Liver Int 33(9):1324–1331. https://doi.org/10.1111/liv.12214

Thies JC, Teklote J, Clauer U, Tox U, Klar E, Hofmann WJ, Herfarth C, Otto G (1998) The efficacy of N-acetylcysteine as a hepatoprotective agent in liver transplantation. Transpl Int 11(Suppl 1):S390–S392

Virlos IT, Mason J, Schofield D, McCloy RF, Eddleston JM, Siriwardena AK (2003) Intravenous n-acetylcysteine, ascorbic acid and selenium-based anti-oxidant therapy in severe acute pancreatitis. Scand J Gastroenterol 38(12):1262–1267

Wang N, Shi XF, Guo SH, Zhang DZ, Ren H (2008) [A clinical study of N-acetylcysteine treatment in chronic hepatitis B patients]. Zhonghua Gan Zang Bing Za Zhi 16(7):487–489

Weigand MA, Plachky J, Thies JC, Spies-Martin D, Otto G, Martin E, Bardenheuer HJ (2001) N-acetylcysteine attenuates the increase in alpha-glutathione S-transferase and circulating ICAM-1 and VCAM-1 after reperfusion in humans undergoing liver transplantation. Transplantation 72(4):694–698

The Clinical Use of N-Acetylcysteine in Other Medical Disorders

Richard Eugene Frye

18.1 Introduction

This chapter will review the clinical trial evidence for the use of NAC for disorders not otherwise reviewed in other chapters in this book, including autoimmune disorders, critical illness, cancer, neonatology, surgery, hearing, infectious disease, diabetes, hematology, ophthalmology, and burns as well as skin, reproductive, bone, and metabolic disorders. Proposed biological mechanisms of action are provided in Table 18.1.

18.2 Methods

A systematic online literature search was conducted to identify all clinical trials using NAC using the filters "human" and "clinical trials." From these the author reviewer screened titles and abstracts of all potentially relevant publications, and high-quality studies were selected for medical disorders that are not discussed in other chapters.

18.3 The Effectiveness of NAC in the Treatment of Other Miscellaneous Medical Disorders

18.3.1 Autoimmune Disorders

18.3.1.1 Lupus

In a medium-sized double-blind placebo-controlled (DBPC) study (level 2b), 2.4 g and 4.8 g, but not 1.2 g, doses of NAC daily for 3 months reduced British Isles Lupus Assessment Group index, the Systemic Lupus Erythematosus (SLE) Disease

R. E. Frye
Barrow Neurological Institute, Phoenix Children's Hospital, University of Arizona
College of Medicine – Phoenix, Phoenix, AZ, USA
e-mail: rfrye@phoenixchildrens.com

© Springer Nature Singapore Pte Ltd. 2019
R. E. Frye, M. Berk (eds.), *The Therapeutic Use of N-Acetylcysteine (NAC) in Medicine*, https://doi.org/10.1007/978-981-10-5311-5_18

Table 18.1 Summary of NAC mechanisms of action across miscellaneous disorder

Disorder	Mechanism of N-Acetylcysteine (NAC)
Autoimmune disorder	Restores glutathione and normalizes mitochondrial membrane potential Restores T-cell regulation
Critical illness	Improves oxygen extraction and tissue oxygenation Decreases neutrophil activation Decreases platelet aggregation Enhances nitric oxide release by the endothelium and enhances endothelium function Inhibition of tumor necrosis factor and pro-inflammatory cytokine production Inhibits cellular apoptosis
Cancer	Restores glutathione and reduces oxidative stress
Neonatology	Reduces the viscosity of meconium Decreases neutrophil activation Inhibition of tumor necrosis factor and pro-inflammatory cytokine production Restores glutathione and reduces oxidative stress
Surgery	Inhibition of tumor necrosis factor and pro-inflammatory cytokine production Restores glutathione and reduces oxidative stress
Burns	Decreases activation of granulocytes, lymphocyte, and monocyte Inhibition of tumor necrosis factor and pro-inflammatory cytokine production Restores glutathione and reduced oxidative stress
Skin disorders	Antiproliferative effect Restores glutathione and reduced oxidative stress Decreases inflammation
Auditory disorders	Restores glutathione and reduced oxidative stress
Infectious disease	Reduces the viscosity of sputum Inhibition of tumor necrosis factor and pro-inflammatory cytokine production
Diabetes	Restores glutathione and reduced oxidative stress
Hematology	Restores red cell glutathione and protects red cell protein and DNA from oxidative stress
Ophthalmology	Mucolytic Restores glutathione and reduces oxidative stress Decreases inflammation
Infertility	Restores glutathione and reduces oxidative stress Improves insulin sensitivity and testosterone levels Improves homocysteine levels
Bone health	Inhibitor of osteoclast differentiation and function
Metabolic disorders	Reduction of oxidative stress

Activity Index, and the Fatigue Assessment Scale in patients with SLE. Although one-third of patients receiving 4.8 g NAC developed nausea, it resolved with discontinuation of NAC (Lai et al. 2012). This provides some very compelling evidence for the role of NAC in the treatment of SLE, but with only one study, more research is needed to further confirm and expand on these findings.

18.3.1.2 Systemic Sclerosis

Two clinical trials have examined the effect of NAC on systemic sclerosis. In a small DPBC study (level 2b), NAC up to 10 g daily for 1 year did not demonstrate any significant changes in a wide variety of clinical measures in patients with progressive systemic sclerosis, leading the authors to suggest that larger studies were needed (Furst et al. 1979). In a medium-sized open-label study (level 2b), intravenous (IV) NAC (15 mg/kg/h for 5 h) significantly reduced the resistance index in the renal artery in patients with low disease severity but increased it in patients with more severe disease (Rosato et al. 2009a). Additionally, NAC also improved mean hepatic flow volume in patients with low disease severity as compared to those with more severe disease (Rosato et al. 2009b). Thus, with two level 2b studies, the GOR is B, but the results are mixed with one study being blinded and the other being open-label, but the positive study also used IV NAC as compared to oral NAC in the negative study. Given the inability to clearly interpret the results, there are no recommendations until further studies provide more evidence.

18.3.1.3 Raynaud's Phenomenon Secondary to Systemic Sclerosis

Three clinical studies, one blinded and two open-label, have examined the therapeutic effect of NAC on Raynaud's phenomenon secondary to systemic sclerosis. In a medium-sized DBPC study (level 2b), oral NAC 600 mg three times a day for 4 weeks did not change microcirculation blood flow before and after cold stimulation (Correa et al. 2014). In an open-label study (level 2b), IV NAC (15 mg/kg/h for 5 h) every 2 weeks for 2 years increased global hands perfusion as measured by laser Doppler perfusion imaging and reduced plasma adrenomedullin levels (Salsano et al. 2005). In a small multicenter open-label study (level 2b), IV NAC (150 mg/kg loading followed by 15 mg/kg/h for 120 h) significantly decreased the severity and frequency of attacks, reduced the number of ulcers, and reduced the recovery time in the cold challenge test (Sambo et al. 2001). Thus, with three level 2b studies, the GOR is B but the results are mixed. The blinded study was negative, but it also used oral NAC, while the open-level studies were positive but used IV NAC. Clearly this is a promising area where NAC therapy could be useful, but further clinical studies are needed.

18.3.1.4 Sjögren's Syndrome

In a small DBPC crossover study (level 2b), oral NAC 200 mg three times a day for 4 weeks improved ocular soreness and irritability, halitosis, daytime thirst, and the van Bijsterveld score but not the Schirmer test in patients with Sjögren's syndrome (Walters et al. 1986).

18.3.1.5 Summary

Thus, several studies of various qualities, none with large samples, have used both oral and IV forms of NAC for autoimmune diseases. Overall there is some promising evidence for the use of NAC for various autoimmune diseases, including lupus (one study), systemic sclerosis (two studies), Raynaud's phenomenon (three studies), and Sjögren's syndrome (one study), with all three of the studies that used IV

NAC, and half of the four studies that used oral NAC demonstrating positive findings. Thus, further studies may be helpful for gaining additional evidence of the therapeutic effectiveness of NAC in autoimmune diseases.

18.3.2 Critical Illness

Several, mostly small- to medium-sized studies have examined the utility of NAC in the intensive care unit (ICU) and critical care setting. These will be reviewed in this section.

18.3.2.1 General Use in the Intensive Care Unit

In a medium-sized DBPC study (level 2b) of patients who stayed in the ICU more than 48 h, IV NAC (150 mg/kg bolus followed by infusion of 12 mg/kg/h) for up to 5 days did not affect the length of inotropic support, mechanical ventilation, or ICU stay (Molnar et al. 1998). In a larger DBPC study (level 2b), the same NAC dose was associated with worse mortality in patients admitted to the ICU after being in the hospital for more than 24 h (Molnar et al. 1999). With two level 2b studies, the GOR is B, but with one study demonstrating worse outcomes, the recommendation needs to be no until more studies are available to demonstrate some benefit. It is likely particularly important that future studies consider the specific etiologies for ICU admission as well as the severity of the illness.

18.3.2.2 Multiple Organ Failure

Two DBPC studies have examined the effect of NAC on multiple organ failure. In a small DBPC crossover study (level 2b) in patients with multiple organ failure and evidence of splanchnic hypoxia, IV NAC (150 mg/kg) increased the cardiac index and systemic vasodilation but decreased arterial oxygen and gastric mucosa pH, providing mixed evidence for a beneficial effect of NAC in patients with multiple organ failure (Agusti et al. 1997). In a small DBPC study (level 2b), IV NAC (40 mg/kg/day) did not affect indices of organ dysfunction, length of ICU stay, days of mechanical ventilation, or mortality (Akinci et al. 2005). Thus, with two level 2b studies, there is GOR B with no clear evidence for the use of NAC in patients in the ICU with multiple organ failure, resulting in a recommendation of no for NAC in this context.

18.3.2.3 Respiratory Insufficiency

Four studies have examined the effect of NAC in patients with respiratory insufficiency in the ICU, with two studies specifically examining whether NAC can prevent the change in whole-body oxygen consumption associated with hyperoxic ventilation.

Two medium-sized placebo-controlled studies (level 2b) examined whether pretreatment with IV NAC (150 mg/kg) could prevent the reduction in whole-body oxygen consumption associated with hyperoxic ventilation. In the first study on ICU patient with cardiac risk factors, NAC improved whole-body oxygen consumption, cardiac index, left ventricular stroke work index, and ST segment depression during hyperoxic ventilation, suggesting improved tissue oxygenation and preservation of myocardial performance during hyperoxia (Spies et al. 1996). In a second study, NAC improved whole-body oxygen consumption and oxygen extraction and gastric intramucosal pH during hyperoxia as well as increased cardiac output and decreased systemic vascular resistance, suggesting that NAC improved tissue oxygenation during hyperoxia (Reinhart et al. 1995). Thus, this evidence provides GOR B for NAC pretreatment prior to hyperoxic ventilation with both studies showing benefit leading to a recommendation of yes for this indication.

Two additional studies have examined the effect of NAC on patients with respiratory insufficiency in the ICU. In a medium-sized DBPC study (level 2b) of long-term ventilated patients in a surgical ICU, 3 g NAC daily for 5 days did not affect measures of lung, liver, or kidney function or coagulation or tracheobronchial mucus (Konrad et al. 1995). In an uncontrolled study (level 2b) of cefuroxime plus acetylcysteine, none of the ICU patient with respiratory insufficiency had any adverse effect or worsened in their clinical status (Testasecca and Mengoni 1985). Thus, with two level 2b studies (GOR B) showing no benefit, there is no recommendation made for NAC use in general respiratory insufficiency in the ICU.

18.3.2.4 Hypotension

In a medium-sized DBPC study (level 2b) of ICU patients with hypotension, IV NAC (50 mg/kg over 4 h followed by 100 mg/kg/d for 48 h) with deferoxamine decreased markers of oxidative damage as well as serum creatinine at hospital discharge (Fraga et al. 2012), suggesting that NAC may have some benefit in ICU patients with hypotension. Since there is only one study, it is not possible to make any recommendations for this indication.

18.3.2.5 Sepsis

Five studies have examined the utility of NAC for treating sepsis in the ICU, with four studies demonstrating a benefit and one study showing worse patient outcomes. In a placebo-controlled study, patients with septic shock receiving IV glutathione (GSH) 70 mg/kg/d and NAC 75 mg/kg/d for 5 days demonstrated significant improvements in clinical scores as compared to patients receiving only IV GSH or no antioxidant treatment (Ortolani et al. 2000). In a small DBPC study, IV NAC (150 mg/kg over 15 min followed by 50 mg/kg over 4 h followed by 2.1 mg/kg/h for 72 h) decreased inflammatory mediators, specifically nuclear factor-kappa B and interleukin-8 in patients with sepsis (Paterson et al. 2003). In a medium-sized DBPC study in patients with septic shock, IV NAC (150 mg/kg over 15 min followed by 12.5 mg/kg/h over 90 min) increased absolute liver blood flow and cardiac index and monoethylglycinexylidide and decreased the difference between arterial and gastric mucosal CO_2 tension (Rank et al. 2000). In a medium-sized DPBC study of patients requiring hemodynamic support due to septic shock, significantly more patients receiving IV NAC (150 mg/kg bolus followed by 12.5 mg/kg over 90 min) demonstrated at least a 10% increase in VO_2 (45% NAC vs 0% placebo). Such patients also demonstrated an increase in gastric intramucosal pH, O_2 delivery, and cardiac, stroke, and left ventricular stroke work indexes and a decrease in systemic vascular resistance and venoarterial pCO_2 and had a higher survival rate. However, the authors suggested that the physiological observations may be simply diagnostic of a response to NAC rather than therapeutic since they were not long lasting after NAC was discontinued (Spies et al. 1994). In a medium-sized placebo-controlled study of patients with severe sepsis, IV NAC (50 mg/kg over 4 h followed by 4.2 mg/kg/h for 40 h) resulted in worsening of the sequential organ failure assessment score, particularly for the cardiovascular failure score (Spapen et al. 2005). The authors question whether this effect of NAC may be potentially detrimental on the immune system. Thus, with at least two level 2b studies, the GOR is B, but the data is not consistently positive. Four studies suggest benefit; one study demonstrates that patients have worse outcomes although that particular study enrolled very sick individuals. Lastly, one study demonstrated some physiological inhibition of the immune system but did not demonstrate that such changes were detrimental to the physiological sepsis state. Thus, recommendations cannot be made because of the one study showing detrimental outcomes. Clearly more research is needed to determine whether NAC is beneficial in patients with sepsis and whether any beneficial effect might be limited to less severe patients.

18.3.2.6 Summary for ICU and Critical Care NAC Use

NAC has been investigated in the general ICU setting (two studies) and for patients with multiple organ failure (two studies), respiratory insufficiency (four studies), hypotension (one study), and sepsis (five studies). Of these 14 studies, 7 of these studies (50%) demonstrated positive effects of NAC, but 2 studies suggested that NAC was detrimental to patients with 1 such study examining patients with severe disease. This data suggested that a subset of critical care patients may benefit from NAC while others may not. Thus, further studies are needed to identify specific subsets that will benefit, and larger studies are needed to confirm such benefit on such subpopulations of critical care patients. Because of the heterogeneity of the uses investigated in the ICU, there is no recommendation for the use of NAC in the ICU in general.

18.3.3 Cancer

18.3.3.1 Treatment

Given its importance as an antidote to acetaminophen, a small open-label study demonstrated the utility of NAC in conjunction with high-dose acetaminophen for advanced cancer treatment (Kobrinsky et al. 1996).

18.3.3.2 Prevention of Chemotherapy Adverse Effects

The protective effect of NAC in combination with chemotherapy has been demonstrated in animal studies, leading the way for clinical studies in patients. There is some evidence that NAC can prevent oxaliplatin-induced neuropathy and ifosfamide-induced hematuria. In a small placebo-controlled study of stage III colon cancer patients, oral NAC 1200 mg given before biweekly oxaliplatin therapy significantly improved the incidence of neuropathy (Lin et al. 2006), while in another small open-label study, patients with advanced non-small cell lung cancer were found to be protected from ifosfamide-induced hematuria with NAC at various doses with 6 g daily appearing to be the optimal dose (Slavik and Saiers 1983). Thus, NAC is a promising treatment to prevention of serious adverse effects (AEs) in these chemotherapies, but further controlled trials would be helpful to support this preliminary evidence.

However, the evidence for NAC preventing doxorubicin cardiomyopathy is unclear. In a small placebo-controlled study (level 2b), oral NAC (140 mg/kg) 1 h before doxorubicin did not change measures of acute myocardial damage (Unverferth et al. 1983). In another medium-sized placebo-controlled study (level 2b), oral NAC (5.5 g/m^2) 1 h before doxorubicin demonstrated some cardioprotective effect early in the treatment course that disappeared as the cumulative doxorubicin dose increased (Myers et al. 1983). Thus, there is mixed but weak evidence for NAC in the protection of doxorubicin cardiomyopathy, so recommendations cannot be made unless there are further supportive research studies for this indication.

In a small open-label controlled case series (level 2b), IV and inhaled NAC were added to radiotherapy treatments but did not appear to change tissue reactions and tumor responses (Maasilta et al. 1992). Thus, the preliminary evidence provides no support for NAC in this context.

18.3.3.3   Cancer Prevention

In a very large (over 2500 patients) study (level 1b) of patients with head, neck, or lung cancer, most of whom had a history of smoking, retinyl palmitate, and/or NAC 600 mg daily did not alter survival, event-free survival, or the development of second primary tumors over a 2-year period (van Zandwijk et al. 2000). In an addition analysis of this aforementioned population, it was found that NAC treatment for 3–9 months did not decrease mutagen sensitivity (Cloos et al. 1996).

In a medium-sized DBPC study (level 2b), oral NAC 800 mg daily for 12 weeks significantly improved the proliferative index of colonic crypts in patients with a history of adenomatous colonic polyps, indicating that NAC may decrease the risk of colon cancer in these high-risk patients (Estensen et al. 1999).

In a medium-sized DBPC trial (level 2b) of healthy smokers, oral NAC 1.2 g over 6 months improved certain cancer-associated biomarkers, including lipophilic DNA and 7,8-dihydro-8-oxo-2'-deoxyguanosine adducts in bronchoalveolar lavage cells, the frequency of micronuclei in mouth floor and in soft palate cells, and plasma antioxidant scavenging capacity, suggesting that NAC could positively impact the carcinogenicity effects of tobacco smoke (Van Schooten et al. 2002).

18.3.3.4   Role of NAC in Cancer Treatment and Prevention

NAC has been investigated in the treatment and prevention of cancer as well as the reduction of AEs of chemotherapy for cancer. There is little evidence for NAC in the direct treatment for cancer. Although there are two studies that suggest that NAC may improve markers of cancer recurrence in patients with color cancer and neoplastic markers of cancer in healthy smokers, NAC did not improve or worsen outcomes in individuals with history of head, neck, or lung cancer, suggesting that there is potential for the role of NAC in the prevention of cancer, but it probably depends on the type, severity, and stage of the cancer. There is some evidence that NAC can be helpful in oxaliplatin-induced neuropathy and ifosfamide-induced hematuria, but the evidence remains preliminary. In contrast, studies of doxorubicin cardiomyopathy have provided limited evidence of its effectiveness, and a small study did not support its use as an adjunct to radiotherapy. Because of the heterogeneity of the uses investigated in cancer, there is no recommendation for the use of NAC in cancer in general.

18.3.4 Neonatology

Few studies have examined the use of NAC as a therapeutic agent in neonatal disorders, even though research in the use of NAC in animal models of neonatal disorders appears to be supportive (Kopincova et al. 2014; Mokra et al. 2015a, b; Mikolka et al. 2016; McAdams and Juul 2016). One study examined the pharmacokinetics of NAC in preterm infants, demonstrating that elimination of NAC is much slower in preterm neonates and is highly dependent on weight and gestational age of the patient (Ahola et al. 1999). In a small DBPC, the pharmacokinetics and placental transfer of IV NAC were studied in the context of chorioamnionitis. Clearance was increased in pregnant mothers as compared to nonpregnant adults, and placental transfer was found to be rapid with a slower rate of clearance in the fetus and was affected by gestational age (Wiest et al. 2014). Thus, this demonstrates some of the complications in the research and treatment of neonates with NAC.

18.3.4.1   Chronic Lung Disease

In a small placebo-controlled, crossover study (level 2b), intratracheal NAC every 4 h for 1 week increased total airway pressure by an average to 59% by the third day of treatment but did not have any beneficial effect in premature infants with chronic lung disease (Bibi et al. 1992). In a very large (level 1b) DBPC study, IV NAC (16–32 mg/kg/d) for 6 days starting before 36 h of life did not affect the incidence of death, bronchopulmonary dysplasia, or oxygen requirement at the age of 28 days in extremely low birth weight neonates (Ahola et al. 2003). Also, NAC did not affect lung mechanics, including compliance and resistance, functional residual capacity, and gas mixing efficiency, in a subset of participants in the aforementioned study (Sandberg et al. 2004). Thus, three studies have examined NAC in relation to chronic lung disease in neonates with none showing benefit. NAC not only did not appear to improve respiration in chronic lung disease but may have worsened respiratory parameters. In addition, NAC does not seem to prevent the development of chronic lung disease in premature infants when given early in life, although no AEs were noted in this context. Thus, NAC does not seem to have a role in the treatment or preventions of chronic lung disease, resulting in a recommendation of no for its use for this indication.

18.3.4.2 Fetal Protection

Preeclampsia

One study examined the therapeutic effect of NAC on preeclampsia. In a medium-sized DBPC study of women with severe preeclampsia and/or HELLP syndrome, oral NAC 600 mg every 8 h until delivery did not change levels of GSH or other thiols, except for plasma homocysteine concentrations which was significantly lowed, nor did it change maternal complications, rate of cesarean section, stay at intensive care unit, postpartum hospital stay, or neonatal morbidity and mortality (Roes et al. 2006). Thus, there is no evidence of improvement in outcomes with NAC treatment in this context, but with only one study, no recommendations can be made.

Chorioamnionitis

In a small DBPC study, IV NAC (100 mg/kg/dose) starting within 4 h of the diagnosis of clinical chorioamnionitis every 6 h until delivery improved cerebrovascular coupling and cytokine profiles in infants (Jenkins et al. 2016). Although this study is promising, it is only a small study, resulting in no recommendation for the use of NAC for chorioamnionitis.

18.3.4.3 Summary of the Use of NAC in Neonates

Only a few clinical studies have been conducted in neonates despite animal models demonstrating the potential effectiveness of NAC in neonatal disorders. However, the studies that have been conducted, in general, are not supportive of the use of NAC in neonatal disorders. For example, there appears to be no support for its benefit for chronic lung disease, and one study has suggested it may adversely affect the airway when given by intratracheal means. Its promise is seen in a small study in chorioamnionitis, but it did not seem to be of benefit for severe preeclampsia and/or HELLP syndrome (although it did not cause AEs). Further research is needed, but no clear recommendations can be made for its use in neonatology due to the preliminary and conflicting results of the current clinical studies.

18.3.5 Surgery

Two studies examined the role of NAC in outcome after abdominal aortic surgery. In a medium-sized DBPC study (level 2b), IV NAC (150 mg/kg bolus over 20 min followed by 150 mg/kg over 24 h) started after the induction of anesthesia did not improve biomarkers of renal injury in patients undergoing abdominal aortic surgery (Hynninen et al. 2006). In another medium-sized DBPC study (level 2b), oral NAC 1200 mg twice a day before surgery and oral NAC 600 mg twice a day after aortic aneurysm surgical repair did not improve the incidence of acute renal failure or other clinical outcomes (Macedo et al. 2006). Thus, with GOR B there appears to be no role for NAC in abdominal aortic surgery.

Two studies have examined the role of NAC in extensive abdominal surgery. In a medium-sized DBPC study (level 2b), IV NAC (150 mg/kg bolus followed by

12 mg/kg/h) during extensive abdominal surgery did not decrease the incidence of organ failure, mortality, length of intensive care stay, or days of mechanical ventilation (Szakmany et al. 2003). In another large DBPC study (level 1b), IV NAC (150 mg/kg bolus followed by 12 mg/kg/h) during extensive abdominal surgery did not improve clinical outcomes (Molnar et al. 2003). Thus, with GOR A there appears to be no role for NAC in extensive abdominal surgery.

Three studies have looked at the effect of NAC on the prevention of atelectasis due to surgery. In a large DBPC study (level 1b), oral NAC 200 mg three times a day did not improve postoperative pulmonary function or the frequency of atelectasis in patients undergoing elective upper laparotomy (Jepsen et al. 1989a). In a large open-label controlled study (level 2b), inhaled 20% NAC did not decrease the incidence of massive atelectasis in thoracotomy patients (Silvola et al. 1967). In a medium-sized DBPC study (level 2b), oral NAC 200 mg three times per day did not change the alveolo-arterial oxygen difference or the incidence of atelectasis or pneumonic infiltration in patients undergoing pulmonary surgery (Jepsen et al. 1989b). Thus, with a GOR A, there is no evidence for the use of NAC for the prevention of atelectasis due to surgery.

In a medium-sized DBPC study (level 2b), preoperative IV NAC (240 mg/kg over 12 h) did not change clinical outcomes in patients undergoing lung resection (Bastin et al. 2016). Thus, NAC does not seem to be helpful with lung resection surgery although studies are limited for this indication (GOR C).

In a small single-blinded crossover study (level 2b), nebulized 20% NAC decreased sputum viscosity and improved expectoration and oxygen saturation and increased sputum weight in thoracotomy patients (Gallon 1996). Thus, improving sputum in this small study (GOR C) is the only area where NAC seems to be helpful in thoracic surgery.

18.3.6 Burns

Two studies have examined the effectiveness of NAC for burn injury. In a small controlled open-label randomized trial (level 2b), IV NAC (150 mg/kg bolus followed by 12 mg/kg/h) reduced the vasopressor and inotropic drugs required for patients with burn injury affecting more than 20% of body surface area (Csontos et al. 2011). In another small controlled open-label randomized trial (level 2b), IV NAC (150 mg/kg bolus followed by 12 mg/kg/h) reduced catecholamine requirements but did not decrease multiple organ dysfunction score in burn patients (Csontos et al. 2012). Thus, there is a GOR of B for the use of IV NAC for burns.

18.3.7 Skin

NAC has been investigated for use in the treatment of acne, lamellar ichthyosis, and photodermatosis.

In a large DBPC study (level 1b), topical 5% NAC gel significantly reduced comedo counts in patients with grade I acne (Montes et al. 2012). Thus, there is promising evidence (GOR B) that topical NAC may be useful for acne treatment.

In a small case series, topical 10% NAC along with 5% urea significantly improved lamellar ichthyosis in children (Bassotti et al. 2011). Similar findings were reported in two case studies (Redondo and Bauza 1999; Davila-Seijo et al. 2014).

Two small DBPC crossover studies have failed to show the benefit of oral NAC 1800 mg daily on decreasing photodermatosis in erythropoietic protoporphyria (Bijlmer-Iest et al. 1992; Norris et al. 1995). Additionally NAC did not decrease skin photosensitivity to photodynamic therapy in a small randomized open-label study (Baas et al. 1995).

18.3.8 Auditory Disorder

As reviewed above, NAC has been investigated of iatrogenic-induced hearing loss, particularly prevention of cisplatin-induced hearing loss and hearing loss caused by antibiotics. Other uses include noise-induced hearing loss.

18.3.8.1 Prevention of Cisplatin-Induced Ototoxicity

Three clinical studies have examined the effectiveness of NAC for preventing cisplatin-induced ototoxicity. In a small controlled study (level 2b), transtympanic 10% NAC infusion into one ear, using the opposite ear as a control, during IV effusion of cisplatin, protected the ear against cisplatin induced changes in auditory thresholds at the 8000 Hz frequency band, although the injection was associated with some acute pain (Riga et al. 2013). In similar smaller study, only 2 of 11 (18%) patients demonstrated protection with a transtympanic 2% NAC infusion, resulting in no statistical significance for the overall group (Yoo et al. 2014). In a medium-sized three-arm study (level 2b), oral NAC 600 mg, but not salicylate, given with cisplatin protected patients from ototoxic damage at 10–12 kHz as determined by audiogram but not as measured by brainstem auditory response (Yildirim et al. 2010). Thus, in three, mostly small, studies, there is some evidence for the effectiveness of NAC for preventing cisplatin-induced ototoxicity. The limited nature of this evidence suggests much more research needs to be performed to determine the optimal route and dose of NAC for this indication. Thus, the recommendation (GOR B) is none and should be based on the expert opinion of the treating physician(s) regarding its use for this indication.

18.3.8.2 Prevention of Antibiotic-Induced Hearing Loss

Three studies have examined the effect of NAC on preventing ototoxicity of antibiotics, particularly in the context of treating dialysis-related infections. In a medium-sized open-label controlled randomized study (level 2b) of hemodialysis patients scheduled to receive gentamicin for dialysis catheter-related bacteremia, oral NAC 600 mg twice daily during and 1 week following gentamicin therapy prevented ototoxicity, especially at high frequencies (Feldman et al. 2007). In a medium-sized placebo-controlled randomized study (level 2b), patients receiving amikacin during their first peritoneal dialysis-related peritonitis were protected from ototoxicity, especially at high frequencies, by oral NAC 600 mg twice daily given with amikacin treatment (Kocyigit et al. 2015). In a medium-sized open-label randomized controlled study (level 2b), patients treated with cephalozine or vancomycin and/or amikacin for their first peritoneal dialysis-related peritonitis were protected from low- and high-frequency hearing loss by oral NAC 600 mg during the antibiotic therapy (Tokgoz et al. 2011). Thus, in three medium-sized open-label randomized controlled studies, oral NAC was protective from antibiotic-related ototoxicity. Thus, with GOR B, the recommendation is yes for the use of NAC for antibiotic-related ototoxicity, particularly for dialysis-related infections.

18.3.8.3 Prevention of Noise-Induced Hearing Loss

Additional studies have examined the use of NAC for noise-induced hearing loss. In a medium-sized DBPC study (level 2b), oral NAC 900 mg did not protect normal-hearing participants from detrimental effects of 2 h of live music in a nightclub (Kramer et al. 2006). In a very large DBPC study (level 1b), oral NAC 900 mg three times per day given to a military population during weapons training did significantly decrease the incidence of a significant threshold shift in the trigger-hand ear from 35% to 27% (Kopke et al. 2015), although this was considered a secondary outcome. Thus, there is limited evidence for a benefit for NAC for preventing noise-induced hearing loss. With GOR A, there is no recommendation for this indication, and more research is needed to define the population and dosing of NAC that could be protective from noise-induced hearing loss.

18.3.8.4 Treatment for Otosclerosis

In a large DBPC multisite study (level 1b), IV NAC (150 mg/kg) just prior to stapedotomy for otosclerosis did not improve outcomes (Bagger-Sjoback et al. 2015). Thus, with a GOR B, there is no evidence for NAC for this indication.

18.3.8.5 Summary for the Use of NAC in Auditory Disorders

There are promising studies suggesting that NAC may be helpful in auditory disorders. There is preliminary evidence that NAC could be helpful in preventing cisplatin-induced ototoxicity and good evidence that it is helpful in preventing antibiotic-induced ototoxicity. There is evidence that NAC may be helpful in noise-induced hearing loss in military individuals exposed to loud gunshots but not a general population exposed to loud music, so there may be specific populations and noise levels that NAC may be most useful for. Clearly, more research is needed. Thus, this is a promising area for NAC treatment.

18.3.9 Infectious Disease

18.3.9.1 HIV

There have been several studies on the use of NAC in patients with human immunodeficiency virus (HIV) infection. Three studies have examined the effect of NAC in improving clinical immune parameters specific to the disease, and two studies have examined its effect for preventing AEs of sulfamethoxazole for *Pneumocystis carinii* pneumonia.

In a medium-sized DBPC study (level 2b) of HIV-positive patients with a CD4+ >200, oral NAC 400 mg twice daily slowed the decline in the CD4 count over the 4 months study period (Akerlund et al. 1996). In a medium-sized randomized cross-over trial (level 2b), NAC 500 mg three times a day along with sodium selenite 500 mcg daily for 6 weeks resulted in an increase in the CD4/CD8 ratio and a decrease in the absolute CD8/CD38 count and percentage of lymphocytes and a trend toward an increase in the percentage of CD4+ lymphocytes but no change in the viral load in asymptomatic HIV-infected patients (Look et al. 1998). Although this beneficial effect was found, this benefit was not considered to be comparable with standard antiretroviral drug therapy. In a small DBPC study (level 2b), oral NAC 600 mg daily in HIV-infected patients resulted in a faster increase in the CD4 count during the initiation of antiretroviral therapy (Spada et al. 2002). Thus, there is evidence that NAC may be helpful for improving immunological function in HIV-infected patients, resulting in a recommendation of yes for it use for this indication (GOR B). However, as noted, the effect may not be comparable with modern HIV treatments, so it should not be used as a substitute for standard treatment, and the question remains whether it would have any additional benefit to standard modern HIV antiretroviral treatments.

Two studies have examined whether NAC can be used to reduce the AEs of trimethoprim-sulfamethoxazole therapy for *Pneumocystis carinii* pneumonia prophylaxis. NAC did not reduce the incidence of AEs in a medium-sized DBPC study (level 2b) of HIV-infected patients with CD4 <200 taking oral NAC 800 mg daily (Akerlund et al. 1997) or in a large multisite placebo-controlled single-blinded controlled study (level 2b) of HIV-infected patient with CD4+ <200 treated with oral NAC 3000 mg daily (Walmsley et al. 1998). Thus, there is no evidence to support the notion that NAC can prevent AEs from the antibiotic combination trimethoprim-sulfamethoxazole in HIV-infected patients.

18.3.9.2 Malaria

Three studies have examined the effectiveness of adding NAC to standard malaria therapy. In a large DBPC study (level 1b), IV NAC (150 mg/kg bolus followed by 50 mg/kg over 4 h followed by 100 mg/kg over 16 h) as an adjunctive to IV artesunate did not improve outcomes in patients with severe falciparum malaria (Charunwatthana et al. 2009). In a medium-sized DBPC study (level 2b), IV NAC (300 mg/kg over 20 h) improved serum lactate more quickly but did not improve cytokines or clinical measures in patients with severe malaria (Watt et al. 2002). In a large open-label placebo-controlled study (level 2b), IV NAC (140 mg/kg) followed by either IV or oral NAC (70 mg/kg every 4 h up to 18 dose) as an adjunctive to IV artesunate did not improve clinical outcomes in patients with severe falciparum malaria (Treeprasertsuk et al. 2003). Thus, there does not appear to be any clear evidence for the use of NAC as an adjunct in the treatment of severe malaria (GOR A).

18.3.9.3 Otitis Media

In a medium-sized DBPC study (level 2b), patients undergoing their first bilateral insertion of ventilation tubes due to otitis media with effusion who also underwent infusion of NAC into one ear were found to have a significant reduction in the recurrence of otitis media with effusion and reinsertion of ventilation tubes and a significant increase in the time until ventilation tube extrusion, number of episodes of ear problems, and visits at the clinic (Ovesen et al. 2000). Thus, this appears to be a promising area of NAC therapy, but more studies are needed.

18.3.9.4 Influenza

In a large DBPC study (level 1b), oral NAC 600 mg twice a day for 6 months significantly decreased the frequency of influenza-like episodes and the severity and length of time confined to bed (De Flora et al. 1997). Interesting, although there was similar seroconversion of A/H1N1 Singapore 6/86 influenza virus, significantly fewer patients in the NAC group were symptomatic. Thus, this appears to be a promising area of NAC therapy, but more studies are needed, and it will be important to understand whether NAC improves the ability to prevent infections or rather prevent symptoms of infections.

18.3.9.5 Pulmonary Infections

Bronchiolitis

In a large prospective randomized, controlled study of very young children (level 2b) with acute viral bronchiolitis, nebulized NAC appeared to be superior to nebulized salbutamol, but formal statistics of this study was inadequate to support this qualitative observation (Naz et al. 2014). Thus, although this seems to be a promising application for NAC, more clinical studies are needed before any recommendation can be made (GOR C).

Chronic Bronchitis

Eight good-quality controlled studies have examined the use of oral NAC in patients with chronic bronchitis with seven (88%) reporting positive effects of NAC. Three large DBPC studies (level 1b) used oral NAC 200 mg three times per day (Brocard et al. 1980; Jackson et al. 1984; Boman et al. 1983) while the other positive studies used different dosing, including 200 mg twice a day (Multicenter Study Group 1980), controlled-release 300 mg twice a day (Rasmussen and Glennow 1988), 600 mg twice a day (Hansen et al. 1994), and 600 mg three times per week (Grassi and Morandini 1976). Overall these studies report improvements on sputum characteristics (Brocard et al. 1980; Multicenter Study Group 1980), expectoration (Jackson et al. 1984; Multicenter Study Group 1980), cough (Brocard et al. 1980; Jackson et al. 1984; Multicenter Study Group 1980), rate of exacerbation and/or sick leave (Boman et al. 1983; Multicenter Study Group 1980; Grassi and Morandini 1976; Rasmussen and Glennow 1988), and scores on the General Health Questionnaire, a measure of well-being (Hansen et al. 1994). These studies are supported by a large open-label uncontrolled study (level 2b) of patients with chronic bronchitis, which showed that oral NAC 200 mg three times per day improved the viscosity and character of sputum, cough severity, pulmonary physical examination, and dyspnea at rest (Tattersall et al. 1984). However, one large DBPC study showed that oral NAC 600 mg and/or vitamin C 500 mg did not improve spirometry or symptoms in patients with chronic bronchitis (Lukas et al. 2005). Additionally, a medium-sized multicenter DBPC study found that inhaled NAC over a 16-week study did not improve subjective symptoms (Dueholm et al. 1992). Thus, this data does support the use of oral NAC (GOR A), but not inhaled NAC, for improving symptoms, sputum, exacerbations, and sick days for patients with chronic bronchitis.

Pneumonia

In a large randomized controlled study (level 2b), different doses of aerosolized NAC were given to mechanically ventilated patients. NAC decreased the biofilm thickness and the rate of culture positive biofilm and ventilator-associated pneumonia (Qu et al. 2016). Although this is a promising study, more research is needed to replicate and extend these findings, so no recommendations can be made at this time (GOR C).

18.3.9.6   Biofilms

Bacteria can grow as independent cells in a planktonic form or organized into aggregates known as biofilms. Biofilms increase resistance to antibiotics and allows bacteria to evade host defense and are implicated in chronic infections (Bjarnsholt 2013). NAC has been shown to inhibit the maintenance of biofilm in many laboratory and a few clinical studies.

Several in vitro studies have demonstrated that NAC many be useful in eradicating endodontic biofilms. Choi et al. (2018) demonstrated that NAC better attenuated *Actinomyces naeslundii, Lactobacillus salivarius, Streptococcus mutans,* and *Enterococcus faecalis* from sterile human dentin blocks as compared to other root canal medicaments with 100 mg/mL NAC disrupting the mature multispecies endodontic biofilms completely. Moon et al. (2016) found that NAC significantly inhibited biofilm formation of monospecies and multispecies bacteria broth of *Actinomyces naeslundii, Lactobacillus salivarius, Streptococcus mutans,* and *Enterococcus faecalis* at minimum concentrations of 0.78–3.13 mg/mL and performed significantly better than other root canal medicaments. Other in vitro studies have confirmed these findings (e.g., Moon et al. 2015; Palaniswamy et al. 2016; Quah et al. 2012; Rasmussen et al. 2016; Silveira et al. 2013; Ulusoy et al. 2016).

There is evidence that NAC can inhibit biofilms of bacteria involved in urinary tract infection. NAC has been shown to inhibit *Proteus mirabilis* (Abdel-Baky et al. 2017; Marchese et al. 2003) and *Escherichia coli* strain (Naves et al. 2010) biofilms in vitro. In another study NAC was found to increase the therapeutic efficacy of ciprofloxacin in inhibiting biofilm formation of *Staphylococcus aureus, Staphylococcus epidermidis, Escherichia coli, Klebsiella pneumoniae, Pseudomonas aeruginosa,* and *Proteus vulgaris* from ureteral stent surfaces by degrading the extracellular polysaccharide biofilm matrix (El-Feky et al. 2009). In a randomized comparison study of 80 patients undergoing urodynamic examination, the combination of D-mannose, NAC, and *Morinda citrifolia* extract was found to have a similar effect in preventing urinary tract infections as compared to prulifloxacin antibiotic therapy (Palleschi et al. 2017).

For orthopedic applications, NAC has been shown to enhance the effect of ciprofloxacin on *Pseudomonas aeruginosa* (Onger et al. 2016) and teicoplanin on *Staphylococcus aureus* (Göçer et al. 2017) biofilm formation in bone cement.

In a clinical study, inhaled NAC was found to reduce endotracheal biofilm thickness as well as the rate of ventilator-associated pneumonia in tracheal intubated patients undergoing mechanical ventilation for 48 h or more in the ICU as compared to placebo (Qu et al. 2016). In an in vitro study, NAC was shown to have a synergistic effect with several antibiotics at reducing nonpigmented rapidly growing mycobacteria biofilms (Muñoz-Egea et al. 2016). In another in vitro study, NAC, alone and in combination with ciprofloxacin, was found to reduce *Pseudomonas aeruginosa* biofilms (Zhao and Liu 2010).

When considering applications of eradication of biofilms on vascular catheter in order to reduce nosocomial infections (Aslam et al. 2007), several studies have examined the effect of NAC on bacteria common for these infections. For *Staphylococcus epidermidis* biofilm, NAC potentiated the effect of linezolid (Leite et al. 2013a), farnesol (Gomes et al. 2012), and rifampicin (Leite et al. 2013b), although it was also effective alone in these studies as well as in other studies (Perez-Giraldo et al. 1997). Other studies have shown the inhibitory effect of NAC alone on disrupting biofilms of Gram-positive human skin and mucous membrane pathogens (Eroshenko et al. 2017). Additionally, NAC also improved the activity of amphotericin-B and anidulafungin against *Candida tropicalis* biofilm formation (Fernández-Rivero et al. 2017).

18.3.9.7 Infectious Disease Summary

Clinical studies have examined the role of NAC in several infectious diseases, such as HIV, malaria, otitis media, influenza, as well as pulmonary infections including bronchiolitis, chronic bronchitis, and pneumonia. In most of these areas, there are limited studies except for HIV and chronic bronchitis. For HIV, there is good evidence to suggest that NAC can help immune parameters, although the practical implication of its use is uncertain given the current advances in HIV treatment. For chronic bronchitis there appears to be good evidence for oral NAC reducing symptoms and improving health and well-being. Other areas that are promising but underdeveloped include prevention of influenza symptoms and recurrent otitis media and treatment of acute viral bronchiolitis and pneumonia. Studies on treatment of malaria and prevention of AEs from trimethoprim-sulfamethoxazole in HIV-infected patients do not support its use for these indications.

18.3.10 Diabetes

In a small open-labeled study (level 2b), oral NAC 600–1200 mg twice daily did not improve glycemic control, glucose tolerance, or insulin release in patients with type 2 diabetes nor did it improve oxidative stress (Szkudlinska et al. 2016). Thus, there is no evidence for the use of NAC for blood glucose control in patients with diabetes, but this small study provides limited evidence. Thus, GOR is C, and there is no recommendation for this indication.

18.3.11   Hematology

18.3.11.1   Anemia

Two studies have examined the effect of NAC on genetic anemia. In laboratory studies, NAC inhibits dense cell and irreversible sickle cell formation in sickle erythrocytes. Thus one clinical study has examined the effectiveness of NAC in patients with sickle cell disease on clinical outcome measures. In a small DBPC study of patient with sickle cell disease or S–β^0 thalassemia, oral NAC 2400 mg daily was found to significantly decrease the percent dense cells and the number of vaso-occlusive episodes (Pace et al. 2003). Another clinical study examined the effect of NAC on children with transfusion-dependent β-thalassemia major. In a medium-sized randomized non-blinded controlled study, oral NAC (10 mg/kg; Max 600 mg) daily increased pre-transfusion hemoglobin after 3 months of treatment (Ozdemir et al. 2014). Thus, there is preliminary evidence that oral NAC can be helpful for genetic anemia. Despite the fact that both studies have some positive outcomes, the outcome measures are different in either study as is the population. Thus, given the preliminary nature of these studies, no recommendation (GOR B) can be made at this time.

18.3.11.2   Epistaxis

In a medium-sized open-label baseline controlled study (level 2b) for the treatment of epistaxis in hereditary hemorrhagic telangiectasia, oral NAC 600 mg three times per day decreased the severity and frequency of epistaxis, particularly in those with an ENDOGLIN mutation (de Gussem et al. 2009). This preliminary study provides some promising data, but this isolated study does not allow recommendations to be made.

18.3.11.3   Platelet-Monocyte Conjugation

In a small randomized placebo-controlled crossover study (level 2b), oral NAC 1200 mg daily decreased platelet-monocyte conjugation in patients with well-controlled type 2 diabetes (Treweeke et al. 2012). This preliminary study provides some promising data, but this isolated study does not allow recommendations to be made.

18.3.11.4   Hematology Summary

Although NAC has been used for several hematological disorders, the studies are limited but promising. More research is needed to further identify the therapeutic role of NAC in hematological disorders.

18.3.12 Ophthalmology

Three clinical studies have examined the effect of topical and oral NAC on different ophthalmological indications. In a small controlled study, topical 5% NAC four times per day significantly improved the fluorescein break-up time and Schirmer scores as compared to preservative-free artificial tears in patients with meibomian gland dysfunction (Akyol-Salman et al. 2010). In a small prospective baseline-controlled open-label study, topical 20% NAC four times daily resulted in a decrease in protein deposition on contact lens and improvement in object visual acuity and subjective improvement in vision in patients with Boston keratoprosthesis type I or trichiasis from Stevens-Johnson syndrome, necessitating full-time contact lens wear (Kruh et al. 2015). In a medium-sized prospective randomized, controlled study, oral NAC 100 mg three times daily significantly improved fluorescein break-up time and the mucous fern pattern in patients with chronic posterior blepharitis (Yalcin et al. 2002). Thus, there are promising but preliminary studies suggesting that NAC could be helpful for several ophthalmological indications.

18.3.13 Fertility

Three studies have examined the role of NAC in improving fertility in patients with polycystic ovary syndrome (PCOS), and one study has examined the role of NAC in male infertility. In a medium-sized randomized placebo-controlled study (level 2b), oral 1800 mg NAC daily significantly decreased the number of immature and abnormal oocytes, leptin, luteinizing hormone, and insulin levels in young women with PCOS (Cheraghi et al. 2016). In a large DBPC study (level 1b), oral NAC 1200 mg daily added to clomiphene citrate increased the number of follicles >18 mm, mean endometrial thickness, and ovulation and pregnancy rates as compared to treatment with clomiphene citrate alone in infertile PCOS women (Salehpour et al. 2012). In a large controlled study (level 1b), oral NAC 600 mg twice daily added to clomiphene citrate increased the average number of ovulatory follicles >18 mm, pregnancy rates and peak endometrial thickness as compared to clomiphene citrate alone and clomiphene citrate plus metformin in women with PCOS (Maged et al. 2015). Thus, with three positive studies, with two of them large, NAC appears to have a therapeutic effect for fertility for women with PCOS. Thus, the recommendation (GOR A) is yes for this indication. Infertility in men has also been examined. In a large randomized placebo-controlled study (level 1b) of men with idiopathic infertility, oral NAC 600 mg daily significantly improved the volume, motility, and viscosity of semen (Ciftci et al. 2009). Thus, NAC appears to be a promising treatment for both male and female infertility.

18.3.14 Bone Health

Studies suggest that NAC prevents bone loss in ovariectomized animals. In a small DBPC study (level 2b), oral NAC 2000 mg daily nonsignificantly reduced the bone resorption marker serum C-telopeptide in early postmenopausal women (Sanders et al. 2007). This is promising but very preliminary findings, resulting in no recommendations.

18.3.15 Mitochondrial and Other Metabolic Diseases

Several expert reviewers have suggested NAC as a treatment for mitochondrial disorders (Niyazov et al. 2016; Frye and Rossignol 2012), and in vitro studies have shown that NAC can protect the mitochondria against oxidative stress (Rose et al. 2014). Interesting a case report has suggested that NAC normalized liver dysfunction and coagulation abnormalities in two patients with mitochondrial disease (Enns and Cohen 2017). In a case series of five subjects, the combination of NAC and metronidazole was found in significantly improve clinical and biochemical indices of disease in patients with ethylmalonic encephalopathy (Viscomi et al. 2010). Thus, small studies and expert opinion suggest that NAC may be helpful for several metabolic disorders, but clearly more studies are needed to investigate this in more detail.

18.4 Summary

In this review we found several clinical trials that examined the effect of NAC in disorders not reviewed in other chapters. These disorders include autoimmune, skin, auditory, hematological, ophthalmological, fertility, metabolic and bone disorders, diabetes, cancer and infectious diseases, as well as care in the ICU, including neonatal ICU, and during surgery. There are ongoing clinical trials (Table 18.2) in some of these areas for the use of NAC, including its use in cancer, preventing hearing loss, treatment of human immunodeficiency virus infection, diabetes, and hematological disorders. The evidence and recommendations for the use of NAC for these various conditions are given in Table 18.3.

There are limited studies for most of the disorders reviewed in this chapter. However, there are some areas where the results of clinical studies are consistently strong to justify a recommendation for use of NAC. These areas include pretreatment in the ICU before hyperoxic ventilation, stabilizing burn patients and preventing antibiotic-induced hearing loss, adjunctive treatment for human immunodeficiency virus infection, and improving outcomes in chronic bronchitis and polycystic ovary syndrome. Other areas have shown promising findings in

Table 18.2 Ongoing clinical trials on N-Acetylcysteine for miscellaneous disorders

Trial title	NCT (#)	Trial status
Effect of acetylcysteine with topotecan hydrochloride on the tumor microenvironment in patients with persistent or recurrent high grade ovarian, primary peritoneal, or fallopian tube cancer	NCT02569957	Ongoing
Acetylcysteine rinse in reducing saliva thickness and mucositis in patients with head and neck cancer undergoing radiation therapy	NCT02123511	Ongoing
NAC to prevent cisplatin-induced hearing loss	NCT02094625	Recruiting
RIPE vs RIPE plus N-Acetylcysteine in patients with HIV/TB coinfection (RIPENACTB)	NCT03281226	Recruiting
N-Acetylcysteine (NAC) for healing of amputation stumps in the setting of diabetes	NCT03253328	Recruiting
Antioxidant use in diabetes to reduce oxidative stress	NCT03056014	Not yet recruiting
A randomized double-blind study to examine the use of N-Acetylcysteine for the prevention and treatment of HAAF in patients with type 1 diabetes (NAC for HAAF)	NCT02206152	Recruiting
A pilot study of N-Acetylcysteine in patients with sickle cell disease (NACinSCD)	NCT01800526	Recruiting
A safety and efficacy study of N-Acetylcysteine in patients with hematopoietic stem cell transplantation associated thrombotic microangiopathy	NCT03252925	Recruiting
Effect of NAC on the hematopoietic reconstitution after haploidentical hematopoietic stem cell transplantation	NCT03236220	Recruiting

clinical trials, but there is not enough evidence to make a recommendation at this time, requiring further studies in these areas. These areas include autoimmune and metabolic disease, prevention and treatment of cancer and cancer therapies, chorioamnionitis, skin disorders such as acne and lamellar ichthyosis, treatment and prevention of otitis media, influenza and bronchiolitis, hematological disorders, and male infertility. In some areas there has been a number of clinical trials performed without any benefit seen, resulting in a recommendation not to use NAC. These areas include general use in the ICU, multiple organ failure, extensive abdominal surgery including aortic aneurysm surgery, photodermatosis or malaria, and preventing atelectasis during surgery, chronic lung disease in neonates, or adverse reaction to sulfamethoxazole.

From this review, we can see that NAC has the potential to be therapeutic in many disorders although the number and quality of the studies are limited in many disorders. Clearly, there are promising areas for the use of NAC as a therapeutic agent. Thus, more studies are needed in these areas to better define the dosing regime and the more precise subpopulation that are optimally responsive to NAC therapy.

Table 18.3 Overall ratings of NAC based on clinical studies presented by condition

Reason for treatment	Uncontrolled studies positive% (positive/total)	Controlled studies positive% (positive/total)	Grade of recommendation	Recommendation for treatment
Autoimmune disorders (overall)	100% (2/2)	50% (2.5/5)	B	Mixed
Lupus		100% (1/1)	C	None
Systemic sclerosis		25% (0.5/2)	B	None
Raynaud's phenomenon	100% (2/2)	0% (0/1)	B	Mixed
Sjögren's syndrome		100% (1/1)	C	None
Critical illness				
General intensive care unit		0% (0/2)	B	No
Multiple organ failure		25% (0.5/2)	B	No
Pretreatment with hyperoxic ventilation		100% (2/2)	B	Yes
Respiratory insufficiency		0%(0/2)	B	None
Hypotension		100%(1/1)	C	None
Sepsis		80% (4/5)	B	None
Cancer				
Treatment	100% (1/1)		C	None
Oxaliplatin-induced neuropathy		100%(1/1)	C	None
Ifosfamide-induced hematuria		100%(1/1)	C	None
Doxorubicin cardiomyopathy		25% (0.5/2)	B	None
Radiotherapy		0% (0/1)	C	None
Prevention		67% (2/3)	A	Mixed
Neonatology				
Chronic lung disease		0% (0/3)	A	No
Preeclampsia		0% (0/1)	C	None
Chorioamnionitis		100% (1/1)	C	None
Surgery				
Aortic aneurysm surgery		0% (0/2)	B	No
Extensive abdominal surgery		0% (0/2)	A	No
Prevention of atelectasis		0% (0/3)	A	No
Lung resection		0% (0/1)	C	None
Thoracotomy		100% (1/1)	C	None

(continued)

Table 18.3 (continued)

Reason for treatment	Uncontrolled studies positive% (positive/total)	Controlled studies positive% (positive/total)	Grade of recommendation	Recommendation for treatment
Burns		100% (2/2)	B	Yes
Skin disorders				
Acne		100% (1/1)	B	None
Lamellar ichthyosis	100% (3/3)		C	None
Photodermatosis		0% (3/3)	B	No
Auditory disorder				
Prevention of cisplatin-induced ototoxicity		67% (2/3)	B	None
Prevention of antibiotic-induced hearing loss		100% (3/3)	B	Yes
Prevention of noise-induced hearing loss		25% (0.5/2)	A	None
Otosclerosis		0% (0/1)	B	None
Infectious disease				
Human immunodeficiency virus treatment		100% (3/3)	B	Yes
Prevention of sulphamethoxazole adverse effects		0% (0/2)	B	No
Malaria		0% (0/3)	A	No
Otitis media		100% (1/1)	C	None
Influenza		100% (1/1)	B	None
Bronchiolitis		100% (1/1)	C	None
Chronic bronchitis (oral NAC)		88% (7/8)	A	Yes
Pneumonia		100%	C	None
Diabetes		0% (0/0)	C	None
Hematology				
Genetic anemia		100% (2/2)	B	None
Epistaxis		100% (1/1)	C	None
Platelet-monocyte conjugation		100% (1/1)	C	None
Ophthalmology		100% (3/3)	B	None
Infertility				
Polycystic ovary syndrome		100% (3/3)	A	Yes
Male idiopathic infertility		100% (1/1)	B	None
Bone health		0% (0/1)	C	None
Mitochondrial disease	100% (2/2)		C	None

References

Abdel-Baky RM, Ali MA, Abuo-Rahma GEAA, AbdelAziz N (2017) Inhibition of urease enzyme production and some other virulence factors expression in Proteus mirabilis by N-acetyl cysteine and Dipropyl disulphide. Adv Exp Med Biol 973:99–113

Agusti AG, Togores B, Ibanez J, Raurich JM, Maimo A, Bergada J, Marse P, Jorda R (1997) Effects of N-acetylcysteine on tissue oxygenation in patients with multiple organ failure and evidence of tissue hypoxia. Eur Respir J 10(9):1962–1966

Ahola T, Fellman V, Laaksonen R, Laitila J, Lapatto R, Neuvonen PJ, Raivio KO (1999) Pharmacokinetics of intravenous N-acetylcysteine in pre-term new-born infants. Eur J Clin Pharmacol 55(9):645–650

Ahola T, Lapatto R, Raivio KO, Selander B, Stigson L, Jonsson B, Jonsbo F, Esberg G, Stovring S, Kjartansson S, Stiris T, Lossius K, Virkola K, Fellman V (2003) N-acetylcysteine does not prevent bronchopulmonary dysplasia in immature infants: a randomized controlled trial. J Pediatr 143(6):713–719. https://doi.org/10.1067/s0022-3476(03)00419-0

Akerlund B, Jarstrand C, Lindeke B, Sonnerborg A, Akerblad AC, Rasool O (1996) Effect of N-acetylcysteine(NAC) treatment on HIV-1 infection: a double-blind placebo-controlled trial. Eur J Clin Pharmacol 50(6):457–461

Akerlund B, Tynell E, Bratt G, Bielenstein M, Lidman C (1997) N-acetylcysteine treatment and the risk of toxic reactions to trimethoprim-sulphamethoxazole in primary Pneumocystis carinii prophylaxis in HIV-infected patients. J Infect 35(2):143–147

Akinci SB, Erden IA, Kanbak M, Aypar U (2005) Lack of effect of N-acetylcysteine treatment to ameliorate the progression of multiple organ failure. Saudi Med J 26(4):651–655

Akyol-Salman I, Azizi S, Mumcu U, Baykal O (2010) Efficacy of topical N-acetylcysteine in the treatment of meibomian gland dysfunction. J Ocul Pharmacol Ther 26(4):329–333

Aslam S, Trautner BW, Ramanathan V, Darouiche RO (2007) Combination of tigecycline and N-acetylcysteine reduces biofilm-embedded bacteria on vascular catheters. Antimicrob Agents Chemother 51(4):1556–1558

Baas P, van Mansom I, van Tinteren H, Stewart FA, van Zandwijk N (1995) Effect of N-acetylcysteine on Photofrin-induced skin photosensitivity in patients. Lasers Surg Med 16(4):359–367

Bagger-Sjoback D, Stromback K, Hakizimana P, Plue J, Larsson C, Hultcrantz M, Papatziamos G, Smeds H, Danckwardt-Lilliestrom N, Hellstrom S, Johansson A, Tideholm B, Fridberger A (2015) A randomised, double blind trial of N-Acetylcysteine for hearing protection during stapes surgery. PLoS One 10(3):e0115657. https://doi.org/10.1371/journal.pone.0115657

Bassotti A, Moreno S, Criado E (2011) Successful treatment with topical N-acetylcysteine in urea in five children with congenital lamellar ichthyosis. Pediatr Dermatol 28(4):451–455. https://doi.org/10.1111/j.1525-1470.2011.01375.x

Bastin AJ, Davies N, Lim E, Quinlan GJ, Griffiths MJ (2016) Systemic inflammation and oxidative stress post-lung resection: effect of pretreatment with N-acetylcysteine. Respirology 21(1):180–187. https://doi.org/10.1111/resp.12662

Bibi H, Seifert B, Oullette M, Belik J (1992) Intratracheal N-acetylcysteine use in infants with chronic lung disease. Acta Paediatr 81(4):335–339

Bijlmer-Iest JC, Baart de la Faille H, van Asbeck BS, van Hattum J, van Weelden H, Marx JJ, Koningsberger JC (1992) Protoporphyrin photosensitivity cannot be attenuated by oral N-acetylcysteine. Photodermatol Photoimmunol Photomed 9(6):245–249

Bjarnsholt T (2013) The role of bacterial biofilms in chronic infections. APMIS Suppl 136:1–58

Boman G, Backer U, Larsson S, Melander B, Wahlander L (1983) Oral acetylcysteine reduces exacerbation rate in chronic bronchitis: report of a trial organized by the Swedish Society for Pulmonary Diseases. Eur J Respir Dis 64(6):405–415

Brocard H, Charpin J, Germouty J (1980) Multicenter, double-blind study of oral acetylcysteine vs. placebo. Eur J Respir Dis Suppl 111:65–69

Charunwatthana P, Abul Faiz M, Ruangveerayut R, Maude RJ, Rahman MR, Roberts LJ, Moore K, Bin Yunus E, Hoque MG, Hasan MU, Lee SJ, Pukrittayakamee S, Newton PN, White NJ, Day NP, Dondorp AM (2009) N-acetylcysteine as adjunctive treatment in severe malaria: a randomized, double-blinded placebo-controlled clinical trial. Crit Care Med 37(2):516–522. https://doi.org/10.1097/CCM.0b013e3181958dfd

Cheraghi E, Mehranjani MS, Shariatzadeh MA, Esfahani MH, Ebrahimi Z (2016) N-Acetylcysteine improves oocyte and embryo quality in polycystic ovary syndrome patients undergoing intracytoplasmic sperm injection: an alternative to metformin. Reprod Fertil Dev 28(6):723–731

Choi YS, Kim C, Moon JH, Lee JY (2018) Removal and killing of multispecies endodontic biofilms by N-acetylcysteine. Braz J Microbiol 49(1):184–188

Ciftci H, Verit A, Savas M, Yeni E, Erel O (2009) Effects of N-acetylcysteine on semen parameters and oxidative/antioxidant status. Urology 74(1):73–76. https://doi.org/10.1016/j.urology.2009.02.034

Cloos J, Bongers V, Lubsen H, Tobi H, Braakhuis BJ, Snow GB (1996) Lack of effect of daily N-acetylcysteine supplementation on mutagen sensitivity. Cancer Epidemiol Biomark Prev 5(11):941–944

Correa MJ, Mariz HA, Andrade LE, Kayser C (2014) Oral N-acetylcysteine in the treatment of Raynaud's phenomenon secondary to systemic sclerosis: a randomized, double-blind, placebo-controlled clinical trial. Rev Bras Reumatol 54(6):452–458. https://doi.org/10.1016/j.rbr.2014.07.001

Csontos C, Rezman B, Foldi V, Bogar L, Bognar Z, Drenkovics L, Roth E, Weber G, Lantos J (2011) Effect of N-acetylcysteine treatment on the expression of leukocyte surface markers after burn injury. Burns 37(3):453–464. https://doi.org/10.1016/j.burns.2010.10.008

Csontos C, Rezman B, Foldi V, Bogar L, Drenkovics L, Roth E, Weber G, Lantos J (2012) Effect of N-acetylcysteine treatment on oxidative stress and inflammation after severe burn. Burns 38(3):428–437. https://doi.org/10.1016/j.burns.2011.09.011

Davila-Seijo P, Florez A, Davila-Pousa C, No N, Ferreira C, De la Torre C (2014) Topical N-acetylcysteine for the treatment of lamellar ichthyosis: an improved formula. Pediatr Dermatol 31(3):395–397. https://doi.org/10.1111/pde.12305

De Flora S, Grassi C, Carati L (1997) Attenuation of influenza-like symptomatology and improvement of cell-mediated immunity with long-term N-acetylcysteine treatment. Eur Respir J 10(7):1535–1541

de Gussem EM, Snijder RJ, Disch FJ, Zanen P, Westermann CJ, Mager JJ (2009) The effect of N-acetylcysteine on epistaxis and quality of life in patients with HHT: a pilot study. Rhinology 47(1):85–88

Dueholm M, Nielsen C, Thorshauge H, Evald T, Hansen NC, Madsen HD, Maltbaek N (1992) N-acetylcysteine by metered dose inhaler in the treatment of chronic bronchitis: a multi-Centre study. Respir Med 86(2):89–92

El-Feky MA, El-Rehewy MS, Hassan MA, Abolella HA, Abd El-Baky RM, Gad GF (2009) Effect of ciprofloxacin and N-acetylcysteine on bacterial adherence and biofilm formation on ureteral stent surfaces. Pol J Microbiol 58(3):261–267

Enns GM, Cohen BH (2017) Clinical trials in mitochondrial disease: an update on EPI-743 and RP103. J Inborn Errors Metab Screen 5:1–7

Eroshenko D, Polyudova T, Korobov V (2017) N-acetylcysteine inhibits growth, adhesion and biofilm formation of gram-positive skin pathogens. Microb Pathog 105:145–152

Estensen RD, Levy M, Klopp SJ, Galbraith AR, Mandel JS, Blomquist JA, Wattenberg LW (1999) N-acetylcysteine suppression of the proliferative index in the colon of patients with previous adenomatous colonic polyps. Cancer Lett 147(1–2):109–114

Feldman L, Efrati S, Eviatar E, Abramsohn R, Yarovoy I, Gersch E, Averbukh Z, Weissgarten J (2007) Gentamicin-induced ototoxicity in hemodialysis patients is ameliorated by N-acetylcysteine. Kidney Int 72(3):359–363

Fernández-Rivero ME, Del Pozo JL, Valentín A, de Diego AM, Pemán J, Cantón E (2017) Activity of amphotericin B and anidulafungin combined with rifampicin, clarithromycin, ethylenediaminetetraacetic acid, N-acetylcysteine, and farnesol against Candida tropicalis biofilms. J Fungi 3(1):E16

Fraga CM, Tomasi CD, Biff D, Topanotti MF, Felisberto F, Vuolo F, Petronilho F, Dal-Pizzol F, Ritter C (2012) The effects of N-acetylcysteine and deferoxamine on plasma cytokine and oxidative damage parameters in critically ill patients with prolonged hypotension: a randomized controlled trial. J Clin Pharmacol 52(9):1365–1372. https://doi.org/10.1177/0091270011418657

Frye RE, Rossignol DA (2012) Treatments for mitochondrial dysfunction associated with autism spectrum disorders. J Pediatr Biochem 2(4):241–249

Furst DE, Clements PJ, Harris R, Ross M, Levy J, Paulus HE (1979) Measurement of clinical change in progressive systemic sclerosis: a 1 year double-blind placebo-controlled trial of N-acetylcysteine. Ann Rheum Dis 38(4):356–361

Gallon AM (1996) Evaluation of nebulised acetylcysteine and normal saline in the treatment of sputum retention following thoracotomy. Thorax 51(4):429–432

Göçer H, Emir D, Önger ME, Dabak N (2017) Effects of bone cement loaded with teicoplanin, N-acetylcysteine or their combination on Staphylococcus aureus biofilm formation: an in vitro study. Eklem Hastalik Cerrahisi 28(1):13–18

Gomes F, Leite B, Teixeira P, Azeredo J, Oliveira R (2012) Farnesol in combination with N-acetylcysteine against Staphylococcus epidermidis planktonic and biofilm cells. Braz J Microbiol 43(1):235–242

Grassi C, Morandini GC (1976) A controlled trial of intermittent oral acetylcysteine in the long-term treatment of chronic bronchitis. Eur J Clin Pharmacol 09(5–6):393–396

Hansen NC, Skriver A, Brorsen-Riis L, Balslov S, Evald T, Maltbaek N, Gunnersen G, Garsdal P, Sander P, Pedersen JZ et al (1994) Orally administered N-acetylcysteine may improve general well-being in patients with mild chronic bronchitis. Respir Med 88(7):531–535

Hynninen MS, Niemi TT, Poyhia R, Raininko EI, Salmenpera MT, Lepantalo MJ, Railo MJ, Tallgren MK (2006) N-acetylcysteine for the prevention of kidney injury in abdominal aortic surgery: a randomized, double-blind, placebo-controlled trial. Anesth Analg 102(6):1638–1645. https://doi.org/10.1213/01.ane.0000219590.79796.66

Jackson IM, Barnes J, Cooksey P (1984) Efficacy and tolerability of oral acetylcysteine (Fabrol) in chronic bronchitis: a double-blind placebo controlled study. J Int Med Res 12(3):198–206. https://doi.org/10.1177/030006058401200312

Jenkins DD, Wiest DB, Mulvihill DM, Hlavacek AM, Majstoravich SJ, Brown TR, Taylor JJ, Buckley JR, Turner RP, Rollins LG, Bentzley JP, Hope KE, Barbour AB, Lowe DW, Martin RH, Chang EY (2016) Fetal and neonatal effects of N-acetylcysteine when used for neuroprotection in maternal chorioamnionitis. J Pediatr 168:67–76.e66. https://doi.org/10.1016/j.jpeds.2015.09.076

Jepsen S, Klaerke A, Nielsen PH, Nielsen ST, Simonsen O (1989a) Systemic administration of N-acetylcysteine has no effect on postoperative lung function following elective upper laparotomy in lung healthy patients. Acta Anaesthesiol Scand 33(3):219–222

Jepsen S, Nielsen PH, Klaerke A, Nielsen ST, Simonsen O (1989b) Peroral N-acetylcysteine as prophylaxis against bronchopulmonary complications of pulmonary surgery. Scand J Thorac Cardiovasc Surg 23(2):185–188

Kobrinsky NL, Hartfield D, Horner H, Maksymiuk A, Minuk GY, White DF, Feldstein TJ (1996) Treatment of advanced malignancies with high-dose acetaminophen and N-acetylcysteine rescue. Cancer Investig 14(3):202–210. https://doi.org/10.3109/07357909609012140

Kocyigit I, Vural A, Unal A, Sipahioglu MH, Yucel HE, Aydemir S, Yazici C, Ilhan Sahin M, Oymak O, Tokgoz B (2015) Preventing amikacin related ototoxicity with N-acetylcysteine in patients undergoing peritoneal dialysis. Eur Arch Otorhinolaryngol 272(10):2611–2620. https://doi.org/10.1007/s00405-014-3207-z

Konrad F, Schoenberg MH, Wiedmann H, Kilian J, Georgieff M (1995) The application of n-acetylcysteine as an antioxidant and mucolytic in mechanical ventilation in intensive care patients. A prospective, randomized, placebo-controlled, double-blind study. Anaesthesist 44(9):651–658

Kopincova J, Mokra D, Mikolka P, Kolomaznik M, Calkovska A (2014) N-acetylcysteine advancement of surfactant therapy in experimental meconium aspiration syndrome: possible mechanisms. Physiol Res 63(Suppl 4):S629–S642

Kopke R, Slade MD, Jackson R, Hammill T, Fausti S, Lonsbury-Martin B, Sanderson A, Dreisbach L, Rabinowitz P, Torre P, Balough B (2015) Efficacy and safety of N-acetylcysteine in prevention of noise induced hearing loss: a randomized clinical trial. Hear Res 323:40–50. https://doi.org/10.1016/j.heares.2015.01.002

Kramer S, Dreisbach L, Lockwood J, Baldwin K, Kopke R, Scranton S, O'Leary M (2006) Efficacy of the antioxidant N-acetylcysteine (NAC) in protecting ears exposed to loud music. J Am Acad Audiol 17(4):265–278

Kruh JN, Kruh-Garcia NA, Foster CS (2015) Evaluation of the effect of N-acetylcysteine on protein deposition on contact lenses in patients with the Boston Keratoprosthesis type I. J Ocul Pharmacol Ther 31(6):314–322. https://doi.org/10.1089/jop.2015.0010

Lai ZW, Hanczko R, Bonilla E, Caza TN, Clair B, Bartos A, Miklossy G, Jimah J, Doherty E, Tily H, Francis L, Garcia R, Dawood M, Yu J, Ramos I, Coman I, Faraone SV, Phillips PE, Perl A (2012) N-acetylcysteine reduces disease activity by blocking mammalian target of rapamycin in T cells from systemic lupus erythematosus patients: a randomized, double-blind, placebo-controlled trial. Arthritis Rheum 64(9):2937–2946. https://doi.org/10.1002/art.34502

Leite B, Gomes F, Teixeira P, Souza C, Pizzolitto E, Oliveira R (2013a) Combined effect of linezolid and N-acetylcysteine against Staphylococcus epidermidis biofilms. Enferm Infecc Microbiol Clin 31(10):655–659

Leite B, Gomes F, Teixeira P, Souza C, Pizzolitto E, Oliveira R (2013b) Staphylococcus epidermidis Biofilms control by N-acetylcysteine and rifampicin. Am J Ther 20(4):322–328

Lin PC, Lee MY, Wang WS, Yen CC, Chao TC, Hsiao LT, Yang MH, Chen PM, Lin KP, Chiou TJ (2006) N-acetylcysteine has neuroprotective effects against oxaliplatin-based adjuvant chemotherapy in colon cancer patients: preliminary data. Support Care Cancer 14(5):484–487. https://doi.org/10.1007/s00520-006-0018-9

Look MP, Rockstroh JK, Rao GS, Barton S, Lemoch H, Kaiser R, Kupfer B, Sudhop T, Spengler U, Sauerbruch T (1998) Sodium selenite and N-acetylcysteine in antiretroviral-naive HIV-1-infected patients: a randomized, controlled pilot study. Eur J Clin Investig 28(5):389–397

Lukas R, Scharling B, Schultze-Werninghaus G, Gillissen A (2005) Antioxidant treatment with N-acetylcysteine and vitamin C in patients with chronic bronchitis. Dtsch Med Wochenschr 130(11):563–567. https://doi.org/10.1055/s-2005-865062

Maasilta P, Holsti LR, Blomqvist P, Kivisaari L, Mattson K (1992) N-acetylcysteine in combination with radiotherapy in the treatment of non-small cell lung cancer: a feasibility study. Radiother Oncol 25(3):192–195

Macedo E, Abdulkader R, Castro I, Sobrinho AC, Yu L, Vieira JM Jr (2006) Lack of protection of N-acetylcysteine (NAC) in acute renal failure related to elective aortic aneurysm repair-a randomized controlled trial. Nephrol Dial Transplant 21(7):1863–1869. https://doi.org/10.1093/ndt/gfl079

Maged AM, Elsawah H, Abdelhafez A, Bakry A, Mostafa WA (2015) The adjuvant effect of metformin and N-acetylcysteine to clomiphene citrate in induction of ovulation in patients with Polycystic Ovary Syndrome. Gynecol Endocrinol 31(8):635–638

Marchese A, Bozzolasco M, Gualco L, Debbia EA, Schito GC, Schito AM (2003) Effect of fosfomycin alone and in combination with N-acetylcysteine on E. coli biofilms. Int J Antimicrob Agents 22:95–100

McAdams RM, Juul SE (2016) Neonatal encephalopathy: update on therapeutic hypothermia and other novel therapeutics. Clin Perinatol 43(3):485–500. https://doi.org/10.1016/j.clp.2016.04.007

Mikolka P, Kopincova J, Mikusiakova LT, Kosutova P, Calkovska A, Mokra D (2016) Anti-inflammatory effect of N-acetylcysteine combined with exogenous surfactant in meconium-induced lung injury. Adv Exp Med Biol 934:63–75. https://doi.org/10.1007/5584_2016_15

Mokra D, Drgova A, Mokry J, Antosova M, Durdik P, Calkovska A (2015a) N-acetylcysteine effectively diminished meconium-induced oxidative stress in adult rabbits. J Physiol Pharmacol 66(1):101–110

Mokra D, Drgova A, Petras M, Mokry J, Antosova M, Calkovska A (2015b) N-acetylcysteine alleviates the meconium-induced acute lung injury. Adv Exp Med Biol 832:59–67. https://doi.org/10.1007/5584_2014_7

Molnar Z, MacKinnon KL, Shearer E, Lowe D, Watson ID (1998) The effect of N-acetylcysteine on total serum anti-oxidant potential and urinary albumin excretion in critically ill patients. Intensive Care Med 24(3):230–235

Molnar Z, Shearer E, Lowe D (1999) N-Acetylcysteine treatment to prevent the progression of multisystem organ failure: a prospective, randomized, placebo-controlled study. Crit Care Med 27(6):1100–1104

Molnar Z, Szakmany T, Koszegi T (2003) Prophylactic N-acetylcysteine decreases serum CRP but not PCT levels and microalbuminuria following major abdominal surgery. A prospective, randomised, double-blinded, placebo-controlled clinical trial. Intensive Care Med 29(5):749–755. https://doi.org/10.1007/s00134-003-1723-1

Montes LF, Wilborn WH, Montes CM (2012) Topical acne treatment with acetylcysteine: clinical and experimental effects. Skinmed 10(6):348–351

Moon JH, Jang EY, Shim KS, Lee JY (2015) In vitro effects of N-acetyl cysteine alone and in combination with antibiotics on Prevotella intermedia. J Microbiol 53(5):321–329

Moon JH, Choi YS, Lee HW, Heo JS, Chang SW, Lee JY (2016) Antibacterial effects of N acetyl-cysteine against endodontic pathogens. J Microbiol 54(4):322–329

Multicenter Study Group (1980) Long-term oral acetylcysteine in chronic bronchitis. A double-blind controlled study. Eur J Respir Dis Suppl 111:93–108

Muñoz-Egea MC, García-Pedrazuela M, Mahillo-Fernandez I, Esteban J (2016) Effect of antibiotics and antibiofilm agents in the ultrastructure and development of biofilms developed by nonpigmented rapidly growing mycobacteria. Microb Drug Resist 22(1):1–6

Myers C, Bonow R, Palmeri S, Jenkins J, Corden B, Locker G, Doroshow J, Epstein S (1983) A randomized controlled trial assessing the prevention of doxorubicin cardiomyopathy by N-acetylcysteine. Semin Oncol 10(1 Suppl 1):53–55

Naves P, del Prado G, Huelves L, Rodríguez-Cerrato V, Ruiz V, Ponte MC, Soriano F (2010) Effects of human serum albumin, ibuprofen and N-acetyl-L-cysteine against biofilm formation by pathogenic Escherichia coli strains. J Hosp Infect 76(2):165–170

Naz F, Raza AB, Ijaz I, Kazi MY (2014) Effectiveness of nebulized N-acetylcysteine solution in children with acute bronchiolitis. J Coll Physicians Surg Pak 24(6):408–411. doi:06.2014/jcpsp.408411

Niyazov DM, Kahler SG, Frye RE (2016) Primary mitochondrial disease and secondary mitochondrial dysfunction: importance of distinction for diagnosis and treatment. Mol Syndromol 7(3):122–137. https://doi.org/10.1159/000446586

Norris PG, Baker CS, Roberts JE, Hawk JL (1995) Treatment of erythropoietic protoporphyria with N-acetylcysteine. Arch Dermatol 131(3):354–355

Onger ME, Gocer H, Emir D, Kaplan S (2016) N-acetylcysteine eradicates Pseudomonas aeruginosa biofilms in bone cement. Scanning 38(6):766–770

Ortolani O, Conti A, De Gaudio AR, Moraldi E, Cantini Q, Novelli G (2000) The effect of glutathione and N-acetylcysteine on lipoperoxidative damage in patients with early septic shock. Am J Respir Crit Care Med 161(6):1907–1911. https://doi.org/10.1164/ajrccm.161.6.9903043

Ovesen T, Felding JU, Tommerup B, Schousboe LP, Petersen CG (2000) Effect of N-acetylcysteine on the incidence of recurrence of otitis media with effusion and re-insertion of ventilation tubes. Acta Otolaryngol Suppl 543:79–81

Ozdemir ZC, Koc A, Aycicek A, Kocyigit A (2014) N-Acetylcysteine supplementation reduces oxidative stress and DNA damage in children with beta-thalassemia. Hemoglobin 38(5):359–364. https://doi.org/10.3109/03630269.2014.951890

Pace BS, Shartava A, Pack-Mabien A, Mulekar M, Ardia A, Goodman SR (2003) Effects of N-acetylcysteine on dense cell formation in sickle cell disease. Am J Hematol 73(1):26–32

Palaniswamy U, Lakkam SR, Arya S, Aravelli S (2016) Effectiveness of N-acetyl cysteine, 2% chlorhexidine, and their combination as intracanal medicaments on Enterococcus faecalis biofilm. J Conserv Dent 19(1):17–20

Palleschi G, Carbone A, Zanello PP, Mele R, Leto A, Fuschi A, Al Salhi Y, Velotti G, Al Rawashdah S, Coppola G, Maurizi A, Maruccia S, Pastore AL (2017) Prospective study to compare antibiosis versus the association of N-acetylcysteine, D-mannose and Morinda citrifolia fruit extract in preventing urinary tract infections in patients submitted to urodynamic investigation. Arch Ital Urol Androl 89(1):45–50

Paterson RL, Galley HF, Webster NR (2003) The effect of N-acetylcysteine on nuclear factor-kappa B activation, interleukin-6, interleukin-8, and intercellular adhesion molecule-1 expression in patients with sepsis. Crit Care Med 31(11):2574–2578

Perez-Giraldo C, Rodriguez-Benito A, Moran FJ, Hurtado C, Blanco MT, Gomez-Garcia AC (1997) Influence of N-acetylcysteine on the formation of biofilm by Staphylococcus epidermidis. J Antimicrob Chemother 39(5):643–646

Qu D, Ren XX, Guo LY, Liang JX, Xu WJ, Han YH, Zhu YM (2016) Effect of N-acetylcysteine inhalation on ventilator-associated pneumonia caused by biofilm in endotracheal tubes. Zhonghua Er Ke Za Zhi 54(4):278–282

Quah SY, Wu S, Lui JN, Sum CP, Tan KS (2012) N-acetylcysteine inhibits growth and eradicates biofilm of Enterococcus faecalis. J Endod 38(1):81–85

Rank N, Michel C, Haertel C, Lenhart A, Welte M, Meier-Hellmann A, Spies C (2000) N-acetylcysteine increases liver blood flow and improves liver function in septic shock patients: results of a prospective, randomized, double-blind study. Crit Care Med 28(12):3799–3807

Rasmussen JB, Glennow C (1988) Reduction in days of illness after long-term treatment with N-acetylcysteine controlled-release tablets in patients with chronic bronchitis. Eur Respir J 1(4):351–355

Rasmussen K, Nikrad J, Reilly C, Li Y, Jones RS (2016) N-acetyl-l-cysteine effects on multi-species oral biofilm formation and bacterial ecology. Lett Appl Microbiol 62(1):30–38

Redondo P, Bauza A (1999) Topical N-acetylcysteine for lamellar ichthyosis. Lancet 354(9193):1880. https://doi.org/10.1016/s0140-6736(99)04245-2

Reinhart K, Spies CD, Meier-Hellmann A, Bredle DL, Hannemann L, Specht M, Schaffartzik W (1995) N-acetylcysteine preserves oxygen consumption and gastric mucosal pH during hyperoxic ventilation. Am J Respir Crit Care Med 151(3 Pt 1):773–779. https://doi.org/10.1164/ajrccm/151.3_Pt_1.773

Riga MG, Chelis L, Kakolyris S, Papadopoulos S, Stathakidou S, Chamalidou E, Xenidis N, Amarantidis K, Dimopoulos P, Danielides V (2013) Transtympanic injections of N-acetylcysteine for the prevention of cisplatin-induced ototoxicity: a feasible method with promising efficacy. Am J Clin Oncol 36(1):1–6. https://doi.org/10.1097/COC.0b013e31822e006d

Roes EM, Raijmakers MT, Boo TM, Zusterzeel PL, Merkus HM, Peters WH, Steegers EA (2006) Oral N-acetylcysteine administration does not stabilise the process of established severe preeclampsia. Eur J Obstet Gynecol Reprod Biol 127(1):61–67. https://doi.org/10.1016/j.ejogrb.2005.09.007

Rosato E, Cianci R, Barbano B, Menghi G, Gigante A, Rossi C, Zardi EM, Amoroso A, Pisarri S, Salsano F (2009a) N-acetylcysteine infusion reduces the resistance index of renal artery in the early stage of systemic sclerosis. Acta Pharmacol Sin 30(9):1283–1288. https://doi.org/10.1038/aps.2009.128

Rosato E, Zardi EM, Barbano B, Menghi G, Cianci R, Amoroso A, Afeltra A, Pisarri S, Salsano F (2009b) N-acetylcysteine infusion improves hepatic perfusion in the early stages of systemic sclerosis. Int J Immunopathol Pharmacol 22(3):763–772. https://doi.org/10.1177/039463200902200322

Rose S, Frye RE, Slattery J, Wynne R, Tippett M, Melnyk S, James SJ (2014) Oxidative stress induces mitochondrial dysfunction in a subset of autistic lymphoblastoid cell lines. Transl Psychiatry 4:e377. https://doi.org/10.1038/tp.2014.15

Salehpour S, Sene AA, Saharkhiz N, Sohrabi MR, Moghimian F (2012) N-acetylcysteine as an adjuvant to clomiphene citrate for successful induction of ovulation in infertile patients with polycystic ovary syndrome. J Obstet Gynaecol Res 38(9):1182–1186. https://doi.org/10.1111/j.1447-0756.2012.01844.x

Salsano F, Letizia C, Proietti M, Rossi C, Proietti AR, Rosato E, Pisarri S (2005) Significant changes of peripheral perfusion and plasma adrenomedullin levels in N-acetylcysteine long term treatment of patients with sclerodermic Raynauds phenomenon. Int J Immunopathol Pharmacol 18(4):761–770

Sambo P, Amico D, Giacomelli R, Matucci-Cerinic M, Salsano F, Valentini G, Gabrielli A (2001) Intravenous N-acetylcysteine for treatment of Raynaud's phenomenon secondary to systemic sclerosis: a pilot study. J Rheumatol 28(10):2257–2262

Sandberg K, Fellman V, Stigson L, Thiringer K, Hjalmarson O (2004) N-acetylcysteine administration during the first week of life does not improve lung function in extremely low birth weight infants. Biol Neonate 86(4):275–279. https://doi.org/10.1159/000080089

Sanders KM, Kotowicz MA, Nicholson GC (2007) Potential role of the antioxidant N-acetylcysteine in slowing bone resorption in early post-menopausal women: a pilot study. Transl Res 150(4):215. https://doi.org/10.1016/j.trsl.2007.03.012

Van Schooten FJ, Besaratinia A, De Flora S, D'Agostini F, Izzotti A, Camoirano A, Balm AJ, Dallinga JW, Bast A, Haenen GR, Van't Veer L, Baas P, Sakai H, Van Zandwijk N (2002) Effects of oral administration of N-acetyl-L-cysteine: a multi-biomarker study in smokers. Cancer Epidemiol Biomark Prev 11(2):167–175

Silveira LF, Baca P, Arias-Moliz MT, Rodríguez-Archilla A, Ferrer-Luque CM (2013) Antimicrobial activity of alexidine alone and associated with N-acetylcysteine against Enterococcus faecalis biofilm. Int J Oral Sci 5(3):146–149

Silvola HJ, Salonen I, Tala P (1967) Acetylcysteine inhalations and postoperative atelectasis in thoracic surgery. Ann Chir Gynaecol Fenn 56(2):233–236

Slavik M, Saiers JH (1983) Phase I clinical study of acetylcysteine's preventing ifosfamide-induced hematuria. Semin Oncol 10(1 Suppl 1):62–65

Spada C, Treitinger A, Reis M, Masokawa IY, Verdi JC, Luiz MC, Silveira MV, Michelon CM, Avila-Junior S, Gil l D, Ostrowskyl S (2002) The effect of N-acetylcysteine supplementation upon viral load, CD4, CD8, total lymphocyte count and hematocrit in individuals undergoing antiretroviral treatment. Clin Chem Lab Med 40(5):452–455. https://doi.org/10.1515/cclm.2002.077

Spapen HD, Diltoer MW, Nguyen DN, Hendrickx I, Huyghens LP (2005) Effects of N-acetylcysteine on microalbuminuria and organ failure in acute severe sepsis: results of a pilot study. Chest 127(4):1413–1419

Spies C, Giese C, Meier-Hellmann A, Specht M, Hannemann L, Schaffartzik W, Reinhart K (1996) The effect of prophylactically administered n-acetylcysteine on clinical indicators for tissue oxygenation during hyperoxic ventilation in cardiac risk patients. Anaesthesist 45(4):343–350

Spies CD, Reinhart K, Witt I, Meier-Hellmann A, Hannemann L, Bredle DL, Schaffartzik W (1994) Influence of N-acetylcysteine on indirect indicators of tissue oxygenation in septic shock patients: results from a prospective, randomized, double-blind study. Crit Care Med 22(11):1738–1746

Szakmany T, Marton S, Molnar Z (2003) Lack of effect of prophylactic N-acetylcysteine on postoperative organ dysfunction following major abdominal tumour surgery: a randomized, placebo-controlled, double-blinded clinical trial. Anaesth Intensive Care 31(3):267–271

Szkudlinska MA, von Frankenberg AD, Utzschneider KM (2016) The antioxidant N-Acetylcysteine does not improve glucose tolerance or beta-cell function in type 2 diabetes. J Diabetes Complicat 30(4):618–622. https://doi.org/10.1016/j.jdiacomp.2016.02.003

Tattersall AB, Bridgman KM, Huitson A (1984) Irish general practice study of acetylcysteine (Fabrol) in chronic bronchitis. J Int Med Res 12(2):96–101. https://doi.org/10.1177/030006058401200206

Testasecca D, Mengoni M (1985) A combination of cefuroxime plus acetylcysteine in the intensive care of patients with respiratory insufficiency. Int J Clin Pharmacol Ther Toxicol 23(2):115–117

Tokgoz B, Ucar C, Kocyigit I, Somdas M, Unal A, Vural A, Sipahioglu M, Oymak O, Utas C (2011) Protective effect of N-acetylcysteine from drug-induced ototoxicity in uraemic patients with CAPD peritonitis. Nephrol Dial Transplant 26(12):4073–4078. https://doi.org/10.1093/ndt/gfr211

Treeprasertsuk S, Krudsood S, Tosukhowong T, Maek ANW, Vannaphan S, Saengnetswang T, Looareesuwan S, Kuhn WF, Brittenham G, Carroll J (2003) N-acetylcysteine in severe falciparum malaria in Thailand. Southeast Asian J Trop Med Public Health 34(1):37–42

Treweeke AT, Winterburn TJ, Mackenzie I, Barrett F, Barr C, Rushworth GF, Dransfield I, MacRury SM, Megson IL (2012) N-acetylcysteine inhibits platelet-monocyte conjugation in patients with type 2 diabetes with depleted intraplatelet glutathione: a randomised controlled trial. Diabetologia 55(11):2920–2928. https://doi.org/10.1007/s00125-012-2685-z

Ulusoy AT, Kalyoncuoğlu E, Reis A, Cehreli ZC (2016) Antibacterial effect of N-acetylcysteine and taurolidine on planktonic and biofilm forms of Enterococcus faecalis. Dent Traumatol 32(3):212–218

Unverferth DV, Jagadeesh JM, Unverferth BJ, Magorien RD, Leier CV, Balcerzak SP (1983) Attempt to prevent doxorubicin-induced acute human myocardial morphologic damage with acetylcysteine. J Natl Cancer Inst 71(5):917–920

van Zandwijk N, Dalesio O, Pastorino U, de Vries N, van Tinteren H (2000) EUROSCAN, a randomized trial of vitamin A and N-acetylcysteine in patients with head and neck cancer or lung cancer. For the EUropean Organization for Research and Treatment of Cancer Head and Neck and Lung Cancer Cooperative Groups. J Natl Cancer Inst 92(12):977–986

Viscomi C, Burlina AB, Dweikat I, Savoiardo M, Lamperti C, Hildebrandt T, Tiranti V, Zeviani M (2010) Combined treatment with oral metronidazole and N-acetylcysteine is effective in ethylmalonic encephalopathy. Nat Med 16(8):869–871. https://doi.org/10.1038/nm.2188

Walmsley SL, Khorasheh S, Singer J, Djurdjev O (1998) A randomized trial of N-acetylcysteine for prevention of trimethoprim-sulfamethoxazole hypersensitivity reactions in Pneumocystis carinii pneumonia prophylaxis (CTN 057). Canadian HIV trials network 057 study group. J Acquir Immune Defic Syndr Hum Retrovirol 19(5):498–505

Walters MT, Rubin CE, Keightley SJ, Ward CD, Cawley MI (1986) A double-blind, cross-over, study of oral N-acetylcysteine in Sjogren's syndrome. Scand J Rheumatol Suppl 61:253–258

Watt G, Jongsakul K, Ruangvirayuth R (2002) A pilot study of N-acetylcysteine as adjunctive therapy for severe malaria. QJM 95(5):285–290

Wiest DB, Chang E, Fanning D, Garner S, Cox T, Jenkins DD (2014) Antenatal pharmacokinetics and placental transfer of N-acetylcysteine in chorioamnionitis for fetal neuroprotection. J Pediatr 165(4):672–677.e672

Yalcin E, Altin F, Cinhuseyinoglue F, Arslan MO (2002) N-acetylcysteine in chronic blepharitis. Cornea 21(2):164–168

Yildirim M, Inancli HM, Samanci B, Oktay MF, Enoz M, Topcu I (2010) Preventing cisplatin induced ototoxicity by N-acetylcysteine and salicylate. Kulak Burun Bogaz Ihtis Derg 20(4):173–183

Yoo J, Hamilton SJ, Angel D, Fung K, Franklin J, Parnes LS, Lewis D, Venkatesan V, Winquist E (2014) Cisplatin otoprotection using transtympanic L-N-acetylcysteine: a pilot randomized study in head and neck cancer patients. Laryngoscope 124(3):E87–E94. https://doi.org/10.1002/lary.24360

Zhao T, Liu Y (2010) N-acetylcysteine inhibit biofilms produced by Pseudomonas aeruginosa. BMC Microbiol 10:140

The Physiological Effects of N-Acetylcysteine in Clinical Studies

Richard Eugene Frye

19.1 Introduction

NAC affects many fundamental physiological processes that are common to many diseases, particularly redox metabolism, oxidative stress, and inflammation. This chapter highlights clinical in vivo studies on humans that have examined these effects, mostly in clinical populations. These studies highlight the validity of the evidence based on basic science studies by providing empirical evidence for the beneficial effects of NAC in humans.

19.2 Methods

A systematic online literature search was conducted to identify all clinical trials using NAC using the filters "human" and "clinical trials." From these the author reviewer screened titles and abstracts of all potentially relevant publications and high-quality studies were selected that investigated the physiological effect of NAC in humans.

19.3 The Effect of NAC on Human Physiology

19.3.1 Redox Metabolism

One major rationale for treatment with NAC is to reduce oxidative stress by increasing the production of glutathione (GSH), the body's major intrinsic antioxidant, as well as improving other measures of oxidative stress by acting as an antioxidant.

R. E. Frye
Barrow Neurological Institute, Phoenix Children's Hospital, University of Arizona College of Medicine – Phoenix, Phoenix, AZ, USA
e-mail: rfrye@phoenixchildrens.com

© Springer Nature Singapore Pte Ltd. 2019
R. E. Frye, M. Berk (eds.), *The Therapeutic Use of N-Acetylcysteine (NAC) in Medicine*, https://doi.org/10.1007/978-981-10-5311-5_19

This assumption has been tested in clinical studies, some of which will be reviewed here.

19.3.1.1 Glutathione and Its Precursors

One major supposition when using NAC therapeutically is that NAC increases GSH levels since NAC can donate the rate-limiting amino acid, cysteine, to the reaction that produces GSH. Several clinical studies have examined whether the GSH and its direct precursors are improved by NAC treatment.

Gastrointestinal Disorders

Studies using NAC in gastrointestinal (GI) disorders have shown variable results with two out of three studies demonstrating increases in GSH with NAC treatment. In a small placebo-controlled study in liver transplant patients, NAC reduced the rise in alpha-glutathione S-transferase after reperfusion of the donor liver, suggesting that it stabilized GSH metabolism (Weigand et al. 2001). In a large double-blind placebo-controlled (DPBC) study of patients undergoing orthotopic liver transplant intravenous (IV), NAC increased GSH in only about 50% of the patients, although the increase was associated with a decreased risk of developing post-op kidney injury (Hilmi et al. 2010). However, in a medium-sized DPBC study, oral NAC did not significantly change cysteine or GSH in chronic hepatitis C patients treated with interferon (Bernhard et al. 1998).

Pulmonary Disorders

Pulmonary studies have also examined change in GSH in clinical populations with some positive, but variable, results with five of eight studies demonstrating some positive changes in GSH with NAC treatment. In a crossover study of patients with chronic obstructive pulmonary disease, 3 months of NAC significantly improved GSH, but most importantly, changes in airway resistance as measured by functional respiratory imaging correlated with changes in GSH (De Backer et al. 2013). Twelve weeks of oral NAC increased intracellular GSH in bronchoalveolar lavage cells from patients with fibrosing alveolitis (Behr et al. 2002). IV NAC for 4 days improved intracellular GSH and outcomes of patients with acute respiratory distress syndrome in the intensive care unit (Soltan-Sharifi et al. 2007). In patients with cystic fibrosis, oral NAC significantly increased neutrophil GSH (Tirouvanziam et al. 2006). Oral NAC for 5 days did not increase the depressed levels of GSH in epithelial lining fluid but did increased GSH levels in bronchoalveolar lavage fluid in patients with idiopathic pulmonary fibrosis (Meyer et al. 1994). However, three studies failed to show a positive effect of NAC on GSH. IV NAC increased postoperative plasma thiol concentration, but not red blood cell (RBC) GSH, in patients undergoing lung resection (Bastin et al. 2016). In patients with chronic bronchitis, oral NAC with or without vitamin C did not change the release of reactive oxygen species or GSH concentration from isolated neutrophilic granulocytes and mononuclear cells (Lukas et al. 2005). Four months of oral NAC did not alter plasma cysteine, cysteinylglycine, or GSH in asymptomatic asbestos-exposed individuals in a DBPC trial (Alfonso et al. 2015).

Cardiovascular Disorders

NAC has been shown to increase GSH in patients with cardiovascular disorders, including those with acute myocardial infarction (AMI). Fifteen grams of IV NAC combined with IV nitroglycerin and streptokinase significantly increased the GSH redox ratio in patients with AMI (Arstall et al. 1995). Oral NAC improved the GSH redox ratio in patients with intermittent claudication during treadmill exercise test (da Silva et al. 2015). NAC added to crystalloid cardioplegia increased myocardial GSH content and reduced myeloperoxidase activity in coronary artery bypass graft (CABG) patients (Vento et al. 2003).

Human Immunodeficiency Virus

Evidence for the ability of NAC to increase GSH in patients infected with human immunodeficiency virus (HIV) is inconsistent. De Rosa et al. (2000) found that GSH levels normalized and T cell GSH improved in patients with HIV infection and low GSH at baseline in a large DBPC trial. In contrast, Look et al. (1998) found that combined NAC and selenite (Se) treatment did not alter RBC GSH peroxidase (GSH-Px) activity, GSH, or oxidized GSH (GSSG) concentrations or the GSH redox ratio in HIV-infected patients.

Healthy Individuals

Lastly, studies on healthy individuals suggest that NAC improves GSH metabolism. Oral NAC for 4 weeks significantly increased cysteine in middle-aged men regardless of lipid or smoking status (Hildebrandt et al. 2015), while oral NAC for 8 days significantly increased GSH in healthy men (Zembron-Lacny et al. 2009).

Effect of NAC on Glutathione and Its Precursors

Thus, there is good evidence that NAC can increase GSH and improve the GSH redox ratio in many diseases with some studies demonstrating a correspondence between positive changes in GSH and outcomes. Thus, NAC is a viable treatment option when GSH production or GSH redox ratio is compromised as part of the disease process. Of course, clinical trials supporting the use of NAC in order to improve outcomes are important for supporting its use in specific disorders.

19.3.1.2 Markers of Oxidative Stress

The effect of NAC on markers of oxidative stress has been studied in several organ systems, which will be considered separately below.

Renal Disease

There are several studies on renal disorders that have examined whether NAC influences oxidative stress. Lipid peroxidation markers have been widely used in NAC treatment studies. Three studies examined these biomarkers in hemodialysis (HD) patients with all studies demonstrating positive results. In a small trial, oral NAC significantly reduced elevated malondialdehyde (MDA) levels associated with end-stage renal disease (ESRD) in HD patients (Trimarchi et al. 2003). In another small DBPC study, NAC pretreatment reduced MDA prior to receiving iron therapy in HD patients (Swarnalatha et al. 2010). Finally, in HD patients being treated with erythropoietin, NAC improved plasma 8-isoprostane and oxidized low-density lipoprotein (Hsu et al. 2010). Thus, NAC seems to be effective in reducing lipid peroxidation markers of oxidative stress in HD patients.

Two studies examined asymmetric dimethylarginine, a metabolite that is increased in uremic patients because of oxidative inhibition of the enzyme that breaks it down, known as dimethylarginine dimethylaminohydrolase. In one study, IV NAC during HD significantly reduced plasma asymmetric dimethylarginine concentration (Thaha et al. 2008), while another study demonstrated that oral NAC did not decrease asymmetric dimethylarginine in patients undergoing peritoneal dialysis (Nascimento et al. 2010).

NAC has also been shown to significantly increase total antioxidant capacity in patients undergoing HD in a small DBPC study (Shahbazian et al. 2016). However, oral NAC did not significantly decrease advanced oxidation protein products in patients undergoing peritoneal dialysis (Nascimento et al. 2010).

Thus, it appears that in patients with renal disease, improvement in oxidative stress may be a viable mechanism of action in which the therapeutic effect of NAC may occur with most studies demonstrating positive findings.

Radiological Contrast

Studies examining the prophylactic use of NAC for angiography have mixed results with less than half of the studies (three of seven) showing improvement in markers of oxidative stress. In a DBPC study, oral NAC prevented the increase in 15-isoprostane F2(t) associated with radiological contrast (Drager et al. 2004). In another placebo-controlled study, oral NAC decreased oxidized low-density lipoprotein (Thiele et al. 2010). Oral NAC given prophylactically in patients undergoing primary angioplasty significantly reduced activated oxygen protein products (Thiele et al. 2010). However, in a controlled clinical trial, oral NAC did not influence urine MDA concentrations in patients undergoing non-coronary angiography (Sandhu et al. 2006). In a small DBPC study, oral NAC did not change F2-isoprostane excretion despite improving kidney function (Efrati et al. 2003). Lastly, in another study oral NAC did not prevent the increase in urinary lipid hydroperoxides associated with radiological contrast (Saitoh et al. 2011). Oral NAC did not affect total antioxidant capacity in patients with coronary artery disease undergoing elective percutaneous coronary procedure with angiography (Buyukhatipoglu et al. 2010). Thus, like the clinical outcome studies on the ability of NAC to prophylactically protect the kidney from radiological contrast, the effect of NAC on oxidative stress in its prophylactic use for radiological contrast shows variable outcome. The significant potential protection against kidney injury with the low incidence of adverse effects has driven its continuing use for this indication. Clearly more research on the mechanism of NAC for renal protection and the optimal population for treatment is needed.

Cardiovascular Disorders

NAC has also been studied in several cardiovascular disorders with regard to its antioxidant ability. Fifteen grams of IV NAC, combined with IV streptokinase with

(Arstall et al. 1995) or without (Yesilbursa et al. 2006) nitroglycerin, significantly reduced plasma MDA in patients with AMI. In patients undergoing CABG, NAC, along with Mg, significantly reduced lipid peroxidation and improved antioxidant enzyme levels, including catalase, GSH-Px, superoxide dismutase, and GSH reductase (Kurian and Paddikkala 2010). NAC infused into the cardiopulmonary bypass prime followed by continuous infusion during bypass significantly improved 8-isoprostaglandin-F(2)alpha and nitrotyrosine staining of left ventricular cardiomyocytes (Tossios et al. 2003). Thus, all studies demonstrate that NAC improves biomarkers of oxidative stress in cardiovascular indications.

Pulmonary Disorders

Three studies on pulmonary disorders suggest a role for NAC in reducing oxidative stress, although the last study illustrates the complicated dynamics of redox metabolism. In a DBPC study, preoperative NAC IV improved postoperative plasma thiols, but not 8-isoprostane or RBC GSH in patients undergoing lung resection (Bastin et al. 2016). IV NAC for 4 days improved extracellular total antioxidant power, total thiols, and the outcome of patients with acute respiratory distress syndrome in the intensive care unit (Soltan-Sharifi et al. 2007). Inhaled nebulized NAC reduced exhaled hydrogen peroxide 30 min after treatment but increased hydrogen peroxide and thiols 3 h following treatment, suggesting a complex influence on redox metabolism (Szkudlarek et al. 2004).

Endocrine Disorders

Two studies have examined endocrine disorders with mixed results. Oral NAC decreased MDA levels in a medium-sized placebo-controlled study of women with polycystic ovary syndrome (Cheraghi et al. 2016). In 13 patients with type 2 diabetes, oral NAC did not improve fasting RBC GSH or GSSG concentrations, plasma thiobarbituric acid reactive substances (TBARS), or urine F2-alpha isoprostanes (Szkudlinska et al. 2016).

Reperfusion Ischemia

NAC appears to have evidence for reducing oxidative stress in reperfusion ischemia. NAC did not change catalase enzyme activity but prevented an increase in MDA and decrease in thiols following reperfusion in patients with lower extremity ischemia (Ege et al. 2006). NAC was found to prevent detrimental changes in MDA, superoxide dismutase (SOD), GSH-Px, total antioxidant capacity (TAC), and total oxidant status (TOS) during reperfusion in patients undergoing tourniquet-induced ischemia during arthroscopic knee surgery (Koca et al. 2011).

Other Disorders

NAC has also been found to improve oxidative stress in several other disorders in isolated studies. Three months of oral NAC significantly improved total serum oxidant status and antioxidant capacity, oxidative stress index, and mononuclear DNA damage in 75 children with transfusion-dependent beta-thalassemia (Ozdemir et al. 2014). In a large randomized placebo-controlled study of men with idiopathic infertility, oral daily NAC significantly improved the serum TAC, total peroxide, and oxidative stress index (Ciftci et al. 2009). NAC was found to improve protein sulfhydryl groups in patients hospitalized for severe burns with a 5-day treatment course (Csontos et al. 2012). Oral NAC was found to reduce lipid peroxidation induced by hyperbaric oxygen therapy (Pelaia et al. 1995).

19.3.1.3 NAC and Redox Metabolism

One of the major biological therapeutic mechanisms of NAC is believed to be an increase in GSH and attenuation of oxidative stress. Interventional studies in gastro-intestinal, pulmonary, cardiovascular disorders as well as studies on healthy individuals verify the ability of NAC to improve GSH in disease and non-disease state, suggesting that improvement in GSH is indeed a major mechanism of therapeutic action of NAC. Additionally, intervention studies on renal, cardiovascular, and pulmonary disorders as well as in reperfusion ischemia suggest NAC reduces oxidative stress in disease states, again supporting an improvement in redox metabolism as a viable therapeutic pathway for NAC.

19.3.2 Homocysteine Metabolism

Four studies found that NAC reduced homocysteine (HCY) in healthy subjects. Oral NAC for 4 weeks significantly lowered plasma HCY in middle-aged men regardless of lipid or smoking status (Hildebrandt et al. 2015). Oral NAC also quickly lowered HCY in young females (Roes et al. 2002). In a crossover study, oral NAC significantly decreased plasma HCY while increasing urinary HCY excretion (Ventura et al. 2003). Interestingly, oral NAC decreased oxidized HCY and improved the free to oxidized HCY ratio resulting from the auto-oxidation of HCY following methionine loading (Raijmakers et al. 2003).

Two studies in clinical populations have shown promising results. In a DBPC crossover trial of patient with high lipoprotein(a), oral NAC significantly decreased plasma HCY but did not alter lipoprotein(a) levels (Wiklund et al. 1996). In a placebo-controlled trial, 8 weeks of oral NAC improved HCY and endothelium-dependent dilation in patients with hyperhomocysteinemia (Yilmaz et al. 2007).

However, NAC did not appear to be effective at lowering HCY levels in several studies on clinical populations. Ten weeks of oral NAC did not alter HCY in stable cardiac transplant recipients in an open-label trial (Miner et al. 2002). A 4-month DBPC trial of oral NAC did not alter plasma HCY in asymptomatic asbestos-exposed individuals (Alfonso et al. 2015). In another study of chronic hepatitis C patients being treated with interferon alpha, oral NAC did not change HCY (Bernhard et al. 1998).

Hyperhomocysteinemia is refractory to standard treatment and persists in a majority of HD patients, prompting the investigation of NAC as a therapeutic agent, although all of these studies have not been positive. In two medium-sized placebo-controlled studies of patients with end-stage renal failure, IV NAC during HD reduced HCY to a greater extent than placebo along with a reduction in blood pressure (Scholze et al. 2004; Thaha et al. 2006). However, three studies on HD patients were negative. In a small controlled study of patients on maintenance HD, oral NAC given as a pretreatment did not change plasma HCY levels (Bostom et al. 1996). In a medium-sized placebo-controlled study, 4 weeks of daily oral NAC did not lower HCY levels in chronic HD patients (Friedman et al. 2003). In a medium-sized placebo-controlled crossover trial of nondiabetic patients with mild renal dysfunction, 8 weeks of oral NAC did not alter plasma HCY levels (Renke et al. 2010).

Thus, these studies suggest that NAC can reduce HCY, although its effectiveness can vary with specific disease state. Clearly this is a fertile area in which research can help define the indications in which NAC can be useful for lowering HCY.

19.3.3 Inflammatory Pathways

Basic science and clinical studies demonstrate that NAC has a positive effect on inflammatory pathways and in inflammatory diseases. Several studies have examined the effect of NAC on biomarkers of inflammation. These studies will be reviewed here.

19.3.3.1 Renal Disease

The effect of NAC on markers of inflammation has been examined in patients with renal disease. Oral NAC twice daily for 8 weeks reduced high-sensitivity C-reactive protein (hsCRP) in peritoneal dialysis (PD) patients with an 8-week treatment course (Purwanto and Prasetyo 2012) and in HD patients with a 3-month treatment course (Saddadi et al. 2014). However, hsCRP was not reduced by the same dose of NAC in a small study on HD patient receiving IV iron therapy for 10 days (Swarnalatha et al. 2010) or in PD patients treated for 8 weeks (Nascimento et al. 2010). One study found a decrease in the erythrocyte sedimentation rate with NAC treatment (Saddadi et al. 2014). Multiple studies demonstrated the positive effect of NAC on IL-6, two studies treating PD patients (Nascimento et al. 2010; Purwanto and Prasetyo 2012) and one study treating HD patients (Saddadi et al. 2014). Two studies using the same NAC treatment regime and similar populations found conflicting effects on tumor necrosis factor-α (TNF-α) (Nascimento et al. 2010; Purwanto and Prasetyo 2012). Thus, in the few studies that have been conducted, there is evidence that NAC can affect biomarkers of inflammation in patients with renal disease, suggesting a potential mechanism of action in these patients although more research is needed to understand the variations in outcomes in these studies.

19.3.3.2 Gastrointestinal Disorders

There is some evidence for NAC reducing markers of liver inflammation. In a small placebo-controlled study, NAC significantly reduced the rise in circulating intercellular adhesion molecule-1 (ICAM-1) and vascular cell adhesion protein-1 (VCAM-1) after reperfusion of the donor liver in orthotopic liver transplant patients (Weigand et al. 2001). IV NAC during the anhepatic phase of liver transplantation significantly increased recipient IL-4 and IL-10 plasma values, suggesting a protective effect against reperfusion injury (Santiago et al. 2008). NAC significantly decreased IL-17 concentrations in patients admitted for non-acetaminophen acute liver failure following liver transplant (Stravitz et al. 2013). Thus, this a promising area of the anti-inflammatory effect of NAC, but with only a few studies, more research is needed to further investigate this therapeutic aspect of NAC.

19.3.3.3 Cardiovascular

In patients undergoing cardiac surgery with extracorporeal circulation, treatment with NAC before and after surgery prevented an increase in plasma neutrophil elastase activity along with improvement in the partial pressure of arterial oxygen, indicating a potential protection against neutrophil-mediated lung injury, although myeloperoxidase, total antigenic human neutrophil elastase, and complex formation were not altered (De Backer et al. 1996). NAC added to crystalloid cardioplegia reduced the number of leukocytes sequestered in the coronary circulation during the first minute after reperfusion in CABG patients (Vento et al. 2003). Oral NAC prevented an increased in TGF-β but did not affect TNF-α in patients with AMI (Talasaz et al. 2013). Oral NAC did not improve markers of inflammation, including VCAM-1, monocyte chemotactic protein-1, and endothelin-1 in patients with intermittent claudication during a treadmill exercise test (da Silva et al. 2015). Thus, NAC was effective in reducing markers of inflammation in patients with cardiac disorders but not in the one study that examined vascular dysfunction. These studies are promising and support the notion that NAC may be useful for cardiac indications, but given the limited number of studies, further research would be helpful to validate these findings.

19.3.3.4 Pulmonary Disorders

Oral NAC was found to decrease neutrophil burden, the number of airway neutrophils actively releasing elastase-rich granules, and sputum IL-8 levels in patients with cystic fibrosis (Tirouvanziam et al. 2006). Four months of oral NAC did not alter markers of inflammation, including IL-8 and TNF-α in bronchoalveolar lavage in asymptomatic asbestos-exposed individuals in a DBPC trial (Alfonso et al. 2015). IV NAC failed to attenuate an increase in IL-6 in patients undergoing lung resection (Bastin et al. 2016). Thus, with mixed results for pulmonary disorders, NAC does seem to have evidence for improving inflammation in cystic fibrosis. Given that there are limited studies on specific disorders, further studies are needed to verify the results of these studies.

19.3.3.5 Human Immunodeficiency Virus

In asymptomatic HIV-infected patients, oral NAC, combined with sodium selenite, improved CD4 counts and the CD4/CD8 and CD8/CD38 ratios (Look et al. 1998). Oral NAC reduced TNF-α but did not affect free radical activity in neutrophils in patients with HIV with low CD4 counts (Akerlund et al. 1996). Thus, in the few studies conducted, NAC was useful in improving biomarkers of inflammation in HIV patients.

19.3.3.6 Systemic Inflammation

NAC has also been shown to improve inflammatory mediators in the face of systemic inflammation. Two studies have examined the effect of NAC in several burns with one demonstrating that NAC reduced the surface expressions of CD11a, CD18, and CD97 on granulocytes, CD49d on lymphocytes, and CD49d and CD97 on monocytes (Csontos et al. 2011) and the other showing that NAC lowered IL-6, IL-8, and IL-10 but not TNF-α (Csontos et al. 2012). In septic patients, IV NAC significantly decreased IL-8 and nuclear factor-kappa β activation in mononuclear leukocytes but not IL-6 or soluble intercellular adhesion molecule-1 (Paterson et al. 2003). In critically ill patients, IV NAC improved polymorphonuclear phagocytosis but reduced oxidative burst activity (Heller et al. 2001). Lastly, in a DBPC study, IV NAC decreased the production of TNF-α induced by IV administration of *Escherichia coli* endotoxin in healthy participants (Schaller et al. 2007). Thus, in these five studies on systemic inflammation, NAC has been shown to have positive effects on reducing biomarkers of inflammation.

19.3.3.7 Other Disorders

There are a few other disorders in which NAC has also been shown to be helpful in reducing inflammatory mediators. IV NAC resulted in higher anti-inflammatory IL-1 receptor antagonist and lower proinflammatory vascular endothelial growth factor in infants who were exposed to maternal chorioamnionitis (Jenkins et al. 2016). Oral NAC reversed expansion and stimulated FoxP3 expression in CD4-CD8-T cells in patients with systemic lupus erythematosus (Lai et al. 2012).

19.3.3.8 NAC and Inflammatory Mediators

Although the studies are limited, the immunomodulatory and anti-inflammatory effect of NAC has been demonstrated for multiple diseases involving multiple organ systems. NAC has been shown to modulate general inflammatory mediators, cytokines, as well as immune cell activity and function. Thus, this is a viable biological mechanism in which NAC may have its biological effect in therapeutically positively influencing disease. However, given the limited number of studies, clearly more research will be needed in this area.

19.3.4 Vascular Physiology

NAC has been used to improve vascular function. Such studies will be reviewed here. The effect of NAC on endothelial function, including its effect on nitric oxide, has been investigated.

19.3.4.1 Endothelial Function

Four studies have demonstrated improvement in endothelial function with NAC treatment in patients with renal disease using noninvasive measurements. In a prospective, randomized, placebo-controlled crossover study in 20 patients with ESRD, IV NAC during HD improved the photoplethysmogram waveform suggesting improved endothelial function (Scholze et al. 2004). In another study a 6-week treatment of oral NAC 600 mg twice a day improved flow-mediated dilatation, a measure of endothelium-dependent vasodilatation, in 30 uremic patients on HD (Sahin et al. 2007). In a randomized, prospective, placebo-controlled crossover study of 24 patients with ESRD 5 g IV NAC was found to significantly decrease the reflective index during reactive hyperemia indicating improved arterial vascular reactivity (Wittstock et al. 2009). Lastly, in a prospective, double-blinded, randomized controlled, crossover trial of 14 adult HD patients, oral NAC 600 mg twice daily for 10 days prior to IV iron therapy improved the digital plethysmography reflection index suggesting an improvement in endothelial function (Swarnalatha et al. 2010).

Two studies have examined the effect of NAC on endothelial function in patients with cardiac disease. In a placebo-controlled study, 8 weeks of daily NAC increased endothelium-dependent dilation of the brachial artery in patients with coronary artery disease (Yilmaz et al. 2007). In stable cardiac transplant recipients, 10 weeks of daily oral NAC did not change flow-mediated dilation of the brachial artery (Miner et al. 2002).

In a small DBPC of patients with type 2 diabetes and hypertension, NAC combined with L-arginine for 6 months improved endothelial function, including intima-media thickness during endothelial postischemic vasodilation (Martina et al. 2008).

Overall these studies suggest NAC may have a therapeutic effect on endothelial function that is mediated through vascular reactivity, particularly in patients with renal disease.

19.3.4.2 Nitric Oxide

NAC also has been shown to improve nitric oxide metabolism, a regulator of vascular tone. In a DBPC trial in patients with renal impairment, 1 g oral NAC twice a day before coronary angiography prevented the reduction in urinary nitric oxide seen in the placebo group (Efrati et al. 2003). Oral NAC enhanced endothelial nitric oxide synthase in patients with intermittent claudication during a treadmill exercise test (da Silva et al. 2015).

19.3.4.3 Vascular Flow

In an uncontrolled study, IV NAC improved the cardiac index, mean arterial pressure, and systemic vascular resistance in patients with acetaminophen-induced fulminant hepatic failure as well as acute liver failure from other causes (Harrison et al. 1991). In a study of women with chorioamnionitis, IV NAC improved cerebrovascular coupling of the infant (Jenkins et al. 2016).

19.3.4.4 NAC and Vascular Physiology

Limited studies have examined the effect of NAC on vascular function through examination of endothelial reactivity, nitric oxide metabolism, and vascular flow with mostly positive results. Although limited in number, these studies support the notion that therapeutic aspects of NAC may include positive changes in vascular function.

19.3.5 Exercise Physiology

A limited number of studies have investigated the ability of NAC to enhance exercise physiology by preventing fatigue, increasing strength, and reducing exercise-induced pathophysiological processes such as oxidative stress and inflammation.

19.3.5.1 Fatigue and Strength

Several studies have shown that that NAC improves fatigue and strength during exercise. In three small placebo-controlled studies, oral NAC extended time to fatigue in a cycling test (Corn and Barstow 2011; McKenna et al. 2006; Medved et al. 2004b) with one study showing that this effect was related to improving potassium regulation and muscle sodium-potassium pump activity (McKenna et al. 2006). Oral NAC was also found to reduce respiratory muscle fatigue during heavy exercise in a small placebo-controlled study (Kelly et al. 2009).

In other studies improvement in exercise was related to improvement in redox status. In one study, oral NAC improved handgrip exercise performance in healthy individuals by improving the cysteine to total cysteine ratio (Ferreira et al. 2011), while another study with IV NAC showed that improvement in severe-intensity exercise tolerance was related to improvement in total plasma sulfhydryl groups (Bailey et al. 2011).

Two studies did not show clear improvements in fatigue during a cycling exercise test (Medved et al. 2003; Medved et al. 2004a). One study suggested that NAC impaired potassium regulation (Medved et al. 2003), while the other demonstrated that it improved potassium regulation (Medved et al. 2004a).

19.3.5.2 Oxidative Stress

Several studies have examined the effect of IV and oral NAC on oxidative stress with exercise with most studies demonstrating positive results. In a DBPC crossover studies, IV NAC improved total and reduced GSH and cysteine in muscle during prolonged, submaximal exercise in endurance athletes (Medved et al. 2004b), attenuated detrimental changes in GSH and GSSG in untrained men during cycling exercise (Medved et al. 2003), and induced gene expression of MnSOD with a cycling test (Petersen et al. 2012). Similar results were found for oral NAC with exercise. Oral NAC improved total antioxidant capacity in a controlled study of sedentary men who performed a graded exercise treadmill test (Leelarungrayub et al. 2011) and in trained athletes with high-intensity interval exercise (Slattery et al. 2014). Also, oral NAC improved markers of oxidative damage in trained athletes with high-intensity interval exercise (Slattery et al. 2014; Trewin et al. 2013) and in healthy men with incremental cycle exercise (Zembron-Lacny et al. 2010). However, in similarly designed studies, oral NAC did not alter measures of oxidative damage after high-intensity eccentric exercise (Silva et al. 2008) or blood GSH concentrations (Trewin et al. 2013). Thus, there is good evidence that NAC can attenuate oxidative stress during exercise in both athletes and nonathletes although there may be some unknown factors that limit its ability to do so in some circumstances.

19.3.5.3   Inflammation

Most studies (four of five) show that oral NAC has at least some positive influence on inflammation during exercise. NAC has been shown to positively affect cytokines with exercise. In a controlled study, oral NAC maintained high levels of IL-10 after high-intensity eccentric exercise (Silva et al. 2008) and attenuated the increase in IL-6 and monocyte chemotactic protein-1 in well-trained triathletes after cycle ergometer race simulation (Slattery et al. 2014). One week of oral daily NAC improved TNF-α in a controlled study of sedentary men who performed a graded exercise treadmill test (Leelarungrayub et al. 2011) while it was not influenced in another study of high-intensity eccentric exercise (Silva et al. 2008). In a small DBPC study of oarsmen during an ergometer rowing test, oral NAC did not influence peripheral lymphocyte counts or subsets, phytohemagglutinin-stimulated lymphocyte proliferation, or natural killer cell activity (Nielsen et al. 1998), while in a similar study performed by the same group, oral NAC suppressed exercise-induced zymosan-stimulated luminol-enhanced chemiluminescence response of neutrophil oxidative burst during a 6-min maximal ergometer row (Nielsen et al. 2001). Thus, in a limited number of studies, mostly in athletes, NAC appears to have a positive effect on inflammation during exercise.

19.3.5.4   Blood Flow

In a placebo-controlled study, oral NAC did not change brachial artery blood flow in eight healthy non-endurance trained men during a constant power handgrip exercise tests (Smith et al. 2016).

19.3.5.5   Energy Metabolism

In a small DBPC crossover study of well-trained male cyclists, oral NAC reduced insulin sensitivity but did not change phosphorylation of AKT, AS160, and mTOR and blunted phosphorylation of p70S6K (Trewin et al. 2015) and elevated fatty acid oxidation and glucose and reduced lactate (Trewin et al. 2013) with exercise. In contrast, in a small DBPC crossover study of healthy men, IV NAC did not influence glucose metabolism or concentrations of lactate, non-esterified fatty acids insulin or skeletal muscle AMPK or acetyl-CoA carboxylase-beta phosphorylation during moderate-intensity exercise (Merry et al. 2010). Thus, two of three studies suggest some influence of NAC on energy metabolism during exercise.

19.3.5.6   The Effect of NAC on Exercise

In a limited number of studies, there is evidence for NAC improving exercise performance in athletes and nonathletes and improving exercise-induced oxidative stress and inflammations with some studies suggesting improvement in exercise performance may be related to the improvements in oxidative stress. There are several studies that implicate improvements in energy metabolism as a result of NAC, but these studies are limited with some inconsistent results. Clearly this is an interesting application of NAC for improving physiology in a non-disease state that deserves further research.

19.3.6 Other Cellular Pathways

In a medium-sized DBPC study, oral NAC increased mitochondrial transmembrane potential and profoundly reduced mTOR activity in patients with systemic lupus erythematosus (Lai et al. 2012). Given the implications of NAC improving mitochondrial function in basic science studies, the application of NAC to diseases which involve mitochondrial dysfunction may be a fruitful area of therapeutic application of NAC in the future.

References

Akerlund B, Jarstrand C, Lindeke B, Sonnerborg A, Akerblad AC, Rasool O (1996) Effect of N-acetylcysteine(NAC) treatment on HIV-1 infection: a double-blind placebo-controlled trial. Eur J Clin Pharmacol 50(6):457–461

Alfonso H, Franklin P, Ching S, Croft K, Burcham P, Olsen N, Reid A, Joyce D, de Klerk N, Musk AB (2015) Effect of N-acetylcysteine supplementation on oxidative stress status and alveolar inflammation in people exposed to asbestos: a double-blind, randomized clinical trial. Respirology (Carlton, Vic) 20(7):1102–1107. https://doi.org/10.1111/resp.12592

Arstall MA, Yang J, Stafford I, Betts WH, Horowitz JD (1995) N-acetylcysteine in combination with nitroglycerin and streptokinase for the treatment of evolving acute myocardial infarction. Safety and biochemical effects. Circulation 92(10):2855–2862

Bailey SJ, Winyard PG, Blackwell JR, Vanhatalo A, Lansley KE, Dimenna FJ, Wilkerson DP, Campbell IT, Jones AM (2011) Influence of N-acetylcysteine administration on pulmonary O(2) uptake kinetics and exercise tolerance in humans. Respir Physiol Neurobiol 175(1):121–129. https://doi.org/10.1016/j.resp.2010.10.002

Bastin AJ, Davies N, Lim E, Quinlan GJ, Griffiths MJ (2016) Systemic inflammation and oxidative stress post-lung resection: effect of pretreatment with N-acetylcysteine. Respirology (Carlton, Vic) 21(1):180–187. https://doi.org/10.1111/resp.12662

Behr J, Degenkolb B, Krombach F, Vogelmeier C (2002) Intracellular glutathione and bronchoalveolar cells in fibrosing alveolitis: effects of N-acetylcysteine. Eur Respir J 19(5):906–911

Bernhard MC, Junker E, Hettinger A, Lauterburg BH (1998) Time course of total cysteine, glutathione and homocysteine in plasma of patients with chronic hepatitis C treated with interferon-alpha with and without supplementation with N-acetylcysteine. J Hepatol 28(5):751–755

Bostom AG, Shemin D, Yoburn D, Fisher DH, Nadeau MR, Selhub J (1996) Lack of effect of oral N-acetylcysteine on the acute dialysis-related lowering of total plasma homocysteine in hemodialysis patients. Atherosclerosis 120(1–2):241–244

Buyukhatipoglu H, Sezen Y, Yildiz A, Bas M, Kirhan I, Ulas T, Turan MN, Taskin A, Aksoy N (2010) N-acetylcysteine fails to prevent renal dysfunction and oxidative stress after noniodine contrast media administration during percutaneous coronary interventions. Pol Arch Med Wewn 120(10):383–389

Cheraghi E, Mehranjani MS, Shariatzadeh MA, Esfahani MH, Ebrahimi Z (2016) N-Acetylcysteine improves oocyte and embryo quality in polycystic ovary syndrome patients undergoing intracytoplasmic sperm injection: an alternative to metformin. Reprod Fertil Dev 28(6):723–731. https://doi.org/10.1071/rd14182

Ciftci H, Verit A, Savas M, Yeni E, Erel O (2009) Effects of N-acetylcysteine on semen parameters and oxidative/antioxidant status. Urology 74(1):73–76. https://doi.org/10.1016/j.urology.2009.02.034

Corn SD, Barstow TJ (2011) Effects of oral N-acetylcysteine on fatigue, critical power, and W' in exercising humans. Respir Physiol Neurobiol 178(2):261–268. https://doi.org/10.1016/j.resp.2011.06.020

Csontos C, Rezman B, Foldi V, Bogar L, Bognar Z, Drenkovics L, Roth E, Weber G, Lantos J (2011) Effect of N-acetylcysteine treatment on the expression of leukocyte surface markers after burn injury. Burns 37(3):453–464. https://doi.org/10.1016/j.burns.2010.10.008

Csontos C, Rezman B, Foldi V, Bogar L, Drenkovics L, Roth E, Weber G, Lantos J (2012) Effect of N-acetylcysteine treatment on oxidative stress and inflammation after severe burn. Burns 38(3):428–437. https://doi.org/10.1016/j.burns.2011.09.011

da Silva ND Jr, Roseguini BT, Chehuen M, Fernandes T, Mota GF, Martin PK, Han SW, Forjaz CL, Wolosker N, de Oliveira EM (2015) Effects of oral N-acetylcysteine on walking capacity, leg reactive hyperemia, and inflammatory and angiogenic mediators in patients with intermittent claudication. Am J Phys Heart Circ Phys 309(5):H897–H905. https://doi.org/10.1152/ajpheart.00158.2015

De Backer J, Vos W, Van Holsbeke C, Vinchurkar S, Claes R, Parizel PM, De Backer W (2013) Effect of high-dose N-acetylcysteine on airway geometry, inflammation, and oxidative stress in COPD patients. Int J Chron Obstruct Pulmon Dis 8:569–579. https://doi.org/10.2147/copd.s49307

De Backer WA, Amsel B, Jorens PG, Bossaert L, Hiemstra PS, van Noort P, van Overveld FJ (1996) N-acetylcysteine pretreatment of cardiac surgery patients influences plasma neutrophil elastase and neutrophil influx in bronchoalveolar lavage fluid. Intensive Care Med 22(9):900–908

De Rosa SC, Zaretsky MD, Dubs JG, Roederer M, Anderson M, Green A, Mitra D, Watanabe N, Nakamura H, Tjioe I, Deresinski SC, Moore WA, Ela SW, Parks D, Herzenberg LA, Herzenberg LA (2000) N-acetylcysteine replenishes glutathione in HIV infection. Eur J Clin Investig 30(10):915–929

Drager LF, Andrade L, Barros de Toledo JF, Laurindo FR, Machado Cesar LA, Seguro AC (2004) Renal effects of N-acetylcysteine in patients at risk for contrast nephropathy: decrease in oxidant stress-mediated renal tubular injury. Nephrol Dial Transplant 19(7):1803–1807. https://doi.org/10.1093/ndt/gfh261

Efrati S, Dishy V, Averbukh M, Blatt A, Krakover R, Weisgarten J, Morrow JD, Stein MC, Golik A (2003) The effect of N-acetylcysteine on renal function, nitric oxide, and oxidative stress after angiography. Kidney Int 64(6):2182–2187. https://doi.org/10.1046/j.1523-1755.2003.00322.x

Ege T, Eskiocak S, Edis M, Duran E (2006) The role of N-acetylcysteine in lower extremity ischemia/reperfusions. J Cardiovasc Surg 47(5):563–568

Ferreira LF, Campbell KS, Reid MB (2011) N-acetylcysteine in handgrip exercise: plasma thiols and adverse reactions. Int J Sport Nutr Exerc Metab 21(2):146–154

Friedman AN, Bostom AG, Laliberty P, Selhub J, Shemin D (2003) The effect of N-acetylcysteine on plasma total homocysteine levels in hemodialysis: a randomized, controlled study. Am J Kidney Dis 41(2):442–446. https://doi.org/10.1053/ajkd.2003.50054

Harrison PM, Wendon JA, Gimson AE, Alexander GJ, Williams R (1991) Improvement by acetylcysteine of hemodynamics and oxygen transport in fulminant hepatic failure. N Engl J Med 324(26):1852–1857. https://doi.org/10.1056/nejm199106273242604

Heller AR, Groth G, Heller SC, Breitkreutz R, Nebe T, Quintel M, Koch T (2001) N-acetylcysteine reduces respiratory burst but augments neutrophil phagocytosis in intensive care unit patients. Crit Care Med 29(2):272–276

Hildebrandt W, Sauer R, Bonaterra G, Dugi KA, Edler L, Kinscherf R (2015) Oral N-acetylcysteine reduces plasma homocysteine concentrations regardless of lipid or smoking status. Am J Clin Nutr 102(5):1014–1024. https://doi.org/10.3945/ajcn.114.101964

Hilmi IA, Peng Z, Planinsic RM, Damian D, Dai F, Tyurina YY, Kagan VE, Kellum JA (2010) N-acetylcysteine does not prevent hepatorenal ischaemia-reperfusion injury in patients undergoing orthotopic liver transplantation. Nephrol Dial Transplant 25(7):2328–2333. https://doi.org/10.1093/ndt/gfq077

Hsu SP, Chiang CK, Yang SY, Chien CT (2010) N-acetylcysteine for the management of anemia and oxidative stress in hemodialysis patients. Nephron Clin Pract 116(3):c207–c216. https://doi.org/10.1159/000317201

Jenkins DD, Wiest DB, Mulvihill DM, Hlavacek AM, Majstoravich SJ, Brown TR, Taylor JJ, Buckley JR, Turner RP, Rollins LG, Bentzley JP, Hope KE, Barbour AB, Lowe DW, Martin

RH, Chang EY (2016) Fetal and neonatal effects of N-acetylcysteine when used for neuroprotection in maternal chorioamnionitis. J Pediatr 168:67–76.e66. https://doi.org/10.1016/j.jpeds.2015.09.076

Kelly MK, Wicker RJ, Barstow TJ, Harms CA (2009) Effects of N-acetylcysteine on respiratory muscle fatigue during heavy exercise. Respir Physiol Neurobiol 165(1):67–72. https://doi.org/10.1016/j.resp.2008.10.008

Koca K, Yurttas Y, Cayci T, Bilgic S, Kaldirim U, Durusu M, Cekli Y, Ozkan H, Hanci V, Purtuloglu T, Akgul EO, Oguz E, Yildiz C, Basbozkurt M (2011) The role of preconditioning and N-acetylcysteine on oxidative stress resulting from tourniquet-induced ischemia-reperfusion in arthroscopic knee surgery. J Trauma 70(3):717–723. https://doi.org/10.1097/TA.0b013e3181f30fb0

Kurian GA, Paddikkala J (2010) N-acetylcysteine and magnesium improve biochemical abnormalities associated with myocardial ischaemic reperfusion in South Indian patients undergoing coronary artery bypass grafting: a comparative analysis. Singap Med J 51(5):381–388

Lai ZW, Hanczko R, Bonilla E, Caza TN, Clair B, Bartos A, Miklossy G, Jimah J, Doherty E, Tily H, Francis L, Garcia R, Dawood M, Yu J, Ramos I, Coman I, Faraone SV, Phillips PE, Perl A (2012) N-acetylcysteine reduces disease activity by blocking mammalian target of rapamycin in T cells from systemic lupus erythematosus patients: a randomized, double-blind, placebo-controlled trial. Arthritis Rheum 64(9):2937–2946. https://doi.org/10.1002/art.34502

Leelarungrayub D, Khansuwan R, Pothongsunun P, Klaphajone J (2011) N-acetylcysteine supplementation controls total antioxidant capacity, creatine kinase, lactate, and tumor necrotic factor-alpha against oxidative stress induced by graded exercise in sedentary men. Oxidative Med Cell Longev 2011:329643. https://doi.org/10.1155/2011/329643

Look MP, Rockstroh JK, Rao GS, Barton S, Lemoch H, Kaiser R, Kupfer B, Sudhop T, Spengler U, Sauerbruch T (1998) Sodium selenite and N-acetylcysteine in antiretroviral-naive HIV-1-infected patients: a randomized, controlled pilot study. Eur J Clin Investig 28(5):389–397

Lukas R, Scharling B, Schultze-Werninghaus G, Gillissen A (2005) Antioxidant treatment with N-acetylcysteine and vitamin C in patients with chronic bronchitis. Dtsch Med Wochenschr (1946) 130(11):563–567. https://doi.org/10.1055/s-2005-865062

Martina V, Masha A, Gigliardi VR, Brocato L, Manzato E, Berchio A, Massarenti P, Settanni F, Della Casa L, Bergamini S, Iannone A (2008) Long-term N-acetylcysteine and L-arginine administration reduces endothelial activation and systolic blood pressure in hypertensive patients with type 2 diabetes. Diabetes Care 31(5):940–944. https://doi.org/10.2337/dc07-2251

McKenna MJ, Medved I, Goodman CA, Brown MJ, Bjorksten AR, Murphy KT, Petersen AC, Sostaric S, Gong X (2006) N-acetylcysteine attenuates the decline in muscle Na+,K+-pump activity and delays fatigue during prolonged exercise in humans. J Physiol 576(Pt 1):279–288. https://doi.org/10.1113/jphysiol.2006.115352

Medved I, Brown MJ, Bjorksten AR, Leppik JA, Sostaric S, McKenna MJ (2003) N-acetylcysteine infusion alters blood redox status but not time to fatigue during intense exercise in humans. J Appl Physiol 94(4):1572–1582. https://doi.org/10.1152/japplphysiol.00884.2002

Medved I, Brown MJ, Bjorksten AR, McKenna MJ (2004a) Effects of intravenous N-acetylcysteine infusion on time to fatigue and potassium regulation during prolonged cycling exercise. J Appl Physiol 96(1):211–217. https://doi.org/10.1152/japplphysiol.00458.2003

Medved I, Brown MJ, Bjorksten AR, Murphy KT, Petersen AC, Sostaric S, Gong X, McKenna MJ (2004b) N-acetylcysteine enhances muscle cysteine and glutathione availability and attenuates fatigue during prolonged exercise in endurance-trained individuals. J Appl Physiol 97(4):1477–1485. https://doi.org/10.1152/japplphysiol.00371.2004

Merry TL, Wadley GD, Stathis CG, Garnham AP, Rattigan S, Hargreaves M, McConell GK (2010) N-Acetylcysteine infusion does not affect glucose disposal during prolonged moderate-intensity exercise in humans. J Physiol 588(Pt 9):1623–1634. https://doi.org/10.1113/jphysiol.2009.184333

Meyer A, Buhl R, Magnussen H (1994) The effect of oral N-acetylcysteine on lung glutathione levels in idiopathic pulmonary fibrosis. Eur Respir J 7(3):431–436

Miner SE, Cole DE, Evrovski J, Forrest Q, Hutchison SJ, Holmes K, Ross HJ (2002) N-acetylcysteine neither lowers plasma homocysteine concentrations nor improves brachial artery endothelial function in cardiac transplant recipients. Can J Cardiol 18(5):503–507

Nascimento MM, Suliman ME, Silva M, Chinaglia T, Marchioro J, Hayashi SY, Riella MC, Lindholm B, Anderstam B (2010) Effect of oral N-acetylcysteine treatment on plasma inflammatory and oxidative stress markers in peritoneal dialysis patients: a placebo-controlled study. Perit Dial Int 30(3):336–342. https://doi.org/10.3747/pdi.2009.00073

Nielsen HB, Kharazmi A, Bolbjerg ML, Poulsen HE, Pedersen BK, Secher NH (2001) N-acetylcysteine attenuates oxidative burst by neutrophils in response to ergometer rowing with no effect on pulmonary gas exchange. Int J Sports Med 22(4):256–260. https://doi.org/10.1055/s-2001-13817

Nielsen HB, Secher NH, Kappel M, Pedersen BK (1998) N-acetylcysteine does not affect the lymphocyte proliferation and natural killer cell activity responses to exercise. Am J Physiol 275(4 Pt 2):R1227–R1231

Ozdemir ZC, Koc A, Aycicek A, Kocyigit A (2014) N-Acetylcysteine supplementation reduces oxidative stress and DNA damage in children with beta-thalassemia. Hemoglobin 38(5):359–364. https://doi.org/10.3109/03630269.2014.951890

Paterson RL, Galley HF, Webster NR (2003) The effect of N-acetylcysteine on nuclear factor-kappa B activation, interleukin-6, interleukin-8, and intercellular adhesion molecule-1 expression in patients with sepsis. Crit Care Med 31(11):2574–2578. https://doi.org/10.1097/01.ccm.0000089945.69588.18

Pelaia P, Rocco M, De Blasi RA, Spadetta G, Alampi D, Araimo FS, Nicolucci S (1995) Assessment of lipid peroxidation in hyperbaric oxygen therapy: protective role of N-acetylcysteine. Minerva Anestesiol 61(4):133–139

Petersen AC, McKenna MJ, Medved I, Murphy KT, Brown MJ, Della Gatta P, Cameron-Smith D (2012) Infusion with the antioxidant N-acetylcysteine attenuates early adaptive responses to exercise in human skeletal muscle. Acta Physiol 204(3):382–392. https://doi.org/10.1111/j.1748-1716.2011.02344.x

Purwanto B, Prasetyo DH (2012) Effect of oral N-acetylcysteine treatment on immune system in continuous ambulatory peritoneal dialysis patients. Acta Med Indones 44(2):140–144

Raijmakers MT, Schilders GW, Roes EM, van Tits LJ, Hak-Lemmers HL, Steegers EA, Peters WH (2003) N-Acetylcysteine improves the disturbed thiol redox balance after methionine loading. Clin Sci (Lond) 105(2):173–180. https://doi.org/10.1042/cs20030052

Renke M, Tylicki L, Rutkowski P, Larczynski W, Neuwelt A, Aleksandrowicz E, Lysiak-Szydlowska W, Rutkowski B (2010) The effect of N-acetylcysteine on blood pressure and markers of cardiovascular risk in non-diabetic patients with chronic kidney disease: a placebo-controlled, randomized, cross-over study. Med Sci Monit 16(7):Pi13–Pi18

Roes EM, Raijmakers MT, Peters WH, Steegers EA (2002) Effects of oral N-acetylcysteine on plasma homocysteine and whole blood glutathione levels in healthy, non-pregnant women. Clin Chem Lab Med 40(5):496–498. https://doi.org/10.1515/cclm.2002.086

Saddadi F, Alatab S, Pasha F, Ganji MR, Soleimanian T (2014) The effect of treatment with N-acetylcysteine on the serum levels of C-reactive protein and interleukin-6 in patients on hemodialysis. Saudi J Kidney Dis Transplant 25(1):66–72

Sahin G, Yalcin AU, Akcar N (2007) Effect of N-acetylcysteine on endothelial dysfunction in dialysis patients. Blood Purif 25(4):309–315. https://doi.org/10.1159/000106103

Saitoh T, Satoh H, Nobuhara M, Machii M, Tanaka T, Ohtani H, Saotome M, Urushida T, Katoh H, Hayashi H (2011) Intravenous glutathione prevents renal oxidative stress after coronary angiography more effectively than oral N-acetylcysteine. Heart Vessel 26(5):465–472. https://doi.org/10.1007/s00380-010-0078-0

Sandhu C, Belli AM, Oliveira DB (2006) The role of N-acetylcysteine in the prevention of contrast-induced nephrotoxicity. Cardiovasc Intervent Radiol 29(3):344–347. https://doi.org/10.1007/s00270-005-0127-8

Santiago FM, Bueno P, Olmedo C, Muffak-Granero K, Comino A, Serradilla M, Mansilla A, Villar JM, Garrote D, Ferron JA (2008) Effect of N-acetylcysteine administration on intraoperative plasma levels of interleukin-4 and interleukin-10 in liver transplant recipients. Transplant Proc 40(9):2978–2980. https://doi.org/10.1016/j.transproceed.2008.08.103

Schaller G, Pleiner J, Mittermayer F, Posch M, Kapiotis S, Wolzt M (2007) Effects of N-acetylcysteine against systemic and renal hemodynamic effects of endotoxin in healthy humans. Crit Care Med 35(8):1869–1875. https://doi.org/10.1097/01.ccm.0000275385.45557.25

Scholze A, Rinder C, Beige J, Riezler R, Zidek W, Tepel M (2004) Acetylcysteine reduces plasma homocysteine concentration and improves pulse pressure and endothelial function in patients with end-stage renal failure. Circulation 109(3):369–374. https://doi.org/10.1161/01.cir.0000109492.65802.ad

Shahbazian H, Shayanpour S, Ghorbani A (2016) Evaluation of administration of oral N-acetylcysteine to reduce oxidative stress in chronic hemodialysis patients: a double-blind, randomized, controlled clinical trial. Saudi J Kidney Dis Transplant 27(1):88–93. https://doi.org/10.4103/1319-2442.174084

Silva LA, Silveira PC, Pinho CA, Tuon T, Dal Pizzol F, Pinho RA (2008) N-acetylcysteine supplementation and oxidative damage and inflammatory response after eccentric exercise. Int J Sport Nutr Exerc Metab 18(4):379–388

Slattery KM, Dascombe B, Wallace LK, Bentley DJ, Coutts AJ (2014) Effect of N-acetylcysteine on cycling performance after intensified training. Med Sci Sports Exerc 46(6):1114–1123. https://doi.org/10.1249/mss.0000000000000222

Smith JR, Broxterman RM, Ade CJ, Evans KK, Kurti SP, Hammer SM, Barstow TJ, Harms CA (2016) Acute supplementation of N-acetylcysteine does not affect muscle blood flow and oxygenation characteristics during handgrip exercise. Physiol Rep 4(7):e12748. https://doi.org/10.14814/phy2.12748

Soltan-Sharifi MS, Mojtahedzadeh M, Najafi A, Reza Khajavi M, Reza Rouini M, Moradi M, Mohammadirad A, Abdollahi M (2007) Improvement by N-acetylcysteine of acute respiratory distress syndrome through increasing intracellular glutathione, and extracellular thiol molecules and anti-oxidant power: evidence for underlying toxicological mechanisms. Hum Exp Toxicol 26(9):697–703. https://doi.org/10.1177/0960327107083452

Stravitz RT, Sanyal AJ, Reisch J, Bajaj JS, Mirshahi F, Cheng J, Lee WM (2013) Effects of N-acetylcysteine on cytokines in non-acetaminophen acute liver failure: potential mechanism of improvement in transplant-free survival. Liver Int 33(9):1324–1331. https://doi.org/10.1111/liv.12214

Swarnalatha G, Ram R, Neela P, Naidu MU, Dakshina Murty KV (2010) Oxidative stress in hemodialysis patients receiving intravenous iron therapy and the role of N-acetylcysteine in preventing oxidative stress. Saudi J Kidney Dis Transplant 21(5):852–858

Szkudlarek U, Zdziechowski A, Witkowski K, Kasielski M, Luczynska M, Luczynski R, Sarniak A, Nowak D (2004) Effect of inhaled N-acetylcysteine on hydrogen peroxide exhalation in healthy subjects. Pulm Pharmacol Ther 17(3):155–162. https://doi.org/10.1016/j.pupt.2004.01.007

Szkudlinska MA, von Frankenberg AD, Utzschneider KM (2016) The antioxidant N-Acetylcysteine does not improve glucose tolerance or beta-cell function in type 2 diabetes. J Diabetes Complicat 30(4):618–622. https://doi.org/10.1016/j.jdiacomp.2016.02.003

Talasaz AH, Khalili H, Jenab Y, Salarifar M, Broumand MA, Darabi F (2013) N-Acetylcysteine effects on transforming growth factor-beta and tumor necrosis factor-alpha serum levels as pro-fibrotic and inflammatory biomarkers in patients following ST-segment elevation myocardial infarction. Drugs R D 13(3):199–205. https://doi.org/10.1007/s40268-013-0025-5

Thaha M, Pranawa W, Yogiantoro M, Tomino Y (2008) Intravenous N-acetylcysteine during hemodialysis reduces asymmetric dimethylarginine level in end-stage renal disease patients. Clin Nephrol 69(1):24–32

Thaha M, Yogiantoro M, Tomino Y (2006) Intravenous N-acetylcysteine during haemodialysis reduces the plasma concentration of homocysteine in patients with end-stage renal disease. Clinical Drug Invest 26(4):195–202

Thiele H, Hildebrand L, Schirdewahn C, Eitel I, Adams V, Fuernau G, Erbs S, Linke A, Diederich KW, Nowak M, Desch S, Gutberlet M, Schuler G (2010) Impact of high-dose N-acetylcysteine versus placebo on contrast-induced nephropathy and myocardial reperfusion injury in unselected patients with ST-segment elevation myocardial infarction undergoing primary percutaneous coronary intervention. The LIPSIA-N-ACC (Prospective, Single-Blind, Placebo-Controlled, Randomized Leipzig Immediate Percutaneous Coronary Intervention Acute Myocardial Infarction N-ACC) Trial. J Am Coll Cardiol 55(20):2201–2209. https://doi.org/10.1016/j.jacc.2009.08.091

Tirouvanziam R, Conrad CK, Bottiglieri T, Herzenberg LA, Moss RB, Herzenberg LA (2006) High-dose oral N-acetylcysteine, a glutathione prodrug, modulates inflammation in cystic fibrosis. Proc Natl Acad Sci U S A 103(12):4628–4633. https://doi.org/10.1073/pnas.0511304103

Tossios P, Bloch W, Huebner A, Raji MR, Dodos F, Klass O, Suedkamp M, Kasper SM, Hellmich M, Mehlhorn U (2003) N-acetylcysteine prevents reactive oxygen species-mediated myocardial stress in patients undergoing cardiac surgery: results of a randomized, double-blind, placebo-controlled clinical trial. J Thorac Cardiovasc Surg 126(5):1513–1520. https://doi.org/10.1016/s0022

Trewin AJ, Lundell LS, Perry BD, Patil KV, Chibalin AV, Levinger I, McQuade LR, Stepto NK (2015) Effect of N-acetylcysteine infusion on exercise-induced modulation of insulin sensitivity and signaling pathways in human skeletal muscle. Am J Phys Endocrinol Metab 309(4):E388–E397. https://doi.org/10.1152/ajpendo.00605.2014

Trewin AJ, Petersen AC, Billaut F, McQuade LR, McInerney BV, Stepto NK (2013) N-acetylcysteine alters substrate metabolism during high-intensity cycle exercise in well-trained humans. Appl Physiol Nutr Metab 38(12):1217–1227. https://doi.org/10.1139/apnm-2012-0482

Trimarchi H, Mongitore MR, Baglioni P, Forrester M, Freixas EA, Schropp M, Pereyra H, Alonso M (2003) N-acetylcysteine reduces malondialdehyde levels in chronic hemodialysis patients – a pilot study. Clin Nephrol 59(6):441–446

Vento AE, Nemlander A, Aittomaki J, Salo J, Karhunen J, Ramo OJ (2003) N-acetylcysteine as an additive to crystalloid cardioplegia increased oxidative stress capacity in CABG patients. Scand Cardiovasc J SCJ 37(6):349–355. https://doi.org/10.1080/14017430310015406

Ventura P, Panini R, Abbati G, Marchetti G, Salvioli G (2003) Urinary and plasma homocysteine and cysteine levels during prolonged oral N-acetylcysteine therapy. Pharmacology 68(2):105–114. https://doi.org/10.1159/000069535

Weigand MA, Plachky J, Thies JC, Spies-Martin D, Otto G, Martin E, Bardenheuer HJ (2001) N-acetylcysteine attenuates the increase in alpha-glutathione S-transferase and circulating ICAM-1 and VCAM-1 after reperfusion in humans undergoing liver transplantation. Transplantation 72(4):694–698

Wiklund O, Fager G, Andersson A, Lundstam U, Masson P, Hultberg B (1996) N-acetylcysteine treatment lowers plasma homocysteine but not serum lipoprotein(a) levels. Atherosclerosis 119(1):99–106

Wittstock A, Burkert M, Zidek W, Tepel M, Scholze A (2009) N-acetylcysteine improves arterial vascular reactivity in patients with chronic kidney disease. Nephron Clin Pract 112(3):c184–c189. https://doi.org/10.1159/000218107

Yesilbursa D, Serdar A, Senturk T, Serdar Z, Sag S, Cordan J (2006) Effect of N-acetylcysteine on oxidative stress and ventricular function in patients with myocardial infarction. Heart Vessel 21(1):33–37. https://doi.org/10.1007/s00380-005-0854-4

Yilmaz H, Sahin S, Sayar N, Tangurek B, Yilmaz M, Nurkalem Z, Onturk E, Cakmak N, Bolca O (2007) Effects of folic acid and N-acetylcysteine on plasma homocysteine levels and endothelial function in patients with coronary artery disease. Acta Cardiol 62(6):579–585. https://doi.org/10.2143/ac.62.6.2024017

Zembron-Lacny A, Slowinska-Lisowska M, Szygula Z, Witkowski K, Szyszka K (2009) The comparison of antioxidant and hematological properties of N-acetylcysteine and alpha-lipoic acid in physically active males. Physiol Res 58(6):855–861

Zembron-Lacny A, Slowinska-Lisowska M, Szygula Z, Witkowski Z, Szyszka K (2010) Modulatory effect of N-acetylcysteine on pro-antioxidant status and haematological response in healthy men. J Physiol Biochem 66(1):15–21. https://doi.org/10.1007/s13105-010-0002-1

Cysteine/Glutathione Deficiency: A Significant and Treatable Corollary of Disease

20

Pietro Ghezzi, Kevin V. Lemley, James P. Andrus,
Stephen C. De Rosa, Arne Holmgren, Dean Jones,
Farook Jahoor, Richard Kopke, Ian Cotgreave,
Teodoro Bottiglieri, Neil Kaplowitz, Hajime Nakamura,
Frank Staal, Stephen W. Ela, Kondala R. Atkuri,
Rabindra Tirouvanziam, Kartoosh Heydari, Bita Sahaf,
Andrew Zolopa, Richard Eugene Frye, John J. Mantovani,
Leonard A. Herzenberg, and Leonore A. Herzenberg

Electronic supplementary material The online version of this article (https://doi.org/10.1007/978-981-10-5311-5_20) contains supplementary material, which is available to authorized users.

The following authors contributed equally: Pietro Ghezzi, Kevin V. Lemley, James P. Andrus and Stephen C. De Rosa

P. Ghezzi
Experimental Medicine, Brighton and Sussex Medical School, Sussex, UK

K. V. Lemley · B. Sahaf
Department of Medicine, Stanford University, Stanford, CA, USA

J. P. Andrus
Department of Pediatrics, Memorial Hospital, Las Vegas, NV, USA

S. C. De Rosa
Fred Hutchinson Cancer Center, Seattle, WA, USA

A. Holmgren
Medical Nobel Institute for Biochemistry, Karolinska Institute, Stockholm, Sweden

D. Jones
Department of Pulmonary, Allergy, Critical Care and Sleep Medicine, Emory University, Atlanta, GA, USA

© Springer Nature Singapore Pte Ltd. 2019
R. E. Frye, M. Berk (eds.), *The Therapeutic Use of N-Acetylcysteine (NAC) in Medicine*, https://doi.org/10.1007/978-981-10-5311-5_20

F. Jahoor
USDA/ARS Children's Nutrition Research Center, Baylor College of Medicine,
Waco, TX, USA

R. Kopke
Hough Ear Institute, Oklahoma City, OK, USA

I. Cotgreave
Division of Biochemical Toxicology, Karolinska Institute, Stockholm, Sweden

T. Bottiglieri
Baylor Institute of Metabolic Disease, Dallas, TX, USA

N. Kaplowitz
Keck School of Medicine, University of Southern California Medical Center,
Los Angeles, CA, USA

H. Nakamura
Institute for Virus Research, Kyoto University, Kyoto, Japan

F. Staal
Department of Immunology, University Rotterdam, Rotterdam, The Netherlands

S. W. Ela
Venture Science Consulting, Paso Robles, CA, USA

K. R. Atkuri · J. J. Mantovani · L. A. Herzenberg · K. Heydari
L. A. Herzenberg (✉)
Department of Genetics, Stanford University, Stanford, CA, USA
e-mail: leeherz@stanford.edu

R. Tirouvanziam
Department of Pediatrics, Emory University School of Medicine, Atlanta, GA, USA

R. E. Frye
Barrow Neurological Institute, Phoenix Children's Hospital, University of Arizona
College of Medicine – Phoenix, Phoenix, AZ, USA

A. Zolopa
Positive Care Clinic, Stanford University, Stanford, CA, USA

20.1   Introduction

Life-threatening hepatotoxicity in the setting of acetaminophen (APAP) overdose is due to depletion of glutathione (GSH), a vital cysteine-containing tripeptide that protects cells and organs against oxidant injury. GSH depletion can occur when supplies of cysteine are inadequate to maintain GSH homeostasis in the face of the increased GSH consumption. Thus, rapid administration of N-Acetylcysteine (NAC), which is converted to cysteine by first-pass metabolism and provides the cysteine necessary to replenish the depleted GSH, is the standard of care for preventing injury in APAP overdose.

GSH deficiency has also been recognized in a variety of apparently unrelated clinical conditions and diseases. NAC has been widely tested in randomized placebo-controlled trials (RPCTs) for efficacy in these diseases and conditions. In this chapter, we systematically review reports from early trials of NAC, which collectively suggest that GSH deficiency may be a common occurrence and that NAC may be a useful therapeutic adjunct for treating or preventing the development of this deficiency.

20.2   Methods

Publications included in this systematic literature review describe results from RPCT testing NAC for efficacy in a variety of disease settings. Publications were located by searching with the keywords "placebo AND N-Acetylcysteine AND NOT animal" as well as "placebo AND N-Acetylcysteine AND human, AND NOT animal." We searched PubMed, the NLM database, the FDA website, Cochrane Database, Google, and subsequent material through 2006 and the references lists of all placebo- and non-placebo-controlled trials that we review here. This search identified nearly 2000 relevant publications. Within these, we identified 102 RPCTs that met the strict criteria for inclusion that we set for this review, i.e., publications reporting results from RPCT in which at least 10 subjects were used to test the efficacy of NAC administered without other drugs. Findings reported for these trials are summarized in tabular form (Online Tables 20.2 and 20.3) and discussed in the text. Trials excluded are listed in Online Table 20.1. Clinical studies relevant to the findings here but not conducted under strictly controlled conditions are found in Online Table 20.4.

20.3   Results

20.3.1 Glutathione (GSH)

Rapid administration of NAC is the standard of care for preventing hepatic injury in APAP overdose. The administered NAC is converted by first-pass metabolism to cysteine, which is needed to replenish the cysteine-containing intracellular tripeptide (L-γ-glutamyl-L-cysteinyl-glycine), commonly known as GSH. GSH is depleted during detoxification of excessive amounts of APAP. If it is not rapidly replenished, severe hepatic injury ensues.

In addition to this well-known use of NAC, at least 102 RPCTs conducted over 25 years have examined the effects of NAC treatment in respiratory, cardiovascular, endocrine, and infectious and other disease settings. Of these, 72 reported beneficial effects (Keays et al. 1991; Jackson et al. 1984; Ardissino et al. 1997; Andersen et al. 1995; Altomare et al. 1996; Aylward et al. 1980; Akerlund et al. 1996; Adair et al. 2001; Bromley et al. 1995; Badaloo et al. 2002; Boesgaard et al. 1992; Brocard et al. 1980; Bernard et al. 1997; Breitkreutz et al. 2000b; Bowles and Goral 1985; Diaz-Sandoval et al. 2002; Drager et al. 2004; De Mattia et al. 1998a, b; Dueholm et al. 1992; De Backer et al. 1996; De Flora et al. 1997; De Rosa et al. 2000; Estensen et al. 1999; Eren et al. 2003; Efrati et al. 2003; Evald et al. 1989; Fischer et al. 2004; Fulghesu et al. 2002; Ferrari 1980; Boman et al. 1983; Grassi 1980; Grassi and Morandini 1976; Horowitz et al. 1988a, b; Hansen et al. 1994; Heinig et al. 1985; Hauer et al. 2003; Herzenberg et al. 1997; Kay et al. 2003; Kasielski and Nowak 2001; McGavin 1985; MacNeill et al. 2003; Olivieri et al. 1985; Ovesen et al. 2000; Pace et al. 2003; Parr and Huitson 1987; Reinhart et al. 1995; Ratjen et al. 1985; Rasmussen and Glennow 1988; Rank et al. 2000; Shyu et al. 2002; Scholze et al. 2004; Spies et al. 1994, 1996; Spapen et al. 1998; Spada et al. 2002; Suter et al. 1994; Svendsen et al. 1989; Stafanger et al. 1988; Stafanger and Koch 1989; Tepel et al. 2000, 2003; Tepel and Zidek 2001; Tossios et al. 2003; Todisco et al. 1985; Verstraeten 1979; Van Schooten et al. 2002; Walters et al. 1986; Watt et al. 2002; Wiklund et al. 1996; Yalcin et al. 2002). Collectively, these findings suggest that cysteine/GSH deficiency contributes to the pathophysiology of a wide range of diseases and that treatment of this deficiency may be important in these diseases.

GSH is a central component of the oxidative-reductive (redox) apparatus of every cell. One of its key functions is to combine with, and thereby inactivate (detoxify), reactive oxygen species (ROS), other oxidative molecules, and certain drugs, exogenous chemicals, and toxins. Because GSH is depleted in these reactions, it must continually be replenished to maintain cell and organ viability and to support normal cellular functions. Drug intoxications resulting in severe GSH depletion, notably APAP overdose, cause extensive hepatic injury if treatment to replenish GSH is not initiated before GSH stores are depleted to below-critical protective levels.

Synthesis of GSH requires cysteine, a conditionally essential amino acid that must be obtained from dietary sources or by conversion of dietary methionine via the cystathionase pathway. If the supply of cysteine is adequate, normal GSH levels are maintained. In contrast, if supplies of cysteine are inadequate to maintain GSH homeostasis in the face of increased GSH consumption, GSH depletion occurs.

GSH depletion impacts a wide variety of cellular processes, ranging from DNA synthesis and gene expression to sugar metabolism and lactate production. The pleiotropic activity of this key intracellular molecule, which arose very early in evolution, derives from its participation in the energy economy and the synthetic and catabolic activities of virtually all cells. In higher animals, it also participates in regulating the expression or activity of extracellular molecules, including many of the cytokines and adhesion molecules implicated in inflammatory reactions and other disease processes.

Acute GSH depletion causes severe—often fatal—oxidative and/or alkylation injury. This injury can be prevented (e.g., in APAP overdose) by rapid treatment with NAC, an efficient nontoxic source of cysteine, which is able to replenish hepatocellular GSH. Chronic or slowly arising GSH deficiency due to administration of GSH-depleting drugs, or to diseases and conditions that deplete GSH, can be similarly debilitating (Taniguchi et al. 1989).

In this chapter, we first review evidence for a cysteine/GSH deficiency in a variety of disease settings and consider the biochemical mechanisms through which this deficiency, and its correction, can impact disease processes. We then consider findings from a large series of RPCT in which the effectiveness of NAC treatment has been investigated and discuss this in terms of cysteine/GSH replenishment.

20.3.2 GSH Deficiency and Disease

A role for GSH deficiency in the clinical manifestations of a broad spectrum of diseases and conditions is suggested either by the direct documentation of low GSH levels in these conditions or by the demonstration of significant improvement in patient condition following NAC administration. Over 70 RPCTs demonstrate beneficial effects of NAC treatment (Online Table 20.2) (Keays et al. 1991; Bromley et al. 1995; Estensen et al. 1999; Reinhart et al. 1995; Ardissino et al. 1997; Badaloo et al. 2002; Boesgaard et al. 1992; Horowitz et al. 1988a, b; Spies et al. 1996, 1994; Svendsen et al. 1989; Andersen et al. 1995; Eren et al. 2003; Fischer et al. 2004; Tossios et al. 2003; Altomare et al. 1996; Diaz-Sandoval et al. 2002; Drager et al. 2004; Efrati et al. 2003; Kay et al. 2003; MacNeill et al. 2003; Shyu et al. 2002; Tepel et al. 2000, 2003; Tepel and Zidek 2001; De Mattia et al. 1998a, b; Fulghesu et al. 2002; Pace et al. 2003; Ratjen et al. 1985; Stafanger et al. 1988; Stafanger and Koch 1989; Scholze et al. 2004; Wiklund et al. 1996; Aylward et al. 1980; Boman et al. 1983; Brocard et al. 1980; Dueholm et al. 1992; Evald et al. 1989; Ferrari 1980; Ferrari and Spinelli 1980; Grassi 1980; Grassi and Morandini 1976; Hansen et al. 1994; Heinig et al. 1985; Jackson et al. 1984; McGavin 1985; Parr and Huitson 1987; Rasmussen and Glennow 1988; Kasielski and Nowak 2001; Verstraeten 1979; Olivieri et al. 1985; Van Schooten et al. 2002; Todisco et al. 1985; Bernard et al. 1997; De Backer et al. 1996; Suter et al. 1994; Rank et al. 2000; Spapen et al. 1998; De Flora et al. 1997; Akerlund et al. 1996; Breitkreutz et al. 2000b; De Rosa et al. 2000; Herzenberg et al. 1997; Spada et al. 2002; Watt et al. 2002; Adair et al. 2001; Hauer et al. 2003; Ovesen et al. 2000; Walters et al. 1986; Yalcin et al. 2002; Bowles and Goral 1985) in diseases and conditions that include systemic inflammatory response syndrome (SIRS), acute respiratory distress syndrome (ARDS), chronic lung disease (CLD), chronic obstructive pulmonary disease (COPD), neurodegenerative disease, cardiovascular disease, alcoholism, infectious disease (e.g., HIV-1 infection and chronic hepatitis), hepatic and renal failure, diabetes, malnutrition, and certain autoimmune diseases.

The mechanisms that underlie the development of GSH deficiency in disease are reasonably well understood, at least in some instances. A wide variety of inflammatory and metabolic stimuli common during active disease increase the production of intracellular oxidants. In addition, neutrophils and other cells present at sites of inflammation release oxidants (reactive oxygen and nitrogen intermediates) that enter other cells and add to the internal oxidant burden. GSH provides the main defense against toxic oxidative intermediates by reducing and thereby inactivating them. However, in so doing, GSH is oxidized to GSH disulfide (GSSG). GSSG is then either rapidly reduced to GSH by GSSG reductase and NADPH or is excreted from the cell and only in part recovered from the circulation.

Factors that may contribute to GSH deficiency include GSH losses that occur when GSH is enzymatically conjugated to exogenous chemicals (drugs, dietary components, and toxins) and excreted from the cell as GSH or acetylcysteine mercapturates (conjugates). In addition, disease processes may decrease the cellular uptake or synthesis of cysteine or cystine, increase GSH efflux (Abrams et al. 1995), or increase the loss of cysteine/GSH sulfur due to accelerated oxidation to the final oxidized forms (sulfate and taurine) (Hortin et al. 1994; Breitkreutz et al. 2000a). Because a balance between cysteine supply and GSH utilization must be maintained, if oxidant production or levels of substrate for GSH conjugation are high and cysteine supplies for GSH replenishment become limiting, severe GSH deficiency may occur.

Importantly, there are significant potential iatrogenic contributions to GSH depletion. Inadvertent treatment with higher doses of APAP than patients can tolerate is perhaps the most common. This can be particularly dangerous for patients with conditions in which GSH depletion tends to occur as a consequence of the disease process or following treatment with drugs that are detoxified by GSH. In addition, long-term maintenance on parenteral nutrition may result in GSH depletion since parenteral nutrition formulations are not necessarily designed to provide adequate cysteine equivalents to meet the metabolic needs of diseased patients. In the absence of adequate attention to maintenance of adequate cysteine supplies, physicians and other caregivers can inadvertently contribute to GSH deficiency.

Patient behavior may also result in the development of GSH deficiency. Chronic over-consumption of alcohol is well known to deplete GSH in certain tissues, particularly the liver, and thus to render patients susceptible to APAP toxicity at doses well below those that cause toxicity in healthy individuals. Indeed, the FDA has issued a warning to this effect (www.fda.gov/ohrms/dockets/ac/02/briefing/3882b1. htm). However, chronic consumption of APAP or other GSH-depleting drugs, even well below toxic dose levels, can gradually deplete GSH to the point where these drugs elicit toxicity. Such practices become more dangerous if patients are malnourished or are GSH deficient for other reasons.

In summary, GSH deficiency occurs more frequently than previously suspected. GSH is readily replenished by de novo synthesis as long as sufficient supplies of cysteine are available, either directly from dietary sources or indirectly by conversion of dietary methionine. However, failure to obtain sufficient dietary cysteine to replace that lost when GSH is oxidized or conjugated to drugs or exogenous chemicals results in a deficiency in cysteine and/or GSH that may necessitate pharmacological intervention.

20.3.3 Dietary Sources of Cysteine

Cysteine utilized in the body is derived from dietary cysteine and methionine, sulfur-containing amino acids (SAAs) that are largely obtained from digested protein. Since mammals obtain cysteine both directly from the diet and by degradation of dietary methionine, the normal cysteine requirement can be satisfied from dietary sources. However, as indicated above, an additional source of cysteine may be required when cysteine loss (e.g., via GSH loss) outstrips the usual dietary supply.

Requirements for SAAs in humans are based upon nitrogen and SAA balance studies conducted with healthy individuals. The average American diet contains about 100 g of protein daily, greater than half of which is animal protein with a relatively high content of SAAs. The recommended daily allowance (RDA) for SAAs for an adult male is about 1 g (200 mg of methionine and an additional 810 mg of methionine that can be replaced by an equivalent amount of cysteine). A healthy, well-fed person will often consume greater than twice the SAA RDA. However, poor appetite and/or a tendency to select fresh food with low SAA content or bioavailability (Hitchins et al. 1989) or processed food depleted of SAAs (Volkin and Klibanov 1987; Schnackenberg et al. 2009; Briganti et al. 2008) can result in cysteine deficiency even in otherwise healthy people. Furthermore, as evidence here indicates, the need for SAAs can be substantially increased in many disease states.

The limited ability of the body to store amino acids is an additional problem. The human liver does contain a reservoir of cysteine (about 1 g) that is largely present in GSH. Since this amount approximates the daily SAA requirement, it provides only a short-term source to maintain a stable cysteine supply despite intermittent methionine and cysteine consumption. Under conditions of excessive cysteine requirements or deficient cysteine/methionine consumption, GSH is released from skeletal muscle and other tissues to supply cysteine. This results in decreased antioxidant and detoxification functions throughout the body. Consequently, even short-term inadequate intake of SAAs can pose a risk to individuals who may consume adequate amounts most of the time (Larsen and Fuller 1996; Shriner and Goetz 1992).

20.3.4 Mechanisms that May Mediate the Clinical Effects of Cysteine/GSH Deficiency

GSH has multiple roles in cells, ranging from neutralization of ROS to acting as a coenzyme in a variety of metabolic processes. The widespread participation of GSH in biochemical reactions of importance to cell growth, differentiation, and function offers mechanistic insights into how interfering with GSH homeostasis could influence the course of varied disease processes. A full discussion of the preclinical data bearing on these issues is beyond the scope of this review. However, to provide a mechanistic context for the clinical findings we discuss, we have summarized some of the key processes regulated by GSH in the following section.

20.3.4.1 Oxidative Reactions

In its best-known role, GSH participates in enzyme-mediated reactions to neutralize ROS, preventing the accumulation of ROS damage to DNA, proteins, and lipids. Glutathione peroxidases play a key role in this process by catalyzing the reaction of GSH with peroxides, including hydrogen peroxide and lipid peroxides. Thus, decreasing GSH can sharply augment oxidative damage and result in cell death or loss of function.

20.3.4.2 DNA Synthesis

Low GSH availability can impair DNA synthesis since GSH acts (via thioredoxin) as a coenzyme for ribonucleotide reductase, an enzyme required for the synthesis of DNA (Holmgren 1985, 1989; Zhong et al. 2000a).

20.3.4.3 Gene Expression and Signal Transduction

GSH has been shown to regulate or influence the expression of several genes, notably inflammatory genes under the control of transcription factor nuclear factor kappa B (NF-κB) and activator protein 1 (AP-1), even in settings where there is no marked overproduction of ROS. In addition, GSH has been shown to regulate T-cell signaling by controlling phosphorylation of phospholipase C γ 1 (PLCg1), which is required to stimulate the calcium flux that occurs early in the T-cell receptor-signaling cascade (Kanner et al. 1992a, b, c; Kanner and Ledbetter 1992; Flescher et al. 1994). Importantly, GSH has also been shown to regulate the expression of vascular cell adhesion molecule-1 (VCAM-1) on vascular endothelial cells, one of the early features in the pathogenesis of atherosclerosis and other inflammatory diseases (Ahmad et al. 2002; De Mattia et al. 1998a, b; Marui et al. 1993; Schmidt et al. 1995; Weigand et al. 2001).

20.3.4.4 Enzymes and Protein Functions

GSH regulates the activity of enzymes and other intracellular molecules by post-translational modifications (glutathionylations) that control the oxidation state of protein-SH groups. When intracellular GSH is at its normal level for a particular cell type in a healthy individual, most of the free protein thiol groups are reduced, i.e., are present as protein-SH. In contrast, when GSH levels are low and/or GSSG levels are increased, GSH is reversibly coupled to many free thiols to create mixed disulfides (protein-S-S-G) (Ghezzi et al. 2002). These *S*-glutathionylated proteins, which may be functionally altered, then persist as such until GSH levels return to normal.

By controlling the activities of a series of enzymes and other intracellular proteins, glutathionylation can rapidly and reversibly alter the metabolic status of cells in response to changes in the redox environment. For example, glutathionylation has been shown to regulate actin polymerization (Wang et al. 2001), to inhibit the activity of several key enzymes (including glyceraldehyde-3-phosphate dehydrogenase, carbonic anhydrase, and protein tyrosine phosphatase), and to activate or stabilize other enzymes (including HIV-1 protease and the NF-κB transcription factor (Pineda-Molina et al. 2001)). Nitrosylation of protein thiols has similarly been shown to increase under oxidative conditions (Galli et al. 2002; Choudhary and Dudley 2002; Estevez and Jordan 2002; Yang et al. 2002) and to alter functions of key enzymes (Arnelle and Stamler 1995) and other molecules (Gow et al. 2002; Marshall et al. 2002). Thus, both glutathionylation and nitrosylation are of central importance to mechanisms through which cysteine/GSH deficiency may impact cell, and hence organ, function.

As indicated above, these types of posttranslational modifications are highly sensitive to shifts in the intracellular redox balance. They are rapidly initiated when GSH is depleted and rapidly reversed when GSH is replenished. As such, they provide the kind of flexible response to oxidative stress necessary for organisms living in an oxidative environment. However, at the extreme, they may underlie some of the pathologic changes that occur when chronic cysteine/GSH deficiency occurs in disease.

20.3.4.5 Glutaredoxin and Thioredoxin

Glutaredoxin (Grx) and thioredoxin (Trx) belong to the two major oxidoreductase enzyme families, which take electrons from GSH and NADPH respectively (Zhong et al. 2000a; Holmgren 1989; Cotgreave et al. 2002; Nakamura et al. 2001; Vlamis-Gardikas and Holmgren 2002). Trx and Grx interact with proteins to regulate functional activity, both directly and via glutathionylation. Intracellular GSH and GSSG levels play a major role in this regulation. The activity of Grx is directly regulated by the amount of intracellular GSH and GSSG, which controls the status of the Grx active site. The active sites in Trx (Cys-Gly-Pro-Cys) and Grx (Cys-Pro-Tyr-Cys) contain a dithiol that can be oxidized when GSH levels are low (or GSSG levels increase) to form an internal disulfide between the two cysteine residues or a mixed disulfide in which GSH is bound to one or both cysteine residues in the active site.

Formation of the Grx mixed disulfide (Casagrande et al. 2002; Cotgreave et al. 2002; Ghezzi et al. 2002) represents a special case of protein glutathionylation since it arms the Grx for glutathionylation of other proteins. Although Trx can also be glutathionylated (Casagrande et al. 2002), current data indicate that glutathionylation is mainly mediated by the Grx mixed disulfide (Daily et al. 2001; Shenton et al. 2002; Song et al. 2002). Oxidation of Grx and Trx active sites can also regulate Trx or Grx functions mediated by direct binding to key intracellular proteins. For example, under reducing conditions, Trx and Grx protect cells from apoptosis by binding to and inactivating apoptosis signaling kinase I (Song et al. 2002; Saitoh et al. 1998), whereas this binding is blocked, and apoptosis induction proceeds at low GSH levels (and/or high GSSG levels; Arner and Holmgren 2000).

20.3.4.6   Selenoenzymes

Decreasing GSH increases the intracellular redox potential of the GSH/GSSG redox couple and puts an additional burden on the Trx-Trx reductase system. This may be quite important in patients who have low selenium levels, since human Trx reductases are selenoenzymes with an essential selenocysteine residue in the active site (Arner and Holmgren 2000; Gladyshev et al. 1996a, b; Sandalova et al. 2001; Zhong et al. 2000a, b; Zhong and Holmgren 2000). Cysteine/GSH deficiency in these patients, in whom Trx reductase activity is compromised, may make them particularly susceptible to cell damage under oxidative stress. Thus, cysteine/GSH deficiency can impact cell and organ function through multiple pathways operating at the same or different sites, depending on the underlying mechanisms responsible for depleting GSH. The fact that multiple different pathways are affected explains why the effects of cysteine/GSH deficiency can affect many diseases and why cysteine/GSH deficiency has not been readily recognizable as a single clinical entity in the past.

20.3.5 N-Acetylcysteine (NAC) Treatment to Relieve Cysteine/GSH Deficiency

Clinical experience in the treatment of APAP toxicity has established that rapid administration of NAC, an essentially nontoxic cysteine source, restores normal GSH levels in solid tissues and the systemic circulation and thus prevents the potentially lethal consequences of severe cysteine/GSH deficiency induced by APAP overdose. In addition to this well-known role for NAC, NAC treatment has been shown to be clinically beneficial in a wide variety of diseases and conditions. In fact, over 70 RPCTs (Online Table 20.2) have reported beneficial effects of NAC treatment. Collectively, these studies demonstrate that cysteine/GSH deficiency is an important emerging clinical entity and that NAC administration offers an effective method for treating this deficiency.

Although various forms of cysteine and its precursors have been used as nutritional and therapeutic sources of cysteine, NAC is the most widely used and extensively studied. NAC is about ten times more stable than cysteine and much more soluble than the stable cysteine disulfide, cystine. L-2-oxothiazolidine-4-carboxylate (procysteine/OTC) has also been used effectively in some studies (Aaseth and Stoa-Birketvedt 2000) as have GSH and GSH monoethyl ester (Meister et al. 1986). In addition, dietary methionine is an effective source of cysteine, as is S-adenosylmethionine (referred to either as SAM or SAM-e) (Castagna et al. 1995). We focus on NAC in this review because NAC is the cysteine source used for correcting cysteine/GSH deficiency in most studies and because NAC is already approved for therapeutic use for treatment of APAP overdose and as a mucolytic agent in cystic fibrosis.

Surprisingly, given the diverse roles that GSH plays in cellular physiology and regulation of enzyme activity and protein function (see above), GSH deficiency has mainly been discussed from a clinical perspective in terms of the loss of intracellular protection against oxidative stress. Similarly, NAC is principally considered to be an antioxidant rather than a source of cysteine for GSH replenishment. However, while antioxidants such as vitamins E and C can spare GSH under conditions of oxidative stress, GSH loss due to oxidative or detoxifying reactions can only be offset by GSH resynthesis, which requires a cysteine source.

In addition to providing the cysteine necessary to replenish GSH, NAC administration improves the cysteine supply for protein synthesis and metabolic purposes. When administered intravenously, it also appears for a short period of time at high levels in blood and can react directly with oxidants and nitric oxide derivatives. However, when administered orally (as in most of the studies), it is rapidly converted by first-pass metabolism to cysteine, which is either incorporated into GSH in the liver or released into the blood in a regulated manner. Thus, orally administered NAC appears in the circulation only transiently and at only minimal levels. Hence, it is effective largely via its ability to increase cysteine supplies and thereby facilitate the GSH replenishment.

In the sections that follow, we discuss examples of RPCTs (Online Table 20.2) which have examined the outcomes of NAC therapy in various medical disorders. We also discuss selected findings from observational studies (Online Table 20.3) that further illuminate clinical aspects of cysteine/GSH deficiency.

20.3.5.1 Acetaminophen Toxicity

APAP overdose is a well-known cause of fulminant hepatic failure. In fact, APAP overdose and idiosyncratic drug reactions have now replaced viral hepatitis as the most frequent causes of acute liver failure in the United States (Ostapowicz and Lee 2000). The toxicity of APAP is due to depletion of GSH in hepatocytes (Mitchell et al. 1974, 1981; Peterson and Rumack 1978; Lauterburg et al. 1983; Smilkstein et al. 1988; Ostapowicz et al. 2002). NAC is extremely effective in preventing liver damage due to APAP toxicity. NAC administered promptly and at a sufficient dose is the standard of care for treatment of APAP poisoning (Mitchell et al. 1974; Lyons et al. 1977; Prescott et al. 1977; Peterson and Rumack 1977a, b, 1978; Marquardt 1977; Maurer and Zeisler 1978; Macy 1979; Stewart et al. 1979; Bailey 1980; Black 1980; Sellers and Freedman 1981; Rumack et al. 1981; Prescott and Critchley 1983; Miller and Rumack 1983; Rumack 1984, 1986, 2002; Davis 1986; Larrauri et al. 1987; Slattery et al. 1987, 1989; Smilkstein et al. 1988, 1991; Burgunder et al. 1989; Beckett et al. 1990, 1985; Harrison et al. 1990; Keays et al. 1991; Bray et al. 1991; Winkler and Halkin 1992; Lee 1993, 1995, 1996; Larsen and Fuller 1996; De Roos and Hoffman 1996; Perry and Shannon 1998; Salgia and Kosnik 1999; Ammenti et al. 1999; Buckley et al. 1999; Broughan and Soloway 2000; Kearns et al. 2000; Woo et al. 2000; Amirzadeh and McCotter 2002; Schmidt et al. 2002; Jones 2002; Kearns 2002; Peterson et al. 1998) and can improve survival (Harrison et al. 1990) and cardiovascular function (Harrison et al. 1991) in those already with hepatic failure.

Interestingly, although the acute dose of APAP likely to cause severe liver toxicity is well established for healthy individuals (Peterson and Rumack 1978), under conditions in which GSH levels are compromised, doses of APAP that are within the usual prescribed range can cause hepatic injury (Peterson and Rumack 1978;

Larsen and Fuller 1996). Thus, usage of APAP and other GSH-depleting drugs may be quite important to overall pathology in diseases and conditions where GSH deficiency is known to occur.

This is especially important in patients with chronic alcohol consumption (Bray et al. 1991; Salgia and Kosnik 1999) because they often have lower GSH levels. In such patients, doses of APAP below those usually considered toxic could deplete GSH below the critical threshold for hepatocellular necrosis (Lauterburg and Velez 1988). Thus, it has been suggested that patients with chronic alcoholism and suspected APAP poisoning should be treated with NAC regardless of risk estimation (Johnston and Pelletier 1997; Ozaras et al. 2003; Moss et al. 2000). This has prompted the FDA to a special warning for individuals with chronic alcohol use in regard to APAP use.

20.3.5.2　Gastrointestinal Disease

Several studies have demonstrated GSH depletion in children with the edematous syndromes of protein-energy malnutrition (PEM), kwashiorkor, and marasmic kwashiorkor (Badaloo et al. 2002; Golden and Ramdath 1987; Jackson 1986; Reid et al. 2000). Children with edematous PEM have biomarkers of oxidant damage (Lenhartz et al. 1998; Fechner et al. 2001). The observation that biomarkers of oxidant damage normalize as soon as clinical signs and symptoms resolve (Lenhartz et al. 1998) suggests that oxidant damage plays an important role in the pathogenesis of the disease.

In a study of children with edematous PEM, Jahoor and colleagues showed that RBC GSH depletion is due to a slower rate of GSH synthesis secondary to inadequate cysteine availability (Reid et al. 2000). In another study of children with edematous PEM, Jahoor and colleagues demonstrated that GSH synthesis rate and concentration can be restored during the early phase of nutritional rehabilitation if diets are supplemented with NAC (Badaloo et al. 2002). The observation that edema is lost at a faster rate by the group whose GSH pools were restored early with NAC suggests that early restoration of GSH homeostasis accelerates recovery. This possibility is supported by another study showing that increases in GSH levels in children with kwashiorkor are associated with recovery (Fechner et al. 2001).

These findings also raise the question of whether the modest malnutrition common in elderly people, who also frequently have low GSH levels (Anderson et al. 1993, 2001), puts the elderly at risk for developing clinically significant cysteine/ GSH deficiency and hence at increased risk of hepatic and other tissue injuries associated with consumption of GSH-depleting pharmaceuticals such as APAP.

20.3.5.3　Kidney Transplantation

Delayed graft function (DGF) after kidney transplantation is probably in large part caused by production of ROS following reperfusion of the transplant organ after a period of warm and cold ischemia. In general, these reactive molecules are detoxified by GSH-dependent mechanisms, including conjugation to GSH by a family of GSH-S-transferase (GST) enzymes, some of which are expressed in large quantity in the proximal tubule of the kidney (Davies et al. 1995). In an observational study of 229 kidney transplant recipients, donor (but not recipient) GST M1B polymorphism was associated with significantly lower rates of DGF after transplantation (Akgul et al. 2012).

20.3.5.4 Diabetes Mellitus

Three RPCTs demonstrate beneficial effects of NAC treatment in insulin-related disease (Online Table 20.2d). One study demonstrates that oral administration of NAC to patients with non-insulin-dependent diabetes mellitus reverses the elevation of soluble vascular cell adhesion molecule-1 (De Mattia et al. 1998b), a substance that promotes accumulation of macrophages and T lymphocytes at sites of inflammation and increases progression of vascular damage (Marui et al. 1993; Schmidt et al. 1995). A second placebo-controlled study by the same group shows that intravenous GSH infusion significantly increases both RBC GSH/GSSG redox ratio and total glucose uptake in these patients and suggests that abnormal intracellular GSH redox status plays an important role in reducing insulin sensitivity (De Mattia et al. 1998a). Consistent with these findings, in an ongoing study in type 2 diabetics, Jahoor and colleagues have demonstrated that 2 weeks of dietary supplementation with NAC elicited significant increases in both RBC GSH concentration and synthesis, suggesting that positive clinical effects of NAC are mediated through improved GSH availability (McKay et al. 2000).

20.3.5.5 Metabolic and Genetic Disease

Genetic defects that impair GSH synthesis or homeostasis are well known (Ristoff and Larsson 2002). The most common defect affects GSH synthetase (GS) and has a wide range of disease manifestations, including hemolytic anemia, progressive neurological symptoms, metabolic acidosis, and, in the most severe form, death during the neonatal period. Data from a small observational study suggests that early supplementation with Vitamins C and E may improve long-term outcome in these patients (Ristoff et al. 2001).

20.3.5.6 Systemic Inflammatory Response Syndrome

Five of seven RPCTs showed a beneficial effect of NAC as an adjunct therapy for acute lung injury and end-organ failure. These studies indicate that oxidative stress and cysteine/GSH depletion play a major role in inflammation leading to capillary leak syndromes and end-organ failure (De Flora et al. 1997; Suter et al. 1994; Rank et al. 2000). These study show that NAC: (a) decreases the cytotoxic effects of TNF-α and other inflammatory cytokines (Zimmerman et al. 1989), (b) decreases neutrophil elastase production in acute lung injury (Borregaard et al. 1987; De Backer et al. 1996; Laurent et al. 1996; Eklund et al. 1988; Moriuchi et al. 1998), and (c) increases neutrophil protection and decreases mortality in septic shock (Villa et al. 2002).

20.3.5.7 HIV Disease

A broad series of studies clearly demonstrates GSH levels in RBCs, lymphocytes, and other peripheral blood mononuclear cells progressively decrease as HIV disease advances (De Rosa et al. 2000; Herzenberg et al. 1997; Akerlund et al. 1996; Droge and Breitkreutz 1999; Clotet et al. 1995; Spada et al. 2002; Verhagen et al. 2001). In addition, careful pharmacokinetic studies demonstrate that the low GSH in HIV-infected individuals is due to limited availability of sufficient cysteine to maintain cellular GSH homeostasis (Droge et al. 1991; Roederer et al. 1990). In fact, a massive peripheral tissue catabolism of sulfur-containing peptides and amino acids has been observed in HIV patients (Hortin et al. 1994; Breitkreutz et al. 2000a).

Five of six RPCTs show beneficial effects of NAC treatment in HIV infection. Several trials collectively demonstrated that NAC administration to HIV-infected subjects with low GSH levels replenishes lymphocyte and erythrocyte GSH (Online Table 20.2g) (De Rosa et al. 2000; Breitkreutz et al. 2000b). Importantly, one of these studies demonstrates that NAC treatment significantly improves T-cell function (Breitkreutz et al. 2000b). This finding supports the idea that cysteine/GSH deficiency contributes to the immunodeficiency in HIV-infected individuals and plays an important and reversible role in the functional impairment of those T cells that are still present at later stages of HIV disease.

Cysteine/GSH deficiency may also contribute to the failure of the innate immune system and the development of opportunistic infections in the final stages of HIV disease. Observational studies have shown that HIV-infected individuals with low CD4 T-cell counts and low cellular and systemic GSH levels frequently have elevated blood levels of Trx, which is an effective chemokine (Bertini et al. 1999). In mice, circulating Trx (like other chemokines) blocks neutrophil migration to infection sites and hence interferes with innate defense against invading pathogens (Villa et al. 2002). Similar interference may occur in HIV infection, since the survival of infected individuals with Trx levels above the normal range is significantly decreased compared to survival of subjects with Trx levels in the normal range (Ghezzi et al. 2002). Since NAC treatment lowers Trx levels (Nakamura et al. 2001, 2002), this may contribute to the observed association between NAC ingestion and prolonged survival in HIV disease (Roederer et al. 1992; De Rosa et al. 2000; Akerlund et al. 1996; Spada et al. 2002).

The improvement in T-cell function observed in HIV-infected subjects treated with NAC (Breitkreutz et al. 2000b) suggests that NAC treatment may be a useful adjunct in HIV vaccination. In addition, this improvement provides a rationale for the strong associations observed between low GSH levels and decreased survival in HIV infection (Herzenberg et al. 1997) and between NAC administration and improved survival in an open-label NAC study (Huengsberg et al. 1998).

20.3.5.8   Otic Disease

Preclinical studies point to the importance of oxidative stress and GSH depletion in the genesis of noise and toxin-induced hearing loss (Kopke et al. 1999, 2001). Medications with inner ear toxicity such as aminoglycoside antibiotics and the chemotherapy agent cisplatin damage the cochlea through the generation of oxygen free radicals. Hearing loss and cochlear damage associated with administration of these compounds have been shown, in animal models, to be greatly reduced by administration of both NAC and methionine (Hoffer et al. 2001; Kopke et al. 2000; Sha and Schacht 2000). Similarly, studies with animal models show that permanent cochlear damage due to acute acoustic overexposure, which induces ischemia reperfusion, glutamate excitotoxicity, free radical generation, and GSH depletion (Kopke et al. 1999, 2000, 2001, 2002), can be almost completely prevented by systemic administration of NAC or methionine (Kopke et al. 2000, 2002).

20.4 Summary

The evidence reviewed here reveals cysteine/GSH deficiency as an emerging clinical entity. The manifestations of this deficiency may vary in different disease settings, as may the biochemical mechanisms that mediate its effects. However, they are united by a common positive response to NAC therapy in RPCTs (Online Table 20.2). The studies we have reviewed collectively argue for consideration of cysteine/GSH deficiency as a significant and treatable clinical entity.

Surprisingly, given the diverse roles that GSH plays in cellular physiology and regulation of enzyme activity and protein function, the consequences of low GSH levels have mainly been discussed from a clinical perspective in terms of the loss of protection against intracellular oxidative stress. However, while antioxidants such as vitamins E and C can spare GSH under conditions of oxidative stress, GSH loss can only be offset by GSH resynthesis, indicating a central role for this molecule over and above its ability to counteract the effects of intracellular oxidants.

Similarly, although NAC is a well-known source of cysteine for GSH replenishment in APAP toxicity, it is principally cast as an antioxidant in other settings. By and large, physicians and the lay public tend to equate NAC with vitamins C and E and other antioxidants. Like GSH, NAC can serve as an antioxidant. However, while other antioxidants can replace NAC and GSH in this role, only NAC or another cysteine source can provide the raw material necessary to replenish GSH and enable GSH-dependent biochemical reactions.

We have pointed out that physicians may find NAC administration useful as adjunct therapy for diseases and conditions in which cysteine/GSH deficiency is likely to play a role. The positive findings in the RPCTs we have discussed support this argument. However, the absence of large multicenter trials testing NAC in various settings leaves this as an open question. The recognition that cysteine/GSH deficiency is an important clinical entity will encourage support for such trials.

In the meantime, the findings we have discussed suggests that patients with diseases or conditions in which cysteine/GSH deficiency has been demonstrated may be well advised to avoid unnecessary exposures to medications that may exacerbate GSH depletion. In fact, when advising such patients, it seems reasonable for physicians to emphasize that alcohol usage be kept at modest levels and that APAP usage should be kept strictly within the recommended dosing.

The availability of OTC NAC, and the low toxicity of this cysteine prodrug in situations where it has been tested, opens the possibility of patient- or physician-initiated therapy. However, if such therapy is elected, we suggest that the NAC preparation(s) used be prepared under Good Manufacturing Practice conditions and packaged to prevent oxidation of the product.

Acknowledgments This presentation would not have been completed without the help from Mr. David Aiello (BioAdvantex Pharma, Mississauga, Ontario, Canada) and Dr. Thilo Messerschmidt (Diamalt B.F. Goodrich, Raubling, Germany). Mr. Aiello helped ferret out and interpret citations of importance for this manuscript and provided key editorial and technical support when we needed it most. Dr. Messerschmidt provided highly valuable technical and biochemical insights in addition to editorial advice concerning NAC synthesis and the mechanisms involved in maintaining the redox balance in cells and organisms. Mr. Onny Chattergee and Mr. Kevin McCaffrey provided unstinting technical help in the organization and handling of the many publications reviewed here, and Ms. Claudia Weber provided the solid administrative support that allowed us to focus on the mammoth job of collecting and reviewing all of these publications. Studies presented here were supported in part by a grant (CA-42509) from the National Cancer Institute of the US National Institutes of Health.

References

Aaseth J, Stoa-Birketvedt G (2000) Glutathione in overweight patients with poorly controlled type 2 diabetes. J Trace Elem Exp Med 13(1):105–111

Abrams D, Cotton D, Mayer K (1995) AIDS/HIV treatment directory, vol 7 #4. American Foundation for AIDS Research (AmFAR), Rockville, MD

Adair JC, Knoefel JE, Morgan N (2001) Controlled trial of N-acetylcysteine for patients with probable Alzheimer's disease. Neurology 57(8):1515–1517

Agusti AG, Togores B, Ibanez J, Raurich JM, Maimo A, Bergada J, Marse P, Jorda R (1997) Effects of N-acetylcysteine on tissue oxygenation in patients with multiple organ failure and evidence of tissue hypoxia. Eur Respir J 10(9):1962–1966

Ahmad M, Zhang Y, Papharalambus C, Alexander RW (2002) Role of isoprenylcysteine carboxyl methyltransferase in tumor necrosis factor-alpha stimulation of expression of vascular cell adhesion molecule-1 in endothelial cells. Arterioscler Thromb Vasc Biol 22(5):759–764

Ahola T, Lapatto R, Raivio KO, Selander B, Stigson L, Jonsson B, Jonsbo F, Esberg G, Stovring S, Kjartansson S, Stiris T, Lossius K, Virkola K, Fellman V (2003) N-acetylcysteine does not prevent bronchopulmonary dysplasia in immature infants: a randomized controlled trial. J Pediatr 143(6):713–719

Akerlund B, Jarstrand C, Lindeke B, Sonnerborg A, Akerblad A-C, Rasool O (1996) Effect of N-acetylcysteine (NAC) treatment on HIV-1 infection: a double-blind placebo-controlled trial. Eur J Clin Pharmacol 50(6):457–461

Akerlund B, Tynell E, Bratt G, Bielenstein M, Lidman C (1997) N-acetylcysteine treatment and the risk of toxic reactions to trimethoprim-sulphamethoxazole in primary Pneumocystis carinii prophylaxis in HIV-infected patients. J Infect 35(2):143–147

Akgul SU, Oguz FS, Caliskan Y, Kekik C, Gurkan H, Turkmen A, Nane I, Aydin F (2012) The effect of glutathione S-transferase polymorphisms and anti-GSTT1 antibodies on allograft functions in recipients of renal transplant. Transplant Proc 44(6):1679–1684. https://doi.org/10.1016/j.transproceed.2012.04.004

Allaqaband S, Tumuluri R, Malik AM, Gupta A, Volkert P, Shalev Y, Bajwa TK (2002) Prospective randomized study of N-acetylcysteine, fenoldopam, and saline for prevention of radiocontrast-induced nephropathy. Catheter Cardiovasc Interv 57(3):279–283. https://doi.org/10.1002/ccd.10323

Allard JP, Aghdassi E, Chau J, Tam C, Kovacs CM, Salit IE, Walmsley SL (1998) Effects of vitamin E and C supplementation on oxidative stress and viral load in HIV-infected subjects. AIDS 12(13):1653–1659

Altomare E, Colonna P, Dagostino C, Castellaneta G, Vendemiale G, Grattagliano I, Cirelli F, Bovenzi F, Colonna L (1996) High-dose antioxidant therapy during thrombolysis in patients with acute myocardial infarction. Curr Ther Res 57(2):131–141

Altomare E, Vendemiale G, Albano O (1988) Hepatic glutathione content in patients with alcoholic and non alcoholic liver disease. Life Sci 43:991–998

Amirzadeh A, McCotter C (2002) The intravenous use of oral acetylcysteine (mucomyst) for the treatment of acetaminophen overdose. Arch Intern Med 162(1):96–97

Ammenti A, Ferrante R, Spagna A (1999) Renal impairment without hepatic damage after acetaminophen overdose. Pediatr Nephrol 13(3):271–272

Andersen LW, Thiis J, Kharazmi A, Rygg I (1995) The role of N-acetylcystein administration on the oxidative response of neutrophils during cardiopulmonary bypass. Perfusion 10(1):21–26

Anderson BB, Giuberti M, Perry GM, Salsini G, Casadio I, Vullo C (1993) Low red blood cell glutathione reductase and pyridoxine phosphate oxidase activities not related to dietary riboflavin: selection by malaria? Am J Clin Nutr 57(5):666–672

Anderson RA, Roussel AM, Zouari N, Mahjoub S, Matheau JM, Kerkeni A (2001) Potential antioxidant effects of zinc and chromium supplementation in people with type 2 diabetes mellitus. J Am Coll Nutr 20(3):212–218

Andrews NP, Prasad A, Quyyumi AA (2001) N-acetylcysteine improves coronary and peripheral vascular function. J Am Coll Cardiol 37(1):117–123

Angulo P, Lindor KD (2001) Treatment of nonalcoholic fatty liver: present and emerging therapies. Semin Liver Dis 21(1):81–88

App EM, Baran D, Dab I, Malfroot A, Coffiner M, Vanderbist F, King M (2002) Dose-finding and 24-h monitoring for efficacy and safety of aerosolized Nacystelyn in cystic fibrosis. Eur Respir J 19(2):294–302

Ardissino D, Merlini PA, Savonitto S, Demicheli G, Zanini P, Bertocchi F, Falcone C, Ghio S, Marinoni G, Montemartini C, Mussini A (1997) Effect of transdermal nitroglycerin or N-acetylcysteine, or both, in the long-term treatment of unstable angina pectoris. J Am Coll Cardiol 29(5):941–947

Arnelle DR, Stamler JS (1995) NO+, NO, and NO- donation by S-nitrosothiols: implications for regulation of physiological functions by S-nitrosylation and acceleration of disulfide formation. Arch Biochem Biophys 318(2):279–285. https://doi.org/10.1006/abbi.1995.1231

Arner ES, Holmgren A (2000) Physiological functions of thioredoxin and thioredoxin reductase. Eur J Biochem 267(20):6102–6109

Aukrust P, Svardal AM, Muller F, Lunden B, Berge RK, Froland SS (1995) Decreased levels of total and reduced glutathione in CD4+ lymphocytes in common variable immunodeficiency are associated with activation of the tumor necrosis factor system: possible immunopathogenic role of oxidative stress. Blood 86(4):1383–1391

Aylward M, Maddock J, Dewland P (1980) Clinical evaluation of acetylcysteine in the treatment of patients with chronic obstructive bronchitis: a balanced double-blind trial with placebo control. Eur J Respir Dis Suppl 111:81–89

Badaloo A, Reid M, Forrester T, Heird WC, Jahoor F (2002) Cysteine supplementation improves the erythrocyte glutathione synthesis rate in children with severe edematous malnutrition. Am J Clin Nutr 76(3):646–652

Bailey BO (1980) Acetaminophen hepatotoxicity and overdose. Am Fam Physician 22(1):83–87

Bains JS, Shaw CA (1997) Neurodegenerative disorders in humans: the role of glutathione in oxidative stress-mediated neuronal death. Brain Res Rev 25(3):335–358

Banaclocha MM (2001) Therapeutic potential of N-acetylcysteine in age-related mitochondrial neurodegenerative diseases. Med Hypotheses 56(4):472–477

Banerjee BD, Seth V, Bhattacharya A, Pasha ST, Chakraborty AK (1999) Biochemical effects of some pesticides on lipid peroxidation and free-radical scavengers. Toxicol Lett 107(1–3):33–47

Barbaro G, Di Lorenzo G, Soldini M, Bellomo G, Belloni G, Grisorio B, Barbarini G (1997) Vagal system impairment in human immunodeficiency virus-positive patients with chronic hepatitis C: does hepatic glutathione deficiency have a pathogenetic role? Scand J Gastroenterol 32(12):1261–1266

Barbaro G, Di Lorenzo G, Soldini M, Parrotto S, Bellomo G, Belloni G, Grisorio B, Barbarini G (1996) Hepatic glutathione deficiency in chronic hepatitis C: quantitative evaluation in patients who are HIV positive and HIV negative and correlations with plasmatic and lymphocytic concentrations and with the activity of the liver disease. Am J Gastroenterol 91(12):2569–2573

Barditch-Crovo P, Noe D, Skowron G, Lederman M, Kalayjian RC, Borum P, Buier R, Rowe WB, Goldberg D, Lietman P (1998) A phase I/II evaluation of oral L-2-oxothiazolidine-4-carboxylic acid in asymptomatic patients infected with human immunodeficiency virus. J Clin Pharmacol 38(4):357–363

Barton AD (1974) Aerosolized detergents and mucolytic agents in the treatment of stable chronic obstructive pulmonary disease. Am Rev Respir Dis 110(6 Pt 2):104–110

Beckett GJ, Chapman BJ, Dyson EH, Hayes JD (1985) Plasma glutathione S-transferase measurements after paracetamol overdose: evidence for early hepatocellular damage. Gut 26(1):26–31

Beckett GJ, Donovan JW, Hussey AJ, Proudfoot AT, Prescott LF (1990) Intravenous N-acetylcysteine, hepatotoxicity and plasma glutathione S-transferase in patients with paracetamol overdosage. Hum Exp Toxicol 9(3):183–186

Behr J, Degenkolb B, Krombach F, Vogelmeier C (2002) Intracellular glutathione and bronchoalveolar cells in fibrosing alveolitis: effects of N-acetylcysteine. Eur Respir J 19(5):906–911

Behr J, Maier K, Degenkolb B, Krombach F, Vogelmeier C (1997) Antioxidative and clinical effects of high-dose N-acetylcysteine in fibrosing alveolitis. Adjunctive therapy to maintenance immunosuppression. Am J Respir Crit Care Med 156(6):1897–1901

Beloqui O, Prieto J, Suarez M, Gil B, Qian CH, Garcia N, Civeira MP (1993) N-acetyl cysteine enhances the response to interferon-alpha in chronic hepatitis-C: a pilot study. J Interf Res 13:279–282

Ben-Ari Z, Vaknin H, Tur-Kaspa R (2000) N-acetylcysteine in acute hepatic failure (Non-paracetamol-induced). Hepatogastroenterology 47(33):786–789

Ben-Menachem E, Kyllerman M, Marklund S (2000) Superoxide dismutase and glutathione peroxidase function in progressive myoclonus epilepsies. Epilepsy Res 40(1):33–39

Bernard GR (1990) Potential of N-acetylcysteine as treatment for the adult respiratory distress syndrome. Eur Respir J Suppl 11:496s–498s

Bernard GR, Wheeler AP, Arons MM, Morris PE, Paz HL, Russell JA, Wright PE, Bernard GR, Arons MM, Wheeler AP, Carmichael LC, Morris PE, Higgins SB, Dupont WD, Edens TR, Swindell BB, Russell JA, Paz HL, Wright PE, Steinberg KP (1997) A trial of antioxidants N-acetylcysteine and procysteine in ARDS. Chest 112(1):164–172

Bernhard MC, Junker E, Hettinger A, Lauterburg BH (1998) Time course of total cysteine, glutathione and homocysteine in plasma of patients with chronic hepatitis C treated with interferon-alpha with and without supplementation with N-acetylcysteine. J Hepatol 28(5):751–755

Bertini R, Howard OM, Dong HF, Oppenheim JJ, Bizzarri C, Sergi R, Caselli G, Pagliei S, Romines B, Wilshire JA, Mengozzi M, Nakamura H, Yodoi J, Pekkari K, Gurunath R, Holmgren A, Herzenberg LA, Ghezzi P (1999) Thioredoxin, a redox enzyme released in infection and inflammation, is a unique chemoattractant for neutrophils, monocytes, and T cells. J Exp Med 189(11):1783–1789

Bianchi G, Bugianesi E, Ronchi M, Fabbri A, Zoli M, Marchesini G (1997) Glutathione kinetics in normal man and in patients with liver cirrhosis. J Hepatol 26(3):606–613

Bibi H, Seifert B, Oullette M, Belik J (1992) Intratracheal N-acetylcysteine use in infants with chronic lung disease. Acta Paediatr 81(4):335–339

Bijlmer-Iest JC, Baart de la Faille H, van Asbeck BS, van Hattum J, van Weelden H, Marx JJ, Koningsberger JC (1992) Protoporphyrin photosensitivity cannot be attenuated by oral N-acetylcysteine. Photodermatol Photoimmunol Photomed 9(6):245–249

Black M (1980) Acetaminophen hepatotoxicity. Gastroenterology 78(2):382–392

Boccalandro F, Amhad M, Smalling RW, Sdringola S (2003) Oral acetylcysteine does not protect renal function from moderate to high doses of intravenous radiographic contrast. Catheter Cardiovasc Interv 58(3):336–341

Boesgaard S, Aldershvile J, Pedersen F, Pietersen A, Madsen JK, Grande P (1991) Continuous oral N-acetylcysteine treatment and development of nitrate tolerance in patients with stable angina pectoris. J Cardiovasc Pharmacol 17(6):889–893

Boesgaard S, Aldershvile J, Poulsen HE (1992) Preventive administration of intravenous N-acetylcysteine and development of tolerance to isosorbide dinitrate in patients with angina pectoris. Circulation 85(1):143–149

Boman G, Backer U, Larsson S, Melander B, Wahlander L (1983) Oral acetylcysteine reduces exacerbation rate in chronic bronchitis: report of a trial organized by the Swedish Society for Pulmonary Diseases. Eur J Respir Dis 64(6):405–415

Bondy SC (1992) Ethanol toxicity and oxidative stress. (Comment). Toxicol Lett 63:231–241

Boon AC, Vos AP, Graus YM, Rimmelzwaan GF, Osterhaus AD (2002) In vitro effect of bioactive compounds on influenza virus specific B- and T-cell responses. Scand J Immunol 55(1):24–32

Borregaard N, Jensen HS, Bjerrum OW (1987) Prevention of tissue damage: inhibition of myeloperoxidase mediated inactivation of alpha 1-proteinase inhibitor by N-acetyl cysteine, glutathione, and methionine. Agents Actions 22(3–4):255–260

Bostom AG, Shemin D, Yoburn D, Fisher DH, Nadeau MR, Selhub J (1996) Lack of effect of oral N-acetylcysteine on the acute dialysis-related lowering of total plasma homocysteine in hemodialysis patients. Atherosclerosis 120(1–2):241–244

Bounous G (2000) Whey protein concentrate (WPC) and glutathione modulation in cancer treatment. Anticancer Res 20(6C):4785–4792

Boushey CJ, Beresford SA, Omenn GS, Motulsky AG (1995) A quantitative assessment of plasma homocysteine as a risk factor for vascular disease. Probable benefits of increasing folic acid intakes. JAMA 274(13):1049–1057

Bowles WH, Goral V (1985) Clinical trial of the anti-plaque activity of a mucolytic agent, N-acetyl cysteine. Dent Hyg (Chic) 59(10):454–456

Bray GP, Mowat C, Muir DF, Tredger JM, Williams R (1991) The effect of chronic alcohol intake on prognosis and outcome in paracetamol overdose. Hum Exp Toxicol 10(6):435–438

Breitkreutz R, Holm S, Pittack N, Beichert M, Babylon A, Yodoi J, Droge W (2000a) Massive loss of sulfur in HIV infection. AIDS Res Hum Retrovir 16(3):203–209

Breitkreutz R, Pittack N, Nebe CT, Schuster D, Brust J, Beichert M, Hack V, Daniel V, Edler L, Droge W (2000b) Improvement of immune functions in HIV infection by sulfur supplementation: two randomized trials. J Mol Med 78(1):55–62

Briganti S, Wlaschek M, Hinrichs C, Bellei B, Flori E, Treiber N, Iben S, Picardo M, Scharffetter-Kochanek K (2008) Small molecular antioxidants effectively protect from PUVA-induced oxidative stress responses underlying fibroblast senescence and photoaging. Free Radic Biol Med 45(5):636–644. https://doi.org/10.1016/j.freeradbiomed.2008.05.006

Briguori C, Manganelli F, Scarpato P, Elia PP, Golia B, Riviezzo G, Lepore S, Librera M, Villari B, Colombo A, Ricciardelli B (2002) Acetylcysteine and contrast agent-associated nephrotoxicity. J Am Coll Cardiol 40(2):298–303

Brocard H, Charpin J, Germouty J (1980) Multicenter, double-blind study of oral acetylcysteine vs. placebo. Eur J Respir Dis Suppl 111:65–69

Brok J, Buckley N, Gluud C (2002) Interventions for paracetamol (acetaminophen) overdoses. Cochrane Database Syst Rev 3:CD003328

Bromley PN, Cottam SJ, Hilmi I, Tan KC, Heaton N, Ginsburg R, Potter DR (1995) Effects of intraoperative N-acetylcysteine in orthotopic liver transplantation. Br J Anaesth 75(3):352–354

Broughan TA, Soloway RD (2000) Acetaminophen hepatoxicity. Dig Dis Sci 45(8):1553–1558

Brown L, Rimm EB, Seddon JM, Giovannucci EL, Chasan-Taber L, Spiegelman D, Willett WC, Hankinson SE (1999) A prospective study of carotenoid intake and risk of cataract extraction in US men. Am J Clin Nutr 70(4):517–524

Buckley NA, Whyte IM, O'Connell DL, Dawson AH (1999) Oral or intravenous N-acetylcysteine: which is the treatment of choice for acetaminophen (paracetamol) poisoning? J Toxicol Clin Toxicol 37(6):759–767

Buhl R, Holroyd KJ, Mastrangeli A, Cantin AM, Jaffe HA, Wells FB, Saltini C, Crystal RG (1989) Systemic glutathione deficiency in symptom-free HIV-seropositive individuals. Lancet 334:1294–1298

Burgunder JM, Varriale A, Lauterburg BH (1989) Effect of N-acetylcysteine on plasma cysteine and glutathione following paracetamol administration. Eur J Clin Pharmacol 36(2):127–131

Bylin G, Hedenstierna G, Lagerstrand L, Wagner PD (1987) No influence of acetylcysteine on gas exchange and spirometry in chronic asthma. Eur J Respir Dis 71(2):102–107

Cantin AM, Hubbard RC, Crystal RG (1989) Glutathione deficiency in the epithelial lining fluid of the lower respiratory tract in idiopathic pulmonary fibrosis. Am Rev Respir Dis 139:370–372

Casagrande S, Bonetto V, Fratelli M, Gianazza E, Eberini I, Massignan T, Salmona M, Chang G, Holmgren A, Ghezzi P (2002) Glutathionylation of human thioredoxin: a possible crosstalk between the glutathione and thioredoxin systems. Proc Natl Acad Sci U S A 99(15):9745–9749. https://doi.org/10.1073/pnas.152168599

Castagna A, Legrazie C, Accordini A, Giulidori P, Cavalli G, Bottiglieri T, Lazzarin A (1995) Cerebrospinal fluid S-adenosylmethionine (SAMe) and glutathione concentrations in HIV infection: effect of parenteral treatment with SAMe. Neurology 45(9):1678–1683

Cayota A, Vuillier F, Gonzalez G, Dighiero G (1996) In vitro antioxidant treatment recovers proliferative responses of anergic CD4+ lymphocytes from human immunodeficiency virus-infected individuals. Blood 87(11):4746–4753

Chasan-Taber L, Willett WC, Seddon JM, Stampfer MJ, Rosner B, Colditz GA, Speizer FE, Hankinson SE (1999) A prospective study of carotenoid and vitamin A intakes and risk of cataract extraction in US women. Am J Clin Nutr 70(4):509–516

Chiao JW, Chung FL, Kancherla R, Ahmed T, Mittelman A, Conaway CC (2002) Sulforaphane and its metabolite mediate growth arrest and apoptosis in human prostate cancer cells. Int J Oncol 20(3):631–636

Chikina S, Iagmurov B, Kopylev ID, Soodaeva SK, Chuchalin AG (2002) N-Acetylcysteine: low and high doses in the treatment of chronic obstructive lung diseases in Chernobyl accident liquidators. Ter Arkh 74(3):62–65

Childs A, Jacobs C, Kaminski T, Halliwell B, Leeuwenburgh C (2001) Supplementation with vitamin C and N-acetyl-cysteine increases oxidative stress in humans after an acute muscle injury induced by eccentric exercise. Free Radic Biol Med 31(6):745–753

Choudhary G, Dudley SC Jr (2002) Heart failure, oxidative stress, and ion channel modulation. Congest Heart Fail 8(3):148–155

Christman BW, Bernard GR (1993) Antilipid mediator and antioxidant therapy in adult respiratory distress syndrome. New Horiz 1(4):623–630

Clotet B, Gomez M, Ruiz L, Sirera G, Romeu J (1995) Lack of short-term efficacy of N-acetyl-L-cysteine in human immunodeficiency virus-positive patients with CD4 cell counts <250/mm(3) {Letter}. J Acquir Immun Defic Syndr Hum Retrovirol 9(1):98–99

Cogo A, Chieffo A, Farinatti M, Ciaccia A (1996) Efficacy of topical tuaminoheptane combined with N-acetyl-cysteine in reducing nasal resistance. A double-blind rhinomanometric study versus xylometazoline and placebo. Arzneimittelforschung 46(4):385–388

Cotgreave IA, Goldschmidt L, Tonkonogi M, Svensson M (2002) Differentiation-specific alterations to glutathione synthesis in and hormonally stimulated release from human skeletal muscle cells. FASEB J 16(3):435–437

Coyle LC, Rodriguez A, Jeschke RE, Simon-Lee A, Abbott KC, Taylor AJ (2006) Acetylcysteine in diabetes (AID): a randomized study of acetylcysteine for the prevention of contrast nephropathy in diabetics. Am Heart J 151(5):1032.e9–1032.e12. https://doi.org/10.1016/j.ahj.2006.02.002

Daily D, Vlamis-Gardikas A, Offen D, Mittelman L, Melamed E, Holmgren A, Barzilai A (2001) Glutaredoxin protects cerebellar granule neurons from dopamine-induced apoptosis by activating NF-kappa B via Ref-1. J Biol Chem 276(2):1335–1344. https://doi.org/10.1074/jbc.M008121200

Davidson SD, Milanesa DM, Mallouh C, Choudhury MS, Tazaki H, Konno S (2002) A possible regulatory role of glyoxalase I in cell viability of human prostate cancer. Urol Res 30(2):116–121

Davies SJ, Reichardt-Pascal SY, Vaughan D, Russell GI (1995) Differential effect of ischaemia-reperfusion injury on anti-oxidant enzyme activity in the rat kidney. Exp Nephrol 3(6):348–354

Davis M (1986) Protective agents for acetaminophen overdose. Semin Liver Dis 6(2):138–147

De Backer WA, Amsel B, Jorens PG, Bossaert L, Hiemstra PS, van Noort P, van Overveld FJ (1996) N-acetylcysteine pretreatment of cardiac surgery patients influences plasma neutrophil elastase and neutrophil influx in bronchoalveolar lavage fluid. Intensive Care Med 22(9):900–908

De Flora S, Grassi C, Carati L (1997) Attenuation of influenza-like symptomatology and improvement of cell-mediated immunity with long-term N-acetylcysteine treatment. Eur Respir J 10(7):1535–1541

De Mattia G, Bravi MC, Laurenti O, Cassone-Faldetta M, Armiento A, Ferri C, Balsano F (1998a) Influence of reduced glutathione infusion on glucose metabolism in patients with non-insulin-dependent diabetes mellitus. Metabolism 47(8):993–997

De Mattia G, Bravi MC, Laurenti O, Cassone-Faldetta M, Proietti A, De Luca O, Armiento A, Ferri C (1998b) Reduction of oxidative stress by oral N-acetyl-L-cysteine treatment decreases plasma soluble vascular cell adhesion molecule-1 concentrations in non-obese, non-dyslipidaemic, normotensive, patients with non-insulin-dependent diabetes. Diabetologia 41(11):1392–1396

de Quay B, Malinverni R, Lauterburg BH (1992) Glutathione depletion in HIV-infected patients: role of cysteine deficiency and effect of oral N-acetylcysteine. AIDS 6(8):815–819

De Roos FJ, Hoffman RS (1996) Drug-induced hepatotoxicity. N Engl J Med 334(13):863. discussion 864

De Rosa SC, Zaretsky MD, Dubs JG, Roederer M, Anderson M, Green A, Mitra D, Watanabe N, Nakamura H, Tjioe I, Deresinski SC, Moore WA, Ela SW, Parks D, Herzenberg LA (2000) N-acetylcysteine replenishes glutathione in HIV infection. Eur J Clin Investig 30(10):915–929

De Stefano N, Matthews PM, Ford B, Genge A, Karpati G, Arnold DL (1995) Short-term dichloroacetate treatment improves indices of cerebral metabolism in patients with mitochondrial disorders. Neurology 45(6):1193–1198

Dean BS, Bricker JD, Krenzelok EP (1996) Outpatient N-acetylcysteine treatment for acetaminophen poisoning: an ethical dilemma or a new financial mandate? Vet Hum Toxicol 38(3):222–224

Demirturk L, Yazgan Y, Tarcin O, Ozel M, Diler M, Oncul O, Yildirim S (2003) Does N-acetyl cystein affect the sensitivity and specificity of Helicobacter pylori stool antigen test? Helicobacter 8(2):120–123

Di Bisceglie AM (1998) Hepatitis C. Lancet 351(9099):351–355

Diaz-Sandoval LJ, Kosowsky BD, Losordo DW (2002) Acetylcysteine to prevent angiography-related renal tissue injury (the APART trial). Am J Cardiol 89(3):356–358

Dick CA, Brown DM, Donaldson K, Stone V (2003) The role of free radicals in the toxic and inflammatory effects of four different ultrafine particle types. Inhal Toxicol 15(1):39–52

Dincer Y, Akcay T, Konukogku D, Hatemi H (1999) Erythrocyte susceptibility to lipid peroxidation in patients with coronary atherosclerosis. Acta Med Okayama 53(6):259–264

Domenighetti G, Suter PM, Schaller MD, Ritz R, Perret C (1997) Treatment with N-acetylcysteine during acute respiratory distress syndrome: a randomized, double-blind, placebo-controlled clinical study. J Crit Care 12(4):177–182

Drager LF, Andrade L, Barros de Toledo JF, Laurindo FR, Machado Cesar LA, Seguro AC (2004) Renal effects of N-acetylcysteine in patients at risk for contrast nephropathy: decrease in oxidant stress-mediated renal tubular injury. Nephrol Dial Transplant 19(7):1803–1807

Droge W, Breitkreutz R (1999) N-acetyl-cysteine in the therapy of HIV-positive patients. Curr Opin Clin Nutr Metab Care 2(6):493–498

Droge W, Breitkreutz R (2000) Glutathione and immune function. Proc Nutr Soc 59(4):595–600

Droge W, Eck H-P, Gmunder H, Mihm S (1991) Modulation of lymphocyte functions and immune responses by cysteine and cysteine derivatives. Am J Med 91(Suppl. 3C):140S–144S

Droge W, Eck H-P, Naher H, Pekar U, Daniel V (1988) Abnormal amino-acid concentrations in the blood of patients with acquired immunodeficiency syndrome (AIDS) may contribute to the immunological deficit. Biol Chem Hoppe Seyler 369:143–148

Droge W, Eck HP, Mihm S (1992) HIV-induced cysteine deficiency and T-cell dysfunction – a rationale for treatment with N-acetylcysteine. Immunol Today 13(6):211–214

Dueholm M, Nielsen C, Thorshauge H, Evald T, Hansen NC, Madsen HD, Maltbaek N (1992) N-acetylcysteine by metered dose inhaler in the treatment of chronic bronchitis: a multi-centre study. Respir Med 86(2):89–92

Durham JD, Caputo C, Dokko J, Zaharakis T, Pahlavan M, Keltz J, Dutka P, Marzo K, Maesaka JK, Fishbane S (2002) A randomized controlled trial of N-acetylcysteine to prevent contrast nephropathy in cardiac angiography. Kidney Int 62(6):2202–2207

Efrati S, Dishy V, Averbukh M, Blatt A, Krakover R, Weisgarten J, Morrow JD, Stein MC, Golik A (2003) The effect of N-acetylcysteine on renal function, nitric oxide, and oxidative stress after angiography. Kidney Int 64(6):2182–2187

Ekberg-Jansson A, Larson M, MacNee W, Tunek A, Wahlgren L, Wouters EF, Larsson S (1999) N-isobutyrylcysteine, a donor of systemic thiols, does not reduce the exacerbation rate in chronic bronchitis. Eur Respir J 13(4):829–834

Eklund A, Eriksson O, Hakansson L, Larsson K, Ohlsson K, Venge P, Bergstrand H, Bjornson A, Brattsand R, Glennow C et al (1988) Oral N-acetylcysteine reduces selected humoral markers of inflammatory cell activity in BAL fluid from healthy smokers: correlation to effects on cellular variables. Eur Respir J 1(9):832–838

Eren N, Cakir O, Oruc A, Kaya Z, Erdinc L (2003) Effects of N-acetylcysteine on pulmonary function in patients undergoing coronary artery bypass surgery with cardiopulmonary bypass. Perfusion 18(6):345–350

Estensen RD, Levy M, Klopp SJ, Galbraith AR, Mandel JS, Blomquist JA, Wattenberg LW (1999) N-acetylcysteine suppression of the proliferative index in the colon of patients with previous adenomatous colonic polyps. Cancer Lett 147(1–2):109–114

Estevez AG, Jordan J (2002) Nitric oxide and superoxide, a deadly cocktail. Ann N Y Acad Sci 962:207–211

Evald T, Hansen M, Balslov S, Brorson-Riis L, Hansen NC, Maltbaek N, Thorshauge H (1989) Steroid response after long-term treatment with oral N-acetylcysteine in patients with chronic obstructive bronchitis. Ugeskr Laeger 151(46):2076–2078

Eylar E, Rivera-Quinones C, Molina C, Baez I, Molina F, Mercado CM (1993) N-acetylcysteine enhances T cell functions and T cell growth in culture. Int Immunol 5(1):97–101

Fechner A, Bohme C, Gromer S, Funk M, Schirmer R, Becker K (2001) Antioxidant status and nitric oxide in the malnutrition syndrome kwashiorkor. Pediatr Res 49(2):237–243

Ferrari V (1980) Safety and drug interactions of oral acetylcysteine related to utilization data. Eur J Respir Dis Suppl 111:151–157

Ferrari V, Spinelli W (1980) Life table analysis of long-term randomised trials in pneumology – a worked example and a plea. Eur J Respir Dis Suppl 110:227–236

Fischer UM, Tossios P, Huebner A, Geissler HJ, Bloch W, Mehlhorn U (2004) Myocardial apoptosis prevention by radical scavenging in patients undergoing cardiac surgery. J Thorac Cardiovasc Surg 128(1):103–108

Flescher E, Ledbetter JA, Schieven GL, Velaroch N, Fossum D, Dang H, Ogawa N, Talal N (1994) Longitudinal exposure of human T lymphocytes to weak oxidative stress suppresses transmembrane and nuclear signal transduction. J Immunol 153(11):4880–4889

Fontana RJ, McCashland TM, Benner KG, Appelman HD, Gunartanam NT, Wisecarver JL, Rabkin JM, Lee WM (1999) Acute liver failure associated with prolonged use of bromfenac leading to liver transplantation. The Acute Liver Failure Study Group. Liver Transpl Surg 5(6):480–484

Freudenthaler SM, Schreeb KH, Wiese A, Pilz J, Gleiter CH (2002) Influence of controlled hypoxia and radical scavenging agents on erythropoietin and malondialdehyde concentrations in humans. Acta Physiol Scand 174(3):231–235

Friedman AN, Bostom AG, Laliberty P, Selhub J, Shemin D (2003) The effect of N-acetylcysteine on plasma total homocysteine levels in hemodialysis: a randomized, controlled study. Am J Kidney Dis 41(2):442–446

Fulghesu AM, Ciampelli M, Muzj G, Belosi C, Selvaggi L, Ayala GF, Lanzone A (2002) N-acetylcysteine treatment improves insulin sensitivity in women with polycystic ovary syndrome. Fertil Steril 77(6):1128–1135

Furst DE, Clements PJ, Harris R, Ross M, Levy J, Paulus HE (1979) Measurement of clinical change in progressive systemic sclerosis: a 1 year double-blind placebo-controlled trial of N-acetylcysteine. Ann Rheum Dis 38(4):356–361

Galli F, Floridi A, Buoncristiani U (2002) Oxidant stress in hemodialysis patients. Contrib Nephrol 137:371–378

Ghezzi P, Romines B, Fratelli M, Eberini I, Gianazza E, Casagrande S, Laragione T, Mengozzi M, Herzenberg LA (2002) Protein glutathionylation: coupling and uncoupling of glutathione to protein thiol groups in lymphocytes under oxidative stress and HIV infection. Mol Immunol 38(10):773–780

Gillissen A, Nowak D (1998) Characterization of N-acetylcysteine and ambroxol in anti-oxidant therapy. Respir Med 92(4):609–623

Giovannucci E, Rimm EB, Stampfer MJ, Colditz GA, Willett WC (1998) Diabetes mellitus and risk of prostate cancer (United States). Cancer Causes Control 9(1):3–9

Gisolf EH, Dreezen C, Danner SA, Weel JL, Weverling GJ (2000) Risk factors for hepatotoxicity in HIV-1-infected patients receiving ritonavir and saquinavir with or without stavudine. Prometheus Study Group. Clin Infect Dis 31(5):1234–1239

Gladyshev VN, Jeang KT, Stadtman TC (1996a) Selenocysteine, identified as the penultimate C-terminal residue in human T-cell thioredoxin reductase, corresponds to TGA in the human placental gene. Proc Natl Acad Sci U S A 93(12):6146–6151

Gladyshev VN, Khangulov SV, Stadtman TC (1996b) Properties of the selenium- and molybdenum-containing nicotinic acid hydroxylase from Clostridium barkeri. Biochemistry 35(1):212–223. https://doi.org/10.1021/bi951793i

Golden MH, Ramdath D (1987) Free radicals in the pathogenesis of kwashiorkor. Proc Nutr Soc 46(1):53–68

Goldenberg I, Shechter M, Matetzky S, Jonas M, Adam M, Pres H, Elian D, Agranat O, Schwammenthal E, Guetta V (2004) Oral acetylcysteine as an adjunct to saline hydration for the prevention of contrast-induced nephropathy following coronary angiography. A randomized controlled trial and review of the current literature. Eur Heart J 25(3):212–218

Gotoh Y, Noda T, Iwakiri R, Fujimoto K, Rhoads CA, Aw TY (2002) Lipid peroxide-induced redox imbalance differentially mediates CaCo-2 cell proliferation and growth arrest. Cell Prolif 35(4):221–235

Gotz M, Kraemer R, Kerrebijn KF, Popow C (1980) Oral acetylcysteine in cystic fibrosis. A co-operative study. Eur J Respir Dis Suppl 111:122–126

Gow AJ, Chen Q, Hess DT, Day BJ, Ischiropoulos H, Stamler JS (2002) Basal and stimulated protein S-nitrosylation in multiple cell types and tissues. J Biol Chem 277(12):9637–9640. https://doi.org/10.1074/jbc.C100746200

Graber R, Farine JC, Fumagalli I, Tatti V, Losa GA (1999) Apoptosis and oxidative status in peripheral blood mononuclear cells of diabetic patients. Apoptosis 4(4):263–270

Grandjean EM, Berthet P, Ruffmann R, Leuenberger P (2000) Cost-effectiveness analysis of oral N-acetylcysteine as a preventive treatment in chronic bronchitis. Pharmacol Res 42(1):39–50

Grant PR, Black A, Garcia N, Prieto J, Garson JA (2000) Combination therapy with interferon-alpha plus N-acetyl cysteine for chronic hepatitis C: a placebo controlled double-blind multi-centre study. J Med Virol 61(4):439–442

Grassi C (1980) Long-term oral acetylcysteine in chronic bronchitis. A double-blind controlled study. Eur J Respir Dis Suppl 111:93–108

Grassi C, Morandini GC (1976) A controlled trial of intermittent oral acetylcysteine in the long-term treatment of chronic bronchitis. Eur J Clin Pharmacol 09(5–6):393–396

Grattagliano I, Vendemiale G, Sabba C, Buonamico P, Altomare E (1996) Oxidation of circulating proteins in alcoholics: role of acetaldehyde and xanthine oxidase. J Hepatol 25(1):28–36

Gringhuis SI, Leow A, Papendrecht-van der Voort EAM, Remans PHJ, Breedveld FC, Verweij CL (2000) Displacement of linker for activation of T cells from the plasma membrane due to redox balance alterations results in hyporesponsiveness of synovial fluid T lymphocytes in rheumatoid arthritis. J Immunol 164(4):2170–2179

Grundman M (2000) Vitamin E and Alzheimer disease: the basis for additional clinical trials. Am J Clin Nutr 71(2):630S–636S

Guan X, Hoffman BN, McFarland DC, Gilkerson KK, Dwivedi C, Erickson AK, Bebensee S, Pellegrini J (2002) Glutathione and mercapturic acid conjugates of sulofenur and their activity against a human colon cancer cell line. Drug Metab Dispos 30(3):331–335

Hammarqvist F, Luo JL, Cotgreave IA, Andersson K, Wernerman J (1997) Skeletal muscle glutathione is depleted in critically ill patients. Crit Care Med 25(1):78–84

Hansen NC, Skriver A, Brorsen-Riis L, Balslov S, Evald T, Maltbaek N, Gunnersen G, Garsdal P, Sander P, Pedersen JZ et al (1994) Orally administered N-acetylcysteine may improve general well-being in patients with mild chronic bronchitis. Respir Med 88(7):531–535

Hansen RM, Csuka ME, McCarty DJ, Saryan LA (1985) Gold induced aplastic anemia. Complete response to corticosteroids, plasmapheresis, and N-acetylcysteine infusion. J Rheumatol 12(4):794–797

Hansen RM, Varma RR, Hanson GA (1991) Gold induced hepatitis and pure red cell aplasia. Complete recovery after corticosteroid and N-acetylcysteine therapy. J Rheumatol 18(8):1251–1253

Harrison PM, Keays R, Bray GP, Alexander GJ, Williams R (1990) Improved outcome of paracetamol-induced fulminant hepatic failure by late administration of acetylcysteine. Lancet 335(8705):1572–1573

Harrison PM, Wendon JA, Gimson AE, Alexander GJ, Williams R (1991) Improvement by acetylcysteine of hemodynamics and oxygen transport in fulminant hepatic failure. N Engl J Med 324(26):1852–1857

Hauer K, Hildebrandt W, Sehl Y, Edler L, Oster P, Droge W (2003) Improvement in muscular performance and decrease in tumor necrosis factor level in old age after antioxidant treatment. J Mol Med 81(2):118–125

Heinig JH, Pedersen B, Andersen I, Dalgaard CE, Rasmussen O, Weeke ER, Enk B (1985) The mucolytic effects of acetylcysteine compared with bromhexine and a placebo in patients with chronic bronchitis. Ugeskr Laeger 147(46):3694–3697

Helbling B, von Overbeck J, Lauterburg BH (1996) Decreased release of glutathione into the systemic circulation of patients with HIV infection. Eur J Clin Investig 26(1):38–44

Henderson A, Hayes P (1994) Acetylcysteine as a cytoprotective antioxidant in patients with severe sepsis: potential new use for an old drug. Ann Pharmacother 28(9):1086–1088

Herzenberg LA, De Rosa SC, Dubs JG, Roederer M, Anderson MT, Ela SW, Deresinski SC (1997) Glutathione deficiency is associated with impaired survival in HIV disease. Proc Natl Acad Sci U S A 94(5):1967–1972

Hitchins AD, McDonough FE, Wells PA (1989) The use of Escherichia coli mutants to measure the bioavailability of essential amino acids in foods. Plant Foods Hum Nutr 39(1):109–120

Hoffer ME, Kopke RD, Weisskopf P, Gottshall K, Allen K, Wester D (2001) Microdose gentamicin administration via the round window microcatheter: results in patients with Meniere's disease. Ann N Y Acad Sci 942:46–51

Hogan JC, Lewis MJ, Henderson AH (1989a) Glyceryl trinitrate and platelet aggregation: effects of N-acetyl-cysteine. Br J Clin Pharmacol 27(5):617–619

Hogan JC, Lewis MJ, Henderson AH (1989b) N-acetylcysteine fails to attenuate haemodynamic tolerance to glyceryl trinitrate in healthy volunteers. Br J Clin Pharmacol 28(4):421–426

Hogan JC, Lewis MJ, Henderson AH (1990) Chronic administration of N-acetylcysteine fails to prevent nitrate tolerance in patients with stable angina pectoris. Br J Clin Pharmacol 30(4):573–577

Holmgren A (1985) Thioredoxin. Annu Rev Biochem 54:237–271

Holmgren A (1989) Thioredoxin and glutaredoxin systems. J Biol Chem 264(24):13963–13966

Holroyd KJ, Buhl R, Borok Z, Roum JH, Bokser AD, Grimes GJ, Czerski D, Cantin AM, Crystal RG (1993) Correction of glutathione deficiency in the lower respiratory tract of HIV seropositive individuals by glutathione aerosol treatment. Thorax 48(10):985–989

Holt S, Goodler D, Marley R, Patch D, Burroughs A, Fernando B, Harry D, Moore K (1999a) Improvement in renal function in hepatorenal syndrome with N-acetylcysteine [letter]. Lancet 353(9149):294–295

Holt S, Marley R, Fernando B, Harry D, Anand R, Goodier D, Moore K (1999b) Acute cholestasis-induced renal failure: effects of antioxidants and ligands for the thromboxane A2 receptor. Kidney Int 55(1):271–277

Horowitz JD, Henry CA, Syrjanen ML, Louis WJ, Fish RD, Antman EM, Smith TW (1988a) Nitroglycerine/N-acetylcysteine in the management of unstable angina pectoris. Eur Heart J 9(Suppl A):95–100

Horowitz JD, Henry CA, Syrjanen ML, Louis WJ, Fish RD, Smith TW, Antman EM (1988b) Combined use of nitroglycerin and N-acetylcysteine in the management of unstable angina pectoris. Circulation 77(4):787–794

Hortin GL, Landt M, Powderly WG (1994) Changes in plasma amino acid concentrations in response to HIV-1 infection. Clin Chem 40:785–789

Huengsberg M, Waring R, Moffitt D, Round R, Winer J, Gompels M, Shahmanesh M (1998) Serum cysteine levels in HIV infection. {LETTER, COMMENT}. AIDS 12(10):1245

Hultberg B, Andersson A, Isaksson A (2001) Interaction of metals and thiols in cell damage and glutathione distribution: potentiation of mercury toxicity by dithiothreitol. Toxicology 156(2–3):93–100

Hurd RW, Wilder BJ, Helveston WR, Uthman BM (1996) Treatment of four siblings with progressive myoclonus epilepsy of the Unverricht-Lundborg type with N-acetylcysteine. Neurology 47(5):1264–1268

Hursting SD, Shen JC, Sun XY, Wang TT, Phang JM, Perkins SN (2002) Modulation of cyclophilin gene expression by N-4-(hydroxyphenyl)retinamide: association with reactive oxygen species generation and apoptosis. Mol Carcinog 33(1):16–24

Iantomasi T, Marraccini P, Favilli F, Vincenzini MT, Ferretti P, Tonelli F (1994) Glutathione metabolism in Crohn's disease. Biochem Med Metab Biol 53(2):87–91

Iversen HK (1992) N-acetylcysteine enhances nitroglycerin-induced headache and cranial arterial responses. Clin Pharmacol Ther 52(2):125–133

Jackson AA (1986) Blood glutathione in severe malnutrition in childhood. Trans R Soc Trop Med Hyg 80(6):911–913

Jackson IM, Barnes J, Cooksey P (1984) Efficacy and tolerability of oral acetylcysteine (Fabrol) in chronic bronchitis: a double-blind placebo controlled study. J Int Med Res 12(3):198–206

Jahoor F, Jackson A, Gazzard B, Philips G, Sharpstone D, Frazer ME, Heird W (1999) Erythrocyte glutathione deficiency in symptom-free HIV infection is associated with decreased synthesis rate. Am J Phys 276(1 Pt 1):E205–E211

Jain SK, Krueger KS, McVie R, Jaramillo JJ, Palmer M, Smith T (1998) Relationship of blood thromboxane-B2 (TxB2) with lipid peroxides and effect of vitamin E and placebo supplementation on TxB2 and lipid peroxide levels in type 1 diabetic patients. Diabetes Care 21(9):1511–1516

Jain SK, Lim G (2000) Lipoic acid decreases lipid peroxidation and protein glycosylation and increases (Na(+) + K(+))- and Ca(++)-ATPase activities in high glucose-treated human erythrocytes. Free Radic Biol Med 29(11):1122–1128

Jain SK, McVie R (1999) Hyperketonemia can increase lipid peroxidation and lower glutathione levels in human erythrocytes in vitro and in type 1 diabetic patients. Diabetes 48(9):1850–1855

Jain SK, McVie R, Jaramillo JJ, Palmer M, Smith T (1996a) Effect of modest vitamin E supplementation on blood glycated hemoglobin and triglyceride levels and red cell indices in type I diabetic patients. J Am Coll Nutr 15(5):458–461

Jain SK, McVie R, Jaramillo JJ, Palmer M, Smith T, Meachum ZD, Little RL (1996b) The effect of modest vitamin E supplementation on lipid peroxidation products and other cardiovascular risk factors in diabetic patients. Lipids 31(Suppl):87–90

Jain SK, McVie R, Smith T (2000) Vitamin E supplementation restores glutathione and malondialdehyde to normal concentrations in erythrocytes of type 1 diabetic children. Diabetes Care 23(9):1389–1394

James JS (1997) Stanford NAC study: glutathione level predicts survival. AIDS Treat News 266:1–5

James LP, Wells E, Beard RH, Farrar HC (2002) Predictors of outcome after acetaminophen poisoning in children and adolescents. J Pediatr 140(5):522–526

Jeannin P, Delneste Y, Lecoanet-Henchoz S, Gauchat J-F, Life P, Holmes D, Bonnefoy J-Y (1995) Thiols decrease human interleukin (IL) 4 production and IL-4-induced immunoglobulin synthesis. J Exp Med 182(6):1785–1792

Jepsen S, Herlevsen P, Knudsen P, Bud MI, Klausen NO (1992) Antioxidant treatment with N-acetylcysteine during adult respiratory distress syndrome: a prospective, randomized, placebo-controlled study. Crit Care Med 20(7):918–923

Jepsen S, Klaerke A, Nielsen PH, Nielsen ST, Simonsen O (1989) Systemic administration of N-acetylcysteine has no effect on postoperative lung function following elective upper laparotomy in lung healthy patients. Acta Anaesthesiol Scand 33(3):219–222

Johnston SC, Pelletier LL Jr (1997) Enhanced hepatotoxicity of acetaminophen in the alcoholic patient. Two case reports and a review of the literature. Medicine (Baltimore) 76(3):185–191

Jones A (2002) Over-the-counter analgesics: a toxicology perspective. Am J Ther 9(3):245–257

Julius M, Lang CA, Gleiberman L, Harburg E, DiFranceisco W, Schork A (1994) Glutathione and morbidity in a community-based sample of elderly. J Clin Epidemiol 47(9):1021–1026

Kanner SB, Damle NK, Blake J, Aruffo A, Ledbetter JA (1992a) CD2/LFA-3 ligation induces phospholipase-C gamma 1 tyrosine phosphorylation and regulates CD3 signaling. J Immunol 148(7):2023–2029

Kanner SB, Deans JP, Ledbetter JA (1992b) Regulation of CD3-induced phospholipase C-gamma 1 (PLC gamma 1) tyrosine phosphorylation by CD4 and CD45 receptors. Immunology 75(3):441–447

Kanner SB, Kavanagh TJ, Grossmann A, Hu SL, Bolen JB, Rabinovitch PS, Ledbetter JA (1992c) Sulfhydryl oxidation down-regulates T-cell signaling and inhibits tyrosine phosphorylation of phospholipase C gamma 1. Proc Natl Acad Sci U S A 89(1):300–304

Kanner SB, Ledbetter JA (1992) CD45 regulates TCR-induced signalling through tyrosine phosphorylation of phospholipase C gamma 1. Biochem Soc Trans 20(1):178–184

Kasielski M, Nowak D (2001) Long-term administration of N-acetylcysteine decreases hydrogen peroxide exhalation in subjects with chronic obstructive pulmonary disease. Respir Med 95(6):448–456

Katsinelos P, Kountouras J, Paroutoglou G, Beltsis A, Mimidis K, Zavos C (2005) Intravenous N-acetylcysteine does not prevent post-ERCP pancreatitis. Gastrointest Endosc 62(1):105–111

Kay J, Chow WH, Chan TM, Lo SK, Kwok OH, Yip A, Fan K, Lee CH, Lam WF (2003) Acetylcysteine for prevention of acute deterioration of renal function following elective coronary angiography and intervention: a randomized controlled trial. JAMA 289(5):553–558

Kearns GL (2002) Acetaminophen poisoning in children: treat early and long enough. J Pediatr 140(5):495–498

Kearns GL, Leeder JS, Wasserman GS (2000) Acetaminophen intoxication during treatment: what you don't know can hurt you. Clin Pediatr (Phila) 39(3):133–144

Keays R, Harrison PM, Wendon JA, Forbes A, Gove C, Alexander GJ, Williams R (1991) Intravenous acetylcysteine in paracetamol induced fulminant hepatic failure: a prospective controlled trial. BMJ 303(6809):1026–1029

Kefer JM, Hanet CE, Boitte S, Wilmotte L, De Kock M (2003) Acetylcysteine, coronary procedure and prevention of contrast-induced worsening of renal function: which benefit for which patient? Acta Cardiol 58(6):555–560

Kelly FJ (1999) Gluthathione: in defence of the lung. Food Chem Toxicol 37(9–10):963–966

Kerr F, Dawson A, Whyte IM, Buckley N, Murray L, Graudins A, Chan B, Trudinger B (2005) The Australasian Clinical Toxicology Investigators Collaboration randomized trial of different loading infusion rates of N-acetylcysteine. Ann Emerg Med 45(4):402–408

Kes P (2000) Hyperhomocysteinemia in end-stage renal failure. Acta Med Croatica 54(4–5):175–181

Kiefer P, Vogt J, Radermacher P (2000) From mucolytic to antioxidant and liver protection: new aspects in the intensive care unit career of N-acetylcysteine. Crit Care Med 28(12):3935–3936

Kim HJ, Liu X, Wang H, Kohyama T, Kobayashi T, Wen FQ, Romberger DJ, Abe S, MacNee W, Rahman I, Rennard SI (2002) Glutathione prevents inhibition of fibroblast-mediated collagen gel contraction by cigarette smoke. Am J Physiol Lung Cell Mol Physiol 283(2):L409–L417

Kinnunen J, Pietila J, Ahovuo J, Mankinen P, Tervahartiala P (1989) Double contrast barium meal and acetylcysteine. Eur J Radiol 9(4):258–259

Knapen MFCM, Mulder TPJ, Van Rooij IALM, Peters WHM, Steegers EAP (1998) Low whole blood glutathione levels in pregnancies complicated by preeclampsia or the hemolysis, elevated liver enzymes, low platelets syndrome. Obstet Gynecol 92(6):1012–1015

Koechlin C, Couillard A, Simar D, Cristol JP, Bellet H, Hayot M, Prefaut C (2004) Does oxidative stress alter quadriceps endurance in chronic obstructive pulmonary disease? Am J Respir Crit Care Med 169(9):1022–1027

Kokcam I, Naziroglu M (1999) Antioxidants and lipid peroxidation status in the blood of patients with psoriasis. Clin Chim Acta 289(1–2):23–31

Konrad F, Schoenberg MH, Wiedmann H, Kilian J, Georgieff M (1995) The application of n-acetylcysteine as an antioxidant and mucolytic in mechanical ventilation in intensive care patients. A prospective, randomized, placebo-controlled, double-blind study. Anaesthesist 44(9):651–658

Konukoglu D, Akcay T, Dincer Y, Hatemi H (1999) The susceptibility of red blood cells to autoxidation in type 2 diabetic patients with angiopathy. Metabolism 48(12):1481–1484

Konukoglu D, Hatemi H, Ozer EM, Gonen S, Akcay T (1997) The erythrocyte glutathione levels during oral glucose tolerance test. J Endocrinol Investig 20(8):471–475

Kopke R, Allen KA, Henderson D, Hoffer M, Frenz D, Van de Water T (1999) A radical demise. Toxins and trauma share common pathways in hair cell death. Ann N Y Acad Sci 884:171–191

Kopke RD, Coleman JK, Liu J, Campbell KC, Riffenburgh RH (2002) Candidate's thesis: enhancing intrinsic cochlear stress defenses to reduce noise-induced hearing loss. Laryngoscope 112(9):1515–1532. https://doi.org/10.1097/00005537-200209000-00001

Kopke RD, Hoffer ME, Wester D, O'Leary MJ, Jackson RL (2001) Targeted topical steroid therapy in sudden sensorineural hearing loss. Otol Neurotol 22(4):475–479

Kopke RD, Weisskopf PA, Boone JL, Jackson RL, Wester DC, Hoffer ME, Lambert DC, Charon CC, Ding DL, McBride D (2000) Reduction of noise-induced hearing loss using L-NAC and salicylate in the chinchilla. Hear Res 149(1–2):138–146

Krenzelok EP (2002) New developments in the therapy of intoxications. Toxicol Lett 127(1–3):299–305

Kretzschmar M, Pfeiffer L, Schmidt C, Schirrmeister W (1998) Plasma levels of glutathione, alpha-tocopherol and lipid peroxides in polytraumatized patients; evidence for a stimulating effect of TNF alpha on glutathione synthesis. Exp Toxicol Pathol 50(4–6):477–483

Kupczyk M, Kuna P (2002) Mucolytics in acute and chronic respiratory tract disorders. II. Uses for treatment and antioxidant properties. Pol Merkuriusz Lek 12(69):248–252

Lamson DW, Brignall MS (2000) The use of nebulized glutathione in the treatment of emphysema: a case report [In Process Citation]. Altern Med Rev 5(5):429–431

Lands LC, Grey VL, Grenier C (2000) Total plasma antioxidant capacity in cystic fibrosis. Pediatr Pulmonol 29(2):81–87

Lang CA, Naryshkin S, Schnieder DL, Mills BJ, Lindeman RD (1992) Low blood glutathione in healthy aging adults. J Lab Clin Med 120(5):720–725

LaRowe SD, Mardikian P, Malcolm R, Myrick H, Kalivas P, McFarland K, Saladin M, McRae A, Brady K (2006) Safety and tolerability of N-acetylcysteine in cocaine-dependent individuals. Am J Addict 15(1):105–110

Larrauri A, Fabra R, Gomez-Lechon MJ, Trullenque R, Castell JV (1987) Toxicity of paracetamol in human hepatocytes. Comparison of the protective effects of sulfhydryl compounds acting as glutathione precursors. Mol Toxicol 1(4):301–311

Larsen LC, Fuller SH (1996) Management of acetaminophen toxicity. Am Fam Physician 53(1):185–190

Laurent T, Markert M, Feihl F, Schaller MD, Perret C (1996) Oxidant-antioxidant balance in granulocytes during ARDS. Effect of N-acetylcysteine. Chest 109(1):163–166

Lauterburg BH, Corcoran GB, Mitchell JR (1983) Mechanism of action of N-acetylcysteine in the protection against the hepatotoxicity of acetaminophen in rats in vivo. J Clin Invest 71(4):980–991

Lauterburg BH, Velez ME (1988) Glutathione deficiency in alcoholics: risk factor for paracetamol hepatotoxicity. Gut 29:1153–1157

Lee WM (1993) Drug-induced hepatotoxicity. Aliment Pharmacol Ther 7(5):477–485

Lee WM (1995) Drug-induced hepatotoxicity. N Engl J Med 333(17):1118–1127

Lee WM (1996) Management of acute liver failure. Semin Liver Dis 16(4):369–378

Lenhartz H, Ndasi R, Anninos A, Botticher D, Mayatepek E, Tetanye E, Leichsenring M (1998) The clinical manifestation of the kwashiorkor syndrome is related to increased lipid peroxidation. J Pediatr 132(5):879–881

Listed NA (1980) Acetylcysteine (Parvolex) for paracetamol poisoning. Drug Ther Bull 18(21):81–82

Listed NA (2000) N-acetylcysteine. Altern Med Rev 5(5):467–471

Loguercio C, Nardi G, Argenzio F, Aurilio C, Petrone E, Grella A, Del Vecchio Blanco C, Coltorti M (1994) Effect of S-adenosyl-L-methionine administration on red blood cell cysteine and glutathione levels in alcoholic patients with and without liver disease. Alcohol Alcohol 29(5):597–604

Lou MF, Dickerson JE Jr, Tung WH, Wolfe JK, Chylack LT Jr (1999) Correlation of nuclear color and opalescence with protein S-thiolation in human lenses. Exp Eye Res 68(5):547–552

Louwerse ES, Weverling GJ, Bossuyt PM, Meyjes FE, de Jong JM (1995) Randomized, double-blind, controlled trial of acetylcysteine in amyotrophic lateral sclerosis. Arch Neurol 52(6):559–564

Lyons L, Studdiford JS, Sommaripa AM (1977) Treatment of acetaminophen overdosage with N-acetylcysteine. N Engl J Med 296(3):174–175

MacNeill BDHS, Bazari H, Patton KK, Colon-Hernadez P, DeJoseph D, Jang IK (2003) Prophylaxis of contrast-induced nephropathy in patients undergoing coronary angiography. Catheter Cardiovas Interv 60(4):458–461

Macy AM (1979) Preventing hepatotoxicity in acetaminophen overdose. Am J Nurs 79(2):301–303

Mangione S, Patel DD, Levin BR, Fiel SB (1994) Erythrocytic glutathione in cystic fibrosis. A possible marker of pulmonary dysfunction. Chest 105(5):1470–1473

Marenzi G, Assanelli E, Marana I, Lauri G, Campodonico J, Grazi M, De Metrio M, Galli S, Fabbiocchi F, Montorsi P, Veglia F, Bartorelli AL (2006) N-acetylcysteine and contrast-induced nephropathy in primary angioplasty. N Engl J Med 354(26):2773–2782

Marini U, Visconti G, Spotti D, Geniram A (1980) Controlled endoscopic study on gastroduodenal safety of acetylcysteine after oral administration. Eur J Respir Dis Suppl 111:147–150

Marquardt ED (1977) Treatment of acetaminophen toxicity. Am J Hosp Pharm 34(8):805–806

Marshall RJ, Scott KC, Hill RC, Lewis DD, Sundstrom D, Jones GL, Harper J (2002) Supplemental vitamin C appears to slow racing greyhounds. J Nutr 132(6 Suppl 2):1616S–1621S

Martin DS, Willis SE, Cline DM (1990) N-acetylcysteine in the treatment of human arsenic poisoning. J Am Board Fam Pract 3(4):293–296

Marui N, Offermann MK, Swerlick R, Kunsch C, Rosen CA, Ahmad M, Alexander RW, Medford RM (1993) Vascular cell adhesion molecule-1 (VCAM-1) gene transcription and expression are regulated through an antioxidant-sensitive mechanism in human vascular endothelial cells. J Clin Invest 92(4):1866–1874. https://doi.org/10.1172/JCI116778

Maurer WG, Zeisler J (1978) Intravenous acetylcysteine as treatment for acetaminophen overdose. Am J Hosp Pharm 35(9):1025, 1030

Maurice MM, Nakamura H, van der Voort EAM, van Vliet AI, Staal FJT, Tak P-P, Breedveld FC, Verweij CL (1997) Evidence for the role of an altered redox state in hyporesponsiveness of synovial T cells in rheumatoid arthritis. J Immunol 158(3):1458–1465

Mayaud C, Lentschner C, Bouchoucha S, Marsac J (1980) Thiamphenicol glycinate acetylcysteinate in the treatment of acute respiratory infections with mucostasis. Eur J Respir Dis Suppl 111:70–73

McGavin C (1985) Oral N-acetylcysteine and exacerbation rates in patients with chronic bronchitis and severe airways obstruction. British Thoracic Society Research Committee. Thorax 40(11):832–835

McKay DL, Perrone G, Rasmussen H, Dallal G, Hartman W, Cao G, Prior RL, Roubenoff R, Blumberg JB (2000) The effects of a multivitamin/mineral supplement on micronutrient status, antioxidant capacity and cytokine production in healthy older adults consuming a fortified diet. J Am Coll Nutr 19(5):613–621

Medved I, Brown MJ, Bjorksten AR, Leppik JA, Sostaric S, McKenna MJ (2003) N-acetylcysteine infusion alters blood redox status but not time to fatigue during intense exercise in humans. J Appl Physiol 94(4):1572–1582

Medved I, Brown MJ, Bjorksten AR, McKenna MJ (2004a) Effects of intravenous N-acetylcysteine infusion on time to fatigue and potassium regulation during prolonged cycling exercise. J Appl Physiol 96(1):211–217

Medved I, Brown MJ, Bjorksten AR, Murphy KT, Petersen AC, Sostaric S, Gong X, McKenna MJ (2004b) N-acetylcysteine enhances muscle cysteine and glutathione availability and attenuates fatigue during prolonged exercise in endurance-trained individuals. J Appl Physiol 97:1477

Meister A, Anderson ME, Hwang O (1986) Intracellular cysteine and glutathione delivery systems. J Am Coll Nutr 5(2):137–151

Melillo G, Chiummariello A, Scala G (1966) On the use of a new molecular combination of acetylcysteine with thiamphenicol glycinate in bronchopulmonary suppurations. G Ital Chemioter 13(1):156–160

Meyer A, Buhl R, Kampf S, Magnussen H (1995) Intravenous N-acetylcysteine and lung glutathione of patients with pulmonary fibrosis and normals. Am J Respir Crit Care Med 152(3):1055–1060

Meyer A, Buhl R, Magnussen H (1994) The effect of oral N-Acetylcysteine on lung glutathione levels in idiopathic pulmonary fibrosis. Eur Respir J 7(3):431–436

Michelet F, Gueguen R, Leroy P, Wellman M, Nicolas A, Siest G (1995) Blood and plasma glutathione measured in healthy subjects by HPLC: relation to sex, aging, biological variables, and life habits. Clin Chem 41(10):1509–1517

Milewski J, Rydzewska G, Degowska M, Kierzkiewicz M, Rydzewski A (2006) N-acetylcysteine does not prevent post-endoscopic retrograde cholangiopancreatography hyperamylasemia and acute pancreatitis. World J Gastroenterol 12(23):3751–3755

Millar AB, Pavia D, Agnew JE, Lopez-Vidriero MT, Lauque D, Clarke SW (1985) Effect of oral N-acetylcysteine on mucus clearance. Br J Dis Chest 79(3):262–266

Miller LF, Rumack BH (1983) Clinical safety of high oral doses of acetylcysteine. Semin Oncol 10(1 Suppl 1):76–85

Miller M (1975) Clinical experimentation using a combination with antibiotic and mucolytic activity in the treatment of respiratory and oto-rhino-laryngologic infections with allergic components. Brux Med 55(6):349–351

Miralles-Barrachina O, Savoye G, Belmonte-Zalar L, Hochain P, Ducrotte P, Hecketsweiler B, Lerebours E, Dechelotte P (1999) Low levels of glutathione in endoscopic biopsies of patients with Crohn's colitis: the role of malnutrition. Clin Nutr 18(5):313–317

Mitchell JR, Corcoran GB, Smith CV, Hughes H, Lauterburg BH (1981) Alkylation and peroxidation injury from chemically reactive metabolites. Adv Exp Med Biol 136(Pt A):199–223

Mitchell JR, Thorgeirsson SS, Potter WZ, Jollow DJ, Keiser H (1974) Acetaminophen-induced hepatic injury: protective role of glutathione in man and rationale for therapy. Clin Pharmacol Ther 16(4):676–684

Moberly JB, Logan J, Borum PR, Story KO, Webb LE, Jassal SV, Mupas L, Rodela H, Alghamdi GA, Moran JE, Wolfson M, Martis L, Oreopoulos DG (1998) Elevation of whole-blood glutathione in peritoneal dialysis patients by L-2-oxothiazolidine-4-carboxylate, a cysteine prodrug (Procysteine(R)). J Am Soc Nephrol 9(6):1093–1099

Molnar Z, MacKinnon KL, Shearer E, Lowe D, Watson ID (1998) The effect of N-acetylcysteine on total serum anti-oxidant potential and urinary albumin excretion in critically ill patients. Intensive Care Med 24(3):230–235

Molnar Z, Shearer E, Lowe D (1999) N-Acetylcysteine treatment to prevent the progression of multisystem organ failure: a prospective, randomized, placebo-controlled study. Crit Care Med 27(6):1100–1104

Molnar Z, Szakmany T, Koszegi T (2003) Prophylactic N-acetylcysteine decreases serum CRP but not PCT levels and microalbuminuria following major abdominal surgery. A prospective, randomised, double-blinded, placebo-controlled clinical trial. Intensive Care Med 29(5):749–755

Montanini S, Sinardi D, Pratico C, Sinardi AU, Trimarchi G (1999) Use of acetylcysteine as the life-saving antidote in Amanita phalloides (Death cap) poisoning – case report on 11 patients. Arzneim Forsch Drug Res 49(12):1044–1047

Moriuchi H, Zaha M, Fukumoto T, Yuizono T (1998) Activation of polymorphonuclear leukocytes in oleic acid-induced lung injury. Intensive Care Med 24(7):709–715

Morrison JA, Jacobsen DW, Sprecher DL, Robinson K, Khoury P, Daniels SR (1999) Serum glutathione in adolescent males predicts parental coronary heart disease. Circulation 100(22):2244–2247

Moss M, Guidot DM, Wong-Lambertina M, Ten Hoor T, Perez RL, Brown LAS (2000) The effects of chronic alcohol abuse on pulmonary glutathione homeostasis. Am J Respir Crit Care Med 161(2):414–419

Murakami K, Kondo T, Ohtsuka Y, Fujiwara Y, Shimada M, Kawakami Y (1989) Impairment of glutathione metabolism in erthrocytes from patients with diabetes mellitus. Metab Clin Exp 38:753–758

Mutimer D, Neuberger J (1993) Acute liver failure: improving outcome despite a paucity of treatment options. Q J Med 86(7):409–411

Mutlu-Turkoglu U, Ademoglu E, Ibrahimoglu L, Aykac-Toker G, Uysal M (1998) Imbalance between lipid peroxidation and antioxidant status in preeclampsia. Gynecol Obstet Investig 46(1):37–40

N'Dow J, Robson CN, Matthews JN, Neal DE, Pearson JP (2001) Reducing mucus production after urinary reconstruction: a prospective randomized trial. J Urol 165(5): 1433–1440

Nakagawa Y, Akao Y, Morikawa H, Hirata I, Katsu K, Naoe T, Ohishi N, Yagi K (2002) Arsenic trioxide-induced apoptosis through oxidative stress in cells of colon cancer cell lines. Life Sci 70(19):2253–2269

Nakamura H, De Rosa SC, Yodoi J, Holmgren A, Ghezzi P, Herzenberg LA (2001) Chronic elevation of plasma thioredoxin: Inhibition of chemotaxis and curtailment of life expectancy in AIDS. Proc Natl Acad Sci U S A 98(5):2688–2693

Nakamura H, Masutani H, Yodoi J (2002) Redox imbalance and its control in HIV infection. Antioxid Redox Signal 4(3):455–464

Nallamothu BK, Shojania KG, Saint S, Hofer TP, Humes HD, Moscucci M, Bates ER (2004) Is acetylcysteine effective in preventing contrast-related nephropathy? A meta-analysis. Am J Med 117(12):938–947

Naziroglu M, Cay M (2001) Protective role of intraperitoneally administered vitamin E and selenium on the antioxidative defense mechanisms in rats with diabetes induced by streptozotocin. Biol Trace Elem Res 79(2):149–159

Nielsen HB (1999) N-acetylcysteine. Ugeskr Laeger 161(31):4424

Nielsen HB, Kharazmi A, Bolbjerg ML, Poulsen HE, Pedersen BK, Secher NH (2001) N-acetylcysteine attenuates oxidative burst by neutrophils in response to ergometer rowing with no effect on pulmonary gas exchange. Int J Sports Med 22(4):256–260

Nuttall SL, Dunne F, Kendall MJ, Martin U (1999) Age-independent oxidative stress in elderly patients with non-insulin-dependent diabetes mellitus. QJM 92(1):33–38

Oldemeyer JB, Biddle WP, Wurdeman RL, Mooss AN, Cichowski E, Hilleman DE (2003) Acetylcysteine in the prevention of contrast-induced nephropathy after coronary angiography. Am Heart J 146(6):E23

Olivieri D, Marsico SA, Del Donno M (1985) Improvement of mucociliary transport in smokers by mucolytics. Eur J Respir Dis Suppl 139:142–145

Ortolani O, Conti A, De Gaudio AR, Moraldi E, Novelli GP (2002) Glutathione and N-acetylcysteine in the prevention of free-radical damage in the initial phase of septic shock. Recenti Prog Med 93(2):125–129

Ostapowicz G, Fontana RJ, Schiodt FV, Larson A, Davern TJ, Han SH, McCashland TM, Shakil AO, Hay JE, Hynan L, Crippin JS, Blei AT, Samuel G, Reisch J, Lee WM (2002) Results of a prospective study of acute liver failure at 17 tertiary care centers in the United States. Ann Intern Med 137(12):947–954

Ostapowicz G, Lee WM (2000) Acute hepatic failure: a western perspective. J Gastroenterol Hepatol 15(5):480–488

Ovesen T, Felding JU, Tommerup B, Schousboe LP, Petersen CG (2000) Effect of N-acetylcysteine on the incidence of recurrence of otitis media with effusion and re-insertion of ventilation tubes. Acta Otolaryngol 120:79–81

Ozaras R, Tahan V, Aydin S, Uzun H, Kaya S, Senturk H (2003) N-acetylcysteine attenuates alcohol-induced oxidative stress in the rat. World J Gastroenterol 9(1):125–128

Pace BS, Shartava A, Pack-Mabien A, Mulekar M, Ardia A, Goodman SR (2003) Effects of N-acetylcysteine on dense cell formation in sickle cell disease. Am J Hematol 73(1):26–32

Pacht ER, Diaz P, Clanton T, Hart J, Gadek JE (1997) Alveolar fluid glutathione decreases in asymptomatic HIV-seropositive subjects over time. Chest 112(3):785–788

Pacht ER, Timerman AP, Lykens MG, Merola AJ (1991) Deficiency of alveolar fluid glutathione in patients with sepsis and the adult respiratory distress syndrome. Chest 100(5):1397–1403

Pannu N, Manns B, Lee H, Tonelli M (2004) Systematic review of the impact of N-acetylcysteine on contrast nephropathy. Kidney Int 65(4):1366–1374

Parr GD, Huitson A (1987) Oral Fabrol (oral N-acetyl-cysteine) in chronic bronchitis. Br J Dis Chest 81(4):341–348

Paterson RL, Galley HF, Webster NR (2003) The effect of N-acetylcysteine on nuclear factor-kappa B activation, interleukin-6, interleukin-8, and intercellular adhesion molecule-1 expression in patients with sepsis. Crit Care Med 31(11):2574–2578. https://doi.org/10.1097/01.ccm.0000089945.69588.18

Peake SL, Moran JL, Leppard PI (1996) N-acetyl-L-cysteine depresses cardiac performance in patients with septic shock. Crit Care Med 24(8):1302–1310

Pena LR, Hill DB, McClain CJ (1999) Treatment with glutathione precursor decreases cytokine activity. J Parenter Enter Nutr 23(1):1–6

Pendyala L, Schwartz G, Bolanowska-Higdon W, Hitt S, Zdanowicz J, Murphy M, Lawrence D, Creaven PJ (2001) Phase I/pharmacodynamic study of N-acetylcysteine/oltipraz in smokers: early termination due to excessive toxicity. Cancer Epidemiol Biomark Prev 10(3):269–272

Perez RS, Zuurmond WW, Bezemer PD, Kuik DJ, van Loenen AC, de Lange JJ, Zuidhof AJ (2003) The treatment of complex regional pain syndrome type I with free radical scavengers: a randomized controlled study. Pain 102(3):297–307

Perry HE, Shannon MW (1998) Efficacy of oral versus intravenous N-acetylcysteine in acetaminophen overdose: results of an open-label, clinical trial [see comments]. J Pediatr 132(1):149–152

Peters WH, Roelofs HM, Hectors MP, Nagengast FM, Jansen JB (1993) Glutathione and glutathione S-transferases in Barrett's epithelium. Br J Cancer 67(6):1413–1417

Peterson JD, Herzenberg LA, Vasquez K, Waltenbaugh C (1998) Glutathione levels in antigen-presenting cells modulate Th1 versus Th2 response patterns. Proc Natl Acad Sci U S A 95(6):3071–3076

Peterson RG, Rumack BH (1977a) N-acetylcysteine for acetaminophen overdosage (cont.) N Engl J Med 296(9):515

Peterson RG, Rumack BH (1977b) Treating acute acetaminophen poisoning with acetylcysteine. JAMA 237(22):2406–2407

Peterson RG, Rumack BH (1978) Toxicity of acetaminophen overdose. J Am Coll Emerg Physicians 7(5):202–205

Pineda-Molina E, Klatt P, Vazquez J, Marina A, Garcia de Lacoba M, Perez-Sala D, Lamas S (2001) Glutathionylation of the p50 subunit of NF-kappaB: a mechanism for redox-induced inhibition of DNA binding. Biochemistry 40(47):14134–14142

Ponnappan U (2002) Ubiquitin-proteasome pathway is compromised in CD45RO+ and CD45RA+ T lymphocyte subsets during aging. Exp Gerontol 37(2–3):359–367

Porsio A, Borgia M (1970) Intravenous administration of acetylcysteine: clinical experience with its tolerance and action. Clin Ter 55(2):123–132

Prasad A, Andrews NP, Padder FA, Husain M, Quyyumi AA (1999) Glutathione reverses endothelial dysfunction and improves nitric oxide bioavailability. J Am Coll Cardiol 34(2):507–514

Prescott LF (1983) New approaches in managing drug overdosage and poisoning. Br Med J (Clin Res Ed) 287(6387):274–276

Prescott LF, Critchley JA (1983) The treatment of acetaminophen poisoning. Annu Rev Pharmacol Toxicol 23:87–101

Prescott LF, Park J, Ballantyne A, Adriaenssens P, Proudfoot AT (1977) Treatment of paracetamol (acetaminophen) poisoning with N- acetylcysteine. Lancet 2(8035):432–434

Pulle DF, Glass P, Dulfano MJ (1970) A controlled study of the safety and efficacy of acetylcysteine-isoproterenol combination. Curr Ther Res Clin Exp 12(8):485–492

Rahman I, Skwarska E, Henry M, Davis M, O'Connor CM, FitzGerald MX, Greening A, MacNee W (1999) Systemic and pulmonary oxidative stress in idiopathic pulmonary fibrosis. Free Radic Biol Med 27(1–2):60–68

Rank N, Michel C, Haertel C, Lenhart A, Welte M, Meier-Hellmann A, Spies C (2000) N-acetylcysteine increases liver blood flow and improves liver function in septic shock patients: results of a prospective, randomized, double-blind study. Crit Care Med 28(12): 3799–3807

Rashid ST, Salman M, Myint F, Baker DM, Agarwal S, Sweny P, Hamilton G (2004) Prevention of contrast-induced nephropathy in vascular patients undergoing angiography: a randomized controlled trial of intravenous N-acetylcysteine. J Vasc Surg 40(6):1136–1141

Rasmussen JB, Glennow C (1988) Reduction in days of illness after long-term treatment with N-acetylcysteine controlled-release tablets in patients with chronic bronchitis. Eur Respir J 1(4):351–355

Ratjen F, Wonne R, Posselt HG, Stover B, Hofmann D, Bender SW (1985) A double-blind placebo controlled trial with oral ambroxol and N-acetylcysteine for mucolytic treatment in cystic fibrosis. Eur J Pediatr 144(4):374–378

Reid M, Badaloo A, Forrester T, Morlese JF, Frazer M, Heird WC, Jahoor F (2000) In vivo rates of erythrocyte glutathione synthesis in children with severe protein-energy malnutrition. Am J Physiol Endocrinol Metab 278(3):E405–E412

Reid M, Jahoor F (2001) Glutathione in disease. Curr Opin Clin Nutr Metab Care 4(1):65–71

Reinhart K, Spies CD, Meier-Hellmann A, Bredle DL, Hannemann L, Specht M, Schaffartzik W (1995) N-acetylcysteine preserves oxygen consumption and gastric mucosal pH during hyperoxic ventilation. Am J Respir Crit Care Med 151(3 Pt 1):773–779

Repetto M, Reides C, Carretero MLG, Costa M, Griemberg G, Llesuy S (1996) Oxidative stress in blood of HIV infected patients. Clin Chim Acta 255(2):107–117

Riise GC, Larsson S, Larsson P, Jeansson S, Andersson BA (1994) The intrabronchial microbial flora in chronic bronchitis patients: a target for N-acetylcysteine therapy? Eur Respir J 7(1):94–101

Ristoff E, Larsson A (2002) Oxidative stress in inborn errors of metabolism: lessons from glutathione deficiency. J Inherit Metab Dis 25(3):223–226

Ristoff E, Mayatepek E, Larsson A (2001) Long-term clinical outcome in patients with glutathione synthetase deficiency. J Pediatr 139(1):79–84. https://doi.org/10.1067/mpd.2001.114480

Rizvi SI, Zaid MA (2001) Intracellular reduced glutathione content in normal and type 2 diabetic erythrocytes: effect of insulin and (-)epicatechin. J Physiol Pharmacol 52(3):483–488

Roederer M, Ela SW, Staal FJT, Herzenberg LA, Herzenberg LA (1992) N-Acetylcysteine: a new approach to anti-HIV therapy. AIDS Res Hum Retroviruses 8(2):209–217

Roederer M, Staal FJ, Raju PA, Ela SW, Herzenberg LA (1990) Cytokine-stimulated human immunodeficiency virus replication is inhibited by N-acetyl-L-cysteine. Proc Natl Acad Sci U S A 87(12):4884–4888

Roederer M, Staal FJT, Osada H, Herzenberg LA, Herzenberg LA (1991) CD4 and CD8 T cells with high intracellular glutathione levels are selectively lost as the HIV infection progresses. Int Immunol 3(9):933–937

Roum JH, Borok Z, McElvaney NG, Grimes GJ, Bokser AD, Buhl R, Crystal RG (1999) Glutathione aerosol suppresses lung epithelial surface inflammatory cell-derived oxidants in cystic fibrosis. J Appl Physiol 87(1):438–443

Roum JH, Buhl R, Mcelvaney NG, Borok Z, Crystal RG (1993) Systemic deficiency of glutathione in cystic fibrosis. J Appl Physiol 75(6):2419–2424

Ruan EA, Rao S, Burdick JS, Stryker SJ, Telford GL, Otterson MF, Opara EC, Koch TR (1997) Glutathione levels in chronic inflammatory disorders of the human colon. Nutr Res 17(3):463–473

Ruffmann R, Wendel A (1991) GSH rescue by N-acetylcysteine. Klin Wochenschr 69(18):857–862

Rumack BH (1984) Acetaminophen overdose in young children. Treatment and effects of alcohol and other additional ingestants in 417 cases. Am J Dis Child 138(5):428–433

Rumack BH (1986) Acetaminophen overdose in children and adolescents. Pediatr Clin N Am 33(3):691–701

Rumack BH (2002) Acetaminophen hepatotoxicity: the first 35 years. J Toxicol Clin Toxicol 40(1):3–20

Rumack BH, Peterson RC, Koch GG, Amara IA (1981) Acetaminophen overdose. 662 cases with evaluation of oral acetylcysteine treatment. Arch Intern Med 141(3 Spec No):380–385

Saitoh M, Nishitoh H, Fujii M, Takeda K, Tobiume K, Sawada Y, Kawabata M, Miyazono K, Ichijo H (1998) Mammalian thioredoxin is a direct inhibitor of apoptosis signal-regulating kinase (ASK) 1. EMBO J 17(9):2596–2606. https://doi.org/10.1093/emboj/17.9.2596

Salgia AD, Kosnik SD (1999) When acetaminophen use becomes toxic. Treating acute accidental and intentional overdose. Postgrad Med 105(4):81–84, 87, 90

Samiec PS, Drews-Botsch C, Flagg EW, Kurtz JC, Sternberg P, Reed RL, Jones DP (1998) Glutathione in human plasma: decline in association with aging, age-related macular degeneration, and diabetes. Free Radic Biol Med 24(5):699–704

Sandalova T, Zhong L, Lindqvist Y, Holmgren A, Schneider G (2001) Three-dimensional structure of a mammalian thioredoxin reductase: implications for mechanism and evolution of a selenocysteine-dependent enzyme. Proc Natl Acad Sci U S A 98(17):9533–9538. https://doi.org/10.1073/pnas.171178698

Sandberg K, Fellman V, Stigson L, Thiringer K, Hjalmarson O (2004) N-acetylcysteine administration during the first week of life does not improve lung function in extremely low birth weight infants. Biol Neonate 86(4):275–279

Sandhu C, Belli AM, Oliveira DB (2006) The role of N-acetylcysteine in the prevention of contrast-induced nephrotoxicity. Cardiovasc Intervent Radiol 29(3):344–347

Sano M, Ernesto C, Thomas RG, Klauber MR, Schafer K, Grundman M, Woodbury P, Growdon J, Cotman CW, Pfeiffer E, Schneider LS, Thal LJ (1997) A controlled trial of selegiline, alpha-tocopherol, or both as treatment for Alzheimer's disease. The Alzheimer's Disease Cooperative Study. N Engl J Med 336(17):1216–1222

Sasazuki S, Kodama H, Yoshimasu K, Liu Y, Washio M, Tanaka K, Tokunaga S, Kono S, Arai H, Doi Y, Kawano T, Nakagaki O, Takada K, Koyanagi S, Hiyamuta K, Nii T, Shirai K, Ideishi M, Arakawa K, Mohri M, Takeshita A (2000) Relation between green tea consumption and the severity of coronary atherosclerosis among Japanese men and women. Ann Epidemiol 10(6):401–408

Sastre J, Pallardo FV, Garcia de la Asuncion J, Vina J (2000) Mitochondria, oxidative stress and aging. Free Radic Res 32(3):189–198

Sastre J, Pallardo FV, Vina J (1996) Glutathione, oxidative stress and aging. Age 19(4):129–139

Saugstad OD (1997) Bronchopulmonary dysplasia and oxidative stress: are we closer to an understanding of the pathogenesis of BPD? Acta Paediatr 86(12):1277–1282

Saxena S, Kumar D, Srivastava P, Khanna VK, Seth PK (1999) Low levels of platelet glutathione in Eales' disease. Med Sci Res 27(9):625–626

Schmidinger M, Budinsky AC, Wenzel C, Piribauer M, Brix R, Kautzky M, Oder W, Locker GJ, Zielinski CC, Steger GG (2000) Glutathione in the prevention of cisplatin induced toxicities. A prospectively randomized pilot trial in patients with head and neck cancer and non small cell lung cancer. Wien Klin Wochenschr 112(14):617–623

Schmidt AM, Hori O, Chen JX, Li JF, Crandall J, Zhang J, Cao R, Yan SD, Brett J, Stern D (1995) Advanced glycation endproducts interacting with their endothelial receptor induce expression of vascular cell adhesion molecule-1 (VCAM-1) in cultured human endothelial cells and in mice. A potential mechanism for the accelerated vasculopathy of diabetes. J Clin Invest 96(3):1395–1403

Schmidt LE, Knudsen TT, Dalhoff K, Bendtsen F (2002) Effect of acetylcysteine on prothrombin index in paracetamol poisoning without hepatocellular injury. Lancet 360(9340): 1151–1152

Schnackenberg LK, Chen M, Sun J, Holland RD, Dragan Y, Tong W, Welsh W, Beger RD (2009) Evaluations of the trans-sulfuration pathway in multiple liver toxicity studies. Toxicol Appl Pharmacol 235(1):25–32. https://doi.org/10.1016/j.taap.2008.11.015

Scholze A, Rinder C, Beige J, Riezler R, Zidek W, Tepel M (2004) Acetylcysteine reduces plasma homocysteine concentration and improves pulse pressure and endothelial function in patients with end-stage renal failure. Circulation 109(3):369–374

Schulz JB, Lindenau J, Seyfried J, Dichgans J (2000) Glutathione, oxidative stress and neurodegeneration. Eur J Biochem 267(16):4904–4911

Seema KR, Mandal RN, Tandon A, Randhawa VS, Mehta G, Batra S, Ray GN, Kapoor AK (1999) Serum TNF-alpha and free radical scavengers in neonatal septicemia. Indian J Pediatr 66(4):511–516

Sellers EM, Freedman F (1981) Treatment of acetaminophen poisoning. Can Med Assoc J 125(8):827–829

Selwa LM (1999) N-acetylcysteine therapy for Unverricht-Lundborg disease. Neurology 52(2):426–427

Sha SH, Schacht J (2000) Antioxidants attenuate gentamicin-induced free radical formation in vitro and ototoxicity in vivo: D-methionine is a potential protectant. Hear Res 142(1–2):34–40

Shan X, Aw TY, Jones DP (1990) Glutathione-dependent protection against oxidative injury. Pharmacol Ther 47:61–71

Shapiro BL, Smith QT, Warick WJ (1975) Serum glutathione reductase and cystic fibrosis. Pediatr Res 9(12):885–888

Shapiro BL, Smith QT, Warwick WJ (1973) Red cell glutathione and glutathione reductase in cystic fibrosis. Proc Soc Exp Biol Med 144(1):181–183

Shenton D, Perrone G, Quinn KA, Dawes IW, Grant CM (2002) Regulation of protein S-thiolation by glutaredoxin 5 in the yeast Saccharomyces cerevisiae. J Biol Chem 277(19):16853–16859. https://doi.org/10.1074/jbc.M200559200

Shriner K, Goetz MB (1992) Severe hepatotoxicity in a patient receiving both acetaminophen and zidovudine. Am J Med 93(1):94–96

Shyu KG, Cheng JJ, Kuan P (2002) Acetylcysteine protects against acute renal damage in patients with abnormal renal function undergoing a coronary procedure. J Am Coll Cardiol 40(8):1383–1388

Sido B, Hack V, Hochlehnert A, Lipps H, Herfarth C, Droge W (1998) Impairment of intestinal glutathione synthesis in patients with inflammatory bowel disease. Gut 42(4):485–492

Skurnick JH, Bogden JD, Baker H, Kemp FW, Sheffet A, Quattrone G, Louria DB (1996) Micronutrient profiles in HIV-1-infected heterosexual adults. J Acquir Immune Defic Syndr 12(1):75–83

Slattery JT, McRorie TI, Reynolds R, Kalhorn TF, Kharasch ED, Eddy AC (1989) Lack of effect of cimetidine on acetaminophen disposition in humans. Clin Pharmacol Ther 46(5):591–597

Slattery JT, Wilson JM, Kalhorn TF, Nelson SD (1987) Dose-dependent pharmacokinetics of acetaminophen: evidence of glutathione depletion in humans. Clin Pharmacol Ther 41:413–418

Smilkstein MJ, Bronstein AC, Linden C, Augenstein WL, Kulig KW, Rumack BH (1991) Acetaminophen overdose: a 48-hour intravenous N-acetylcysteine treatment protocol. Ann Emerg Med 20(10):1058–1063

Smilkstein MJ, Knapp GL, Kulig KW, Rumack BH (1988) Efficacy of oral N-acetylcysteine in the treatment of acetaminophen overdose. Analysis of the national multicenter study (1976 to 1985). N Engl J Med 319(24):1557–1562

Smith CV, Hansen TN, Martin NE, McMicken HW, Elliott SJ (1993) Oxidant stress responses in premature infants during exposure to hyperoxia. Pediatr Res 34(3):360–365

Smith CV, Rogers LK, Rabin RL, Maldonado YA, Herzenberg LA, Herzenberg LA, Petru A (1994) Effects of human immunodeficiency virus (HIV) infection on plasma glutathione status in children. Pediatr Res 35:196A. (Abstract #1163)

Sochman J (2002) N-acetylcysteine in acute cardiology: 10 years later: what do we know and what would we like to know? J Am Coll Cardiol 39(9):1422–1428

Song JJ, Rhee JG, Suntharalingam M, Walsh SA, Spitz DR, Lee YJ (2002) Role of glutaredoxin in metabolic oxidative stress. Glutaredoxin as a sensor of oxidative stress mediated by H2O2. J Biol Chem 277(48):46566–46575. https://doi.org/10.1074/jbc.M206826200

Spada C, Treitinger A, Reis M, Masokawa IY, Verdi JC, Luiz MC, Silveira MV, Michelon CM, Avila-Junior S, Gil DO, Ostrowskyl S (2002) The effect of N-acetylcysteine supplementation upon viral load, CD4, CD8, total lymphocyte count and hematocrit in individuals undergoing antiretroviral treatment. Clin Chem Lab Med 40(5):452–455

Spapen H, Zhang H, Demanet C, Vleminckx W, Vincent JL, Huyghens L (1998) Does N-acetyl-L-cysteine influence cytokine response during early human septic shock? Chest 113(6):1616–1624

Spies C, Giese C, Meier-Hellmann A, Specht M, Hannemann L, Schaffartzik W, Reinhart K (1996) The effect of prophylactically administered n-acetylcysteine on clinical indicators for tissue oxygenation during hyperoxic ventilation in cardiac risk patients. Anaesthesist 45(4):343–350

Spies CD, Reinhart K, Witt I, Meier-Hellmann A, Hannemann L, Bredle DL, Schaffartzik W (1994) Influence of N-acetylcysteine on indirect indicators of tissue oxygenation in septic shock patients: results from a prospective, randomized, double-blind study. Crit Care Med 22(11):1738–1746

Sprietsma JE (1999) Modern diets and diseases: NO-zinc balance. Under Th1, zinc and nitrogen monoxide (NO) collectively protect against viruses, AIDS, autoimmunity, diabetes, allergies, asthma, infectious diseases, atherosclerosis and cancer. Med Hypotheses 53(1):6–16

Sprince H (1985) Protective action of sulfur compounds against aldehyde toxicants of cigarette smoke. Eur J Respir Dis Suppl 139:102–112

Sprince H, Parker CM, Smith GG, Gonzales LJ (1975) Protective action of ascorbic acid and sulfur compounds against acetaldehyde toxicity: implications in alcoholism and smoking. Agents Actions 5(2):164–173

Staal FJ, Ela SW, Roederer M, Anderson MT, Herzenberg LA (1992a) Glutathione deficiency and human immunodeficiency virus infection. Lancet 339(8798):909–912

Staal FJ, Roederer M, Herzenberg LA (1990) Intracellular thiols regulate activation of nuclear factor kappa B and transcription of human immunodeficiency virus. Proc Natl Acad Sci U S A 87(24):9943–9947

Staal FJ, Roederer M, Israelski DM, Bubp J, Mole LA, McShane D, Deresinski SC, Ross W, Sussman H, Raju PA et al (1992b) Intracellular glutathione levels in T cell subsets decrease in HIV-infected individuals. AIDS Res Hum Retrovir 8(2):305–311

Stafanger G, Garne S, Howitz P, Morkassel E, Koch C (1988) The clinical effect and the effect on the ciliary motility of oral N-acetylcysteine in patients with cystic fibrosis and primary ciliary dyskinesia. Eur Respir J 1(2):161–167

Stafanger G, Koch C (1989) N-acetylcysteine in cystic fibrosis and Pseudomonas aeruginosa infection: clinical score, spirometry and ciliary motility. Eur Respir J 2(3):234–237

Stewart DM, Dillman RO, Kim HS, Stewart K (1979) Acetaminophen overdose: a growing health care hazard. Clin Toxicol 14(5):507–513

Stey C, Steurer J, Bachmann S, Medici TC, Tramer MR (2000) The effect of oral N-acetylcysteine in chronic bronchitis: a quantitative systematic review [In Process Citation]. Eur Respir J 16(2):253–262

Stiksa G, Nemcek K, Melin S (1984) Effects of inhaled N-acetylcysteine in combination with terbutaline. Eur J Respir Dis 65(4):278–282

Straface E, Rivabene R, Masella R, Santulli M, Paganelli R, Malorni W (2002) Structural changes of the erythrocyte as a marker of non-insulin-dependent diabetes: protective effects of N-acetylcysteine. Biochem Biophys Res Commun 290(5):1393–1398

Suarez M, Beloqui O, Ferrer JV, Gil B, Qian C, Garcia N, Civeira P, Prieto J (1993) Glutathione depletion in chronic hepatitis C. Int Hepatol Commun 1:215–221

Sulkowski MS, Thomas DL, Chaisson RE, Moore RD (2000) Hepatotoxicity associated with anti-retroviral therapy in adults infected with human immunodeficiency virus and the role of hepatitis C or B virus infection. JAMA 283(1):74–80

Sung L, Simons JA, Dayneka NL (1997) Dilution of intravenous N-acetylcysteine as a cause of hyponatremia. Pediatrics 100(3 Pt 1):389–391

Suter PM, Domenighetti G, Schaller M-D, Laverriere M-C, Ritz R, Perret C (1994) N-acetylcysteine enhances recovery from acute lung injury in man. A randomized, double-blind, placebo-controlled clinical study. Chest 105:190–194

Svendsen JH, Klarlund K, Aldershvile J, Waldorff S (1989) N-acetylcysteine modifies the acute effects of isosorbide-5-mononitrate in angina pectoris patients evaluated by exercise testing. J Cardiovasc Pharmacol 13(2):320–323

Szakmany T, Marton S, Molnar Z (2003) Lack of effect of prophylactic N-acetylcysteine on postoperative organ dysfunction following major abdominal tumour surgery: a randomized, placebo-controlled, double-blinded clinical trial. Anaesth Intensive Care 31(3):267–271

Taniguchi N, Higashi T, Sakamoto Y, Meister A (eds) (1989) Glutathione centennial: molecular perspectives and clinical applications. Academic Press, New York

Tatebe S, Sinicrope FA, Kuo MT (2002) Induction of multidrug resistance proteins MRP1 and MRP3 and gamma-glutamylcysteine synthetase gene expression by nonsteroidal anti-inflammatory drugs in human colon cancer cells. Biochem Biophys Res Commun 290(5):1427–1433

Tenenbein M (1984) Hypersensitivity-like reactions to N-acetylcysteine. Vet Hum Toxicol 26(Suppl 2):3–5

Tepel M, van der Giet M, Schwarzfeld C, Laufer U, Liermann D, Zidek W (2000) Prevention of radiographic-contrast-agent-induced reductions in renal function by acetylcysteine. N Engl J Med 343:180–184

Tepel M, van der Giet M, Statz M, Jankowski J, Zidek W (2003) The antioxidant acetylcysteine reduces cardiovascular events in patients with end-stage renal failure. A randomized, controlled trial. Circulation 107:992

Tepel M, Zidek W (2001) Acetylcysteine for radiocontrast nephropathy. Curr Opin Crit Care 7(6):390–392

Tessier D, Khalil A, Fulop T (1999) Effects of an oral glucose challenge on free radicals/antioxidants balance in an older population with type II diabetes. J Gerontol A Biol Sci Med Sci 54(11):M541–M545

Tice JA, Ross E, Coxson PG, Rosenberg I, Weinstein MC, Hunink MG, Goldman PA, Williams L, Goldman L (2001) Cost-effectiveness of vitamin therapy to lower plasma homocysteine levels for the prevention of coronary heart disease: effect of grain fortification and beyond. JAMA 286(8):936–943

Todisco T, Polidori R, Rossi F, Iannacci L, Bruni B, Fedeli L, Palumbo R (1985) Effect of N-acetylcysteine in subjects with slow pulmonary mucociliary clearance. Eur J Respir Dis Suppl 139:136–141

Tossios P, Bloch W, Huebner A, Raji MR, Dodos F, Klass O, Suedkamp M, Kasper SM, Hellmich M, Mehlhorn U (2003) N-acetylcysteine prevents reactive oxygen species-mediated myocardial stress in patients undergoing cardiac surgery: results of a randomized, double-blind, placebo-controlled clinical trial. J Thorac Cardiovasc Surg 126(5):1513–1520

Travaline JM, Sudarshan S, Roy BG, Cordova F, Leyenson V, Criner GJ (1997) Effect of N-acetylcysteine on human diaphragm strength and fatigability. Am J Respir Crit Care Med 156(5):1567–1571

Treeprasertsuk S, Krudsood S, Tosukhowong T, Maek ANW, Vannaphan S, Saengnetswang T, Looareesuwan S, Kuhn WF, Brittenham G, Carroll J (2003) N-acetylcysteine in severe falciparum malaria in Thailand. Southeast Asian J Trop Med Public Health 34(1):37–42

Tripi S, Di Gaetano G, Soresi M, Carroccio A, Bonfissuto G, Savi A, Vuturo O, Montalto G (1998) Acetylcysteine therapy for chronic hepatitis C: are its effects synergistic with interferon alpha? A pilot study. Clin Drug Invest 16(4):297–302

Uden S, Bilton D, Guyan PM, Kay PM, Braganza JM (1990) Rationale for antioxidant therapy in pancreatitis and cystic fibrosis. Adv Exp Med Biol 264:555–572

Unverferth DV, Jagadeesh JM, Unverferth BJ, Magorien RD, Leier CV, Balcerzak SP (1983) Attempt to prevent doxorubicin-induced acute human myocardial morphologic damage with acetylcysteine. J Natl Cancer Inst 71(5):917–920

Upritchard JE, Sutherland WH, Mann JI (2000) Effect of supplementation with tomato juice, vitamin E, and vitamin C on LDL oxidation and products of inflammatory activity in type 2 diabetes. Diabetes Care 23(6):733–738

Usal A, Acarturk E, Yuregir GT, Unlukurt I, Demirci C, Kurt HI, Birand A (1996) Decreased glutathione levels in acute myocardial infarction. Jpn Heart J 37(2):177–182

van Bakel MM, Printzen G, Wermuth B, Wiesmann UN (2000) Antioxidant and thyroid hormone status in selenium-deficient phenylketonuric and hyperphenylalaninemic patients. Am J Clin Nutr 72(4):976–981

van Dalen EC, Caron HN, Dickinson HO, Kremer LC (2005) Cardioprotective interventions for cancer patients receiving anthracyclines. Cochrane Database Syst Rev 1:CD003917

Van Schooten FJ, Nia AB, De Flora S, D'Agostini F, Izzotti A, Camoirano A, Balm AJ, Dallinga JW, Bast A, Haenen GR, Van't Veer L, Baas P, Sakai H, Van Zandwijk N (2002) Effects of oral administration of N-acetyl-L-cysteine: a multi-biomarker study in smokers. Cancer Epidemiol Biomark Prev 11(2):167–175

Vecchiarelli A, Dottorini M, Pietrella D, Cociani C, Eslami A, Todisco T, Bistoni F (1994) Macrophage activation by N-acetyl-cysteine in COPD patients. Chest 105(3):806–811

Verhagen H, Hageman GJ, Rauma AL, Versluis-de Haan G, van Herwijnen MH, de Groot J, Torronen R, Mykkanen H (2001) Biomonitoring the intake of garlic via urinary excretion of allyl mercapturic acid. Br J Nutr 86(Suppl 1):S111–S114

Verhulst M-L, Van Oijen AHAM, Roelofs HMJ, Peters WHM, Jansen JBMJ (2000) Antral glutathione concentration and glutathione S-transferase activity in patients with and without Helicobacter pylori. Dig Dis Sci 45(3):629–632

Verjee ZH, Behal R (1976) Protein-calorie malnutrition: a study of red blood cell and serum enzymes during and after crisis. Clin Chim Acta 70(1):139–147

Verstraeten JM (1979) Mucolytic treatment in chronic obstructive pulmonary disease. Double-blind comparative clinical trial with N-acetylcysteine, bromhexine and placebo. Acta Tuberc Pneumol Belg 70(1):71–80

Villa P, Saccani A, Sica A, Ghezzi P (2002) Glutathione protects mice from lethal sepsis by limiting inflammation and potentiating host defense. J Infect Dis 185(8):1115–1120

Vita JA, Frei B, Holbrook M, Gokce N, Leaf C, Keaney Jr JF (1998) L-2-oxothiazolidine-4-carboxylic acid reverses endothelial dysfunction in patients with coronary artery disease. J Clin Invest 101(6):1408–1414

Vlamis-Gardikas A, Holmgren A (2002) Thioredoxin and glutaredoxin isoforms. Methods Enzymol 347:286–296

Volkin DB, Klibanov AM (1987) Thermal destruction processes in proteins involving cystine residues. J Biol Chem 262(7):2945–2950

Wagdi P, Fluri M, Aeschbacher B, Fikrle A, Meier B (1996) Cardioprotection in patients undergoing chemo- and/or radiotherapy for neoplastic disease. A pilot study. Jpn Heart J 37(3):353–359

Wagdi P, Rouvinez G, Fluri M, Aeschbacher B, Thoni A, Schefer H, Meier B (1995) Cardioprotection in chemo- and radiotherapy for malignant diseases – an echocardiographic pilot study. Schweiz Rundsch Med Prax 84(43):1220–1223

Walmsley SL, Winn LM, Harrison ML, Uetrecht JP, Wells PG (1997) Oxidative stress and thiol depletion in plasma and peripheral blood lymphocytes from HIV-infected patients: toxicological and pathological implications. AIDS 11(14):1689–1697

Walters MT, Rubin CE, Keightley SJ, Ward CD, Cawley MI (1986) A double-blind, cross-over, study of oral N-acetylcysteine in Sjogren's syndrome. Scand J Rheumatol Suppl 61:253–258

Wang J, Boja ES, Tan W, Tekle E, Fales HM, English S, Mieyal JJ, Chock PB (2001) Reversible Glutathionylation Regulates Actin Polymerization in A431 Cells. J Biol Chem 276(51):47763–47766

Ward KP, Arthur JR, Russell G, Aggett PJ (1984) Blood selenium content and glutathione peroxidase activity in children with cystic fibrosis, coeliac disease, asthma, and epilepsy. Eur J Pediatr 142(1):21–24

Watt G, Jongsakul K, Ruangvirayuth R (2002) A pilot study of N-acetylcysteine as adjunctive therapy for severe malaria. QJM 95(5):285–290

Weber S, Auclert L, Touiza K, Pellois A, Guerin C, Blin P, Guerin F (1992) Evaluation of tolerance during intravenous administration of low dose of isosorbide dinitrate in the treatment of unstable angina. Arch Mal Coeur Vaiss 85(1):59–65

Weigand MA, Plachky J, Thies JC, Spies-Martin D, Otto G, Martin E, Bardenheuer HJ (2001) N-acetylcysteine attenuates the increase in alpha-glutathione S-transferase and circulating ICAM-1 and VCAM-1 after reperfusion in humans undergoing liver transplantation. Transplantation 72(4):694–698

Weikert LF, Bernard GR (1996) Pharmacotherapy of sepsis. Clin Chest Med 17(2):289–305

White AC, Thannickal VJ, Fanburg BL (1994) Glutathione deficiency in human disease. J Nutr Biochem 5:218–226

Whitekus MJ, Li N, Zhang M, Wang M, Horwitz MA, Nelson SK, Horwitz LD, Brechun N, Diaz-Sanchez D, Nel AE (2002) Thiol antioxidants inhibit the adjuvant effects of aerosolized diesel exhaust particles in a murine model for ovalbumin sensitization. J Immunol 168(5):2560–2567

Wiklund O, Fager G, Andersson A, Lundstam U, Masson P, Hultberg B (1996) N-acetylcysteine treatment lowers plasma homocysteine but not serum lipoprotein(a) levels. Atherosclerosis 119(1):99–106

Winkler E, Halkin H (1992) Paracetamol overdose in Israel–1992. Isr J Med Sci 28(11):811–812

Winklhofer-Roob BM (2000) Cystic fibrosis: nutritional status and micronutrients [In Process Citation]. Curr Opin Clin Nutr Metab Care 3(4):293–297

Winterbourn CC, Peskin AV, Parsons-Mair HN (2002) Thiol oxidase activity of copper, zinc superoxide dismutase. J Biol Chem 277(3):1906–1911

Woo OF, Mueller PD, Olson KR, Anderson IB, Kim SY (2000) Shorter duration of oral N-acetylcysteine therapy for acute acetaminophen overdose. Ann Emerg Med 35(4):363–368

Xu D, Finkel T (2002) A role for mitochondria as potential regulators of cellular life span. Biochem Biophys Res Commun 294(2):245–248

Yalcin E, Altin F, Cinhuseyinoglue F, Arslan MO (2002) N-acetylcysteine in chronic blepharitis. Cornea 21(2):164–168

Yang ES, Richter C, Chun JS, Huh TL, Kang SS, Park JW (2002) Inactivation of NADP(+)-dependent isocitrate dehydrogenase by nitric oxide. Free Radic Biol Med 33(7):927–937

Yiengpruksawan A, Lightdale CJ, Gerdes H, Botet JF (1991) Mucolytic-antifoam solution for reduction of artifacts during endoscopic ultrasonography: a randomized controlled trial. Gastrointest Endosc 37(5):543–546

Yoshida K, Hirokawa J, Tagami S, Kawakami Y, Urata Y, Kondo T (1995) Weakened cellular scavenging activity against oxidative stress in diabetes mellitus: regulation of glutathione synthesis and efflux. Diabetologia 38(2):201–210

Yucel D, Aydogdu S, Cehreli S, Saydam G, Canatan H, Senes M, Topkaya BC, Nebioglu S (1998) Increased oxidative stress in dilated cardiomyopathic heart failure. Clin Chem 44(1):148–154

Zhong L, Arner ES, Holmgren A (2000a) Structure and mechanism of mammalian thioredoxin reductase: the active site is a redox-active selenolthiol/selenenylsulfide formed from the conserved cysteine-selenocysteine sequence. Proc Natl Acad Sci U S A 97(11):5854–5859

Zhong L, Holmgren A (2000) Essential role of selenium in the catalytic activities of mammalian thioredoxin reductase revealed by characterization of recombinant enzymes with selenocysteine mutations. J Biol Chem 275(24):18121–18128

Zhong L, Persson K, Sandalova T, Schneider G, Holmgren A (2000b) Purification, crystallization and preliminary crystallographic data for rat cytosolic selenocysteine 498 to cysteine mutant thioredoxin reductase. Acta Crystallogr D Biol Crystallogr 56(Pt 9):1191–1193

Zimmerman RJ, Marafino BJ Jr, Chan A, Landre P, Winkelhake JL (1989) The role of oxidant injury in tumor cell sensitivity to recombinant human tumor necrosis factor in vivo. Implications for mechanism of action. J Immunol 142:1405–1409

Pharmacology, Formulations, and Adverse Effects

Richard Eugene Frye, James P. Andrus, Kevin V. Lemley,
Stephen C. De Rosa, Pietro Ghezzi, Arne Holmgren,
Dean Jones, Farook Jahoor, Richard Kopke, Ian Cotgreave,
Teodoro Bottiglieri, Neil Kaplowitz, Hajime Nakamura,
Frank Staal, Stephen W. Ela, Kondala R. Atkuri,
Rabindra Tirouvanziam, Kartoosh Heydari, Bita Sahaf,
Andrew Zolopa, John J. Mantovani,
Leonard A. Herzenberg, and Leonore A. Herzenberg

R. E. Frye (✉)
Barrow Neurological Institute, Phoenix Children's Hospital, University of Arizona
College of Medicine – Phoenix, Phoenix, AZ, USA
e-mail: rfrye@phoenixchildrens.com

J. P. Andrus
Department of Pediatrics, Lucile Packard Children's Hospital, Stanford University,
Stanford, CA, USA

K. V. Lemley
Department of Medicine, Stanford University, Stanford, CA, USA

S. C. De Rosa
Fred Hutchinson Cancer Center, Seattle, WA, USA

P. Ghezzi
Laboratory of Neuroimmunology, Mario Negri Institute, Milano, Italy

A. Holmgren
Medical Nobel Institute for Biochemistry, Karolinska Institute, Stockholm, Sweden

D. Jones
Department of Biochemistry, Emory University, Atlanta, GA, USA

F. Jahoor
USDA/ARS Children's Nutrition Research Center, Baylor College of Medicine,
Waco, TX, USA

R. Kopke
Department of Defense Spatial Orientation Center, Naval Medical Center,
San Diego, CA, USA

I. Cotgreave
Division of Biochemical Toxicology, Karolinska Institute, Stockholm, Sweden

© Springer Nature Singapore Pte Ltd. 2019
R. E. Frye, M. Berk (eds.), *The Therapeutic Use of N-Acetylcysteine (NAC)
in Medicine*, https://doi.org/10.1007/978-981-10-5311-5_21

T. Bottiglieri
Baylor Institute of Metabolic Disease, Dallas, TX, USA

N. Kaplowitz
Keck School of Medicine, University of Southern California Medical Center,
Los Angeles, CA, USA

H. Nakamura
Institute for Virus Research, Kyoto University, Kyoto, Japan

F. Staal
Department of Immunology, University Rotterdam, Rotterdam, The Netherlands

S. W. Ela
Venture Science Consulting, Paso Robles, CA, USA

K. R. Atkuri · R. Tirouvanziam · K. Heydari · B. Sahaf ·
J. J. Mantovani · L. A. Herzenberg · L. A. Herzenberg
Department of Genetics, Stanford University, Stanford, CA, USA

A. Zolopa
Positive Care Clinic, Stanford University, Stanford, CA, USA

21.1 Introduction

Besides understanding the effectiveness of N-Acetylcysteine (NAC) for the treatment of disease and the positive effect on physiological systems, other considerations of NAC are important, including the pharmacology, formulations, and adverse effects of NAC. This chapter will review these important aspects of NAC.

21.2 Methods

A systematic online literature search was performed to identify all clinical trials using NAC using the filters "human" and "clinical trials." From these the author reviewer screened titles and abstracts of all potentially relevant publications and high-quality studies were selected which discussed the pharmacology, formulations and adverse effects of NAC.

21.3 Pharmacological Studies of NAC

Studies have shown that a single oral dose of 200 mg NAC increased endogenous levels of NAC about 20-fold (Gabard and Mascher 1991). One study investigated the pharmacokinetics of three oral doses of NAC, 200, 600, and 1200 mg, in healthy individuals. Although the maximal plasma concentration increased with dose, the 200 mg dose was significantly lower than the 600 and 1200 mg dose, but the 600 and 1200 mg doses were not statistically significantly different from each other (Borgstrom and Kagedal 1990). There was no difference in the pharmacokinetic parameters if 600 mg NAC was given once or twice a day (Borgstrom and Kagedal

1990). Sustained-release oral NAC was compared between 600 mg and 1200 mg. Dose-related increases in plasma concentrations were observed; a doubling of the dose resulted in a doubling of the area under the curve without a change in clearance (Nolin et al. 2010). One study compared intravenous (IV) NAC 200 mg and oral 400 mg, finding that the half-life was 5.6 h with IV NAC and 6.3 h with oral NAC. Oral bioavailability of total NAC was 9.1% (Olsson et al. 1988).

Changes in pharmacokinetics have been studied in some specific physiological conditions. One study demonstrated that chronic liver disease altered the pharmacokinetics of IV NAC. The area under the curve was increased by 50%, and clearance was decreased by about 30% in patients with biopsy-proven cirrhosis as compared to healthy patients (Jones et al. 1997). NAC clearance was reduced by 90% in end-stage renal disease (ESRD) patients (Nolin et al. 2010). Another study demonstrated that dialysis increased clearance by over 400% (Soldini et al. 2005). In premature neonates the plasma clearance and volume of distribution of IV NAC correlated with weight and gestational age (Ahola et al. 1999). Vigorous cycling exercise reduced the whole-body clearance of IV NAC by about 25% (Brown et al. 2004).

Lastly, clinical studies have demonstrated that NAC can be administered with antibiotics amoxicillin, cefadroxil, cefpodoxime, doxycycline, erythromycin, loracarbef, and thiamphenicol without significant change in concentration (Barkworth et al. 1991; Kees et al. 1996; Roller et al. 1992).

21.4 NAC formulations

The best known NAC formulation in the United States (US), Mucomyst™ (or the generic version thereof), is available as a 10% or 20% solution of NAC sodium salt that is typically administered orally for treatment of acetaminophen (APAP) overdose. Since Mucomyst™ has a strong, disagreeable flavor, it is usually mixed with fruit juice or a soft drink before consumption. Still, as many physicians can attest, patients commonly find it very difficult to tolerate orally, thereby requiring administration via nasogastric tube. Mucomyst™ is also administered IV in some settings, particularly when patients are unconscious or unable to retain the orally administered drug.

To overcome problems with oral administration, European manufacturers produce NAC in pill and capsule formulations. It is also produced and packaged in a variety of effervescent formulations ("fizzy tabs") that can be dissolved in water, juice, or carbonated drinks to create a pleasant tasting, readily tolerated beverage. Formulations produced under European Good Manufacturing Practice (GMP) standards are designed to minimize NAC oxidation to its dimeric form ("di-NAC"), which is pharmacologically active at very low concentrations with immunologic effects opposite to those of NAC (Sandstrom et al. 1998). In general, di-NAC constitutes less than 0.1% of the European GMP NAC formulations, which are intended for oral administration and have qualified for health insurance reimbursement (Grandjean et al. 2000).

Several US nutraceutical dealers manufacture and sell unbuffered (acidic) NAC. Since the Food and Drug Administration (FDA) does not tightly regulate the production and packaging of nutraceutical products in the United States, neither the content nor the purity of the NAC formulations currently produced and marketed in the US can be reliably judged. Manufacturing methods for these NAC preparations may not prevent formation of NAC by-products (e.g., di-NAC) and may not have been validated for stability during storage. The authors are concerned that some of the variability in clinical trials is due to the formulation of NAC as many non-GMP products have been used in various clinical trials (e.g., Weisbord et al., 2018).

21.5 Potential Adverse Effects of NAC

NAC is the clinically accepted cysteine source used to treat GSH deficiency due to APAP overdose and can be administered by IV, enteral, and rectal routes. Oral NAC dosages for APAP overdose start with a loading dose of 140 mg/kg body weight followed by doses of 70 mg/kg body weight administered every 4 h over a period of 3 days (Miller and Rumack 1983). Smaller dosages (600 mg to 8 g daily) have been administered for substantially longer periods in many clinical trials.

Although NAC has been administered orally at quite high dosages, little if any toxicity has been associated with NAC ingestion. In one study with a particular high long-term NAC dosage (an average of 6.9 g/day administered in three to four divided doses) administered to 60 HIV-infected subjects for 8 weeks and to over 50 subjects for up to 6 months in an open-label continuation, no adverse events (AEs) requiring physician intervention were observed (Herzenberg et al. 1997). Current evidence suggests that 600–900 mg/day, the common daily dosage in Europe for cough and cold relief, may be a reasonable maximum dose for healthy individuals who wish to routinely take NAC.

21.5.1 Symptomatic Adverse Effects

21.5.1.1 Gastrointestinal Discomfort

In another study of patients being treated for APAP overdose, the incidence of emesis from 33 to 51%, and diarrhea from 0 to 44% with treatment of 30 g of oral NAC daily for 3 days with the incidence of these AEs proportional to the total dose given (Miller and Rumack 1983). In one study that used high doses of oral NAC, gastric distress was not infrequently reported similar to that reported elsewhere (De Rosa et al. 2000; Herzenberg et al. 1997). However, half of these subjects were in the placebo arm, suggesting that the distress was related to ingestion of the excipient that may have contained significant amounts of lactose. Thus, gastrointestinal AEs are not uncommon with NAC treatment, particularly with high oral doses of NAC, but could be related to the additives or vehicle in which the NAC is formulated.

21.5.1.2 Headache

NAC has been shown to potentiate nitroglycerin-induced headache in two studies, one in healthy volunteers (Iversen 1992) and one study in patients with unstable angina

(Ardissino et al. 1997). In the former study, it was suggested that the headache was caused by prolonged dilation of the temporal artery (Iversen 1992).

21.5.1.3 Allergic Reaction

There are several reports of anaphylactoid and allergic responses in response to IV NAC (Schmidt and Dalhoff 1999; Walton et al. 1979; Vale and Wheeler 1982; Flanagan and Meredith 1991; Bonfiglio et al. 1992; Stavem 1997; Bailey and McGuigan 1998; Huitema et al. 1998; Bateman et al. 1984). These AEs may in part be explained by findings from preclinical studies demonstrating inflammatory-type responses in animals treated with the oxidized (di-NAC) form of NAC (Sandstrom et al. 1998) which can contaminate NAC preparations that have not been protected against oxidation. In any event, the anaphylactoid reactions to IV NAC are easily treated (Bailey and McGuigan 1998).

21.5.1.4 Delirium

In a large open-label study of patients undergoing liver resection, NAC did not change the incidence of AEs or liver failure but was associated with a higher incidence of delirium (2.7 and 9.8%), resulting in early trial termination. A multivariate analysis suggested an association between NAC and postoperative complications (Grendar et al. 2016).

21.5.2 Adverse Physiological Effects

21.5.2.1 Renal Function

Although dozens of studies demonstrate that NAC improves or at least does not worsen indices of kidney function in populations with various disorders and studies performed on healthy humans demonstrate that it improves kidney function (Hoffmann et al. 2004), there is one study that suggests that NAC worsened a measure of proximal tubular damage. In a small study of patients undergoing tourniquet-induced ischemia during knee arthroplasty, NAC was found to be associated with an increase in the urine N-acetyl-beta-D-glucosaminidase to creatinine ratio at reperfusion suggesting an increase in proximal tubular damage with NAC treatment (Laisalmi-Kokki et al. 2009).

21.5.2.2 Coagulation

In a triple-blind trial high-dose study, intracoronary NAC did not reduce the level of platelet activation biomarkers in patients undergoing percutaneous coronary intervention (Eshraghi et al. 2016). However, NAC was associated with decreased prothrombin time and adenosine diphosphate-induced platelet aggregation in patients undergoing abdominal aortic reconstruction (Niemi et al. 2006), and in a large cardiac surgery study, IV NAC resulted in increased chest tube blood loss and a greater transfusion volume (Wijeysundera et al. 2009). However, several other studies in which NAC was used in surgery have not reported increased bleeding, blood loss, or need for transfusion.

21.5.2.3   Hypotension

In patients with severe drug-resistant unstable angina pectoris, 5 g IV NAC reduced the incidence of acute myocardial infarction but increased the incidence of symptomatic hypotension when added to IV nitroglycerin in a small study (Horowitz et al. 1988). In rodent studies, NAC significantly reduced the pressor effect of angiotensin and reduced angiotensin converting enzyme activity (Boesgaard et al. 1993).

21.5.2.4   Hepatic Protein Catabolism

Caution may be indicated concerning the routine consumption of NAC and other sulfur-containing amino acid (SAA) precursors in the absence of diseases or conditions leading to cysteine/GSH deficiency, particularly in the American populations in which the intake of animal protein tends to be high and individuals may be ingesting two to three times the recommended daily allowance for SAAs on a daily basis.

However, recent observational studies showing that colonic hydrogen sulfide production increases in proportion to consumption of animal protein raises questions (Magee et al. 2000). Since the long-term effects of SAAs are not known, it is important to consider this in individuals with high animal protein intake.

In a small controlled study, NAC was found to reduce amino acid loss and increased urea nitrogen release from the liver graft. These findings are believed to signal increased net protein catabolism in the liver, possibly suggesting increase of the energy and oxygen demand of the liver, potentially putting the liver under increased metabolic stress because of increased amino acid metabolism (Taut et al. 2001).

21.5.2.5   Endothelial Damage

Although several studies suggest that NAC improves endothelial function (Scholze et al. 2004; Sahin et al. 2007; Wittstock et al. 2009; Swarnalatha et al. 2010), a medium-sized randomized placebo-controlled trial in the intensive care unit of patient with organ dysfunction in severe clinical sepsis found that NAC treatment was associated with worsening of the cardiovascular sequential organ failure assessment score, leading the authors to conclude that NAC did not attenuate endothelial damage in this specific patient population (Spapen et al. 2005).

References

Ahola T, Fellman V, Laaksonen R, Laitila J, Lapatto R, Neuvonen PJ, Raivio KO (1999) Pharmacokinetics of intravenous N-acetylcysteine in pre-term new-born infants. Eur J Clin Pharmacol 55(9):645–650

Ardissino D, Merlini PA, Savonitto S, Demicheli G, Zanini P, Bertocchi F, Falcone C, Ghio S, Marinoni G, Montemartini C, Mussini A (1997) Effect of transdermal nitroglycerin or N-acetylcysteine, or both, in the long-term treatment of unstable angina pectoris. J Am Coll Cardiol 29(5):941–947

Bailey B, McGuigan MA (1998) Management of anaphylactoid reactions to intravenous N-acetylcysteine. Ann Emerg Med 31(6):710–715

Barkworth MF, Mangold B, Rehm KD, Schmieder G, Toberich H, Vinchenzo A, Weber J, Rubartsch C (1991) The biological availability of cefadroxil given simultaneously with N-acetylcysteine. Arzneimittel-Forschung 41(8):839–843

Bateman DN, Woodhouse KW, Rawlins MD (1984) Adverse reactions to N-acetylcysteine. Hum Toxicol 3(5):393–398

Boesgaard S, Aldershvile J, Poulsen HE, Christensen S, Dige-Petersen H, Giese J (1993) N-acetylcysteine inhibits angiotensin converting enzyme in vivo. J Pharmacol Exp Ther 265(3):1239–1244

Bonfiglio MF, Traeger SM, Hulisz DT, Martin BR (1992) Anaphylactoid reaction to intravenous acetylcysteine associated with electrocardiographic abnormalities. Ann Pharmacother 26(1):22–25

Borgstrom L, Kagedal B (1990) Dose dependent pharmacokinetics of N-acetylcysteine after oral dosing to man. Biopharm Drug Dispos 11(2):131–136

Brown M, Bjorksten A, Medved I, McKenna M (2004) Pharmacokinetics of intravenous N-acetylcysteine in men at rest and during exercise. Eur J Clin Pharmacol 60(10):717–723. https://doi.org/10.1007/s00228-004-0862-9

De Rosa SC, Zaretsky MD, Dubs JG, Roederer M, Anderson M, Green A, Mitra D, Watanabe N, Nakamura H, Tjioe I, Deresinski SC, Moore WA, Ela SW, Parks D, Herzenberg LA (2000) N-acetylcysteine replenishes glutathione in HIV infection. Eur J Clin Invest 30(10):915–929

Eshraghi A, Talasaz AH, Salamzadeh J, Salarifar M, Pourhosseini H, Nozari Y, Bahremand M, Jalali A, Boroumand MA (2016) Evaluating the Effect of Intracoronary N-Acetylcysteine on Platelet Activation Markers After Primary Percutaneous Coronary Intervention in Patients With ST-Elevation Myocardial Infarction. Am J Ther 23(1):e44–e51. https://doi.org/10.1097/mjt.0000000000000309

Flanagan RJ, Meredith TJ (1991) Use of N-acetylcysteine in clinical toxicology. Am J Med 91(3C):131S–139S

Gabard B, Mascher H (1991) Endogenous plasma N-acetylcysteine and single dose oral bioavailability from two different formulations as determined by a new analytical method. Biopharm Drug Dispos 12(5):343–353

Grandjean EM, Berthet P, Ruffmann R, Leuenberger P (2000) Cost-effectiveness analysis of oral N-acetylcysteine as a preventive treatment in chronic bronchitis. Pharmacol Res 42(1):39–50

Grendar J, Ouellet JF, McKay A, Sutherland FR, Bathe OF, Ball CG, Dixon E (2016) Effect of N-acetylcysteine on liver recovery after resection: A randomized clinical trial. J Surg Oncol 114(4):446–450. https://doi.org/10.1002/jso.24312

Herzenberg LA, De Rosa SC, Dubs JG, Roederer M, Anderson MT, Ela SW, Deresinski SC (1997) Glutathione deficiency is associated with impaired survival in HIV disease. Proc Natl Acad Sci USA 94(5):1967–1972

Hoffmann U, Fischereder M, Kruger B, Drobnik W, Kramer BK (2004) The value of N-acetylcysteine in the prevention of radiocontrast agent-induced nephropathy seems questionable. J Am Soc Nephrol: JASN 15(2):407–410

Horowitz JD, Henry CA, Syrjanen ML, Louis WJ, Fish RD, Antman EM, Smith TW (1988) Nitroglycerine/N-acetylcysteine in the management of unstable angina pectoris. Eur Heart J 9(Suppl A):95–100

Huitema AD, Soesan M, Meenhorst PL, Koks CH, Beijnen JH (1998) A dose-dependent delayed hypersensitivity reaction to acetaminophen after repeated acetaminophen intoxications. Hum Exp Toxicol 17(7):406–408

Iversen HK (1992) N-acetylcysteine enhances nitroglycerin-induced headache and cranial arterial responses. Clin Pharmacol Ther 52(2):125–133

Jones AL, Jarvie DR, Simpson D, Hayes PC, Prescott LF (1997) Pharmacokinetics of N-acetylcysteine are altered in patients with chronic liver disease. Aliment Pharmacol Ther 11(4):787–791

Kees F, Wellenhofer M, Brohl K, Grobecker H (1996) Bioavailability of cefpodoxime proxetil with co-administered acetylcysteine. Arzneimittel-Forschung 46(4):435–438

Laisalmi-Kokki M, Pesonen E, Kokki H, Valta P, Pitkanen M, Teppo AM, Honkanen E, Lindgren L (2009) Potentially detrimental effects of N-acetylcysteine on renal function in knee arthroplasty. Free Rad Res 43(7):691–696. https://doi.org/10.1080/10715760902998206

Magee EA, Richardson CJ, Hughes R, Cummings JH (2000) Contribution of dietary protein to sulfide production in the large intestine: an in vitro and a controlled feeding study in humans. Am J Clin Nutr 72(6):1488–1494

Miller LF, Rumack BH (1983) Clinical safety of high oral doses of acetylcysteine. Semin Oncol 10(1 Suppl 1):76–85

Niemi TT, Munsterhjelm E, Poyhia R, Hynninen MS, Salmenpera MT (2006) The effect of N-acetylcysteine on blood coagulation and platelet function in patients undergoing open repair of abdominal aortic aneurysm. Blood Coagul Fibrinolysis 17(1):29–34

Nolin TD, Ouseph R, Himmelfarb J, McMenamin ME, Ward RA (2010) Multiple-dose pharmaco-kinetics and pharmacodynamics of N-acetylcysteine in patients with end-stage renal disease. Clin J Am Soc Nephrol 5(9):1588–1594. https://doi.org/10.2215/CJN.00210110

Olsson B, Johansson M, Gabrielsson J, Bolme P (1988) Pharmacokinetics and bioavailability of reduced and oxidized N-acetylcysteine. Eur J Clin Pharmacol 34(1):77–82

Roller S, Lode H, Stelzer I, Deppermann KM, Boeckh M, Koeppe P (1992) Pharmacokinetics of loracarbef and interaction with acetylcysteine. Eur J Clin Microbiol Infect Dis 11(9):851–855

Sahin G, Yalcin AU, Akcar N (2007) Effect of N-acetylcysteine on endothelial dysfunction in dialysis patients. Blood Purif 25(4):309–315. https://doi.org/10.1159/000106103

Sandstrom PA, Murray J, Folks TM, Diamond AM (1998) Antioxidant defenses influence HIV-1 replication and associated cytopathic effects. Free Radic Biol Med 24(9):1485–1491

Schmidt LE, Dalhoff KP (1999) Side-effects of N-acetylcysteine treatment in patients with paracetamol poisoning. Ugeskr Laeger 161(18):2669–2672

Scholze A, Rinder C, Beige J, Riezler R, Zidek W, Tepel M (2004) Acetylcysteine reduces plasma homocysteine concentration and improves pulse pressure and endothelial function in patients with end-stage renal failure. Circulation 109(3):369–374

Soldini D, Zwahlen H, Gabutti L, Marzo A, Marone C (2005) Pharmacokinetics of N-acetylcysteine following repeated intravenous infusion in haemodialysed patients. Eur J Clin Pharmacol 60(12):859–864

Spapen HD, Diltoer MW, Nguyen DN, Hendrickx I, Huyghens LP (2005) Effects of N-acetylcysteine on microalbuminuria and organ failure in acute severe sepsis: results of a pilot study. Chest 127(4):1413–1419

Stavem K (1997) Anaphylactic reaction to N-acetylcysteine after poisoning with paracetamol. Tidsskr Nor Laegeforen 117(14):2038–2039

Swarnalatha G, Ram R, Neela P, Naidu MU, Dakshina Murty KV (2010) Oxidative stress in hemo-dialysis patients receiving intravenous iron therapy and the role of N-acetylcysteine in prevent-ing oxidative stress. Saudi J Kidney Dis Transpl 21(5):852–858

Taut FJ, Breitkreutz R, Zapletal CM, Thies JC, Babylon A, Martin E, Droge W (2001) Influence of N-acetylcysteine on hepatic amino acid metabolism in patients undergoing orthotopic liver transplantation. Transpl Int 14(5):329–333

Vale JA, Wheeler DC (1982) Anaphylactoid reaction to acetylcysteine. Lancet 2(8305):988

Walton NG, Mann TA, Shaw KM (1979) Anaphylactoid reaction to N-acetylcysteine. Lancet 2(8155):1298

Weisbord SD, Gallagher M, Jneid H, Garcia S, Cass A, Thwin S-S, Conner TA, Chertow GM, Bhatt DL, Shunk K, Parikh CR, McFalls EO, Brophy M, Ferguson R, Hongsheng W, Androsenko M, Myles J, Kaufman J, Palevsky PM (2018) Outcomes after angiography with sodium bicarbon-ate and acetylcysteine. New Eng J Med 378(7):603–614

Wijeysundera DN, Karkouti K, Rao V, Granton JT, Chan CT, Raban R, Carroll J, Poonawala H, Beattie WS (2009) N-acetylcysteine is associated with increased blood loss and blood product utilization during cardiac surgery. Crit Care Med 37(6):1929–1934. https://doi.org/10.1097/CCM.0b013e31819ffed4

Wittstock A, Burkert M, Zidek W, Tepel M, Scholze A (2009) N-acetylcysteine improves arterial vascular reactivity in patients with chronic kidney disease. Nephron Clin Pract 112(3):c184–c189. https://doi.org/10.1159/000218107

Printed by Printforce, the Netherlands